Neuropsychopharmacology and Therapeutics

Neuropsychopharmacology and Therapeutics

Editor: Elsa Armstrong

AMERICAN
MEDICAL PUBLISHERS
www.americanmedicalpublishers.com

AMERICAN
MEDICAL PUBLISHERS
www.americanmedicalpublishers.com

Cataloging-in-Publication Data

Neuropsychopharmacology and therapeutics / edited by Elsa Armstrong.
p. cm.
Includes bibliographical references and index.
ISBN 979-8-88740-319-9
1. Neuropsychopharmacology. 2. Therapeutics. 3. Neuropharmacology. 4. Psychopharmacology.
5. Clinical medicine. 6. Clinical pharmacology. I. Armstrong, Elsa.
RM315 .N483 2023
615.78--dc23

American Medical Publishers,
41 Flatbush Avenue,
1st Floor, New York,
NY 11217, USA

ISBN 979-8-88740-319-9 (Hardback)

Contents

Preface

Every book is a source of knowledge and this one is no exception. The idea that led to the conceptualization of this book was the fact that the world is advancing rapidly; which makes it crucial to document the progress in every field. I am aware that a lot of data is already available, yet, there is a lot more to learn. Hence, I accepted the responsibility of editing this book and contributing my knowledge to the community.

Neuropsychopharmacology is an interdisciplinary science that is related to psychopharmacology and fundamental neuroscience. It is the study of the neural mechanisms on which drugs act upon for influencing behavior. It investigates the mechanisms of neuropathology, pharmacodynamics, psychiatric disease, and states of consciousness. It explains the effects that drugs have at the behavioral and molecular levels. Integration and synthesis of knowledge from numerous disciplines, such as neuroanatomy, physiology, molecular biology, pharmacology, and behavioral sciences are required in neuropsychopharmacology. It is assumed in this field that all the states of mind: diseases involving cognitive or mental dysfunction, or normal and drug-induced altered states, have a neurochemical basis and as well as certain pathways in the central nervous system. Thus, understanding of neurons and nerve cells is important for understanding the mind. This will help in developing and devising prescriptions for various psychiatric disorders and neuropathological conditions. This book covers in detail some existent theories and innovative concepts revolving around the therapeutic perspectives on neuropsychopharmacology. Its aim is to present researches that have transformed this discipline and aided its advancement. This book will help new researchers by foregrounding their knowledge in neuropsychopharmacology.

While editing this book, I had multiple visions for it. Then I finally narrowed down to make every chapter a sole standing text explaining a particular topic, so that they can be used independently. However, the umbrella subject sinews them into a common theme. This makes the book a unique platform of knowledge.

I would like to give the major credit of this book to the experts from every corner of the world, who took the time to share their expertise with us. Also, I owe the completion of this book to the never-ending support of my family, who supported me throughout the project.

Editor

1

Pharmacological Interventions for the MATRICS Cognitive Domains in Schizophrenia: What's the Evidence?

Wilhelmina A. M. Vingerhoets [1,2] ****, Oswald J. N. Bloemen*** [1] ***, Geor Bakker*** [1,2] ***and Therese A. M. J. van Amelsvoort*** [1]

[1] *Department of Psychiatry and Psychology, Maastricht University, Maastricht, Netherlands*
[2] *Department of Nuclear Medicine, Academic Medical Centre, University of Amsterdam, Amsterdam, Netherlands*

***Correspondence:**
Wilhelmina A. M. Vingerhoets, Department of Psychiatry and Psychology, Maastricht University, Vijverdalseweg 1, Maastricht 6226 NB, Netherlands
e-mail: claudia.vingerhoets@maastrichtuniversity.nl

Schizophrenia is a disabling, chronic psychiatric disorder with a prevalence rate of 0.5–1% in the general population. Symptoms include positive (e.g., delusions, hallucinations), negative (e.g., blunted affect, social withdrawal), as well as cognitive symptoms (e.g., memory and attention problems). Although 75–85% of patients with schizophrenia report cognitive impairments, the underlying neuropharmacological mechanisms are not well understood and currently no effective treatment is available for these impairments. This has led to the Measurement and Treatment Research to Improve Cognition in Schizophrenia (MATRICS) initiative, which established seven cognitive domains that are fundamentally impaired in schizophrenia. These domains include verbal learning and memory, visual learning and memory, working memory, attention and vigilance, processing speed, reasoning and problem solving, and social cognition. Recently, a growing number of studies have been conducted trying to identify the underlying neuropharmacological mechanisms of cognitive impairments in schizophrenia patients. Specific cognitive impairments seem to arise from different underlying neuropharmacological mechanisms. However, most review articles describe cognition in general and an overview of the mechanisms involved in these seven separate cognitive domains is currently lacking. Therefore, we reviewed the underlying neuropharmacological mechanisms focusing on the domains as established by the MATRICS initiative which are considered most crucial in schizophrenia.

Keywords: pharmacology, schizophrenia, cognition, MATRICS, neurotransmitters

INTRODUCTION

Schizophrenia is a disabling, chronic psychiatric disorder with a prevalence rate of 0.5–1% in the general population. Symptoms include positive and negative symptoms and disorganization. Approximately 75–85% of the schizophrenia patients report cognitive impairments as well (1). Although this aspect of schizophrenia was already described by Kraepelin nearly a century ago, cognitive impairments have long been under-identified as a symptom of schizophrenia and relatively little research has been conducted on this topic. Previous research showed that cognitive functioning is strongly associated with functional outcome in schizophrenia [e.g., skill acquisition in psychosocial rehabilitation treatment, demonstration of ability to solve simulated interpersonal problems, and community functioning (2, 3)]. Cognitive impairments often precede the onset of other symptoms and persist after other psychotic symptoms have been effectively treated (4). Furthermore, severity of cognitive impairments is predictive of poorer medication compliance (5), treatment adherence (6), and increased tendency for relapse in first-episode patients (7). At present, no effective treatment is available as existing (antipsychotic) medication mainly targets positive symptoms and does not improve cognition. Although it is sometimes assumed by clinicians (possibly due to marketing) that atypical antipsychotics are superior to typical antipsychotics, results from recent studies contradict this theory. Presently available guidelines for treatment of schizophrenia, such as the NICE (8), PORT (9), and WFSBP (10) guidelines, indicate that there is no superiority of atypical antipsychotics on positive symptoms with the exception of clozapine, and instead state that use of antipsychotics should be evaluated based on their side effects. Since cognitive dysfunction is associated with functional outcome, development of an effective intervention strategy for these symptoms and corresponding guidelines is essential, as such guidelines are currently still lacking.

Lack of effective treatment strategies has over recent years led to an increase in studies investigating underlying neurobiological mechanisms of cognitive impairments and potential new pharmacological targets to enhance cognition in schizophrenia. Research has mainly focused on the role of neurotransmitters such as dopamine, serotonin, γ-aminobutyric acid (GABA), glutamate, and acetylcholine. Previous research indicated that specific cognitive impairments seem to arise from different underlying neurobiological mechanisms (11). For example, the prefrontal cortex (PFC) has been implicated in the executive functioning aspect of cognition (12) whereas the hippocampus has been linked to, e.g., episodic memory (13). This suggests that specific pharmacological agents could enhance domains of cognition differentially. Nonetheless, still little is known about the underlying neurobiology of cognition. Knowledge about these neurobiological mechanisms is highly necessary for development of new pharmacological intervention strategies.

Table 1 | Pharmacological agents used and their main mechanism of action.

General pharmacological domain	Pharmacological agent	Agents main mechanism of action
Antipsychotics	Haloperidol	D_2 antagonist
	Chlorprothixene	D_2 antagonist
	Perazine	D_2 antagonist
	Flupenthixol	D_2 antagonist
	Amisulpride	D_2/D_3 antagonist
	Risperidone	D_2 and 5-HT_{2a} antagonist
	Paliperidone	D_2 and 5-HT_{2a} antagonist (active metabolite of risperidone)
	Olanzapine	D_2 and 5-HT_{2a} antagonist
	Loxapine	D_2 and 5-HT_{2a} antagonist
	Sertindole	D_2 and 5-HT_{2a} antagonist
	Ziprasidone	D_2 and 5-HT_{2a} antagonist
	Quetiapine	D_2 and 5-HT_{2a} antagonist partial 5-HT_{1a} agonist
	Aripiprazole	5-HT_{2a} antagonist and partial D_2 agonist and partial 5-HT_{1a} agonist
	Perospirone	D_2 and 5-HT_{2a} antagonist and 5-HT_{1a} agonist
	Clozapine	D_2, D_4, and 5-HT_{2a} antagonist partial 5-HT_{1a} agonist (metabolite shows weak partial agonistic effects on D_2 and D_3)
	BL-1020	D_2 and 5-HT_{2a} antagonist $GABA_A$ agonist
Dopaminergic	Dihydrexidine	D_1 agonist
Serotonergic	Ondansetron	5-HT_{3a} antagonist
	Tandospirone	5-HT_{1a} agonist
	Tropisetron	5-HT_{3a} antagonist
	Fluvoxamine	Reuptake inhibition and sigma-1 receptor agonist
	Citalopram	Reuptake inhibition
Cholinergic	AZD3480	nicotinic $\alpha_4\beta_2$ agonist
	DMXB-A	Partial nicotinic α_7 agonist
	Donepezil	Acetylcholinesterase inhibition
	Galantamine	Acetylcholinesterase inhibition
	Rivastigmine	Acetylcholinesterase inhibition
Glutamatergic	Minocycline	(Mainly used as antibiotic) blocks nitric oxide induced neurotoxicity
	D-Cycloserine	NMDA partial agonist
	Lamotrigine	Glutamate release regulation
	Topiramate	AMPA/kainite antagonist
GABAergic	MK-0777	GABA α_2/α_3 agonist
	Lorazepam	$GABA_A$ agonist
	Flumazenil	$GABA_A$ antagonist
Noradrenergic	Atomoxetine	Reuptake inhibition
Stimulants	D-Amphetamine	Dopamine/norepinephrine releaser thus indirect dopamine agonist
	Modafinil	Unknown
	Armodafinil	Unknown
Other domains	Mifepristone	Glucocorticoid receptor antagonist
	Sildenafil	PDE5 inhibition

To improve cognition research in schizophrenia the Measurement and Treatment to Improve Cognition in Schizophrenia (MATRICS) was developed. The MATRICS identified seven cognitive domains that are fundamentally impaired in schizophrenia: verbal learning and memory, visual learning and memory, working memory, attention and vigilance, processing speed, reasoning and problem solving, and social cognition (14). It was decided that cognition research in schizophrenia should mainly focus on these domains in order to identify the neurobiological mechanisms, ultimately to facilitate development of new pharmacological treatment strategies.

Although specific domains of cognition have been identified, most studies tend to describe cognition in general terms using a composite score. Currently, a review differentiating between separate MATRICS domains is lacking. Therefore, the aim of this review is to provide an outline of the underlying neuropharmacological mechanisms of each individual cognitive domain. We will focus on pharmacological intervention studies which used validated instruments to measure the effect on the MATRICS cognitive domains.

METHODS

SEARCH STRATEGY

A literature search was conducted in medical database PubMed. The following keywords were used: "pharmacology," "schizophrenia," and "Cognition." Subsequently, a separate search was conducted for each individual domain combining the keywords "pharmacology" and "schizophrenia" with the following keywords: "verbal learning," "verbal memory," "visual learning," "visual memory," "working memory," "attention," "vigilance," "processing speed," "reasoning," "problem solving," and "social cognition."

INCLUSION AND EXCLUSION CRITERIA

Papers that met the following inclusion criteria were included: (1) original research papers, both single challenge and clinical trials (full text available); (2) published in English; (3) use of a pharmacological intervention (pharmacological interventions used and their main mechanism of action are displayed in **Table 1**); (4) use of validated cognitive tests to measure one or more of the MATRICS domains; (5) subjects were patients with schizophrenia;

and (6) were published between January 2000 and May 2013. Papers were excluded if: (1) only healthy subjects were included; (2) also schizoaffective disorders and other psychotic disorders were included; (3) cognitive domains were measured with non-validated tests; (4) cognitive domains other than the MATRICS domains were measured; and (5) only a composite score of cognition was reported.

RESULTS

In total, the search strategy yielded 938 articles of which 293 articles were found using the keywords "pharmacology," "cognition," and "schizophrenia." The separate searches yielded 158 articles for verbal learning and memory, 85 for visual learning and memory, 100 for working memory, 234 for attention and vigilance, 22 for processing speed, 17 for reasoning and problem solving, and 29 for social cognition. After final screening 44 articles were included for verbal learning and memory, 26 for visual learning and memory, 43 for working memory, 22 for attention and vigilance, 31 for processing speed, 30 for reasoning and problem solving, and 7 for social cognition. Study characteristics and specifics are shown in **Table 2** (studies investigating antipsychotics) and **Table 3** (studies investigating non-antipsychotic intervention strategies).

VERBAL LEARNING AND MEMORY

It has been proposed that impairments in verbal learning and memory are one of the most consistent cognitive deficits seen in schizophrenia (15) and is one of the most examined cognitive domains in these patients. A majority of the 44 included studies investigated the effects of typical and atypical antipsychotic medication on verbal learning and memory.

In the past, it was assumed that atypical antipsychotics are superior to typical antipsychotics in enhancing cognition in schizophrenia due to their affinity for both dopamine D_2 receptors and serotonin 5-HT_{2A} receptors (16, 17). However large studies such as the Clinical Antipsychotic Trials of Intervention Effectiveness (CATIE) (18) and the European First Episode Schizophrenia Trial (EUFEST) (19) did not find differences between typical and atypical antipsychotics in cognitive enhancing effects. This theory was tested by Wagner et al. (16) who compared olanzapine, a dopamine D_2, and serotonin 5-HT_{2A} antagonist, to amisulpride, a dopamine D_2/D_3 antagonist in 52 patients. No significant differences were found after 8 weeks between the two groups in terms verbal memory; both groups improved on verbal learning and memory tasks. Olanzapine was compared to risperidone and haloperidol by Purdon et al. (20). Although not significant after corrections for multiple comparisons, olanzapine was found to be superior to risperidone and haloperidol in enhancing verbal learning and memory.

The atypical antipsychotic ziprasidone was found to improve verbal learning and memory after 12 weeks of monotherapy (21). However, the study did not include a control group and practice effects were not adequately controlled for. Therefore the results have to be interpreted with caution. A study comparing the effects of risperidone and haloperidol on verbal memory found that performance on a verbal memory task remained essentially unchanged in both groups (22). Since the authors did not include a non-medicated schizophrenia group but included a healthy group as control this mainly provides evidence that there is no difference between risperidone and haloperidol. Nevertheless it suggests that both medications did not cause a clinically relevant enhancement of verbal memory. However, Harvey et al. (23) compared the effects of risperidone and quetiapine and found improvement in verbal memory in both treatment groups. The dropout rate of 57% in this trial was high which may have caused a selection bias. These results are not consistent with other findings. A small study with substantial methodological shortcomings by Purdon et al. (24) found no effect of haloperidol and quetiapine. Velligan et al. (25) also compared quetiapine to haloperidol and found that patients in the quetiapine group improved to a greater extent than the patients in the haloperidol group. However, these findings were not significant after correction for multiple comparisons. Moreover, Kivircik Akdede et al. (26) did not find improvement on a verbal learning and memory task after 8 weeks of quetiapine treatment.

Kim et al. (27) found that switching from oral atypical antipsychotics to depot risperidone led to significant improvement in verbal learning and memory. However, they also did not include a control group and did not correct for possible practice effects. Furthermore a high percentage of the patients dropped out in an early stage of the study which could have caused a bias in the sample. Despite these limitations, their results are supported by Suzuki and Gen (28) who also found an improvement in verbal learning and memory in patients treated with depot risperidone compared to patients who received haloperidol treatment (depot). However, the differences between these two treatments might be caused by the high rate of anticholinergic co-medication in the haloperidol group which is well known for its adverse effects on cognition (29). Additionally, improvement in verbal learning and memory was found by Surguladze et al. (30) with both depot risperidone and typical antipsychotics (depot). Performance did not significantly differ between the groups. However, they did not control for practice effects. Therefore improvement cannot reliably be attributed to medication effects. In addition, Kim et al. (31) found that compared to patients using risperidone, verbal memory improved more in patients using paliperidone extend release (ER), an active metabolite of risperidone with an extended delivery system that decreases fluctuations in serum drug concentrations.

Hence, the theory that atypical antipsychotic medications are superior to typical antipsychotics in enhancing verbal learning and memory is not supported by these findings. Nonetheless, some of the atypical antipsychotics, especially risperidone depot, have shown beneficial effects on this aspect of cognition.

Results regarding the effects of clozapine on verbal learning and memory are inconclusive. Three studies which investigated the effects of clozapine on verbal learning and memory were found. Purdon et al. (32) reported significant improvement in verbal learning and memory after treatment with clozapine. Their results were not replicated by Ertugrul et al. (33) and Sumiyoshi et al. (34) as both of these studies did not find improvement in verbal memory in clozapine-treated patients. This discrepancy in findings could be due to methodological differences such as different test batteries and trial duration.

Table 2 | Summary of included studies using antipsychotics.

Study	Agent(s)	Sample size (in analyses)	Design	MATRICS domains measured	Main results
Wagner et al. (16)	Olanzapine and amisulpride	$N = 36$	8-week randomized clinical trial	Ver. I and m; wm; attention; ps	No difference between treatments conditions in ver. I and m, wm, attention, and ps. Both the olanzapine and the amisulpride group improved on ver. I and m and wm. Attention and ps did not improve in both treatment conditions
Tyson et al. (17)	Risperidone, olanzapine, clozapine, quetiapine, and amisulpride	$N = 44$	18-month clinical trial	Vis. I and m; wm; r and ps	Vis. I and m, wm, and r and ps improved in the low affinity group (quetiapine and amisulpride) whereas vis. I and m and r and ps declined in the high-affinity group (risperidone, olanzapine, and clozapine)
Purdon et al. (20)	Risperidone, olanzapine, and haloperidol	$N = 55$	54-week randomized, double-blind trial	Ver. I and m; vis. I and m; wm; ps; r and ps	After Bonferroni correction, none of the cognitive domains improved in any of the treatment conditions
Malhotra et al. (21)	Ziprasidone	$N = 10$	12-week open-label clinical trial	Ver. I and m; ps	Significant improvement in ver. I and m. Ps did not improve significantly
Rémillard et al. (22)	Risperidone and haloperidol	$N = 28$	12-month randomized	Ver. I and m	Both types of antipsychotics did not improve ver. I and m
Harvey et al. (23)	Quetiapine and risperidone	$N = 289$	8-week, randomized, double-blind clinical trial	Ver. I and m; attention; ps	Both treatment conditions improved on ver. I and m. Although no differences were found between treatment conditions, attention, and ps improved only in the risperidone group
Purdon et al. (24)	Quetiapine and haloperidol	$N = 22$	6-month, randomized, double-blind clinical trial	Ver. I and m; vis. I and m; ps; r and ps	Ver. I and m, vis. I and m, and r and ps did not improve in both treatment conditions. Ps was found to improve in both treatment conditions but this was not significant after corrections for multiple testing
Velligan et al. (25)	Quetiapine and haloperidol	$N = 58$	24-week, randomized, double-blind clinical trial	Ver. I and m; ps	After Bonferroni correction, no significant improvement on ver. I and m and ps in all treatment conditions
Kivircik Akdede et al. (26)	Quetiapine	$N = 14$	8-week clinical trial	Ver. I and m; wm; ps	Improvement was found in wm and ps. Ver. I and m did not improve
Kim et al. (27)	Risperidone depot	$N = 36$	26-week, open-label trial	Ver. I and m; attention; ps; r and ps	Significant improvement in ver. I and m, attention, and r and ps. Ps did not improve
Suzuki and Gen (28)	Risperidone and haloperidol depot	$N = 20$	24-week, open-label trial	Ver. I and m; r and ps	Compared to the haloperidol group, ver. I and m and r and ps improved in the risperidone depot group
Surguladze et al. (30)	Risperidone depot and typical antipsychotics depot (haloperidol, fluphenazine, flupenthixol, zuclopenthixol)	$N = 32$ patients and 8 healthy controls	4-month clinical trial	Ver. I and m; vis. I and m	Although no differences were found between treatment conditions, both groups improved on ver. I and m and vis. I and m

(Continued)

Table 2 | Continued

Study	Agent(s)	Sample size (in analyses)	Design	MATRICS domains measured	Main results
Kim et al. (31)	Paliperidone and risperidone	$N = 58$	12-week, randomized open-label clinical trial	Ver. l and m; wm; attention; ps	Compared to the risperidone group, ver. l and m improved more in the paliperidone group. No differences between treatment conditions were found in wm, attention, and ps
Purdon et al. (32)	Clozapine	$N = 18$	6-week clinical trial	Ver. l and m; vis. l and m; wm; ps; r and ps	Significant improvement in ver. l and m, vis. l and m, and ps. No improvement in wm and r and ps
Ertugrul et al. (33)	Clozapine	$N = 20$ patients and 20 healthy controls	8-week clinical trial	Ver. l and m; vis. l and m; wm; r and ps	No significant improvement in ver. l and m, vis. l and m, and r and ps. Performance on one of the wm tasks improved
Sumiyoshi et al. (34)	Clozapine	$N = 27$	6-week clinical trial	Ver. l and m	No significant improvement in ver. l and m
Geffen et al. (35)	BL-1020 and risperidone	$N = 363$	6-week, randomized, double-blind, placebo-controlled clinical trial	Ver. l and m; wm; ps; r and ps	Compared to placebo, improvement in ver. l and m and wm was found with a high dose of BL-1020. Ps and r and ps did not improve
Riedel et al. (39)	Aripiprazole	$N = 56$	8-week, open-label clinical trial	Ver. l and m; vis. l and m; wm; ps	Improvement in ver. l and m and ps. Vis. l and m and wm did not improve
Bervoets et al. (40)	Aripiprazole	$N = 238$	12-week, open-label clinical trial	Ver. l and m	Ver. l and m improved significantly
Suzuki et al. (41)	Aripiprazole, perospirone, and olanzapine	$N = 31$	8-week, clinical trial	Ver. l and m; r and ps	None of the treatment conditions showed improved on ver. l and m and r and ps. No differences were found between groups
Yasui-Furukori et al. (42)	Aripiprazole (added to risperidone or olanzapine)	$N = 36$	12-week, randomized, double-blind placebo-controlled trial	Ver. l and m; wm; ps; r and ps	None of the cognitive domains measured improved significantly after adjunctive aripiprazole treatment
Rollnik et al. (69)	Atypical (olanzapine, risperidone, clozapine) and typical antipsychotics (haloperidol, chlorprothixene, perazine, flupenthixol)	$N = 20$ patients and 14 healthy controls	12-week, clinical trial	Vis. l and m; wm; ps	No significant differences were found between typical and atypical antipsychotics for all cognitive domains
McGurk et al. (70)	Risperidone and haloperidol	$N = 27$	4-week, randomized double-blind clinical trial	Vis. l and m; wm	After corrections for anticholinergic co-medication, no differences were found between risperidone and haloperidol on vis. l and m and wm
Mori et al. (75)	Risperidone, olanzapine, perospirone; quetiapine	$N = 77$	8-week, randomized clinical trial	wm	Wm improved in the risperidone group and declined in the quetiapine group. Wm performance did not change in the olanzapine and perospirone group

(Continued)

Table 2 | Continued

Study	Agent(s)	Sample size (in analyses)	Design	MATRICS domains measured	Main results
Papageorgiou et al. (76)	Olanzapine and clozapine	$N = 16$	6-week, randomized, double-blind clinical trial	wm	Wm improved in both groups. No significant differences between treatment conditions
Nielsen et al. (77)	Sertindole (added to clozapine)	$N = 41$	12-week, randomized, double-blind, placebo-controlled trial	Wm; r and ps	Adjunctive sertindole did not improve wm and r and ps
Molina et al. (85)	Olanzapine	$N = 17$	24-week clinical? Trial	Attention	No improvement in attention
Liu et al. (86)	Risperidone and haloperidol	$N = 38$	12-week, randomized, double-blind clinical trial	Attention	No improvement in attention
Mizrahi et al. (97)	Clozapine, risperidone, olanzapine, and loxapine	$N = 71$	6-week, clinical trial	sc	Improvement in sc
Sumiyoshi et al. (100)	Perospirone	$N = 5$	6-month, clinical trial	sc	Improvement in sc
Behere et al. (101)	Risperidone	$N = 25$ patients and 30 healthy controls	Mean duration 38 days, clinical trial	sc	Improvement in sc

Ver. l and m, verbal learning and memory; vis. l and m, visual learning and memory; wm, working memory; ps, processing speed; r and ps, reasoning and problem solving; sc, social cognition.

Moreover, the study by Purdon et al. (32) did not correct for possible practice effects and since they did not include a control group, improvement in verbal memory cannot be reliably attributed to the effects of clozapine. Thus, although results are inconclusive, at present no convincing evidence is available for the effectiveness of clozapine in enhancing verbal learning and memory in schizophrenia.

Geffen et al. (35) compared the effects of 10 and 20–30 mg of BL-1020, a new antipsychotic drug, to risperidone and placebo. BL-1020 is an antagonist for D_2 en $5\text{-}HT_{2a}$ receptors and agonist for $GABA_A$ receptors (35). Post-mortem studies have found altered GABAergic transmission in schizophrenia, predominantly in the PFC (36, 37). Treatment with 20–30 mg BL-1020 was found to improve performance on a verbal learning memory task compared to placebo, whereas 10 mg of BL-1020 and risperidone did not have enhancing effects compared to placebo. A substantial number of patients, especially in the risperidone group, received anticholinergics as well, which could have influenced the results.

Although the findings described above do not support the theory that blocking the $5\text{-}HT_{2A}$ receptors improves verbal learning and memory, a role for serotonin in this domain of cognition cannot be ruled out. Sumiyoshi et al. (38) found a significant improvement on verbal memory after adjunctive tandospirone (a $5\text{-}HT_{1a}$ agonist) treatment compared to patients who did not receive adjunctive tandospirone. Riedel et al. (39) and Bervoets et al. (40) both found a significant improvement in verbal memory in patients treated with aripiprazole, an atypical antipsychotic drug with partial D_2 agonistic and antagonistic and $5\text{-}HT_{2a}$ antagonistic properties in addition to partial agonistic activity at the $5\text{-}HT_{1a}$ receptors. However, this is contradicted by Suzuki et al. (41) who compared the effects of aripiprazole, olanzapine, and perospirone on verbal memory. None of the three conditions showed significant changes in verbal memory scores and no differences were found between the three treatment conditions. Moreover, aripiprazole added to atypical antipsychotics did not improve verbal learning and memory in a trial by Yasui-Furukori et al. (42). This discrepancy in findings could be due to practice effects in the studies of Riedel et al. (39) and Bervoets et al. (40), since both studies did not include a control group and did not correct for possible practice effects. Furthermore, different tasks were used which makes it difficult to directly compare the results.

The role of the serotonin $5\text{-}HT_{3a}$ receptor in verbal learning and memory has been examined as well. Akhondzadeh et al. (43) and Levkovitz et al. (44) investigated the effects of ondansetron, a serotonin $5\text{-}HT_{3a}$ receptor antagonist, added to respectively risperidone and clozapine treatment, and found no enhancing effects on verbal learning and memory. However, the sample size of both studies was small. In contrast to these results, Zhang et al. (45) did find improvement in verbal memory after add-on tropisetron (a $5\text{-}HT_{3a}$ receptor antagonist and nicotinic α_7 agonist) to risperidone treatment compared to placebo. This discrepancy in findings could be explained by the fact that the two studies used different pharmacological interventions. Both Akhondzadeh et al. (43) and Levkovitz et al. (44) administered ondansetron whereas Zhang et al. (45) used tropisetron. Since ondansetron has been found to have low affinity for the nicotinic α_7 receptors (46), the positive effects of tropisetron on verbal learning and memory

Table 3 | Summary of included studies using non-antipsychotic interventions.

Study	Agent	Mechanism of action	Sample size (in analyses)	Design	MATRICS domains measured	Results
George et al. (48)	Dihydrexidine	D_1 agonist	$N=20$	Single-challenge, randomized placebo-controlled cross-over trial	Ver. l and m; wm; attention; ps	No improvement in any of the measured domains
Pietrzak et al. (72)	D-Amphetamine	Indirect D_1 agonist	$N=32$	Single-challenge, double-blind, placebo-controlled cross-over trial	Vis. l and m; ps; r and ps	Improvement in ps and r and ps. No improvement in vis. l and m
Sumiyoshi et al. (38)	Tandospirone	5-HT_{1a} agonist	$N=31$	4-week, clinical trial	Ver. l and m; vis. l and m	Ver. l and m improved after adjunctive tandospirone treatment. Vis. l and m did not improve
Akhondzadeh et al. (43)	Ondansetron	5-HT_{3a} antagonist	$N=30$	12-week, randomized double-blind placebo-controlled trial	Ver. l and m; vis. l and m; wm; r and ps	Vis. l and m improved significantly after adjunctive ondansetron treatment. None of the other domains improved
Levkovitz et al. (44)	Ondansetron	5-HT_{3a} antagonist	$N=21$	2-week, double-blind placebo-controlled cross-over trial	Ver. l and m; vis. l and m; wm; ps	Significant improvement in vis. l and m in the ondansetron group. None of the others domains improved significantly
Zhang et al. (45)	Tropisetron	5-HT_{3a} antagonist	$N=38$	10-day, randomized double-blind, placebo-controlled trial	Ver. l and m; vis. l and m; wm	Ver. l and m improved significantly after adjunctive tropisetron treatment. Other domains did not improve significantly
Niitsu et al. (71)	Fluvoxamine	σ-1 Agonist	$N=47$	12-week, randomized double-blind placebo-controlled trial	Vis. l and m; wm; r and ps	None of the cognitive domains measured improved significantly after adjunctive fluvoxamine treatment
Friedman et al. (47)	Citalopram	Serotonin reuptake inhibition	$N=18$	24-week, randomized double-blind placebo-controlled cross-over trial	Ver. l and m; wm; attention; ps; r and ps	None of the cognitive domains measured improved significantly after adjunctive citalopram treatment
Velligan et al. (51)	AZD3480	Nicotinic $\alpha_4\beta_2$ agonist	$N=440$	12-week, randomized double-blind placebo-controlled trial	Ver. l and m; vis. l and m; wm; attention; ps; r and ps	None of the cognitive domains measured improved
Freedman et al. (52)	DMXB-A	Nicotinic α_7 agonist	$N=31$	4-week, double-blind placebo-controlled cross-over trial	Ver. l and m; vis. l and m; wm; attention; ps; r and ps	No significant improvement in any of the cognitive domains over three treatment arms. After 4 weeks (one treatment arm) attention improved in both DMXB-A conditions compared to placebo
Tugal et al. (50)	Donepezil	Acetylcholinesterase inhibition	$N=12$	12-week randomized double-blind placebo-controlled cross-over trial	Ver. l and m; vis. l and m; wm; ps; r and ps	None of the cognitive domains measured improved after adjunctive donepezil treatment
Akhondzadeh et al. (53)	Donepezil	Acetylcholinesterase inhibition	$N=30$	12-week randomized double-blind placebo-controlled trial	Ver. l and m; vis. l and m; wm; r and ps	None of the cognitive domains measured improved after adjunctive donepezil treatment
Friedman et al. (58)	Donepezil	Acetylcholinesterase inhibition	$N=34$	12-week randomized double-blind placebo-controlled trial	Ver. l and m; wm; attention; ps; r and ps	None of the cognitive domains measured improved after adjunctive donepezil treatment

(Continued)

Table 3 | Continued

Study	Agent	Mechanism of action	Sample size (in analyses)	Design	MATRICS domains measured	Results
Freudenreich et al. (57)	Donepezil	Acetylcholinesterase inhibition	$N = 30$	8-week double-blind placebo-controlled trial	Ver. l and m; wm; ps	None of the cognitive domains measured improved after adjunctive donepezil treatment
Fagerlund et al. (55)	Donepezil	Acetylcholinesterase inhibition	$N = 11$ patients and 11 healthy controls	12-week randomized double-blind placebo-controlled trial	Ver. l and m; vis. l and m; wm; ps; r and ps	None of the cognitive domains measured improved after adjunctive donepezil treatment
Lee et al. (54)	Galantamine	Acetylcholinesterase inhibition	$N = 24$	12-week, randomized double-blind placebo-controlled trial	Ver. l and m; vis. l and m; ps	Visual recognition improved in the galantamine group. None of the other measures improved significantly
Sharma et al. (56)	Rivastigmine	Acetylcholinesterase inhibition	$N = 21$	24-week, randomized double-blind placebo-controlled trial	Ver. l and m; wm; attention; ps; r and ps	No significant improvement in any of the measured cognitive domains after adjunctive rivastigmine treatment
Lenzi et al. (88)	Rivastigmine	Acetylcholinesterase inhibition	$N = 10$	52-week clinical trial	Ver. l and m; wm; attention; ps; r and ps	No significant improvement in any of the cognitive domains after adjunctive rivastigmine treatment
Duncan et al. (81)	D-Cycloserine	NMDA partial agonist	$N = 22$	4-week, randomized double-blind placebo-controlled trial	Wm; attention	Both domains did not improve significantly after adjunctive D-cycloserine treatment
Muscatello et al. (92)	Topiramate	AMPA/kainite antagonist	$N = 43$	24-week randomized double-blind placebo-controlled trial	Attention; r and ps	Both domains did not improve significantly after adjunctive topiramate treatment
Zoccali et al. (93)	Lamotrigine	Glutamate release regulation	$N = 51$	24-week randomized double-blind placebo-controlled trial	Attention; r and ps	After Bonferroni correction, no significant improvement was found in both domains
Levkovitz et al. (73)	Minocycline	Blockade nitric oxide induced neurotoxicity	$N = 21$	22-week randomized double-blind placebo-controlled trial	Vis. l and m; wm; r and ps	Vis. l and m, wm and r and ps improved after adjunctive minocycline treatment.
Buchanan et al. (59)	MK-0777	GABA α_2/α_3 agonist	$N = 53$	4-week randomized, double-blind placebo-controlled trial	Ver. l and m; vis. l and m; wm; attention; ps; r and ps; sc	After correction for multiple testing, none of the domains improved significantly after adjunctive MK-077 treatment
Menzies et al. (80)	Lorazepam and attention flumazenil	$GABA_A$ agonist and $GABA_A$ antagonist	$N = 11$ patients and 11 healthy controls	Single-challenge randomized double-blind placebo-controlled cross-over trial	wm	Wm performance declined significantly after lorazepam administration whereas no significant differences were found in the flumazenil group
Friedman et al. (60)	Atomoxetine	Norepinephrine reuptake inhibition	$N = 20$	8-week randomized, double-blind placebo-controlled trial	Ver. l and m; wm; ps; r and ps	No significant improvement in any of the cognitive domains after adjunctive atomoxetine treatment.

(Continued)

Table 3 | Continued

Study	Agent	Mechanism of action	Sample size (in analyses)	Design	MATRICS domains measured	Results
Turner et al. (63)	Modafinil	Unknown	$N = 20$	Single-challenge, randomized, double-blind placebo-controlled cross-over trial	Ver. l and m; vis. l and m; wm; attention; ps; r and ps	Wm improved in the modafinil condition compared to placebo. Response latency on a r and ps task was significantly lower in the modafinil condition. No differences were found in number of attempts on the same task
Spence et al. (82)	Modafinil	Unknown	$N = 17$	Single-challenge, randomized, double-blind placebo-controlled cross-over trial	wm	No significant difference between the modafinil and placebo condition
Kane et al. (61)	Armodafinil	unknown	$N = 49$	4-week, randomized double-blind placebo-controlled trial	Ver. l and m; vis. l and m; wm; attention; ps; r and ps; sc	No significant improvement in any of the cognitive domains after adjunctive armodafinil treatment
Gallagher et al. (66)	Mifepristone	Glucocorticoid antagonist	$N = 19$	2-week, randomized double-blind placebo-controlled cross-over trial	Ver. l and m; vis. l and m; wm; attention	No significant improvement in any of the cognitive domains after adjunctive mifepristone treatment.
Goff et al. (67)	Sildenafil	PDE5 inhibition	$N = 15$	Single-challenge randomized placebo-controlled cross-over trial	Ver. l and m; wm; attention	No significant improvement in any of the cognitive domains after adjunctive sildenafil treatment

Ver. l and m, verbal learning and memory; vis. l and m, visual learning and memory; wm, working memory; ps, processing speed; r and ps, reasoning and problem solving; sc, social cognition.

could be due to its nicotinic α_7 agonistic properties rather than its antagonistic effects on the 5-HT_{3a} receptors.

Effects of a selective serotonin reuptake inhibitor (SSRI) were examined by Friedman et al. (47) who added citalopram to treatment with atypical antipsychotics but found no improvement in verbal learning and memory.

Thus, although results are inconclusive there is preliminary evidence of positive effects of 5-HT_{1a} agonists, but not 5-HT_{3a} antagonists on verbal learning and memory in schizophrenia.

One study examined the effects of a dopamine D_1 *agonist* on verbal learning and memory in schizophrenia. George et al. (48) administered dihydrexidine as a pharmacological challenge and found no effects of dihydrexidine on verbal learning and memory.

The role of the neurotransmitter acetylcholine in cognition has been widely investigated and established (36). Post-mortem, a correlation was found between cognitive impairment and decreased levels of brain choline acetyltransferase in schizophrenia (49). Post-mortem studies have shown changes in both muscarinic and nicotinic acetylcholine receptors in patients with schizophrenia (50). Velligan et al. (51) conducted a trial to assess the effects adjunctive therapy with the selective nicotinic $\alpha_4\beta_2$ receptor agonist AZD3480 on verbal learning and memory in patients but found no improvement. An important limitation of this study is that only patients who smoked were included. Therefore, the lack of effect could be due to desensitization of the nicotinic receptors caused by chronic tobacco use. However, Freedman et al. (52) also did not find an improvement in verbal learning and memory after administration of the partial nicotinic α_7 agonist DMXB-A, added to antipsychotic treatment in patients, who abstained from nicotine at least 1 month prior to participation. Studies using acetylcholinesterase (enzyme that breaks down acetylcholine, thereby increasing acetylcholine levels) inhibitors (AChE-Is) as adjunctive therapy to antipsychotic medication also found no improvement on verbal learning and memory (53–58). These results suggest that acetylcholinesterase inhibitors do not effectively enhance verbal memory in patients with schizophrenia. However, all studies used a small sample size and one study included patients who were taking anticholinergic medication as well. This could have influenced the outcome of the study. Another important limitation is that none of these studies controlled for the effects of smoking. Hence, although there is theoretical evidence for a role of acetylcholine in cognition, various (possibly underpowered) intervention studies have not yielded positive results. Since Zhang et al. (45) found improvement in verbal learning and memory after adjunctive tropisetron treatment, it remains possible that enhancement of verbal learning and memory can be achieved with nicotinic α_7 agonists while simultaneously blocking the 5-HT_{3a} receptors.

The role of the neurotransmitters GABA and norepinephrine in verbal learning in memory has also been investigated. Buchanan et al. (59) found no improvement in verbal learning and memory with adjunctive MK-0777, a partial GABA α_2/α_3 agonist, therapy to antipsychotics. However, the authors argue that a lack of effect may be due to the fact that MK-0777 is a weak GABA α_2/α_3 agonist. A pilot study by Friedman et al. (60) found no effects of the norepinephrine reuptake inhibitor atomoxetine, on verbal memory when added to treatment with atypical antipsychotics.

Hence, although positive effects were found with the antipsychotic BL-1020 with $GABA_A$ agonistic properties, the available studies were not able to detect positive effects of both a partial GABA α_2/α_3 agonist and a norepinephrine reuptake inhibitor on verbal learning and memory. Nonetheless, these results suggest that $GABA_A$ receptors may be a potential target for future studies in verbal learning and memory.

Effects of the psychostimulant armodafinil were investigated by Kane et al. (61). Armodafinil is a longer-lasting isomer of modafinil, which is an alertness-promoting medication with mechanisms of action different from those of amphetamine (62) and has been found to improve cognition in healthy subjects and adults with ADHD (63). However, the exact mechanisms of action are complex and not entirely understood (64). Armodafinil, added to atypical antipsychotics, did not enhance verbal learning and memory.

The effects of several other pharmacological interventions on verbal learning and memory in schizophrenia have been investigated. Six months of daily creatine administration added to antipsychotic treatment did not have beneficial effects on verbal learning and memory (65). Effects of adjunctive mifepristone, a glucocorticoid receptor (GR) antagonist, on verbal learning and memory was examined by Gallagher et al. (66). They found no improvement in this domain of cognition. Goff et al. (67) examined the effects of sildenafil, a phosphodiesterase 5 (PDE5) inhibitor used to treat erectile dysfunction, on verbal learning and memory. PDE5 inhibitors increase cyclic guanine monophosphate (cGMP) which is thought to modulate long-term potentiation. They found single dose of 50 and 100 mg not to improve verbal learning and memory. On the other hand, Feifel et al. (15) found that patients who received intranasal oxytocin for 3 weeks performed better on a verbal learning and memory task. Additionally, Stone et al. (68) found that additional glucose administration in patients who were stable on clozapine, enhanced verbal learning and memory. All studies used a small sample and the dropout rate in the study by Feifel et al. (15) was 25%. Moreover, the majority of the patients in the study of Stone et al. (68) received additional medication besides clozapine. Therefore the effect cannot be attributed to a unique interaction of clozapine and glucose.

To summarize, the proposed superior effect on verbal learning and memory of atypical to typical antipsychotics, is not supported by the available data and any effect does not result from blocking the 5-HT_{2a} receptors. Despite the fact that multiple studies describe a role of acetylcholine in cognition, nicotinic receptor agonist and acetylcholinesterase inhibitors do not seem to effectively improve verbal learning and memory in schizophrenia. However, some positive results have been found with risperidone depot, possibly because of medication compliance. In addition, serotonin 5-HT_{1a} receptors and $GABA_A$ receptors may be molecular targets for enhancing this aspect of cognition. Additionally, there is preliminary evidence that adjunctive oxytocin and glucose treatment may be beneficial in enhancing verbal learning and memory. However, results have to be interpreted with care as the available studies are mostly pilot studies which, although important in early stages of research, inherently suffer from methodological shortcomings.

VISUAL LEARNING AND MEMORY

Compared to verbal learning and memory, considerably less research has been conducted regarding visual learning and memory in schizophrenia. Results of studies that examined the effects of antipsychotic medication on visual learning and memory are, similar to verbal learning and memory, indecisive. Tyson et al. (17) compared the effects of atypical antipsychotic medication with high and low affinity for the 5-HT_{2a} receptors on visual learning and memory. Patients treated with risperidone, olanzapine, and clozapine were assigned to the high-affinity group and patients using quetiapine and amisulpride were assigned to the low affinity group. Performance on visual memory tasks improved in patients in the low affinity group whereas performance in the high-affinity group declined. A limitation is that the authors did not correct for multiple testing. However, the effects were already present after 9 months of treatment and show a consistent pattern. Since performance declined in the high-affinity group, it is not likely that the improvement in the low affinity group is driven by practice effects. However, Rollnik et al. (69) found atypical antipsychotics (olanzapine, risperidone, or clozapine) to be superior to typical antipsychotics (haloperidol, chlorprothixene, perazine, or flupenthixol) in improving visual learning and after 3 weeks of treatment, although at the final assessment, this difference was no longer significant. Purdon et al. (20) compared the effects of olanzapine, risperidone, and haloperidol. After correction for multiple comparisons, no significant differences were found between the three treatment conditions; visual learning and memory did not improve in all three groups. As mentioned earlier, lack of effect could be caused by concomitant anticholinergic treatment and the small sample size.

Two studies compared the effects of haloperidol to respectively quetiapine (24) and risperidone (70). In both studies haloperidol and both quetiapine and risperidone were found not to enhance visual learning and memory. However, a substantial number of patients in both studies were treated with anticholinergics in addition to antipsychotics, which could have influenced the results. Surguladze et al. (30) found no differences in visual learning and memory between depot risperidone and a typical antipsychotic depot treatment, although performance in both groups improved. As discussed earlier, it cannot be ruled out that this improvement is caused by practice effects rather than the effects of medication.

Although results are inconclusive, clozapine does not seem to effectively enhance visual learning and memory. A study by Ertugrul et al. (33) did not find improvement with clozapine whereas Purdon et al. (32) found significant improvement on performance on one of three assessed visual memory subtests. However, this study has important limitations, which were described earlier.

Treatment with aripiprazole did not significantly improve visual learning and memory in the study by Riedel et al. (39). Tandospirone, which like aripiprazole has serotonin 5-HT_{1a} agonistic properties, also did not significantly enhance visual learning and memory in the study of Sumiyoshi et al. (38). These findings suggest that stimulating the serotonin 5-HT_{1a} receptors does not enhance visual learning and memory in schizophrenia. However, the serotonin 5-HT_{3a} receptors may play a role in visual memory in schizophrenia. Both Akhondzadeh et al. (43) and Levkovitz et al. (44) found visual learning and memory to improve with adjunctive ondansetron treatment. Although both studies did not correct for multiple testing and possible practice effects, visual memory was the only aspect of the cognitive domains measured that improved in both studies. Adjunctive tropisetron treatment on the other hand did not enhance visual memory (45). As mentioned earlier, tropisetron is both a 5-HT_{3a} antagonist and partial nicotinic α_7 agonist whereas ondansetron has low affinity for the nicotinic α_7 receptors (46). Hence, the 5-HT_{3a} receptors may play a role in visual learning and memory. However, enhancement of this aspect of cognition may depend on blockade of nicotinic α_7 receptors. The 5-HT_{1a} receptor does not seem to be a promising target for enhancing visual learning and memory.

A preliminary study by Niitsu et al. (71) investigated the effect of the SSRI fluvoxamine, a sigma-1 receptor agonist, on cognition and found it not to enhance visual learning and memory. These preliminary results indicate sigma-1 receptor agonism does not enhance visual learning and memory in schizophrenia patients.

Studies investigating the role acetylcholine in visual learning and memory in schizophrenia have not yielded positive results. Selective nicotinic $\alpha_4\beta_2$ receptor agonist AZD3480 and partial nicotinic α_7 agonist DMXB-A both did not enhance visual learning and memory when added to antipsychotic treatment (51, 52). As mentioned earlier, the lack of effect in the study of Velligan et al. (51) could be due to desensitization of the nicotinic receptors caused by chronic tobacco use since only smokers were included. Studies conducted with acetylcholinesterase inhibitors do not report positive results either. Although Lee et al. (54) found improvement on the recognition subtest of Rey Complex Figure Test (RCTF) with galantamine, the other aspects of the task did not improve. Studies using donepezil also did not find improvement in visual learning and memory (50, 53, 55). Hence, both nicotinic receptor agonists and acetylcholinesterase inhibitors do not seem to effectively enhance visual learning and memory in schizophrenia.

Based on preliminary results of Buchanan et al. (59), GABA does not seem to enhance visual learning and memory in schizophrenia as they found no improvement with partial $GABA_A$ α_2/α_3 agonist MK-0777. However, this is the only study investigating the role of GABA in visual learning and memory and MK-0777 is a weak GABA α_2/α_3 agonist.

The possible enhancing effect of psychostimulant drugs on visual learning and memory has been investigated in schizophrenia as well. A single dose of D-amphetamine, an indirect dopamine D_1 agonist, did not improve visual learning and memory (72). A single administration of modafinil did not significantly enhance visual memory either (63). In addition, adjunctive armodafinil treatment did not improve visual learning and memory (61). Hence, based on these findings D-amphetamine and modafinil do not seem to be promising intervention strategies for enhancing visual learning and memory.

Results of other pharmacological interventions on visual learning and memory are mixed. Gallagher et al. (66) found no improvement after adjunctive mifepristone (a GR antagonist) treatment. The effect of adjunctive creatine treatment was investigated by Kaptsan et al. (65) but they found it not to enhance visual learning and memory. Levkovitz et al. (73) investigated the effects of minocycline, a second generation tetracycline with anti-inflammatory and antimicrobial effects. Minocycline modulates the glutamate pathway by blocking nitric oxide induced neurotoxicity. Hyperactivity of glutamatergic neurotransmission [possibly caused by hypofunction of N-methyl-D-aspartate (NMDA) receptors] has been found in schizophrenia (36). Stimulated by glutamate, the NMDA receptors activate production of nitric oxide. The authors found improvement on a spatial recognition memory task after minocycline administration, added to antipsychotic treatment. Task performance showed a decrease after 10 weeks, but compared to baseline, performance improved at the final assessment. The drop-out rate in this study was high (due to adverse events and non-adherence) and although it did not differ between the two treatment groups, this could have biased the results.

To summarize, results regarding visual learning and memory are inconclusive. At present, there is some evidence for a role of the serotonin 5-HT_{3a} receptors in this cognitive domain. 5-HT_{1a} and sigma-1 receptor agonist on the other hand, did not yield promising results. Additionally, minocycline was found to have positive effects on visual learning memory when added to antipsychotic treatment. Both typical and atypical antipsychotics do not seem to enhance visual learning and memory. Studies investigating nicotinic receptor agonist, acetylcholinesterase inhibitors, GABA α_2/α_3 agonist, psychostimulants, and GR antagonist did not yield positive results but are in need of replication as they were possibly underpowered. Overall, results need be interpreted with care as the described studies are often small pilot studies with inherent limitations.

WORKING MEMORY

Working memory refers to a system with limited capacity for temporary storage and manipulation of information, necessary for cognitive tasks (74), and has been the subject of many studies investigating cognition in schizophrenia. Most of these studies focused on the effects of antipsychotic medication on working memory.

Although results are inconclusive at present, both typical and atypical antipsychotics show little beneficial effects on working memory. Rollnik et al. (69) compared the effectiveness of typical and atypical antipsychotics and found no differences between the two groups. Quetiapine and amisulpride, which both have low affinity for the 5-HT_{2a} receptors, improved performance on a verbal working memory task compared to risperidone, olanzapine, and clozapine (high affinity for 5-HT_{2a}) treatment (17). However, performance on a visual working memory tasks did not significantly improve in both groups. No differences were found in working memory performance between amisulpride and olanzapine by Wagner et al. (16). However, working memory performance did improve in both groups. Effects of olanzapine, risperidone, and haloperidol were compared by Purdon et al. (20). After correction for multiple comparisons, no significant differences were found between the three treatment conditions and working memory did not improve in any group. Mori et al. (75) examined the effects of switching from typical antipsychotics to olanzapine, quetiapine, risperidone, or perospirone on working memory and found improvement in working memory with risperidone, while working memory performance of the patients treated with quetiapine decreased. Working memory performance did not change in the olanzapine and perospirone group. It must be noted that the mean age in the sample was high (59.9 years) and correlated negatively with working memory scores. Therefore age related cognitive decline may have confounded these results. On the contrary, Kivircik Akdede et al. (26) found improvement on working memory with quetiapine. However, this study did not include a control group and did not correct for possible practice effects. Risperidone treatment was found to be superior to haloperidol in the study by McGurk et al. (70), but after correcting for anticholinergic co-medication, this effect was no longer significant. Working memory performance did not improve in both groups. Paliperidone treatment was not superior to risperidone treatment in enhancing working memory in the study by Kim et al. (31) and working memory did not improve in both groups.

Results regarding clozapine are inconclusive. Papageorgiou et al. (76) compared the effects of clozapine and olanzapine on working memory and found that working memory improved in both groups. No differences were found between the two treatment conditions. Ertugrul et al. (33) conducted two working memory tasks (Digit Span Test and the Auditory Consonant Trigram Test) and found that performance on the Digit Span test improved with clozapine treatment, whereas performance on the Auditory Consonant Trigram Test did not. Both studies did not correct for possible practice effects or multiple testing. These results are contradicted by Purdon et al. (32) who did not find improvement in working memory with clozapine treatment. This discrepancy in findings could be due to methodological shortcomings and differences such as different test batteries and trial duration.

Riedel et al. found that aripiprazole did not significantly enhance working memory (39). Aripiprazole also did not improve working memory when added to atypical antipsychotics (42). Adjunctive sertindole, an atypical antipsychotic with high affinity for the D_2 and 5-HT_{2a} receptors, did not improve working memory in patients treated with clozapine (77). Finally, working memory did improve after 20–30 mg of the novel antipsychotic BL-1020 (a dopamine antagonist with GABA agonistic properties) compared to placebo whereas 10 mg BL-1020 and risperidone did not (35).

Hence, although results are preliminary and inconclusive, at present no convincing evidence is available for the effectiveness of both typical and atypical antipsychotics on working memory in schizophrenia. However, the antipsychotic BL-1020 was found to improve working memory, possibly through its $GABA_A$ agonistic properties.

Single administration of the dopamine D_1 agonist dihydrexidine did not enhance working memory in a trial by George et al. (48). Given the small sample size and the fact that dihydrexidine was only administered a single time, beneficial effects of long term dihydrexidine administration on working memory cannot be ruled out.

Serotonin 5-HT_{3a} receptors seem to be less important for working memory functioning. Both Akhondzadeh et al. (43) and Levkovitz et al. (44) found no improvement in working memory with adjunctive ondansetron (5-HT_{3a} antagonist) treatment. Moreover, adjunctive tropisetron treatment also did not enhance working memory (45).

In addition, Niitsu et al. (71) found no improvement in working memory after adjunctive fluvoxamine treatment. Moreover, 12 weeks of adjunctive citalopram treatment did not enhance working memory (47). Hence, these results suggest that serotonin modulation pharmacological agents do not significantly enhance working memory in schizophrenia.

Both the selective nicotinic $\alpha_4\beta_2$ receptor agonist AZD3480 and the partial nicotinic α_7 agonist DMXB-A did not enhance working memory performance (51, 52). Acetylcholinesterase inhibitors donepezil and rivastigmine did not enhance working memory either (50, 53–55, 57, 58, 77). Jacobsen et al. (78) examined the effects of a single administration of nicotine [nicotinic acetylcholine receptor agonist (79)] on working memory in tobacco using patients and tobacco using healthy subjects. Although patients performed significantly worse on the N-back task compared to healthy controls, nicotine administration did improve performance on the two-back in patients while performance of the healthy controls declined. Thus, although the acetylcholinesterase inhibitors donepezil and rivastigmine and nicotinic receptor agonists do not show positive effects on working memory in schizophrenia, positive results were found with a single dose of nicotine administration. Therefore, a role of acetylcholine and nicotinic receptors in enhancing working memory cannot be ruled out.

Working memory did not improve in a study by Buchanan et al. (59) after 4 weeks of treatment with partial GABA α_2/α_3 agonist MK-0777. Menzies et al. (80) studied the effects of lorazepam, a $GABA_A$ receptor agonist, and flumazenil, a $GABA_A$ receptor antagonist, on working memory in patients and healthy subjects. Working memory performance declined after a single dose of lorazepam whereas performance did not change significantly after flumazenil. Thus, although results are inconclusive, there is some evidence that in $GABA_A$ agonists may lower working memory. However positive effects on working memory were found with an antipsychotic with additional $GABA_A$ agonistic properties.

Friedman et al. (60) found no effects of atomoxetine (norepinephrine reuptake inhibitor) on working memory in patients. A lack of effect could be due to insufficient power.

Glutamatergic pathways have been examined by Duncan et al. (81). They added 50 mg of D-cycloserine, an antituberculous drug which, at low doses has agonistic properties at the NDMA receptors, to typical antipsychotics. After 4 weeks of treatment, working memory did not improve. However, these results need to be replicated before the role of NMDA receptors in working memory can be established.

Armodafinil, a longer-lasting isomer of modafinil, did not enhance performance on working memory task when added to atypical antipsychotics for 4 weeks (61). However, Turner et al. (63) found that a single dose of modafinil improved performance on a verbal working memory task compared to placebo. Performance on a spatial working memory task did not differ between modafinil condition and placebo condition. These results were not replicated by Spence et al. (82) who did not find differences in performance on a (verbal) working memory task after a single administration of modafinil compared to placebo. This discrepancy in findings could be due to differences in modafinil dose (200 and 100 mg, respectively). Moreover, both studies used different tasks which make direct comparison of results difficult. Nonetheless, a single dose of modafinil might enhance working memory in schizophrenia patients, although recurrent treatment with a longer-lasting variant showed no effect.

Add-on intranasal oxytocin treatment did not improve working memory (15). Furthermore, adjunctive mifepristone (GR antagonist) treatment did not enhance working memory (66). Goff et al. (67) did not find improvement in working memory after both 50 and 100 mg sildenafil administration. Furthermore, daily creatine administration added to antipsychotic treatment did not have beneficial effects on working memory either (65). Add-on minocycline treatment on the other hand, improved working memory in a study by Levkovitz et al. (73); the number of errors on a working memory task decreased significantly in the minocycline group whereas the number of errors in the placebo group increased. However, this study has some limitations which are described earlier. Thus, apart from minocycline, other lines of research did not identify possible new intervention strategies for working memory enhancement in schizophrenia.

To summarize, even though some positive results were found with minocycline, nicotine, and modafinil, the presently available studies did not identify promising molecular targets for enhancement of working memory in schizophrenia. GABA agonists have shown mixed results. Most of the studies examined the effects of antipsychotic treatment on working memory and only a limited number of studies used other pharmacological interventions, which makes it difficult to draw definite conclusions. More research needs to be conducted, especially on the potential role of GABA, norepinephrine, acetylcholine, glutamate, and psychostimulants.

ATTENTION AND VIGILANCE

The construct of attention refers to a core cognitive function that relates to the ability to select, filter, focus, and process different stimuli in the environment. Attention is closely related to working memory and executive functioning (83) and therefore, it is difficult to distinguish between these constructs. Because of the broad definition, impairment in virtually any task can be considered as impairment in attention (83). Therefore, in this review, we only included articles which used the Continuous Performance Test (CPT) to specifically measure attention as this test is recommended by the MATRICS (84).

Studies using antipsychotics to enhance attention report little beneficial effects. The theory that atypical antipsychotics are superior to typical antipsychotics in enhancing cognition was tested for attention as well. A trial comparing olanzapine to amisulpride did not find differences in effects on attention; attention did not significantly improve in both groups (16). Olanzapine did not enhance attention in a study by Molina et al. (85), who examined the effects of switching from typical antipsychotics or risperidone to olanzapine. Attention did not improve with olanzapine treatment.

The effects of risperidone on attention were compared to the effects of respectively haloperidol (86) and quetiapine (23). In the study of Liu et al. (86) no improvement was found in both the haloperidol and the risperidone group. Additionally, although no differences were found between the risperidone and quetiapine in the study by Harvey et al. (23), within group analyses showed significant improvement in attention in the risperidone group, whereas the quetiapine group did not improve. Kim et al. (27) reported improvement with depot risperidone. However, paliperidone did not improve attention (31). To summarize, both typical and atypical antipsychotics have shown little beneficial effects on attention in schizophrenia patients.

The possible role of dopamine and serotonin in attention has also been examined with intervention strategies other than antipsychotic treatment. George et al. (48) examined the effects of a full dopamine D_1 agonist, dihydrexidine but found it not to enhance attention.

Studies using serotonin intervention strategies have not yielded positive results either. Golightly et al. (87) examined the role of serotonin in attention by using acute tryptophan, a precursor for serotonin, depletion. Depletion had no effect on performance on the CPT. Niitsu et al. (71) investigated the effect of adjunctive fluvoxamine treatment on attention and found no improvement in attention either. The effects of citalopram, added to treatment with atypical antipsychotics was examined by Friedman et al. (47). They found that adjunctive citalopram treatment did not enhance attention. Thus, although serotonin has been implicated in both verbal and visual memory, it does not seem to play a prominent role in attention.

Based on results of mostly preliminary studies, acetylcholine does not seem to play an important role in attention. Selective nicotinic $\alpha_4\beta_2$ receptor agonist AZD3480, did not enhance attention in a study by Velligan et al. (51). Nonetheless, Freedman et al. (52) found some beneficial effects of partial nicotinic α_7 agonist DMXB-A on attention. In their cross-over study, patients were treated with 75, 150 mg DMXB-A, and placebo. All treatment arms lasted 4 weeks, followed by a 1-week washout period. Over the course of the trial, attention improved in all treatment groups. The authors suggested that possible practice effects had obscured the potential effect of treatment, and therefore also examined the scores after the first 4 weeks of treatment. They found that attention improved with both doses of DMXB-A compared to the placebo. Two types of acetylcholinesterase inhibitors, rivastigmine, and donepezil, did not enhance attention in schizophrenia (56, 58, 88). On the other hand, a single nicotine administration improved attention in schizophrenia patients but not in healthy controls (89). Thus, despite negative results with acetylcholinesterase inhibitors, some promising results have been obtained with nicotine and a partial nicotinic α_7 agonist. These preliminary results suggest that the nicotinic receptors are a potential target for enhancement of attention in schizophrenia.

Partial GABA α_2/α_3 agonist MK-0777 did not enhance attention when added to antipsychotic treatment (59). However, as mentioned earlier, MK-0777 is a weak GABA α_2/α_3 agonist and this is the only study investigating the potential role of GABA in attention in schizophrenia. Therefore, these results need to be replicated using specific and more potent GABA modulatory agents.

Other lines of research have not yielded positive results. The psychostimulant drug armodafinil did not enhance attention (61). Furthermore, adjunctive mifepristone (GR antagonist) therapy did not improve attention (66). Duncan et al. (81) found no improvement in attention with adjunctive D-cycloserine treatment. Also, sildenafil (PDE5 inhibitor) did not enhance attention in schizophrenia in a trial by Goff et al. (67). Stone et al. (68) compared the effects of single administration of glucose to placebo in clozapine-treated patients and found attention to be significantly worse in the glucose condition. Thus, several other lines of research did not identify potential new intervention strategies enhancement of attention in schizophrenia.

To summarize, at present only a few pharmacological intervention strategies have been effective in enhancing attention in schizophrenia. Although results are not consistent, positive results have been found with both oral and depot risperidone treatment. Furthermore, a partial nicotinic α_7 agonist, and a single administration of nicotine did improve attention in schizophrenia, suggesting a role for acetylcholine and nicotinic receptors in attention. Overall, results need to be considered preliminary and more research needs to be conducted to replicate these findings as these studies have some important limitations.

PROCESSING SPEED

Processing speed is considered a core cognitive function and refers to the speed at which the brain processes information. It can be measured as the number of correct responses during a task within a given amount of time (90).

As for other domains of cognition, a majority of the studies examined the effects of antipsychotic medication on processing speed. The theory that atypical antipsychotics are superior to typical antipsychotics in improving cognition in patients was tested for processing speed as well. A study comparing amisulpride with olanzapine found that processing speed did not improve in both groups (16). Moreover, performance on a processing speed task did not differ between patients treated with different typical antipsychotics and atypical antipsychotics and performance did not improve in both groups (69). Purdon et al. (20) compared the effects of olanzapine, risperidone, and haloperidol on processing speed. After correction for multiple comparisons, no significant differences were found between the three treatment conditions and processing speed did not improve in any of the groups. Thus, atypical antipsychotics do not appear to be superior to typical antipsychotics. Furthermore, no beneficial effects of the atypical antipsychotic ziprasidone were found on processing speed (21). Anticholinergics were allowed during the trial which might have influenced the results. Risperidone depot treatment did not enhance processing speed in the study by Kim et al. (27). Moreover, paliperidone ER was not found to be superior to risperidone (31). Unfortunately, within group comparisons were not reported. However, although no significant differences were found between two treatment groups, risperidone was found to improve processing speed whereas quetiapine did not in a study comparing these two antipsychotics (23). Contrary to those results, quetiapine was found to enhance processing speed in a trial by Kivircik Akdede et al. (26). As described earlier, this study did not include a control group and did not correct for possible practice effects. These results were not replicated by Purdon et al. (24). Although processing speed improved in both the quetiapine and haloperidol group, these results were not significant after correcting for multiple comparisons. Velligan et al. (25) compared the effectiveness on processing speed between quetiapine and haloperidol treatment. They found no differences between the two treatment groups. Purdon et al. (32) found that processing speed improved with clozapine treatment. However, this improvement cannot reliably be attributed to the effects of clozapine as the study did not include a control group en they did not correct for possible practice effects. Beneficial effects of aripiprazole on processing speed were found by Riedel et al. (39). Yasui-Furukori et al. (42) found no improvement in processing speed with adjunctive aripiprazole treatment to olanzapine or risperidone. Furthermore, a new antipsychotic with $GABA_A$ receptor agonistic properties in addition to dopamine D_2 and serotonin $5\text{-}HT_{2a}$ receptor blockade (BL-1020) did not improve processing speed (35).

To summarize, both typical and atypical antipsychotics do not seem to effectively enhance processing speed in schizophrenia patients. Although some studies reported positive effects of clozapine, quetiapine, and risperidone, these results should be interpreted with care as these studies have important limitations.

Studies examining the role of serotonin in processing speed did not yield positive results. Adjunctive ondansetron ($5\text{-}HT_{3a}$ receptor antagonist) therapy to antipsychotic medication did not enhance processing speed in a study by Levkovitz et al. (44). Adding citalopram to atypical antipsychotic treatment also did not enhance processing speed in the study by Friedman et al. (47). In addition, tryptophan depletion did not affect processing speed in the study by Golightly et al. (87). Thus, the available studies do not provide evidence for a prominent role of serotonin in processing speed in schizophrenia. However, all studies used small samples and the study of Golightly et al. (87) allowed concomitant anticholinergics which could have influenced the results.

Studies using acetylcholine related intervention strategies did not yield positive results either. Both the selective nicotinic $\alpha_4\beta_2$ receptor agonist AZD3480 and the partial nicotinic α_7 agonist DMXB-A did not enhance processing speed (51, 52). Moreover, three types of acetylcholinesterase inhibitors, donepezil, galantamine, and rivastigmine, did not improve processing speed (50, 54–58). Thus, although the role of acetylcholine in memory and attention has been well established, it does not seem to be a potential target in enhancing processing speed in schizophrenia. However, these studies have limitations such as small sample sizes.

Effects of GABA and norepinephrine on processing speed were also examined. Processing speed did not improve after adjunctive treatment with partial α_2/α_3 agonist MK-0777 (59). As mentioned earlier, BL-1020 (antipsychotic with $GABA_A$ agonistic properties) enhanced antipsychotic also did not enhance processing speed (35). In the pilot study of Friedman et al. (60), processing speed did not improve after adjunctive treatment with the norepinephrine reuptake inhibitor atomoxetine. Thus, norepinephrine and GABA α_2/α_3 receptors do not seem to play an important role in processing speed in schizophrenia as the available studies were not able to detect positive effects. However, lack of effect could be due to the small sample size of both studies.

Processing speed did increase after a single dose of D-amphetamine in the study of Pietrzak et al. (72). Adjunctive armodafinil treatment had no beneficial effects on processing speed in the study by Kane et al. (61). Hence, since D-amphetamine is an indirect dopamine D_1 agonist, dopamine D_1 receptors could be a possible target for enhancing processing speed in schizophrenia although the study by Pietrzak et al. (72) needs replication.

Lastly, there are some studies of agents that have no direct (known) effect on neurotransmission. Processing speed did not improve after single dose of 50 and 100 mg sildenafil (a PDE5 inhibitor commonly used for erectile dysfunction) in the crossover trial by Goff et al. (67). Furthermore, adjunctive dehydroepiandrosterone (DHEA) therapy, a corticosteroid that serves as a precursor for both androgenic and estrogenic steroids, did not enhance processing speed (91). Thus, other lines of research did not identify promising intervention strategies for enhancement of processing speed in schizophrenia.

To summarize, at present no convincing evidence exist for the effectiveness of both typical and atypical antipsychotics on processing speed in schizophrenia. Although, positive results were found with quetiapine, risperidone, clozapine, and aripiprazole, these studies have important limitations and therefore the effects cannot be reliably attributed to the effects of the medication. One positive result was found with single dose D-amphetamine, suggesting a potential role of dopamine D_1 receptors in processing speed. Studies investigating 5-HT_{3a} receptor antagonist, SSRI, nicotinic receptor agonist, acetylcholinesterase inhibitors, a GABA α_2/α_3 agonist, and a norepinephrine reuptake inhibitor did not find clinically relevant improvement in processing speed but are in need for replication as the described studies used small samples and were possibly underpowered.

REASONING AND PROBLEM SOLVING

We found 30 studies that measured reasoning and problem solving after a pharmacological intervention. Reasoning and problem solving is considered an aspect of executive functioning. As for the other cognitive domains, a relatively large number of studies investigated the effects of antipsychotics on reasoning and problem solving.

Tyson et al. (17) compared antipsychotics with low affinity for 5-HT_{2a} receptors to antipsychotics with high affinity for these receptors. Response latency on a reasoning and problem solving task decreased in the low affinity group, whereas latency increased in the high-affinity group. The authors did not correct for multiple comparisons. Since response latency increased in the high-affinity group, it is not likely that the improvement in the low affinity group is (only) driven by practice effects. Purdon et al. (20) compared the effects of olanzapine, risperidone, and haloperidol and found that olanzapine was superior in enhancing reasoning and problem solving. However, after correcting for multiple comparisons, none of the medications improved reasoning and problem solving. On the contrary, both Kim et al. (27) and Suzuki and Gen (28) found improvement in performance on a reasoning and problem solving task. However, Kim et al. (27) did not include a control group and did not correct for possible practice effects. Therefore, improvement cannot be reliably attributed to the effects of medication. Moreover, in the study of Suzuki and Gen (28) a high percentage of the patients in the haloperidol group was using concomitant anticholinergics whereas in the risperidone group anticholinergics were tapered during the first weeks of the trial. Therefore improvement in this group could be due to effects of diminishing anticholinergics.

Purdon et al. (24) investigated the effects of haloperidol and quetiapine and found that reasoning and problem solving did not improve in both groups. Olanzapine, perospirone, and aripiprazole did not improve reasoning and problem solving either (41). Moreover, adding aripiprazole to atypical antipsychotics also did not yield positive results (42). Furthermore, no improvement was found with clozapine by Ertugrul et al. (33) and Purdon et al. (32). Nielsen et al. (77) added sertindole to clozapine but found no improvement in reasoning and problem solving either. Finally, the new antipsychotic with GABA agonistic properties BL-1020 also did not improve reasoning and problem solving (35). Hence, although positive results were found with risperidone depot, both typical and atypical antipsychotics have shown little clinically relevant effects on reasoning and problem solving.

Serotonergic intervention strategies have not yielded positive results. Adjunctive ondansetron (5-HT_3 antagonist) treatment had no beneficial effects on reasoning and problem solving (43). Fluvoxamine and citalopram both did not enhance reasoning and problem solving either (47, 71). On the contrary, Golightly et al. (87) found that patients who underwent tryptophan depletion during the first session performed significantly worse on the Wisconsin Card Sorting Test (WCST) compared to placebo. However, this effect was not present during the second session. The WCST requires subjects to sort cards by a certain parameter. The subject is not told which parameter. The sorting principle changes after 10 correct responses in a row. Thus subjects have to acquire a certain strategy to sort the cards. The authors concluded that tryptophan depletion only affected strategy acquisition and that once this is learned; tryptophan depletion did not interfere with application of this strategy. Thus, based on the results described above, 5-HT_{3a} antagonist and SSRI's did not effectively enhance reasoning and problem solving. However, a role for serotonin in this aspect of cognition cannot be ruled out since tryptophan depletion did interfere with strategy acquisition.

Partial nicotinic α_7 agonist DMXB-A had no enhancing effects on reasoning and problem solving in the study by Freedman et al. (52). In addition, studies investigating the effects of the acetylcholinesterase inhibitors donepezil and rivastigmine did not find improvement in performance on a reasoning and problem solving task either (50, 53, 56, 58). Hence, based on these results, nicotinic α_7 agonists and acetylcholinesterase inhibitors do not appear to significantly enhance reasoning and problem solving in schizophrenia.

In line with the results of Geffen et al. (35) described earlier, no positive results were obtained with other GABAergic interventions strategies. Adjunctive therapy with partial GABA α_2/α_3 agonist MK-0777 did not enhance reasoning and problem solving abilities in the study by Buchanan et al. (59). In addition, adjunctive topiramate (an antiepileptic drug which potentiates GABAergic transmission probably through its AMPA/kainite receptor antagonistic properties) treatment did not enhance reasoning and problem solving either (92). Zoccali et al. (93) examined the effects of adjunctive lamotrigine, an anticonvulsant drug which reduces excessive glutamate release in the brain via inhibition of voltage-gated sodium and calcium channels (94). Reasoning and problem solving did not improve.

The potential role of norepinephrine in reasoning and problem solving in schizophrenia was examined in a pilot study by Friedman et al. (60) by adding atomoxetine to antipsychotic treatment. They found no improvement in this aspect of cognition.

In conclusion, the available evidence suggests that modulation of GABA and glutamate transmission and norepinephrine reuptake inhibition does not have enhancing effects on reasoning and problem solving abilities in schizophrenia.

Some positive results have been found with psychostimulant drugs. Compared to placebo, performance on a reasoning and problem solving task improved after a single dose of D-amphetamine [indirect dopamine D_1 agonist, (72)]. Contrary to these results, Turner et al. (63) found that, compared to placebo, response latency on the Tower of London task was significantly lower after modafinil administration. The number of attempts to obtain the correct solution did not differ between the two groups. Armodafinil, the longer-lasting isomer of modafinil, did not affect reasoning and problem solving abilities (61). Thus, although armodafinil and modafinil did not enhance reasoning and problem solving, D-amphetamine did improve this aspect of cognition. This suggests that dopamine D_1 agonists are a potential area of research for further study of reasoning and problem solving in schizophrenia.

Pharmacological intervention strategies that do not directly influence neurotransmission were also investigated. Levkovitz et al. (73) found that reasoning and problem solving abilities improved after add-on minocycline treatment whereas performance in the placebo group did not change. Both creatine and glucose had no enhancing effects on reasoning and problem solving; daily creatine administration in addition to antipsychotic treatment did not have beneficial effects on working memory in the study by Kaptsan et al. (65). Stone et al. (68) found no improvement in reasoning and problem solving after a single dose of glucose. Hence, despite of the study's limitations, minocycline's putative ability to improve reasoning and problem solving abilities should be studied further.

In conclusion, although positive results were found with depot risperidone treatment in studies with important limitations, antipsychotics do not seem to effectively improve reasoning and problem solving in schizophrenia. The available studies did not show enhancing effects of the neurotransmitters serotonin, acetylcholine, GABA, or norepinephrine on reasoning and problem solving. However, dopamine D_1 agonists may have potential in this cognitive domain since one positive result was found with a single dose D-amphetamine. Finally, minocycline had enhancing effects on reasoning and problem solving abilities. However, this study has important limitations. Therefore these results are in need for replication.

SOCIAL COGNITION

In general terms, social cognition refers to the cognitive processes used to decode and encode the social world (95). Of all the MATRICS cognitive domains, social cognition has received the least attention in research. This is probably due to the fact that it is a relatively new area in schizophrenia research (96) and that the boundaries of this domain are not entirely clear (96). Final screening yielded no more than seven articles on social cognition and pharmacology using validated outcome measures.

A study by Mizrahi et al. (97) examined the effects of antipsychotic treatment on social cognition in schizophrenia. They investigated the effects of clozapine, risperidone, olanzapine, and loxapine on Theory of Mind (TOM). TOM is an aspect of social cognition which refers to the ability to understand intentions of others and to recognize that their actions are guided by beliefs about the world (97). They found that TOM improved after 2 weeks of medication use and continued to improve during the rest of the trial. Unfortunately, the authors did not differentiate between the four different antipsychotics. However, all four types of medication have high affinity for dopamine D_2 receptors as well as the 5-HT_{2a} receptors (98, 99). These results are in line with the results of Sumiyoshi et al. (100) who found that perospirone treatment improved performance on a social cognition task. Nonetheless, both studies did not include a control group and used small samples. Hence, given the longitudinal design of this study, natural progression and practice effects cannot be excluded. Additionally, the high drop-out rate in the study of Sumiyoshi et al. (100) could have led to a bias in the sample. Behere et al. (101) found that performance on an emotion recognition task improved after risperidone treatment. However, it must be noted that they did not include a control group and that time of follow-up assessment was not equal for all patients. Opposed to these results, the study by Harvey et al. (23) discussed earlier did not find improvement in performance on an emotional recognition task in patients treated with either quetiapine or risperidone.

Hence, these results imply preliminary evidence that dopamine and serotonin are important for TOM related aspects of social cognition but not for emotion recognition.

The possible role of GABA in social cognition was investigated by Buchanan et al. (59). They found no improvement with the partial GABA α_2/α_3 agonist MK-0777 when added to antipsychotic treatment. The psychostimulant armodafinil also did not improve social cognition (61). Hence, GABA α_2/α_3 receptors are not prime candidates for enhancing social cognition in schizophrenia.

Another line of research focused on the role of oxytocin in social cognition. This neuropeptide is known for its role in positive social behavior (102). Pedersen et al. (103) found that intranasal oxytocin administration improved social cognition. This implicates a role for oxytocin in social cognition. Since previous research showed that plasma oxytocin levels are lower in schizophrenia compared to controls (104), it could be hypothesized that increasing oxytocin levels improves social cognition in schizophrenia. However, the study of Pedersen et al. (103) has some important limitations. First, the sample size was small. Moreover, they carried out multiple tests in this small sample; therefore the results have to be interpreted with caution. Studies investigating the role of oxytocin in social cognition are sparse. Therefore, to determine the exact role of oxytocin in social cognition more research needs to be conducted on this topic.

In conclusion, the available seven studies suggest preliminary evidence for a role of dopamine, serotonin, and oxytocin in social cognition in schizophrenia patients. GABA does not seem to be a promising target for enhancement of social cognition. However, these studies have important limitations. Therefore future research needs to confirm the role of these transmitters in social cognition.

DISCUSSION

With this review we aimed to provide an outline of the underlying neuropharmacological mechanisms of the separate MATRICS domains. Although some potential targets were identified, overall, results of previous studies attempting to identify potential pharmacological targets for cognitive enhancement have been unsatisfactory. This review has shown that dysfunction in separate cognitive domains seems to arise from different underlying neuropharmacological mechanisms. This suggests that schizophrenia patients with different cognitive impairments could benefit from different (adjunctive) pharmacological agents. The identified potential molecular targets, which include dopamine D_1 receptors, serotonin 5-HT_{1a} and 5-HT_{3a} receptors, nicotinic α_7 receptors, $GABA_A$ receptors, and NMDA receptors, are described more extensively below.

DOPAMINE D_1

Although George et al. (48) were not able to detect positive results with a single dose of D_1 agonist dihydrexidine, Pietrzak et al. (72) found improvement in both processing speed and reasoning and problems solving abilities (both aspects of executive functioning) after a single dose of D-amphetamine, an indirect D_1 agonist. Decreased dopaminergic neurotransmission in the PFC has been hypothesized to be associated with cognitive dysfunction in schizophrenia (36). Since D_1 receptors are highly abundant in the PFC (105), this receptor subtype has been particularly associated with executive function and working memory. A PET study by Okubo et al. (106) found decreased D_1 receptors in the PFC in schizophrenia which was indeed associated with poorer executive functioning. Animal studies provide additional evidence for cognitive enhancing effects of D_1 receptor agonists as low doses of several D_1 agonists were found to enhance cognition in non-human primates (107, 108). Because a majority of dopamine receptors in the PFC belong to the D_1 subtype, and not to the D_2 subtype (109), which is related to psychotic symptom severity, D_1 receptors may be a feasible molecular target for enhancement of executive function related aspects of cognition without exacerbation of psychotic symptoms.

SEROTONIN 5-HT_{1a} AND 5-HT_{3a} RECEPTORS

(Partial) 5-HT_{1a} receptor agonism was found to improve verbal learning and memory (38–40). These enhancing effects may be due to the high density of 5-HT_{1a} receptors in the hippocampus (36), which is an area in the brain well known for its role in memory. In addition, preclinical studies showed that both 5-HT_{1a} agonists and antagonist enhanced cognition in rats (110, 111). 5-HT_{3a} receptor antagonism was associated with improvement in visual learning and memory (43, 44). Contrary to other subtypes of serotonin receptors, the 5-HT_{3a} receptor is the only ligand-gated ion channel subtype (43). To date, not many studies investigated the potential role of 5-HT_{3a} receptors in cognition. However, since both Akhondzadeh et al. (43) and Levkovitz et al. (44) found improvement in visual learning and memory with the 5-HT_{3a} receptor antagonist ondansetron, these receptors might be a promising molecular target for enhancement of visual learning and memory in schizophrenia.

ACETYLCHOLINE NICOTINIC α_7 RECEPTORS

The role of acetylcholine in cognition (particularly in learning, memory, and attention) has been widely established and central dysfunction of the cholinergic system has been found to be associated with cognitive symptoms in neurological diseases as Alzheimer and Parkinson's disease (112–114). However, with the exception of positive results found with nicotine and a partial nicotinic α_7 agonist on attention (52, 89), cholinergic interventions strategies did not affect any of the cognitive domains in the available studies. However, all the available studies that met the inclusion criteria used acetylcholinesterase inhibitors or nicotinic agonists. Although (mostly post-mortem) both nicotinic and muscarinic receptor abnormalities have been repeatedly found in schizophrenia (115–120), nicotinic receptor antagonists do not appear to impair cognition in the same manner as antimuscarinic drugs (121). This might explain the lack of improvement in the described studies. Indeed, a small pilot study by Shekar et al. (122) found that the muscarinic receptor agonist xanomeline improves verbal, visual, and working memory in patients with schizophrenia or schizoaffective disorder. Moreover, xanomeline improved cognition in Alzheimer disease (123). Thus, although positive effects on attention were found with nicotine and a partial nicotinic α_7 agonist, future studies should focus on muscarinic agents.

$GABA_A$ RECEPTORS

Both $GABA_A$ receptor antagonists and agonists were found to affect working memory and verbal learning and memory (35, 80). Multiple studies have shown reduced GABAergic transmission, especially in the PFC, in schizophrenia (124). The PFC is strongly involved in working memory functioning (125) and animal studies have shown that appropriate GABA transmission in the dorsolateral prefrontal cortex (DPFC) is essential to adequate working memory functioning (36, 126). Lewis et al. (37) showed that altered GABA transmission in the DPFC is possibly limited to certain cell classes, such as the chandelier cells, which synchronize the activation of the pyramidal neurons via the $GABA_A$ receptor subtypes. Therefore, $GABA_A$ receptors may be a promising molecular target for enhancement of working memory.

GLUTAMATE NMDA RECEPTORS

Glutamate, the primary excitatory neurotransmitter in the mammalian brain, has been linked to learning and memory because of its principal role in modulating long-term potentiation (127), and hyperactivity of glutamatergic neurotransmission has been implicated in schizophrenia (36). It has been hypothesized that cognitive dysfunction in schizophrenia is due to hypofunction of the NMDA receptor (81). Small increases in NMDA-dependent glutamate transmission might enhance cognition, whereas excessive stimulation might have neurodegenerative consequences (36). Activation of the NMDA receptors leads to synthesis of nitric oxide, which is able to further increase the excitotoxicity by increasing glutamate release from presynaptic neurons and inhibition of glial glutamate transporters (73). Indeed, minocycline (which blocks nitric oxide induced neurotoxicity) was found to improve visual learning and memory, working memory, and reasoning and problem solving abilities (73). Although D-cycloserine (which non-competitively enhances NMDA neurotransmission) was not found to improve attention and working memory (81), pharmacological agents reducing the neurotoxic effects of extensive glutamate might still be a promising intervention strategy for cognitive enhancement.

CAN THE NEGATIVE RESULTS BE EXPLAINED BY STUDIES LIMITATIONS?

A substantial number of the studies evaluated in this review addressing pharmacological cognitive enhancement in schizophrenia report negative results. It is debatable whether this is due to ineffectiveness of the agents used, or that potential results were obscured by methodological shortcomings as cognition research in schizophrenia deals with pertinent limitations. First, in many of the studies included in this review, cognition was not the primary outcome parameter. As a result, the design of these studies was not always optimal to measure cognitive enhancement. Second, the sample sizes are often too small to detect clinically relevant effects. Third, concurrent medications may interfere with the investigated pharmacological agents. Patients with schizophrenia are generally treated with antipsychotics. Because the entire mechanism of action of these medications is not completely understood, it cannot be ruled out that antipsychotics alter the effects of the added agents (62). Moreover, patients often use concomitant medications such as benzodiazepines, antidepressants, and anticholinergics, which could influence the effects of the adjunctive pharmacological agents as well. Especially anticholinergic medication is well known for its adverse effects on cognition (29). Therefore, studies including only medication-naïve patients at early stages of the disease are necessary. Fourth, studies often do not use fixed doses. It is possible that certain agents are only effective in a certain dose. If studies do use a fixed dose, this dose is often established for treating the illness or symptoms it was originally used for. However, it is not necessarily so that the same dose is required for cognitive enhancement in schizophrenia. Fifth, research seems to focus on the direct or semi-direct enhancing effect of modulating certain receptors while cognitive decline has most often been a process of a longer period of time possibly implying that enhancement studies should equally allow for more time to yield effects. Also, different paradigms could focus on neuroprotective targets and preventing cognitive decline early in the disorder in contrast to enhancing cognition after impairment. Sixth, not all studies report information about substance use of the participants. Patients with schizophrenia often abuse substances as tobacco, alcohol and cannabis, and epidemiological studies found high co-morbidity rates of substance abuse (40–60%) (128, 129). Particularly tobacco use can interfere with nicotinic receptor agents as it causes desensitization of this receptor subtype. Although most of the studies excluded patients with a (recent) co-morbid diagnosis of alcohol or drug abuse/dependence, tobacco using patients are almost never excluded. Seventh, studies often use different neuropsychological tasks to measure the same aspects of cognition which makes it difficult to compare the results. Therefore, studies should use a standardized cognitive battery, such as the MATRICS Consensus Cognitive Battery [MCCB; (84)] or the CANTAB cognitive battery (130). The MCCB in particular, has been composed to reliably assess cognition in schizophrenia patients. At present, only three of the reported studies used this battery to measure cognition (50, 52, 59). Finally, not all studies used a control group and repeatedly conducted the same test battery without adequately correcting for potential practice effects. Therefore, improvement often cannot be reliably attributed to the effect of the pharmacological agent. Future research should take these limitations in to account in experimental setup and optimize their design for cognition measurement. Ideally, future studies should include a placebo or other control group and should ensure sufficient power by including enough participants. Furthermore, medication-naïve patients should be recruited, preferably non-smokers who do not use other substances as cannabis and alcohol. Regarding the design, future studies should choose cognition as primary outcome measure and optimize the design by using a fixed dose and make sure to choose a dose suitable for schizophrenia patients. Finally, future studies should make sure to choose sufficient trial duration and to use a standardized cognitive test battery which covers all the MATRICS domains. In this manner, studies will be better comparable and the effects of possible confounding variables will be limited. To summarize, the negative results of "pharmacological cognitive enhancement studies" could partially be explained by studies' limitations.

CONCLUSION

Although some potential targets were identified, overall, results of previous studies attempting to identify potential pharmacological targets for cognitive enhancement have been disappointing. This review has shown that dysfunction in separate cognitive domains may arise from different underlying neuropharmacological mechanisms which suggests that schizophrenia patients with different cognitive impairments could benefit from different intervention strategies. Although development of effective cognitive enhancers is a complex process, it is an exciting challenge for this area of research as improvement of cognition contributes significantly to the quality of life of these patients.

AUTHOR CONTRIBUTIONS

Wilhelmina A. M. Vingerhoets wrote the first draft of the manuscript. All authors contributed to and have approved the final manuscript.

REFERENCES

1. Reichenberg A, Weiser M, Caspi A, Knobler HY, Lubin G, Harvey PD, et al. Premorbid intellectual functioning and risk of schizophrenia and spectrum disorders. *J Clin Exp Neuropsychol* (2006) **28**:193–207. doi:10.1080/13803390500360372
2. Green MF, Kern RS, Heaton RK. Longitudinal studies of cognition and functional outcome in schizophrenia: implications for MATRICS. *Schizophr Res* (2004) **72**:41–51. doi:10.1016/j.schres.2004.09.009
3. Green MF. What are the functional consequences of neurocognitive deficits in schizophrenia? *Am J Psychiatry* (1996) **153**:321–30.
4. Heinrichs RW. The primacy of cognition in schizophrenia. *Am Psychol* (2005) **60**:229–42. doi:10.1037/0003-066X.60.3.229
5. Burton SC. Strategies for improving adherence to second-generation antipsychotics in patients with schizophrenia by increasing ease of use. *J Psychiatr Pract* (2005) **11**:369–78. doi:10.1097/00131746-200511000-00003

6. Prouteau A, Verdoux H, Briand C, Lesage A, Lalonde P, Nicole L, et al. Cognitive predictors of psychosocial functioning outcome in schizophrenia: a follow-up study of subjects participating in a rehabilitation program. *Schizophr Res* (2005) **77**:343–53. doi:10.1016/j.schres.2005.03.001
7. Chen EY, Hui CL, Dunn EL, Miao MY, Yeung WS, Wong CK, et al. A prospective 3-year longitudinal study of cognitive predictors of relapse in first-episode schizophrenic patients. *Schizophr Res* (2005) **77**:99–104. doi:10.1016/j.schres.2005.02.020
8. National Institute for Health and Clinical Excellence. *Schizophrenia: Core Interventions in the Treatment and Management of Schizophrenia in Adults in Primary and Secondary Care* (2009). Available from: http://guidance.nice.org.uk/CG82 (Clinical guideline 82).
9. Buchanan RW, Kreyenbuhl J, Kelly DL, Noel JM, Boggs DL, Fischer BA, et al. The 2009 schizophrenia PORT psychopharmacological treatment recommendations and summary statements. *Schizophr Bull* (2010) **36**:71–93. doi:10.1093/schbul/sbp116
10. Hasan A, Falkai P, Wobrock T, Lieberman J, Glenthoj B, Gattaz WF, et al. World Federation of Societies of Biological Psychiatry (WFSBP) guidelines for biological treatment of schizophrenia, part 1: update 2012 on the acute treatment of schizophrenia and the management of treatment resistance. *World J Biol Psychiatry* (2012) **13**:318–78. doi:10.3109/15622975.2012.696143
11. Stip E, Chouinard S, Boulay LJ. On the trail of a cognitive enhancer for the treatment of schizophrenia. *Prog Neuropsychopharmacol Biol Psychiatry* (2005) **29**:219–32. doi:10.1016/j.pnpbp.2004.11.004
12. Volk DW, Lewis DA. Impaired prefrontal inhibition in schizophrenia: relevance for cognitive dysfunction. *Physiol Behav* (2002) **77**:501–5. doi:10.1016/S0031-9384(02)00936-8
13. Cohen NJ, Ryan J, Hunt C, Romine L, Wszalek T, Nash C. Hippocampal system and declarative (relational) memory: summarizing the data from functional neuroimaging studies. *Hippocampus* (1999) **9**:83–98. doi:10.1002/(SICI)1098-1063(1999)9:1<83::AID-HIPO9>3.0.CO;2-7
14. Nuechterlein KH, Barch DM, Gold JM, Goldberg TE, Green MF, Heaton RK. Identification of separable cognitive factors in schizophrenia. *Schizophr Res* (2004) **72**:29–39. doi:10.1016/j.schres.2004.09.007
15. Feifel D, Macdonald K, Cobb P, Minassian A. Adjunctive intranasal oxytocin improves verbal memory in people with schizophrenia. *Schizophr Res* (2012) **139**:207–10. doi:10.1016/j.schres.2012.05.018
16. Wagner M, Quednow BB, Westheide J, Schlaepfer TE, Maier W, Kühn K-U. Cognitive improvement in schizophrenic patients does not require a serotonergic mechanism: randomized controlled trial of olanzapine vs amisulpride. *Neuropsychopharmacology* (2005) **30**:381–90. doi:10.1038/sj.npp.1300626
17. Tyson PJ, Roberts KH, Mortimer AM. Are the cognitive effects of atypical antipsychotics influenced by their affinity to 5HT-2A receptors? *Int J Neurosci* (2004) **114**:593–611. doi:10.1080/00207450490430552
18. Keefe RS, Bilder RM, Davis SM, Harvey PD, Palmer BW, Gold JM, et al. Neurocognitive effects of antipsychotic medications in patients with chronic schizophrenia in the CATIE trial. *Arch Gen Psychiatry* (2007) **64**:633–47. doi:10.1001/archpsyc.64.6.633
19. Davidson M, Galderisi S, Weiser M, Werbeloff N, Ph D, Fleischhacker WW, et al. Cognitive effects of antipsychotic drugs in first-episode schizophrenia and schizophreniform disorder: a randomized, open-label clinical trial (EUFEST). *Am J Psychiatry* (2009) **166**:675–82. doi:10.1176/appi.ajp.2008.08060806
20. Purdon SE, Jones BD, Stip E, Labelle A, Addington D, David SR, et al. Neuropsychological change in early phase schizophrenia during 12 months of treatment with olanzapine, risperidone, or haloperidol. *Arch Gen Psychiatry* (2000) **57**:249–58. doi:10.1001/archpsyc.57.3.249
21. Malhotra AK, Burdick KE, Razi K, Bates JA, Sanders M, Kane JM. Ziprasidone-induced cognitive enhancement in schizophrenia: specificity or pseudospecificity? *Schizophr Res* (2006) **87**:181–4. doi:10.1016/j.schres.2006.05.015
22. Rémillard S, Pourcher E, Cohen H. Long-term effects of risperidone versus haloperidol on verbal memory, attention, and symptomatology in schizophrenia. *J Int Neuropsychol Soc* (2008) **14**:110–8. doi:10.1017/S1355617708080090
23. Harvey PD, Patterson TL, Potter LS, Zhong K, Brecher M. Improvement in social competence with short-term double-blind comparison of quetiapine versus and neuropsychological functioning. *Am J Psychiatry* (2006) **163**:1918–25. doi:10.1176/appi.ajp.163.11.1918
24. Purdon SE, Malla A, Labelle A, Lit W. Neuropsychological change in patients with schizophrenia after treatment with quetiapine or haloperidol. *J Psychiatry Neurosci* (2001) **26**:137–49.
25. Velligan DI, Newcomer J, Pultz J, Csernansky J, Hoff AL, Mahurin R, et al. Does cognitive function improve with quetiapine in comparison to haloperidol? *Schizophr Res* (2002) **53**:239–48. doi:10.1016/S0920-9964(01)00268-7
26. Kivircik Akdede BB, Alptekin K, Kitis A, Arkar H, Akvardar Y. Effects of quetiapine on cognitive functions in schizophrenia. *Prog Neuropsychopharmacol Biol Psychiatry* (2005) **29**:233–8. doi:10.1016/j.pnpbp.2004.11.005
27. Kim S, Shin I, Kim J, Lee S, Lee Y, Yang S, et al. Effects of switching to long-acting injectable risperidone from oral atypical antipsychotics on cognitive function in patients with schizophrenia. *Hum Psychopharmacol* (2009) **24**:565–73. doi:10.1002/hup.1057
28. Suzuki H, Gen K. The influence of switching from haloperidol decanoate depot to risperidone long-acting injection on the clinical symptoms and cognitive function in schizophrenia. *Hum Psychopharmacol* (2012) **27**:470–5. doi:10.1002/hup.2249
29. Campbell N, Boustani M, Limbil T, Ott C, Fox C, Maidment I, et al. The cognitive impact of anticholinergics: a clinical review. *Clin Interv Aging* (2009) **4**:225–33.
30. Surguladze SA, Chu EM, Evans A, Anilkumar AP, Patel MX, Timehin C, et al. The effect of long-acting risperidone on working memory in schizophrenia: a functional magnetic resonance imaging study. *J Clin Psychopharmacol* (2007) **27**:560–70. doi:10.1097/jcp.0b013e31815a256c
31. Kim S-W, Chung Y-C, Lee Y-H, Lee J-H, Kim S-Y, Bae K-Y, et al. Paliperidone ER versus risperidone for neurocognitive function in patients with schizophrenia: a randomized, open-label, controlled trial. *Int Clin Psychopharmacol* (2012) **27**:267–74. doi:10.1097/YIC.0b013e328356acad
32. Purdon SE, Labelle A, Boulay L. Neuropsychological change in schizophrenia after 6 weeks of clozapine. *Schizophr Res* (2001) **48**:57–67. doi:10.1016/S0920-9964(00)00101-8
33. Ertugrul A, Ucar G, Basar K, Demir B, Yabanoglu S, Ulug B. Influence of clozapine on platelet serotonin, monoamine oxidase and plasma serotonin levels. *Psychiatry Res* (2007) **149**:49–57. doi:10.1016/j.psychres.2005.12.009
34. Sumiyoshi T, Roy A, Kim C-H, Jayathilake K, Lee MA, Sumiyoshi C, et al. Prediction of changes in memory performance by plasma homovanillic acid levels in clozapine-treated patients with schizophrenia. *Psychopharmacology* (2004) **177**:79–83. doi:10.1007/s00213-004-1924-5
35. Geffen Y, Keefe R, Rabinowitz J, Anand R, Davidson M. Bl-1020, a new γ-aminobutyric acid-enhanced antipsychotic: results of 6-week, randomized, double-blind, controlled, efficacy and safety study. *J Clin Psychiatry* (2012) **73**:1168–74. doi:10.4088/JCP.12m07642
36. Gray JA, Roth BL. Molecular targets for treating cognitive dysfunction in schizophrenia. *Schizophr Bull* (2007) **33**:1100–19. doi:10.1093/schbul/sbm074
37. Lewis DA, Pierri JN, Volk DW, Melchitzky DS, Woo TU. Altered GABA neurotransmission and prefrontal cortical dysfunction in schizophrenia. *Biol Psychiatry* (1999) **46**:616–26. doi:10.1016/S0006-3223(99)00061-X
38. Sumiyoshi T, Matsui M, Yamashita I, Nohara S, Kurachi M, Uehara T, et al. The effect of tandospirone, a serotonin1A agonist, on memory function in schizophrenia. *Biol Psychiatry* (2001) **49**:861–8. doi:10.1016/S0006-3223(00)01025-8
39. Riedel M, Spellmann I, Schennach-Wolff R, Musil R, Dehning S, Cerovecki A, et al. Effect of aripiprazole on cognition in the treatment of patients with schizophrenia. *Pharmacopsychiatry* (2010) **43**:50–7. doi:10.1055/s-0029-1239539
40. Bervoets C, Morrens M, Vansteelandt K, Kok F, de Patoul A, Halkin V, et al. Effect of aripiprazole on verbal memory and fluency in schizophrenic patients: results from the ESCAPE study. *CNS Drugs* (2012) **26**:975–82. doi:10.1007/s40263-012-0003-4
41. Suzuki H, Gen K, Inoue Y. An unblinded comparison of the clinical and cognitive effects of switching from first-generation antipsychotics to aripiprazole, perospirone or olanzapine in patients with chronic schizophrenia. *Prog Neuropsychopharmacol Biol Psychiatry* (2011) **35**:161–8. doi:10.1016/j.pnpbp.2010.10.021
42. Yasui-Furukori N, Kaneda A, Sugawara N, Tomita T, Kaneko S. Effect of adjunctive treatment with aripiprazole to atypical antipsychotics on cognitive function in schizophrenia patients. *J Psychopharmacol* (2012) **26**:806–12. doi:10.1177/0269881111405555

43. Akhondzadeh S, Mohammadi N, Noroozian M, Karamghadiri N, Ghoreishi A, Jamshidi A-H, et al. Added ondansetron for stable schizophrenia: a double blind, placebo controlled trial. *Schizophr Res* (2009) **107**:206–12. doi:10.1016/j.schres.2008.08.004
44. Levkovitz Y, Arnest G, Mendlovic S, Treves I, Fennig S. The effect of Ondansetron on memory in schizophrenic patients. *Brain Res Bull* (2005) **65**:291–5. doi:10.1016/j.brainresbull.2003.09.022
45. Zhang XY, Liu L, Liu S, Hong X, Chen DC, Xiu MH, et al. Short-term tropisetron treatment and cognitive and P50 auditory gating deficits in schizophrenia. *Am J Psychiatry* (2012) **169**:974–81. doi:10.1176/appi.ajp.2012.11081289
46. Ishikawa M, Sakata M, Toyohara J, Oda K, Ishii K, Wu J, et al. Occupancy of α7 nicotinic acetylcholine receptors in the brain by tropisetron: a positron emission tomography study using [(11)C]CHIBA-1001 in healthy human subjects. *Clin Psychopharmacol Neurosci* (2011) **9**:111–6. doi:10.9758/cpn.2011.9.3.111
47. Friedman JI, Ocampo R, Elbaz Z, Parrella M, White L, Bowler S, et al. The effect of citalopram adjunctive treatment added to atypical antipsychotic medications for cognitive performance in patients with schizophrenia. *J Clin Psychopharmacol* (2005) **25**:237–42. doi:10.1097/01.jcp.0000161499.58266.51
48. George MS, Molnar CE, Grenesko EL, Anderson B, Mu Q, Johnson K, et al. A single 20 mg dose of dihydrexidine (DAR-0100), a full dopamine D1 agonist, is safe and tolerated in patients with schizophrenia. *Schizophr Res* (2007) **93**:42–50. doi:10.1016/j.schres.2007.03.011
49. Karson CN, Mrak RE, Husain MM, Griffin WS. Decreased mesopontine choline acetyltransferase levels in schizophrenia. *Mol Chem Neuropathol* (1996) **29**:181–91. doi:10.1007/BF02815001
50. Tugal O, Yazici KM, Anil Yagcioglu AE, Gögüs A. A double-blind, placebo controlled, cross-over trial of adjunctive donepezil for cognitive impairment in schizophrenia. *Int J Neuropsychopharmacol* (2004) **7**:117–23. doi:10.1017/S1461145703004024
51. Velligan D, Brenner R, Sicuro F, Walling D, Riesenberg R, Sfera A, et al. Assessment of the effects of AZD3480 on cognitive function in patients with schizophrenia. *Schizophr Res* (2012) **134**:59–64. doi:10.1016/j.schres.2011.10.004
52. Freedman R, Olincy A, Buchanan RW, Harris JG, Gold JM, Johnson L, et al. Initial phase 2 trial of a nicotinic agonist in schizophrenia. *Am J Psychiatry* (2008) **165**:1040–7. doi:10.1176/appi.ajp.2008.07071135
53. Akhondzadeh S, Gerami M, Noroozian M, Karamghadiri N, Ghoreishi A, Abbasi S-H, et al. A 12-week, double-blind, placebo-controlled trial of donepezil adjunctive treatment to risperidone in chronic and stable schizophrenia. *Prog Neuropsychopharmacol Biol Psychiatry* (2008) **32**:1810–5. doi:10.1016/j.pnpbp.2008.08.001
54. Lee S, Lee J, Lee B, Hoon Y. Galantamine adjunctive treatment to conventional antipsychotics for the cognitive impairments in chronic schizophrenia. *Int Clin Psychopharmacol* (2007) **22**:63–8. doi:10.1097/YIC.0b013e328011 7feb
55. Fagerlund B, Søholm B, Fink-Jensen A, Lublin H, Glenthøj BY. Effects of donepezil adjunctive treatment to ziprasidone on cognitive deficits in schizophrenia: a double-blind, placebo-controlled study. *Clin Neuropharmacol* (2007) **30**:3–12. doi:10.1097/01.WNF.0000240940.67241.F6
56. Sharma T, Reed C, Aasen I, Kumari V. Cognitive effects of adjunctive 24-weeks rivastigmine treatment to antipsychotics in schizophrenia: a randomized, placebo-controlled, double-blind investigation. *Schizophr Res* (2006) **85**:73–83. doi:10.1016/j.schres.2006.03.037
57. Freudenreich O, Herz L, Deckersbach T, Evins AE, Henderson DC, Cather C, et al. Added donepezil for stable schizophrenia: a double-blind, placebo-controlled trial. *Psychopharmacology* (2005) **181**:358–63. doi:10.1007/s00213-005-2235-1
58. Friedman JI, Adler DN, Howanitz E, Harvey PD, Brenner G, Temporini H, et al. A double blind placebo controlled trial of donepezil adjunctive treatment to risperidone for the cognitive impairment of schizophrenia. *Biol Psychiatry* (2002) **51**:349–57. doi:10.1016/S0006-3223(01)01342-7
59. Buchanan RW, Keefe RS, Lieberman JA, Barch DM, Csernansky JG, Goff DC, et al. A randomized clinical trial of MK-0777 for the treatment of cognitive impairments in people with schizophrenia. *Biol Psychiatry* (2011) **69**:442–9. doi:10.1016/j.biopsych.2010.09.052
60. Friedman JI, Carpenter D, Lu J, Fan J, Tang CY, White L, et al. A pilot study of adjunctive atomoxetine treatment to second-generation antipsychotics for cognitive impairment in schizophrenia. *J Clin Psychopharmacol* (2008) **28**:59–63. doi:10.1097/jcp.0b013e318161318f
61. Kane JM, D'Souza DC, Patkar AA, Youakim JM, Tiller JM, Yang R, et al. Armodafinil as adjunctive therapy in adults with cognitive deficits associated with schizophrenia: a 4-week, double-blind, placebo-controlled study. *J Clin Psychiatry* (2010) **71**:1475–81. doi:10.4088/JCP.09m05950gry
62. Harvey PD. Pharmacological cognitive enhancement in schizophrenia. *Neuropsychol Rev* (2009) **19**:324–35. doi:10.1007/s11065-009-9103-4
63. Turner DC, Clark L, Pomarol-Clotet E, McKenna P, Robbins TW, Sahakian BJ. Modafinil improves cognition and attentional set shifting in patients with chronic schizophrenia. *Neuropsychopharmacology* (2004) **29**:1363–73. doi:10.1038/sj.npp.1300457
64. Ballon JS, Feifel D. A systematic review of modafinil: potential clinical uses and mechanisms of action. *J Clin Psychiatry* (2006) **67**:554–66. doi:10.4088/JCP.v67n0406
65. Kaptsan A, Odessky A, Osher Y, Levine J. Lack of efficacy of 5 grams daily of creatine in schizophrenia: a randomized, double-blind, placebo-controlled trial. *J Clin Psychiatry* (2007) **68**:881–4. doi:10.4088/JCP.v68n0609
66. Gallagher P, Watson S, Smith MS, Ferrier IN, Young AH. Effects of adjunctive mifepristone (RU-486) administration on neurocognitive function and symptoms in schizophrenia. *Biol Psychiatry* (2005) **57**:155–61. doi:10.1016/j.biopsych.2004.10.017
67. Goff DC, Cather C, Freudenreich O, Henderson DC, Evins AE, Culhane MA, et al. A placebo-controlled study of sildenafil effects on cognition in schizophrenia. *Psychopharmacology* (2009) **202**:411–7. doi:10.1007/s00213-008-1278-5
68. Stone WS, Seidman LJ, Wojcik JD, Green AI. Glucose effects on cognition in schizophrenia. *Schizophr Res* (2003) **62**:93–103. doi:10.1016/S0920-9964(02)00406-1
69. Rollnik JD, Borsutzky M, Huber TJ, Mogk H, Seifert J, Emrich HM, et al. Short-term cognitive improvement in schizophrenics treated with typical and atypical neuroleptics. *Neuropsychobiology* (2002) **45**:74–80. doi:10.1159/000048680
70. McGurk SR, Green MF, Wirshing WC, Wirshing DA, Marder SR, Mintz J, et al. Antipsychotic and anticholinergic effects on two types of spatial memory in schizophrenia. *Schizophr Res* (2004) **68**:225–33. doi:10.1016/S0920-9964(03)00123-3
71. Niitsu T, Fujisaki M, Shiina A, Yoshida T, Hasegawa T, Kanahara N, et al. A randomized, double-blind, placebo-controlled trial of fluvoxamine in patients with schizophrenia: a preliminary study. *J Clin Psychopharmacol* (2012) **32**:593–601. doi:10.1097/JCP.0b013e3182664cfc
72. Pietrzak RH, Snyder PJ, Maruff P. Use of an acute challenge with d-amphetamine to model cognitive improvement in chronic schizophrenia. *Hum Psychopharmacol* (2010) **25**:353–8. doi:10.1002/hup.1118
73. Levkovitz Y, Mendlovich S, Riwkes S, Braw Y, Levkovitch-Verbin H, Gal G, et al. A double-blind, randomized study of minocycline for the treatment of negative and cognitive symptoms in early-phase schizophrenia. *J Clin Psychiatry* (2010) **71**:138–49. doi:10.4088/JCP.08m04666yel
74. Hasselmo ME, Stern CE. Mechanisms underlying working memory for novel information. *Trends Cogn Sci* (2006) **10**:487–93. doi:10.1016/j.tics.2006.09.005
75. Mori K, Nagao M, Yamashita H, Morinobu S, Yamawaki S. Effect of switching to atypical antipsychotics on memory in patients with chronic schizophrenia. *Prog Neuropsychopharmacol Biol Psychiatry* (2004) **28**:659–65. doi:10.1016/j.pnpbp.2004.01.019
76. Papageorgiou C, Oulis P, Vasios C, Kontopantelis E, Uzunoglu N, Rabavilas A, et al. P300 alterations in schizophrenic patients experiencing auditory hallucinations. *Eur Neuropsychopharmacol* (2004) **14**:227–36. doi:10.1016/S0924-977X(03)00147-0
77. Nielsen RE, Levander S, Thode D, Nielsen J. Effects of sertindole on cognition in clozapine-treated schizophrenia patients. *Acta Psychiatr Scand* (2012) **126**:31–9. doi:10.1111/j.1600-0447.2012.01840.x
78. Jacobsen LK, D'Souza DC, Mencl WE, Pugh KR, Skudlarski P, Krystal JH. Nicotine effects on brain function and functional connectivity in schizophrenia. *Biol Psychiatry* (2004) **55**:850–8. doi:10.1016/j.biopsych.2003.12.023
79. Rezvani AH, Levin ED. Cognitive effects of nicotine. *Biol Psychiatry* (2001) **49**:258–67. doi:10.1016/S0006-3223(00)01094-5
80. Menzies L, Ooi C, Kamath S, Suckling J, McKenna P, Fletcher P, et al. Effects of γ-aminobutyric acid-modulating drugs on working memory and brain

function in patients with schizophrenia. *Arch Gen Psychiatry* (2007) **64**:156–67. doi:10.1001/archpsyc.64.2.156

81. Duncan EJ, Szilagyi S, Schwartz MP, Bugarski-Kirola D, Kunzova A, Negi S, et al. Effects of D-cycloserine on negative symptoms in schizophrenia. *Schizophr Res* (2004) **71**:239–48. doi:10.1016/j.schres.2004.03.013
82. Spence SA, Green RD, Wilkinson ID, Hunter MD. Modafinil modulates anterior cingulate function in chronic schizophrenia. *Br J Psychiatry* (2005) **187**:55–61. doi:10.1192/bjp.187.1.55
83. Luck SJ, Gold JM. The construct of attention in schizophrenia. *Biol Psychiatry* (2008) **64**:34–9. doi:10.1016/j.biopsych.2008.02.014
84. Nuechterlein KH, Green MF, Kern RS, Baade LE, Barch DM, Cohen JD, et al. The MATRICS consensus cognitive battery, part 1: test selection, reliability, and validity. *Am J Psychiatry* (2008) **165**:203–13. doi:10.1176/appi.ajp.2007.07010042
85. Molina V, Gispert JD, Reig S, Pascau J, Martinez R, Sanz J, et al. Olanzapine-induced cerebral metabolic changes related to symptom improvement in schizophrenia. *Pharmacopsychiatry* (2003) **20**:13–8.
86. Liu SK, Chen WJ, Chang CJ, Lin HN. Effects of atypical neuroleptics on sustained attention deficits in schizophrenia: a trial of risperidone versus haloperidol. *Neuropsychopharmacology* (2000) **22**:311–9. doi:10.1016/S0893-133X(99)00137-2
87. Golightly KL, Lloyd JA, Hobson JE, Gallagher P, Mercer G, Young AH. Acute tryptophan depletion in schizophrenia. *Psychol Med* (2001) **31**:75–84. doi:10.1017/S0033291799003062
88. Lenzi A, Maltinti E, Poggi E, Fabrizio L, Coli E. Effects of rivastigmine on cognitive function and quality of life in patients with schizophrenia. *Clin Neuropharmacol* (2003) **26**:317–21. doi:10.1097/00002826-200311000-00011
89. Dépatie L, O'Driscoll GA, Holahan AL, Atkinson V, Thavundayil JX, Kin NN, et al. Nicotine and behavioral markers of risk for schizophrenia: a double-blind, placebo-controlled, cross-over study. *Neuropsychopharmacology* (2002) **27**:1056–70. doi:10.1016/S0893-133X(02)00372-X
90. Knowles EE, David AS, Reichenberg A. Processing speed deficits in schizophrenia: reexamining the evidence. *Am J Psychiatry* (2010) **167**:828–35. doi:10.1176/appi.ajp.2010.09070937
91. Strous RD, Stryjer R, Maayan R, Gal G, Viglin D, Katz E, et al. Analysis of clinical symptomatology, extrapyramidal symptoms and neurocognitive dysfunction following dehydroepiandrosterone (DHEA) administration in olanzapine treated schizophrenia patients: a randomized, double-blind placebo controlled trial. *Psychoneuroendocrinology* (2007) **32**:96–105. doi:10.1016/j.psyneuen.2006.11.002
92. Muscatello MR, Bruno A, Pandolfo G, Micò U, Bellinghieri PM, Scimeca G, et al. Topiramate augmentation of clozapine in schizophrenia: a double-blind, placebo-controlled study. *J Psychopharmacol* (2011) **25**:667–74. doi:10.1177/0269881110372548
93. Zoccali R, Muscatello M, Bruno A, Cambria R. The effect of lamotrigine augmentation of clozapine in a sample of treatment-resistant schizophrenic patients: a double-blind, placebo-controlled study. *Schizophr Res* (2007) **93**:109–16. doi:10.1016/j.schres.2007.02.009
94. Kalyoncu A, Mirsal H, Pektas O, Unsalan N, Tan D, Beyazyürek M. Use of lamotrigine to augment clozapine in patients with resistant schizophrenia and comorbid alcohol dependence: a potent anti-craving effect? *J Psychopharmacol* (2005) **19**:301–5. doi:10.1177/0269881105051542
95. Beer JS, Ochsner KN. Social cognition: a multi level analysis. *Brain Res* (2006) **1079**:98–105. doi:10.1016/j.brainres.2006.01.002
96. Adolphs R. The neurobiology of social cognition. *Curr Opin Neurobiol* (2001) **11**:231–9. doi:10.1016/S0959-4388(00)00202-6
97. Mizrahi R, Korostil M, Starkstein SE, Zipursky RB, Kapur S. The effect of antipsychotic treatment on theory of mind. *Psychol Med* (2007) **37**:595–601. doi:10.1017/S0033291706009342
98. Burns MJ. The pharmacology and toxicology of atypical antipsychotic agents. *Clin Toxicol* (2001) **39**:1–14.
99. Singh AN, Barlas C, Saeedi H, Mishra RK. Effect of loxapine on peripheral dopamine-like and serotonin receptors in patients with schizophrenia. *J Psychiatry Neurosci* (2003) **28**:39–47.
100. Sumiyoshi T, Higuchi Y, Itoh T, Matsui M, Arai H, Suzuki M. Effect of perospirone on P300 electrophysiological activity and social cognition in schizophrenia: a three-dimensional analysis with sloreta. *Psychiatry Res* (2009) **172**:180–3. doi:10.1016/j.pscychresns.2008.07.005
101. Behere RV, Venkatasubramanian G, Arasappa R, Reddy N, Gangadhar BN. Effect of risperidone on emotion recognition deficits in antipsychotic-naïve schizophrenia: a short-term follow-up study. *Schizophr Res* (2009) **113**:72–6. doi:10.1016/j.schres.2009.05.026
102. Kosfeld M, Heinrichs M, Zak PJ, Fischbacher U, Fehr E. Oxytocin increases trust in humans. *Nature* (2005) **435**:673–6. doi:10.1038/nature03701
103. Pedersen CA, Gibson CM, Rau SW, Salimi K, Smedley KL, Casey RL, et al. Intranasal oxytocin reduces psychotic symptoms and improves theory of mind and social perception in schizophrenia. *Schizophr Res* (2011) **132**:50–3. doi:10.1016/j.schres.2011.07.027
104. Kéri S, Kiss I, Kelemen O. Sharing secrets: oxytocin and trust in schizophrenia. *Soc Neurosci* (2009) **4**:287–93. doi:10.1080/17470910802319710
105. Takahashi H, Yamada M, Suhara T. Functional significance of central D1 receptors in cognition: beyond working memory. *J Cereb Blood Flow Metab* (2012) **32**:1248–58. doi:10.1038/jcbfm.2011.194
106. Okubo Y, Suhara T, Suzuki K, Kobayashi K, Inoue O, Terasaki O, et al. Decreased prefrontal dopamine D1 receptors in schizophrenia revealed by PET. *Nature* (1997) **385**:634–6. doi:10.1038/385634a0
107. Cai JX, Arnsten AF. Dose-dependent effects of the dopamine D1 receptor agonists A77636 or SKF81297 on spatial working memory in aged monkeys. *J Pharmacol Exp Ther* (1997) **283**:183–9.
108. Arnsten AF, Cai JX, Murphy BL, Goldman-Rakic PS. Dopamine D1 receptor mechanisms in the cognitive performance of young adult and aged monkeys. *Psychopharmacology* (1994) **116**:143–51. doi:10.1007/BF02245056
109. Galletly C. Recent advances in treating cognitive impairment in schizophrenia. *Psychopharmacology* (2009) **202**:259–73. doi:10.1007/s00213-008-1302-9
110. Winstanley CA, Chudasama Y, Dalley JW, Theobald DE, Glennon JC, Robbins TW. Intra-prefrontal 8-OH-DPAT and M100907 improve visuospatial attention and decrease impulsivity on the five-choice serial reaction time task in rats. *Psychopharmacology* (2003) **167**:304–14. doi:10.1007/s00213-003-1398-x
111. Boast C, Bartolomeo AC, Morris H, Moyer JA. 5HT antagonists attenuate MK801-impaired radial arm maze performance in rats. *Neurobiol Learn Mem* (1999) 71:259–71. doi:10.1006/nlme.1998.3886
112. Van der Zee EA, Platt B, Riedel G. Acetylcholine: future research and perspectives. *Behav Brain Res* (2011) **221**:583–6. doi:10.1016/j.bbr.2011.01.050
113. Lieberman JA, Javitch JA, Moore H. Cholinergic agonists as novel treatments for schizophrenia: the promise of rational. *Am J Psychiatry* (2008) **165**:931–6. doi:10.1176/appi.ajp.2008.08050769
114. Friedman JI. Cholinergic targets for cognitive enhancement in schizophrenia: focus on cholinesterase inhibitors and muscarinic agonists. *Psychopharmacology* (2004) **174**:45–53. doi:10.1007/s00213-004-1794-x
115. Raedler TJ, Knable MB, Jones DW, Urbina RA, Gorey JG, Lee KS, et al. In vivo determination of muscarinic acetylcholine receptor availability in schizophrenia. *Am J Psychiatry* (2003) **160**:118–27. doi:10.1176/appi.ajp.160.1.118
116. Crook JM, Tomaskovic-Crook E, Copolov DL, Dean B. Low muscarinic receptor binding in prefrontal cortex from subjects with schizophrenia: a study of Brodmann's areas 8, 9, 10, and 46 and the effects of neuroleptic drug treatment. *Am J Psychiatry* (2001) **158**:918–25. doi:10.1176/appi.ajp.158.987.918
117. Crook JM, Tomaskovic-Crook E, Copolov DL, Dean B. Decreased muscarinic receptor binding in subjects with schizophrenia: a study of the human hippocampal formation. *Biol Psychiatry* (2000) **48**:381–8. doi:10.1016/S0006-3223(00)00918-5
118. Breese CR, Lee MJ, Adams CE, Sullivan B, Logel J, Gillen KM, et al. Abnormal regulation of high affinity nicotinic receptors in subjects with schizophrenia. *Neuropsychopharmacology* (2000) **23**:351–64. doi:10.1016/S0893-133X(00)00121-4
119. Dean B, Crook J, Opeskin K, Hill C, Keks N, Copolov D. The density of muscarinic M1 receptors is decreased in the caudate-putamen of subjects with schizophrenia. *Mol Psychiatry* (1996) **1**:54–8.
120. Freedman R, Hall M, Adler LE, Leonard S. Evidence in postmortem brain tissue for decreased numbers of hippocampal nicotinic receptors in schizophrenia. *Biol Psychiatry* (1995) **38**:22–33. doi:10.1016/0006-3223(94)00252-X
121. Everitt BJ, Robbins TW. Central cholinergic systems and cognition. *Annu Rev Psychol* (1997) **48**:649–84. doi:10.1146/annurev.psych.48.1.649
122. Shekhar A, Potter WZ, Lightfoot J, Lienemann J, Dubé S, Mallinckrodt C, et al. Selective muscarinic receptor agonist xanomeline as a novel treatment approach for schizophrenia. *Am J Psychiatry* (2008) **165**:1033–9. doi:10.1176/appi.ajp.2008.06091591

123. Bodick NC, Offen WW, Levey AI, Cutler NR, Gauthier SG, Satlin A, et al. Effects of xanomeline, a selective muscarinic receptor agonist, on cognitive function and behavioral symptoms in Alzheimer disease. *Arch Neurol* (1997) **54**:465–73. doi:10.1001/archneur.1997.00550160091022
124. Blum BP, Mann JJ. The GABAergic system in schizophrenia. *Int J Neuropsychopharmacol* (2002) **5**:159–79. doi:10.1017/S1461145702002894
125. Kane MJ, Engle RW. The role of prefrontal cortex in working-memory capacity, executive attention, and general fluid intelligence: an individual-differences perspective. *Psychon Bull Rev* (2002) **9**:637–71.
126. Lewis DA, Volk DW, Hashimoto T. Selective alterations in prefrontal cortical GABA neurotransmission in schizophrenia: a novel target for the treatment of working memory dysfunction. *Psychopharmacology* (2004) **174**:143–50. doi:10.1007/s00213-003-1673-x
127. Javitt DC. Glutamate as a therapeutic target in psychiatric disorders. *Mol Psychiatry* (2004) **9**:984–97. doi:10.1038/sj.mp.4001551
128. Malchow B, Hasan A, Fusar-Poli P, Schmitt A, Falkai P, Wobrock T. Cannabis abuse and brain morphology in schizophrenia: a review of the available evidence. *Eur Arch Psychiatry Clin Neurosci* (2013) **263**:3–13. doi:10.1007/s00406-012-0346-3
129. Lubman DI, King JA, Castle DJ. Treating comorbid substance use disorders in schizophrenia. *Int Rev Psychiatry* (2010) **22**:191–201. doi:10.3109/09540261003689958
130. Levaux M-N, Potvin S, Sepehry AA, Sablier J, Mendrek A, Stip E. Computerized assessment of cognition in schizophrenia: promises and pitfalls of CANTAB. *Eur Psychiatry* (2007) **22**:104–15. doi:10.1016/j.eurpsy.2006.11.004

2

Targeting Neural Synchrony Deficits is Sufficient to Improve Cognition in a Schizophrenia-Related Neurodevelopmental Model

Heekyung Lee[1†‡], *Dino Dvorak*[2‡] *and André A. Fenton*[3,4]*

[1] *Graduate Program in Neural and Behavioral Science, Downstate Medical Center, State University of New York, Brooklyn, NY, USA*
[2] *Graduate Program in Biomedical Engineering, Downstate Medical Center, State University of New York and New York University Polytechnic School of Engineering, Brooklyn, NY, USA*
[3] *The Robert F. Furchgott Center for Neural and Behavioral Science, Downstate Medical Center, State University of New York, Brooklyn, NY, USA*
[4] *Center for Neural Science, New York University, New York, NY, USA*

Correspondence:
André A. Fenton, Center for Neural Science, New York University, 4 Washington Place, New York, NY 10003, USA
e-mail: afenton@nyu.edu

*[†]**Present address:***
Heekyung Lee, Krieger Mind/Brain Institute, Johns Hopkins University, Baltimore, MD, USA

[‡]Heekyung Lee and Dino Dvorak have contributed equally to this work.

Cognitive symptoms are core features of mental disorders but procognitive treatments are limited. We have proposed a "discoordination" hypothesis that cognitive impairment results from aberrant coordination of neural activity. We reported that neonatal ventral hippocampus lesion (NVHL) rats, an established neurodevelopmental model of schizophrenia, have abnormal neural synchrony and cognitive deficits in the active place avoidance task. During stillness, we observed that cortical local field potentials sometimes resembled epileptiform spike-wave discharges with higher prevalence in NVHL rats, indicating abnormal neural synchrony due perhaps to imbalanced excitation–inhibition coupling. Here, within the context of the hypothesis, we investigated whether attenuating abnormal neural synchrony will improve cognition in NVHL rats. We report that: (1) inter-hippocampal synchrony in the theta and beta bands is correlated with active place avoidance performance; (2) the anticonvulsant ethosuximide attenuated the abnormal spike-wave activity, improved cognitive control, and reduced hyperlocomotion; (3) ethosuximide not only normalized the task-associated theta and beta synchrony between the two hippocampi but also increased synchrony between the medial prefrontal cortex and hippocampus above control levels; (4) the antipsychotic olanzapine was less effective at improving cognitive control and normalizing place avoidance-related inter-hippocampal neural synchrony, although it reduced hyperactivity; and (5) olanzapine caused an abnormal pattern of frequency-independent increases in neural synchrony, in both NVHL and control rats. These data suggest that normalizing aberrant neural synchrony can be beneficial and that drugs targeting the pathophysiology of abnormally coordinated neural activities may be a promising theoretical framework and strategy for developing treatments that improve cognition in neurodevelopmental disorders such as schizophrenia.

Keywords: neural synchrony, oscillations, schizophrenia, neurodevelopmental models, hippocampus, local field potentials, cognitive control, spike-wave discharge

INTRODUCTION

Cognitive impairment is a core feature of schizophrenia but treatments to improve cognition are limited, in part because the physiological mechanisms of cognitive dysfunction are unclear. Recent interest has been directed toward understanding the abnormal synchrony of neural oscillations as a pathophysiological mechanism that underlies the cognitive impairments in schizophrenia (1–4). Dysfunctional neural synchrony in a wide range of frequencies, including the delta (5), theta (6), beta (7), and gamma ranges (8, 9), have been characterized in patients with schizophrenia. In animal models, disruption of long-range hippocampal–prefrontal synchrony has been reported while performing a working memory task in a genetic mouse model of schizophrenia (10) and during an open-field task in the maternal immune activation (MIA) neurodevelopmental model of schizophrenia (11). Abnormal hippocampal–prefrontal synchrony was also observed in the neonatal ventral hippocampus lesion (NVHL) neurodevelopmental model but this synchrony abnormality was not itself associated with cognitive impairment (12). In fact, aberrant neural synchrony may be a common pathophysiology responsible for impaired cognition in a variety of disorders (2, 13). Indeed, treatments that normalize neural network dysfunction without addressing the underlying cellular pathology have been sufficient to improve cognitive function in animal models of neurodegenerative diseases (14, 15). Such studies demonstrate it may be a feasible strategy to improve cognitive functional outcomes by normalizing aberrant neural network synchrony in cases where the network dysfunction is part of the causal chain from the disease etiology to the manifest cognitive symptoms.

We previously reported that NVHL rats, an established neurodevelopmental animal model of schizophrenia (16), have a cognitive control impairment that was associated with abnormal synchrony between the two hippocampi (12). We also detected hippocampal–prefrontal synchrony abnormalities in these rats during home-cage resting behaviors, but these abnormalities were absent during place avoidance training, and so not related to performance on the cognitive test. Clinically, the presence of hippocampal dysfunction is apparent in schizophrenia. Postmortem and neuroimaging studies indicate that the hippocampus is one of the brain regions most consistently altered in schizophrenia (17–22). Furthermore, functional magnetic resonance imaging studies show dysfunctional hippocampal activities are associated with poor cognitive performance in schizophrenia patients (23–25). Perhaps similar to the findings in NVHL rats, reduced inter-hippocampal functional coupling has also been observed between the left- and right-hippocampus areas in healthy carriers of the CACNA1C risk variant in bipolar disorder (26), but to our knowledge these measurements have not been carried out in schizophrenia subjects. Because neuroimaging studies do not have sufficient temporal resolution to detect functional synchrony at the 100-ms or faster timescales of the electrophysiological synchrony that underlies information processing between neural networks, it is unclear whether or not the inter-hippocampal abnormalities in NVHL rats mimics abnormalities in schizophrenia. Regardless, it is our opinion that animal models used to study schizophrenia do not sensibly mimic disease features, instead they are better thought of as being models for testing hypotheses that are relevant to understanding schizophrenia. Thus, we hypothesized that the abnormal hippocampal synchrony plays a role in the pathophysiology of cognitive control impairment in a schizophrenia-related neurodevelopmental animal model. As outlined below, in the present study, we tested the idea that attenuating this pathophysiology can improve cognition.

We, like others, have proposed the discoordination hypothesis, which asserts that cognitive impairment arises because of aberrant coordination of what may otherwise be normal neural activities (12, 27). The discoordination hypothesis is rooted in the idea that disrupted physiological coordination and synchronization of unitary neural processes impair the ability to selectively and dynamically activate and suppress information for organizing knowledge and perception into useable representations (1, 2, 27, 28). We use the term (dis)coordination to refer to the collective temporal organization of unitary neural activity such as action and synaptic and local field potentials (LFPs) at individual sites. Thus, (dis)coordination can be measured at different temporal and spatial scales. In the present work, we examined inter-hippocampal synchrony of LFP oscillations. These oscillations are an example of a long-range spatial scale neural interaction that involves an approximate order of 10^5 neurons. These oscillations result from the multiple timescales of excitation–inhibition neural activity cycles that govern spiking within these networks (29). The discoordination hypothesis predicts that in the NVHL model, restoring the abnormal neural synchrony to normal will attenuate the cognitive control deficit. Accordingly, we took advantage of the hippocampal synchrony abnormality in NVHL rats, specifically the inter-hippocampal synchrony that was associated with cognitive performance, to evaluate the prediction. We examined whether normalizing the abnormal synchrony can attenuate the cognitive control deficit in the NVHL rats. We observed that hippocampal and neocortical LFPs in the NVHL rats sometimes resembled spike-wave discharges (SWDs), a sign of network hyperexcitability. We hypothesized that these aberrant neural activities arise from an excitation–inhibition imbalance that may underlie abnormal neural synchrony in the NVHL rats. Since SWD in epilepsy patients is treated with ethosuximide (2-ethyl-2-methylsuccinimide), an anticonvulsant that acts by blocking T-type Ca^{2+} channels, we studied whether ethosuximide would attenuate the abnormal SWD-like synchrony as well as impaired cognitive behavior and the associated neural synchrony that we have previously described in the NVHL model (12). We stress that our goal is to test the prediction of the discoordination hypothesis, not to suggest the use of ethosuximide as an antipsychotic. For comparison, we also examined the effects of the atypical antipsychotic olanzapine on neural synchrony and cognitive abnormalities in NVHL rats. Given that antipsychotics are not known to improve cognitive symptoms, the hypothesis predicts that olanzapine will not correct either the neural synchrony or cognitive abnormalities in NVHL rats.

We report that in NVHL rats, ethosuximide treatment attenuated the abnormal spike-wave activity, and most importantly, ethosuximide normalized the cognition-associated synchrony of theta and beta oscillations between the two hippocampi, and improved cognitive control in the place avoidance task. Olanzapine was less effective at reducing the abnormal spike-wave activity and normalizing the synchrony of oscillations between the two hippocampi and it did not improve cognitive control in NVHL rats, although it attenuated hyperlocomotion during the cognitive testing. These data are consistent with the discoordination hypothesis, and support the idea that drugs targeting the abnormal neural synchrony may be sufficient to rescue the cognitive deficits in schizophrenia-related neurodevelopmental animal models.

MATERIALS AND METHODS

All procedures were in compliance with National Institutes of Health guidelines and were approved by Downstate Medical Center's Institutional Animal Care and Use Committee.

NEONATAL VENTRAL HIPPOCAMPAL LESION

The procedure followed the manual provided by Lipska and Weinberger. We used the exact protocol that is published in our prior work (12). Briefly, timed-pregnant (13 or 14 days in gestation) female Long-Evans rats were obtained from Charles River Laboratories (Wilmington, MA, USA). Pups were born at the Downstate animal facility. On postnatal day 7 (P7), male pups were anesthetized by hypothermia. Bilateral puncture holes (relative to bregma AP: −3.0 mm, ML: ±3.5 mm) were made in the skull with a 30-Ga injection needle. A bilateral infusion (0.3 μl/side) of ibotenic acid solution (10 μg/μl) was delivered to each ventral hippocampus (relative to the skull surface DV: −5.0 mm). Control animals were treated identically except saline was injected instead of ibotenic acid. A subset of the NVHL and control rats were given drug treatments as described below. The behavioral and neural synchrony measurements from these rats were compared to untreated NVHL and control rats, the data from which were reported previously (12), although all data collection was concurrent amongst the different treatment groups.

DRUGS

Ibotenic acid, purchased from Sigma (St. Louis, MO, USA), was dissolved in artificial cerebrospinal fluid (ACSF) to a final concentration of 10 μg/μl, pH 7.6. Ethosuximide, purchased from Sigma (St. Louis, MO, USA), was dissolved in sterile 0.9% NaCl and a concentration of 100 mg/kg was injected i.p. Olanzapine, purchased from Toronto Research Chemicals Inc. (Toronto, ON, Canada), was dissolved in dimethyl sulfoxide (DMSO) and 1 mg/kg was injected i.p. Both ethosuximide and olanzapine were administered just prior to the start of behavioral training (see below) and based on published work, they were expected to have been bioactive for several hours, beyond the duration of behavioral training.

TWO-FRAME AVOIDANCE TASK

Five adult rats (P65) per group were trained on the two-frame task. The rat was placed on a circular 82 cm diameter, stainless steel rotating arena (Bio-Signal Group Corp., Brooklyn, NY, USA). The rat's position was tracked using an overhead camera and software (Tracker, Bio-Signal Group Corp., Brooklyn, NY, USA). All animals were habituated to the rotating arena the day before the start of active place avoidance training during two 10-min sessions without any shocks. On the following training trials, whenever the rat on the rotating arena entered a 60° shock zone that was defined in room coordinates, a mild constant current (60 Hz, <0.4 mA, 500 ms) foot shock was delivered. Foot shock was repeated every 1.5 s until the rat left the shock zone. Each place avoidance trial was 10 min and the interval between the trials was at least 10 min. A total of eight training trials were given on the training day. The drugs were injected i.p. just prior to the first avoidance training trial. Avoidance was measured by counting the number of times the rat entered the shock zone.

LOCAL FIELD POTENTIAL AND ELECTROENCEPHALOGRAM RECORDINGS

All rats were housed individually, exposed to a 12-h light/dark circadian cycle, and had *ad libitum* access to water and food. When rats were P55-57, electrodes were surgically implanted bilaterally. Rats were given post-operative Ketofen (5 mg/kg) for 2 days after surgery and allowed to recover from the surgical procedure for 7 days. LFPs in the dorsal hippocampus (AP: −4 mm; ML: ±2.5 mm; DV: 3 mm) and in the medial prefrontal cortex (mPFC; AP: +3 mm; ML: ±1 mm; DV: 4 mm) were recorded by implanting 75-μm Nichrome wires that were attached to a Millmax connector. The epidural cortical electroencephalogram (EEG) was recorded with a screw electrode in the frontal and parietal bones of each hemisphere. All electrodes were referred to an electrode implanted in the cerebellar white matter (AP: −10 mm; ML: +2 mm; DV: 3 mm), which seemed to be normal in NVHL rats. Recordings were made with a wireless digital telemetry system (Bio-Signal Group, Brooklyn, NY, USA). Recordings were made while the rats were performing the two-frame avoidance task and in the home-cage (for 2–3 h) during the light cycle.

The signals at the electrode connector were amplified (300 times), low-pass filtered (6 kHz) and digitized (24-bits, 12 kHz using delta-sigma analog-digital convertors). The digital signals were transmitted wirelessly to a recording system (dacqUSB, Axona Ltd., St. Albans, UK) for band-pass filtering (1–500 Hz), digital amplification and down-sampling (16-bits, 2000 Hz) using digital signal processors. The digital electrophysiological data were stored on computer hard drives for off-line analysis. The channels were marked if they had saturated signals and were excluded from further analysis if the proportion was substantial. At the end of training and recording, the rats were trans-cardially perfused and the brains removed for histological verification of the electrode locations.

POWER SPECTRA

Power spectra measure the amplitude of frequency-specific oscillations that arise when spatially patterned synaptic potentials are coincident in time. These oscillations are locally generated phenomena. As such, an oscillation itself may not be a strong indication of neural synchrony as it relates to the concept of neural coordination (1, 27). Instead, power spectra are an estimate of the amount and magnitude of patterns of oscillation-generating synaptic potentials that are the fundamental components of neural coordinating processes. The patterns of synaptic potentials must themselves be temporally and spatially coordinated within and between neural networks to mediate the neural computations and information processing upon which cognition is based (29).

To compute power spectra, LFP signals were first normalized by dividing the signal by its RMS value. This step minimized electrode-specific signal properties caused by variability in electrode location or impedance. The signal was processed using 5 s long non-overlapping windows. For each window power spectral density (PSD) was computed using the "pwelch" Matlab function. The spectral peak at 60 Hz was removed and the PSD was interpolated between 58 and 62 Hz. The resulting PSD was normalized by dividing it by its sum so the total power was equal to 1. Based on the spectral profile, we then defined bands of interest for frequency-specific phase-locking analysis. We excluded the delta band (0–3 Hz) because of its attenuation by the hardware DC-removal filter (**Figure 1**). We defined the theta band as 5–15 Hz, beta as 20–30 Hz in order to exclude the strong second theta harmonic (**Figure 1**), slow gamma 30–55 Hz and fast gamma as 65–100 Hz (excluding the 60-Hz region). **Figure 1** shows that the left and right hippocampal spectra are similar, as expected, and that the spectra are attenuated in NVHL rats. Both ethosuximide and olanzapine only caused a marginal increase in the broad-band spectral power. This confirmation of stable spectral power provides the starting point for the present study, which focuses on measuring how these component oscillations are coordinated between brain regions.

PHASE-LOCKING VALUE

The coordination of neural signals at a pair of electrodes was estimated by computing the phase-locking value (PLV). Eight LFP channel pairs were selected for PLV analysis. They were the left- and right-hippocampi; left- and right-mPFC; left-hippocampus and left-mPFC; right-hippocampus and right-mPFC, as well as the inter-hemispheric and associational epidural electrode pairs. The PLV at a pair of electrodes was computed using custom software written in Matlab, based on a published algorithm (31). The phase of a signal at time t and sample n $\phi(t, n)$ was obtained by filtering the signal with a narrow-band finite input response (FIR)

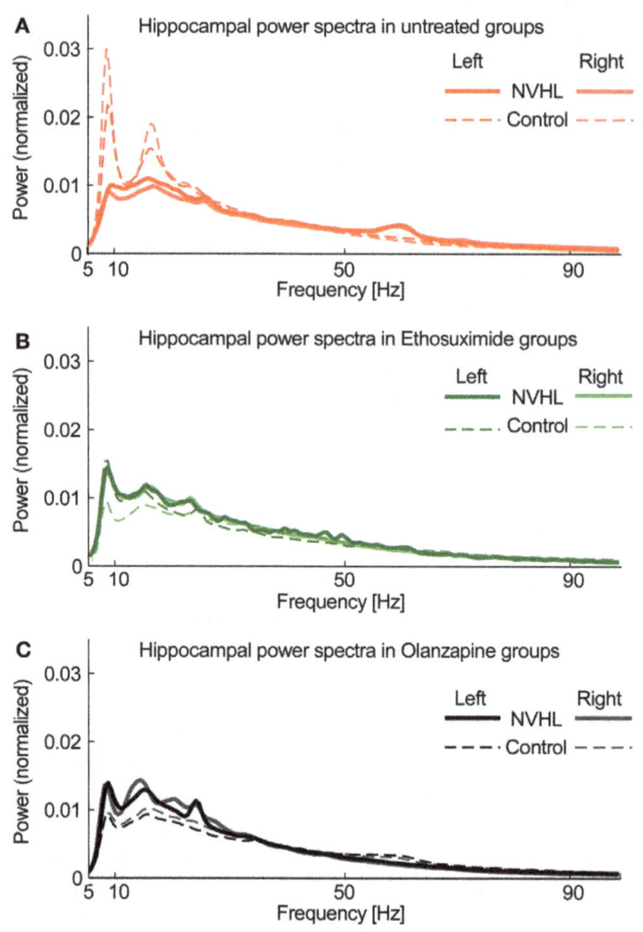

FIGURE 1 | Hippocampal power spectra. (A) Power spectra density plot for untreated groups averaged across all subjects for NVHL (thick line) and control (thin line) computed independently for left (opaque line) and right (semi-transparent line) hippocampi. **(B)** Power spectral density plot for Ethosuximide-treated animals. **(C)** Power spectra density plot for Olanzapine-treated animals. The similarities between the corresponding left and right spectra is a common observation, is independent of phase synchrony, and is only indirectly related to neural coordination in that neural oscillations are the fundamental, unitary components of neural coordination processes such as phase synchrony and cross-frequency coupling (30).

filter using a zero phase-shift filtering algorithm followed by the Hilbert Transform. The filters were designed using the Matlab filter design toolbox. Filters in the range 0–100 Hz had fixed bandwidth of 5 Hz. For bands of interest extending over several 5 Hz bands the PLV across all such bands were averaged. Given a pair of LFP signals of N samples, the PLV was defined as follows:

$$\mathrm{PLV} = \frac{1}{N}\left|\sum_{n=0}^{N} \exp\left[i\theta\left(t, n\right)\right]\right|,$$

where $\theta(t, n)$ is the phase difference $\phi_1(t, n) - \phi_2(t, n)$ between the two signals at time t sample n; N is the total number of samples; and i is the imaginary unit. Prior work showed that the intracranial electrode-pair specific PLVs at the four (theta, beta, slow gamma, fast gamma) frequency bands were different between NVHL and control rats (12). We made these comparisons between the NVHL and control treatment groups to determine if the drug treatment normalized neural synchrony between the particular electrode pairs. In addition, the PLVs for the full set of electrode pairs were studied to look for neural synchrony patterns that distinguished the NVHL and control and the drug-treatment groups. The set of electrode-pair and frequency-specific PLVs for each recording session was treated as a vector with dimension 32 (8 electrode pairs × 4 bands). Principal component analysis (PCA) was performed to reduce the dimensionality and identify the most useful measures of synchrony. Each session vector of PLVs (eight sessions per rat) was plot in the coordinate system of the first three principal components to visualize the group patterns. The first six principal components explained over 90% of the variance and so for quantification we only considered the first six principal components. We quantified the distance between the vectors in each session group by computing the 6-D Euclidean distance between all pairs of data points within a treatment group, and also between all pairs of data points against a reference treatment group. The untreated control and untrained NVHL groups as well as the ethosuximide-treated NVHL and the olanzapine-NVHL groups each served as reference groups for the comparisons. These pair-wise group distances were compared by two-sample Student's t-tests that were adjusted for multiple comparisons using the Bonferroni method.

AUTOMATIC DETECTION OF SPIKE-WAVE ACTIVITY

We used an algorithm to identify activity that resembled epileptiform SWDs, but are observed in normal Long-Evans rats without seizures (32). Each channel was first examined for signal saturation and only data segments with brief (<50 ms) saturations were considered for further analysis. Brief saturations in the LFP were allowed so spike-wave complexes with a large spike component were not removed from the analysis. We manually marked epochs of spike-wave events using the EEGLAB toolbox for Matlab. These epochs were used to calculate and optimize the detection parameters for the automatic classifier of spike-wave events. The classifier is a modified version of a published algorithm (33).

The algorithm worked in several steps (**Figure 2**):

(1) Local field potential signals (**Figure 2A**) were transformed (**Figure 2B**) using the continuous wavelet transform (CWT) from the Wavelet Toolbox in Matlab (Morlet wavelets, scales 5–50 with step of 5 corresponding to pseudo-frequencies 16–160 Hz).
(2) The sliding variance (50 ms long window) was computed for each scale and all variances were summed across all scales resulting in a single variance profile over time.
(3) Candidate spike-wave events were marked as threshold crossings (red line in **Figure 2C**) of the summed variance series.
(4) Gaps between individual marked segments shorter than 0.75 s were filled to create longer segments.
(5) After filling the gaps, all marked segments that were shorter than 1 s were removed from further analysis.
(6) Each marked segment was tested for periodic spiking activity by detecting local maxima (red dots in **Figure 2C**) in the summed variance signal with 50 ms smoothing applied. The

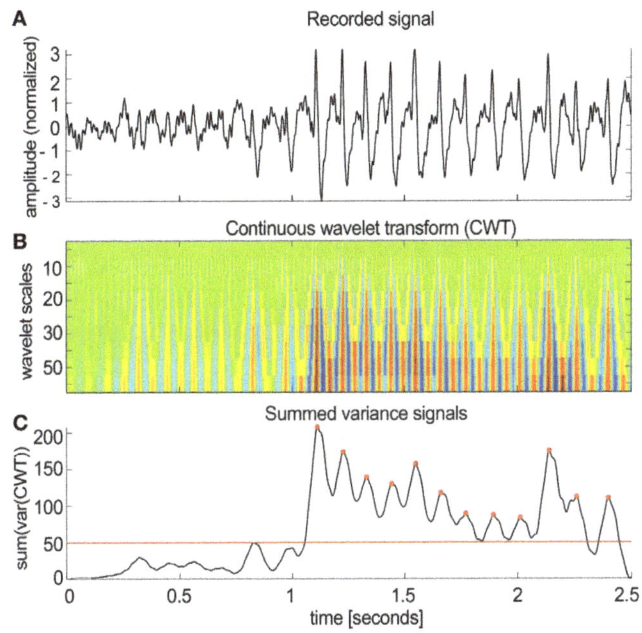

FIGURE 2 | Spike-wave activities in NVHL and control rats.
(A) A segment of the cortical EEG with spike-wave activity. An automatic classifier was used to detect these events. **(B)** The first step in the classifier was to transform the recorded signal using the continuous wavelet transform (CWT). **(C)** Then a sliding variance was computed for each wavelet scale. All the variances were summed across all scales resulting in a single variance profile over time (50 ms smoothing was applied to the resulting signal). SWD candidates were detected as threshold crossings [red line in **(C)**]. Each marked segment was tested for periodic spiking activity by detecting local maxima [red dots in **(C)**]. Only the detected segments that contained at least 50% of inter-spike intervals in the range of 2–10 Hz were included in further analysis.

inter-spike intervals for each pair of sequential maxima were computed. Only those marked segments that contained at least 50% of inter-spike intervals in the range of 2–10 Hz (the typical range of SWDs) were considered as spike-wave segments.

(7) The process was repeated several times with different parameters and the classified event segments were compared with manually marked events to tune the classifier.

ANALYSIS OF SPIKE-WAVE EVENT FEATURES

Only manually marked segments were included in this analysis to avoid distortion by borderline spike-wave-like events that were detected by the automatic algorithm but did not necessarily share all the features such as clear spike and wave components. The subjectively selected events were identified on the basis of the classic spike-wave morphology, by an observer blind to the origin of the EEG. Thus the manual selection of spike-wave events resulted in a dataset of events with a bias to less specificity and more selectivity.

The manually marked events were first low-pass filtered with a cut-off frequency of 100 Hz. The filter removed the high frequency components that could cause errors in feature extraction. Local maxima were then detected in the signal and for each maximum, its preceding and following local minima were found. The spike components of the events were then defined as local maxima, surrounded by local minima with a maxima–minima amplitude of at least 400 μV and with a spike width (defined below) of at least 50 ms. Spike sequences (for computing the inter-spike time) were defined as continuous spikes with a frequency between 5 and 13 Hz. The feature analysis was repeated several times to optimize the parameters for the component detection.

The following features were computed for both NVHL and control rats (**Figure 3**):

(1) Spike duration: the duration of the spike measured at the level of either the preceding or the following local minimum with the higher voltage.
(2) Spike-to-valley voltage: the voltage between the spike peak and the following local minimum (valley).
(3) Inter-spike time: the time between two successive spikes.
(4) Wave duration: the duration of the wave component measured from the local minimum (valley) following the spike component and the local minimum preceding the next spike component.
(5) Wave energy: the energy of the wave component computed as the sum of squares of amplitudes.
(6) Spike-wave event prevalence: only the automatically classified segments were included in this analysis. Prevalence was estimated as the total time spike-wave events were detected and divided by the total amount of time that was analyzed.

STATISTICAL ANALYSIS

Group differences were compared by ANOVA or Student's t-test. The PLV between groups and across frequency bands were compared by two-way ANOVA. Repeated-measures were not used because the data were independently and differentially filtered for computing the synchrony estimates at each frequency band. Significance was set at $p < 0.05$, and Tukey's HSD *post hoc* tests were used as appropriate. The two-sample Kolmogorov–Smirnov test was used to compare the probability distributions of spike-wave event features in the NVHL and control groups. The distributions were generated by selecting a constant subsample of spike-wave events from each animal such that each subject contributed equally to the distribution. The resulting distribution was then divided by its sum to generate probability distributions that are normalized against different numbers of subjects in the NVHL and control groups.

RESULTS

ABNORMAL SPIKE-WAVE ACTIVITIES IN THE EEG OF NVHL RATS

Before focusing on the main aim of this study, to investigate cognition-related inter-hippocampal phase synchrony during active place avoidance cognitive behavior, we began by monitoring the field potential recordings from NVHL and control rats as they behaved in their home-cage. In the home-cage, both groups of rats were still or moving <0.5 cm/s about 80% of the time based on estimates from concurrent video tracking. The most conspicuous feature was the occasional presence of a large amplitude series of spike-wave events. We were surprised to find

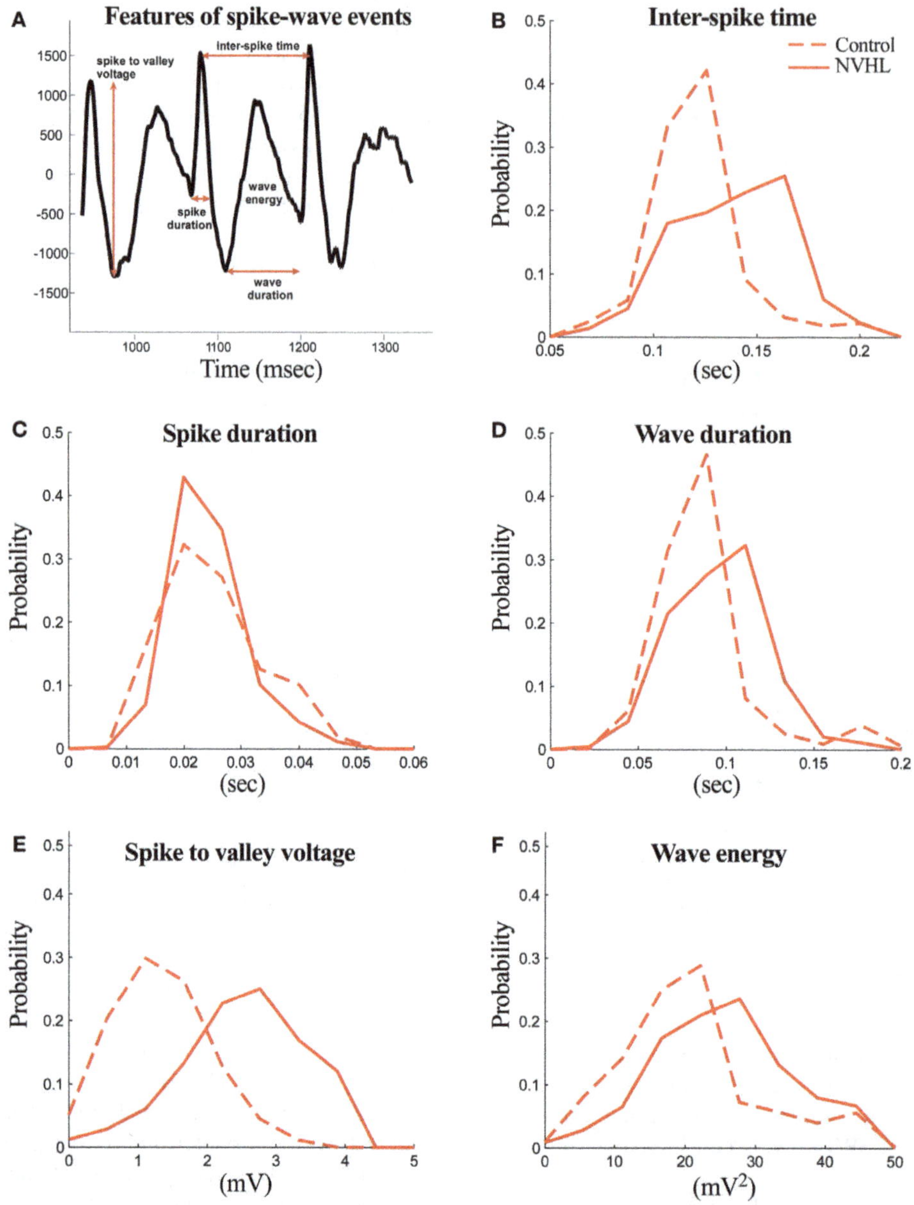

FIGURE 3 | Abnormal features of the spike-wave activities in NVHL rats. **(A)** Three spike-wave cycles are shown to illustrate the features that were measured. The analyzed features include spike duration, inter-spike time, wave duration, spike-to-valley voltage, and inter-spike time. Comparison of the spike-wave complex features in NVHL and control rats: **(B)** inter-spike time, **(C)** spike duration, **(D)** wave duration, **(E)** spike-to-valley voltage, and **(F)** wave energy. Distributions in each feature looked distinct, except in spike duration, and this was confirmed statistically by the two-sample Kolmogorov–Smirnov test in which the null hypothesis that the control and NVHL distributions were drawn from the same underlying distribution was rejected ($p < 0.05$).

these events and will call them spike-wave activity. They typically occurred in trains of ~6 Hz (**Figure 2A**). These events have been observed in the cortical EEG of normal Long-Evans rats during stillness and are a sign of heightened synchrony of cortical neural activity, perhaps the rat analog of the human alpha-like mu rhythm (32, 34). We automatically detected the individual events and confirmed by visual inspection that the algorithm properly detected the events (**Figures 2B,C**). Recordings from the epidural cortical screw electrodes were used for analysis because signals from the epidural cortical electrodes showed the strongest spike-wave waveforms across all animals. We analyzed a total of nine NVHL and seven control rats during home-cage behavior to estimate the prevalence of the spike-wave activity. Each rat was recorded for 3–5 h in the home-cage. The spike-wave activity was detected in six of nine NVHL rats and three of seven control rats. The prevalence was 3% across all the NVHL rats and 2% in all the control rats. In total, 1514 spike-wave events were detected in NVHL rats and 397 spike-wave events were detected in control rats, suggesting that these events were more common in NVHL rats.

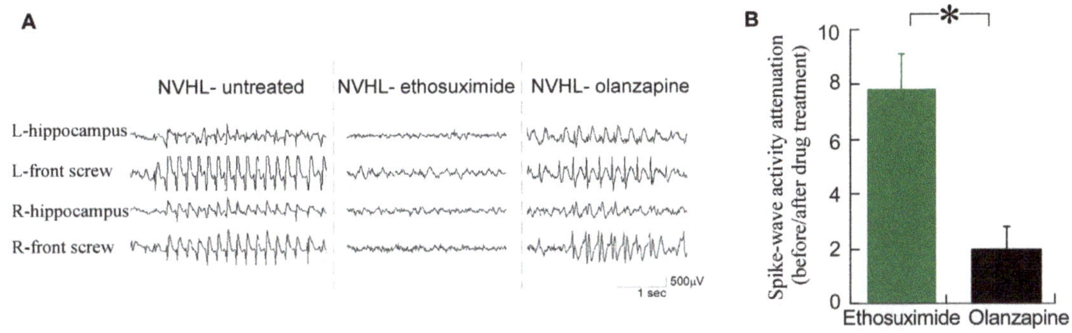

FIGURE 4 | Ethosuximide reduced the prevalence of abnormal spike-wave activities in NVHL rats. (A) Raw EEG traces. Ethosuximide reduced the occurrence of spike-wave activity while olanzapine did not. **(B)** Quantification of the spike-wave activity prevalence before and after drug treatment. There was an eightfold reduction of the prevalence after ethosuximide treatment, while only a twofold attenuation of the prevalence after olanzapine treatment in NVHL rats ($t_4 = 3.79$, $p = 0.02$).

We then measured various features of the spike-wave events in both NVHL and control rats (**Figures 3A–F**). The distributions of NVHL and control groups looked distinct in all the features except in spike duration. These were confirmed statistically by the two-sample Kolmogorov–Smirnov test because the null hypothesis that the control and NVHL distributions are drawn from the same underlying distribution was rejected ($p < 0.05$) for all features. These events tended to be larger amplitude and more frequent in NVHL rats in comparison to the control rats. Since we have previously characterized a cognition-related abnormality in neural synchrony in NVHL rats, in the framework of the discoordination hypothesis, these observations of abnormal synchrony suggested to us that reducing the spike-wave activities could improve cognition and related neural activity in NVHL rats.

ETHOSUXIMIDE REDUCED THE PREVALENCE OF ABNORMAL SPIKE-WAVE ACTIVITIES

We then evaluated whether the spike-wave activities could be attenuated by ethosuximide, an anticonvulsant that is an antagonist of T-type calcium channels (35). It is used mainly to treat absence seizures. Given the framework that animal models are best utilized to test hypotheses about schizophrenia and that it is unwise to assume that models themselves mimic the disease (36), we reasoned that since ethosuximide is effective at suppressing epileptiform SWDs, then it may be also be effective on the spike-wave activities in the NVHL rats. Since it might suppress this specific form of abnormal neural synchrony by rebalancing excitation and inhibition, it occurred to us that ethosuximide could also act to reduce the cognition-related abnormal neural synchrony, which according to the discoordination hypothesis would attenuate the cognitive deficit observed in these rats.

For comparison, we also chose to study the effects of olanzapine, a compound with antagonist actions at dopaminergic, muscarinic, adrenergic, GABAergic, and histaminergic receptors. It is one of the most widely used second-generation antipsychotic drugs. These drugs were designed to suppress hyperlocomotion in animal models and are prescribed to reduce the positive symptoms of psychosis, but are not considered to be effective on cognitive symptoms.

We observed that ethosuximide reduced the spike-wave activity much more than olanzapine (**Figure 4A**). There was an eightfold reduction in the prevalence of spike-wave activity after ethosuximide (100 mg/kg i.p.) treatment, while only a twofold reduction in spike-wave activity in the NVHL rats (**Figure 4B**) after a dose of olanzapine (1 mg/kg i.p.) that is sufficient to attenuate sensorimotor deficits such as hyperlocomotion in the NVHL (see **Figure 7C** below) and acute PCP animal models (37). These observations motivated us to test whether ethosuximide can attenuate the abnormal cognition-related neural synchrony that we have previously characterized in NVHL rats (12).

ETHOSUXIMIDE ATTENUATED ABNORMAL INTER-HIPPOCAMPAL SYNCHRONY

We then turned to the main effort of this research. We recorded LFPs while the rats performed the two-frame active place avoidance task. We previously identified that oscillations in the theta and beta ranges was less synchronized between the left and right dorsal hippocampi in NVHL rats than in control rats and that this inter-hippocampal synchrony was correlated with effective place avoidance behavior (12). Inter-hippocampal theta and beta synchrony was weaker in the NVHL rats compared to the controls (**Figure 5A**), which was already shown in prior work (12). We administered ethosuximide and olanzapine just prior to the first place avoidance training trials in new NVHL and control groups. The difference in inter-hippocampal synchrony between the NVHL and control rats was attenuated by ethosuximide (**Figure 5B**), suggesting that ethosuximide normalized inter-hippocampal synchrony in NVHL rats. Following olanzapine, inter-hippocampal synchrony was different between the NVHL and control groups (**Figure 5C**). However, this difference appeared because the drug increased synchrony in the NVHL rats and decreased synchrony in the control group, especially in the theta and beta bands. Indeed, after olanzapine, synchrony in the NVHL rats was greater than in the treated control rats. Olanzapine also increased inter-hippocampal synchrony in the faster frequency gamma bands. This increase was in excess of the synchrony seen in untreated control rats, which in contrast to ethosuximide, is why olanzapine did not restore normal synchrony.

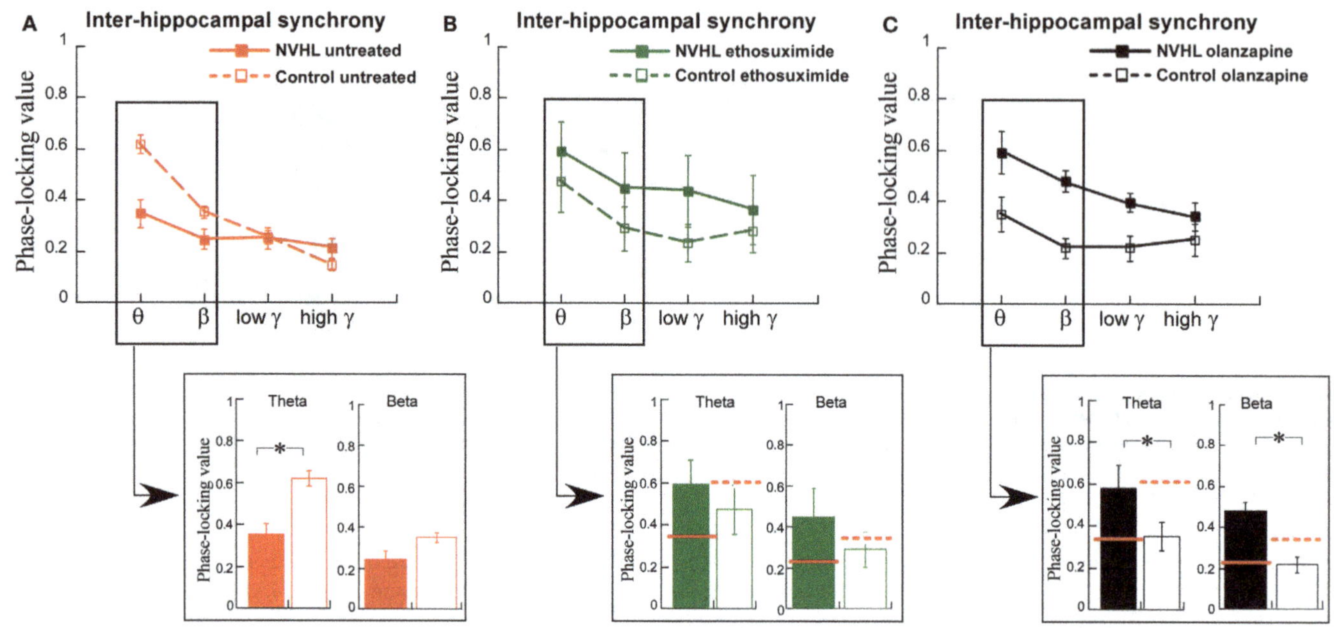

FIGURE 5 | Ethosuximide attenuated abnormal cognitive control-associated inter-hippocampal synchrony. (A) Adult NVHL rats had lower inter-hippocampal synchrony compared to control rats (two-way ANOVA group: $F_{1,32} = 8.87$, $p = 0.006$; frequency: $F_{3,32} = 23.6$, $p < 0.0001$; interaction: $F_{3,32} = 7.68$, $p = 0.0005$). Inter-hippocampal theta ($t_8 = 3.98$, $p = 0.004$) and beta ($t_8 = 2.30$, $p = 0.05$) synchrony was weaker in the NVHL rats compared to the controls. **(B)** Ethosuximide treatment attenuated the inter-hippocampal synchrony difference between the NVHL and control rats (two-way ANOVA group: $F_{1,32} = 3.05$, $p = 0.09$; frequency: $F_{3,32} = 1.42$, $p = 0.25$; interaction: $F_{3,32} = 0.10$, $p = 0.96$). There was no theta ($t_8 = 0.73$, $p = 0.49$) or beta ($t_8 = 0.94$, $p = 0.37$) synchrony difference. **(C)** Olanzapine treatment increased synchrony in NVHL rats and decreased synchrony in control rats, resulting in an inter-hippocampal synchrony difference between the groups (two-way ANOVA group: $F_{1,28} = 28.2$, $p < 0.0001$; frequency: $F_{3,28} = 6.20$, $p = 0.002$; interaction: $F_{3,28} = 1.53$, $p = 0.23$). Inter-hippocampal theta ($t_7 = 2.94$, $p = 0.02$) and beta ($t_7 = 4.43$, $p = 0.003$) synchrony was higher in the NVHL rats compared to the controls.

We also examined inter-hemispheric synchrony between electrodes in the mPFC (**Figure 6A**). The synchrony of LFP oscillations between the left and right-mPFC was greater for slower frequencies than faster frequencies but not different between the NVHL and control groups. After ethosuximide, the frequency dependence on the magnitude of synchrony between the left and right-mPFC was no longer observed. This was in large part because ethosuximide increased synchrony at the faster gamma frequencies, almost to the level of the slower beta frequencies. This effect was more pronounced in the NVHL animals. Olanzapine had a similar effect on synchrony between the left and right-mPFC sites such that there was no longer a detectable difference in the magnitude of synchrony in the different frequency bands and the NVHL and control groups were also indistinguishable.

Finally, we examined synchrony between the mPFC and dorsal hippocampus of one hemisphere (**Figure 6B**). Synchrony was generally less than it was between the two hippocampi or between the two mPFC. There was greater synchrony in slower frequency bands than the faster gamma bands. There was, however, no difference between NVHL and control animals. After ethosuximide, synchrony increased, especially in the faster bands, for both the NVHL and control animals. This removed the effect that synchrony was greater at slow frequencies. The NVHL and control groups were also indistinguishable after ethosuximide. Olanzapine increased synchrony in both NVHL and control rats but the increase was greater for the NVHL rats. Synchrony increased in all bands so there was no effect of the frequency band. Clearly, both ethosuximide and olanzapine altered the synchrony of oscillations in the LFPs of control and NVHL rats.

ETHOSUXIMIDE ATTENUATED THE COGNITIVE CONTROL IMPAIRMENT OF NVHL RATS

We examined whether these changes in synchrony were associated with changes in behavior using the active place avoidance task variant that allows evaluation of the ability to use relevant information and ignore irrelevant information, what is known as cognitive control. We first examined the effects of the drugs on locomotor hyperactivity (**Figure 7A**), which is a feature of NVHL rats that we have previously observed during the place avoidance task (12). Indeed, hyperactivity has been widely used to model the positive symptoms of schizophrenia and the effect of olanzapine in reducing hyperactivity has been shown in a variety of schizophrenia-related animal models (38, 39). Ethosuximide significantly reduced hyperactivity in NVHL rats compared to control rats (**Figure 7B**). As expected, olanzapine also reduced hyperactivity in NVHL rats compared to controls rats, so that the two groups were indistinguishable (**Figure 7C**).

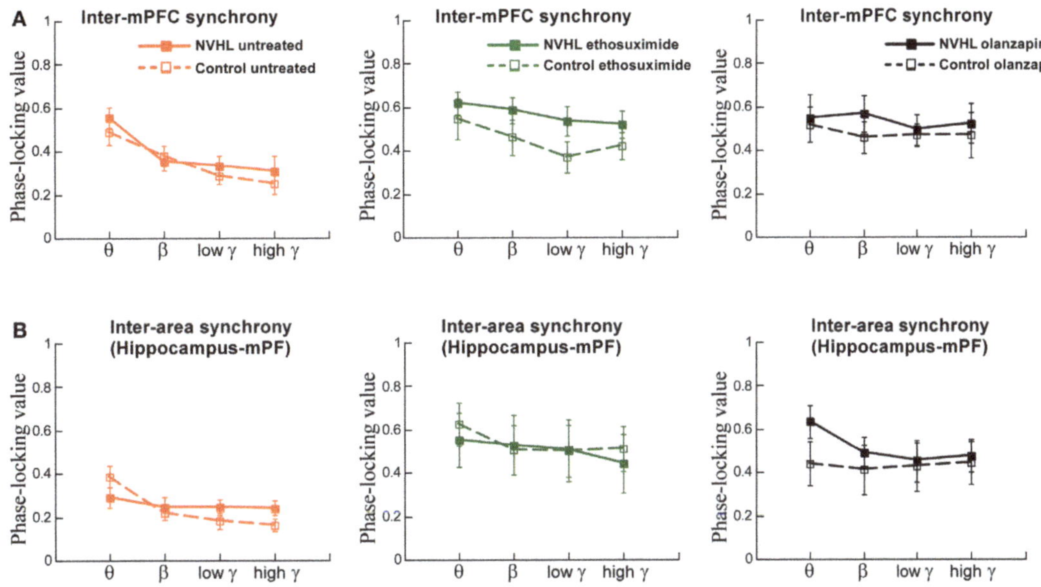

FIGURE 6 | Inter-mPFC or inter-hippocampus-mPFC phase synchrony was not different in the NVHL and control groups during active place avoidance. (A) Inter-mPFC synchrony was frequency-dependent but not different between the NVHL and control rats in the untreated groups (two-way ANOVA group: $F_{1,32}=0.92$, $p=0.34$; frequency: $F_{3,32}=8.97$, $p=0.0001$; interaction: $F_{3,32}=0.33$, $p=0.81$). The inter-mPFC synchrony was greater in the NVHL rats in the ethosuximide-treated group and the frequency dependence was lost due to increased synchrony at the gamma frequencies (middle: two-way ANOVA group: $F_{1,32}=5.42$, $p=0.03$; frequency: $F_{3,32}=1.41$, $p=0.26$; interaction: $F_{3,32}=0.16$, $p=0.92$). In the olanzapine-treated rats, the group and frequency dependencies were no longer observed because the drug increased synchrony at all frequencies we assessed (right: two-way ANOVA group: $F_{1,28}=1.43$, $p=0.24$; frequency: $F_{3,28}=0.40$, $p=0.76$; interaction: $F_{3,28}=0.11$, $p=0.95$) groups. **(B)** Inter-area synchrony (between mPFC and hippocampus) was frequency-dependent but not different between the NVHL and control rats in the untreated group (left: two-way ANOVA group: $F_{1,32}=0.43$, $p=0.51$; frequency: $F_{3,32}=5.29$, $p=0.005$; interaction: $F_{3,32}=2.05$, $p=0.13$). There were no group or frequency dependencies in the ethosuximide-treated rats because the drug increased synchrony at all frequencies to the level of the maximal (theta) inter-hippocampal synchrony (middle: two-way ANOVA group: $F_{1,32}=0.11$, $p=0.74$; frequency: $F_{3,32}=0.30$, $p=0.83$; interaction: $F_{3,32}=0.07$, $p=0.97$). The olanzapine-treated NVHL rats had greater synchrony at all frequencies and there was no frequency dependence because the drug also increased synchrony at all frequencies (right: two-way ANOVA group: $F_{1,28}=1.22$, $p=0.28$; frequency: $F_{3,28}=0.26$, $p=0.85$; interaction: $F_{3,28}=0.19$, $p=0.90$) groups.

We then examined the effects on cognitive behavior. NVHL rats were slower to learn the place avoidance (**Figure 8A**), as we have previously reported (12). Ethosuximide attenuated the deficit because under ethosuximide NVHL rats performed at a level that was statistically indistinguishable from control rats, although there was a trend for them to be slower to learn in the initial trials (**Figure 8B**). The olanzapine treatment did not improve the cognitive performance of NVHL rats, which remained impaired compared to control rats (**Figure 8C**). In fact, olanzapine seemed to slightly impair avoidance of the control rats during the initial trials. This was confirmed by comparing the three groups of control rats from **Figure 7** by two-way ANOVA (treatment: $F_{2,96}=9.70$, $p=0.0001$; trials: $F_{7,96}=33.86$, $p<0.0001$; interaction: $F_{14,96}=1.24$, $p=0.26$; *post hoc* tests: only olanzapine-treated control rats differed from ethosuximide-treated and untreated control rats).

Next we investigated the relationship between place avoidance performance and inter-hippocampal synchrony in the theta and beta bands. In the untreated NVHL and control rats, greater phase-locking at theta and beta frequencies was significantly correlated (r's >0.8; p's <0.01) with better place avoidance measured as lower total entrances (**Figure 9A**) but not with hyperactivity, measured as running speed (**Figure 9B**). The relationship between higher synchrony and lower entrances was apparent but not significant in the ethosuximide-treated animals (theta: $r=0.37$; $p>0.1$; beta: $r=0.14$; $p>0.1$). Because performance was good in most of these rats, there was limited variability in behavior for the synchrony measures to explain. The trend of a relationship between synchrony and cognition was reversed in the olanzapine-treated rats. Greater synchrony was associated with worse performance, but this trend was not significant (theta: $r=0.50$; $p>0.1$; beta: $r=0.35$; $p>0.1$).

Finally, in the effort to describe neural coordination during the place avoidance task, we examined the full set of 32 synchrony measures (8 electrode pairs × 4 frequency bands) as a pattern to investigate if there were group specific patterns of synchrony (**Figure 10**). The 32-dimensional space defined by the synchrony vectors (**Figure 10A**) was reduced to a 3-dimensional space to visualize the data using the first three principal components (**Figure 10B**). The data formed several clusters instead of filling the parameter space, which suggests neural activity may preferentially occupy preferred locales of this parameter state space. The untreated NVHL and control animals appeared to form two clusters. The ethosuximide and olanzapine-treated groups occupied distinct regions of the space away from the untreated groups. To estimate how distinct the groups might be, we computed the average distance amongst all pairs of vectors within a treatment group. The first six principal components accounted

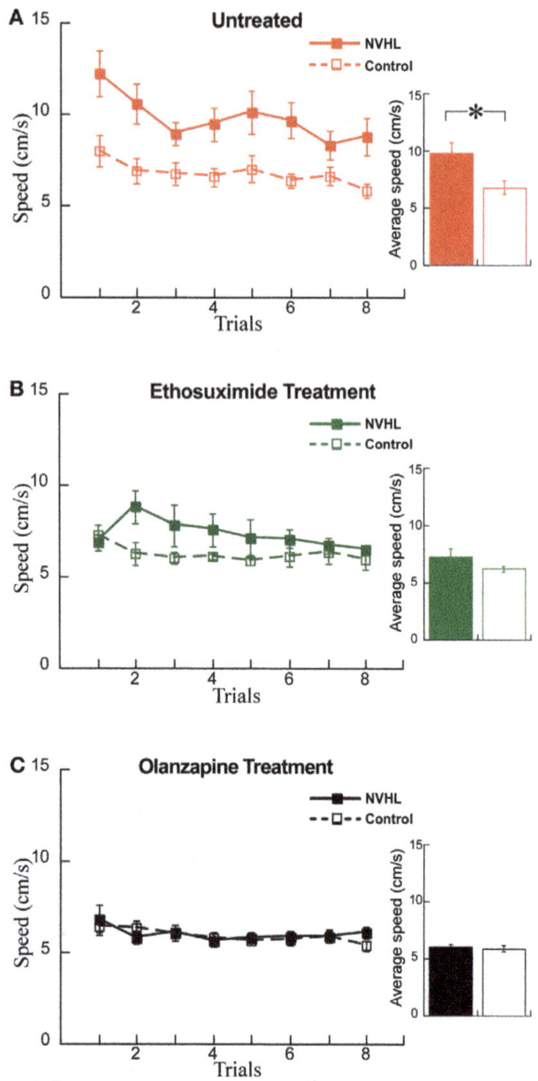

FIGURE 7 | Olanzapine and ethosuximide reduced hyperactivity in NVHL rats. (A) In the untreated group, the NVHL rats were hyperactive compared to control rats while performing the two-frame avoidance task (performance curve: two-way repeated-measures ANOVA group: $F_{1,64} = 53.34$, $p < 0.0001$; trial: $F_{7,64} = 2.37$, $p = 0.03$; interaction: $F_{7,64} = 0.46$, $p = 0.86$); inset: average speed: $t_8 = 2.78$, $p = 0.02$). **(B)** Ethosuximide treatment reduced hyperactivity in the NVHL rats compared to untreated NVHL rats, and showed a statistical difference when compared to control rats (performance curve: two-way repeated-measures ANOVA group: $F_{1,64} = 11.68$, $p = 0.001$; trial: $F_{7,64} = 0.86$, $p = 0.54$; interaction: $F_{7,64} = 1.09$, $p = 0.38$); inset: average speed: $t_8 = 1.5$, $p = 0.17$). **(C)** Olanzapine treatment reduced hyperactivity so there was no longer a difference from control rats (performance curve: two-way repeated-measures ANOVA group: $F_{1,64} = 0.36$, $p = 0.55$; trial: $F_{7,64} = 1.37$, $p = 0.23$; interaction: $F_{7,64} = 0.48$, $p = 0.85$); inset: average speed: $t_8 = 0.30$, $p = 0.77$).

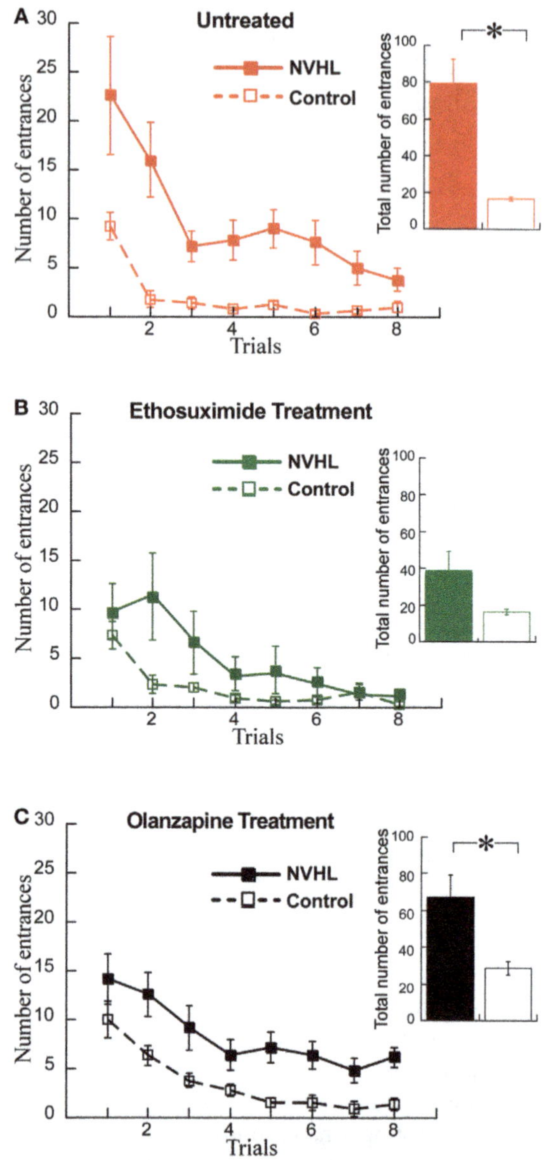

FIGURE 8 | Ethosuximide attenuated the cognitive control impairment of NVHL rats. (A) In the untreated group, the NVHL rats were slower to learn the two-frame task and showed an impairment when compared to the control rats (learning curve: two-way repeated-measures ANOVA group: $F_{1,64} = 53.84$, $p < 0.0001$; trial: $F_{7,64} = 8.80$, $p < 0.0001$; interaction: $F_{7,64} = 1.79$, $p = 0.10$); inset: total number of entrances: $t_8 = 4.69$, $p = 0.002$). **(B)** Ethosuximide treatment attenuated the learning impairment in the NVHL rats when compared to control rats (learning curve: two-way repeated-measures ANOVA group: $F_{1,64} = 5.86$, $p = 0.02$; trial: $F_{7,64} = 9.79$, $p < 0.0001$; interaction: $F_{7,64} = 2.40$, $p = 0.03$); inset: total number of entrances: $t_8 = 1.87$, $p = 0.10$). **(C)** Olanzapine treatment did not improve performance of the NVHL rats on the two-frame task (learning curve: two-way repeated-measures ANOVA group: $F_{1,64} = 42.87$, $p < 0.0001$; trial: $F_{7,64} = 9.66$, $p < 0.0001$; interaction: $F_{7,64} = 0.19$, $p = 0.99$); inset: total number of entrances: $t_8 = 3.10$, $p = 0.02$).

for over 90% of the variance in the data set (**Figure 10C**), so we computed the pair-wise distances as the 6-D Euclidean distance. The average distance from the untreated NVHL group was significantly greater for each group than it was for the vectors in the untreated NVHL group (**Figure 10D**). Similarly, the distances from the untreated control vectors were significantly greater for all other groups except the control group treated with ethosuximide, suggesting that ethosuximide did not significantly

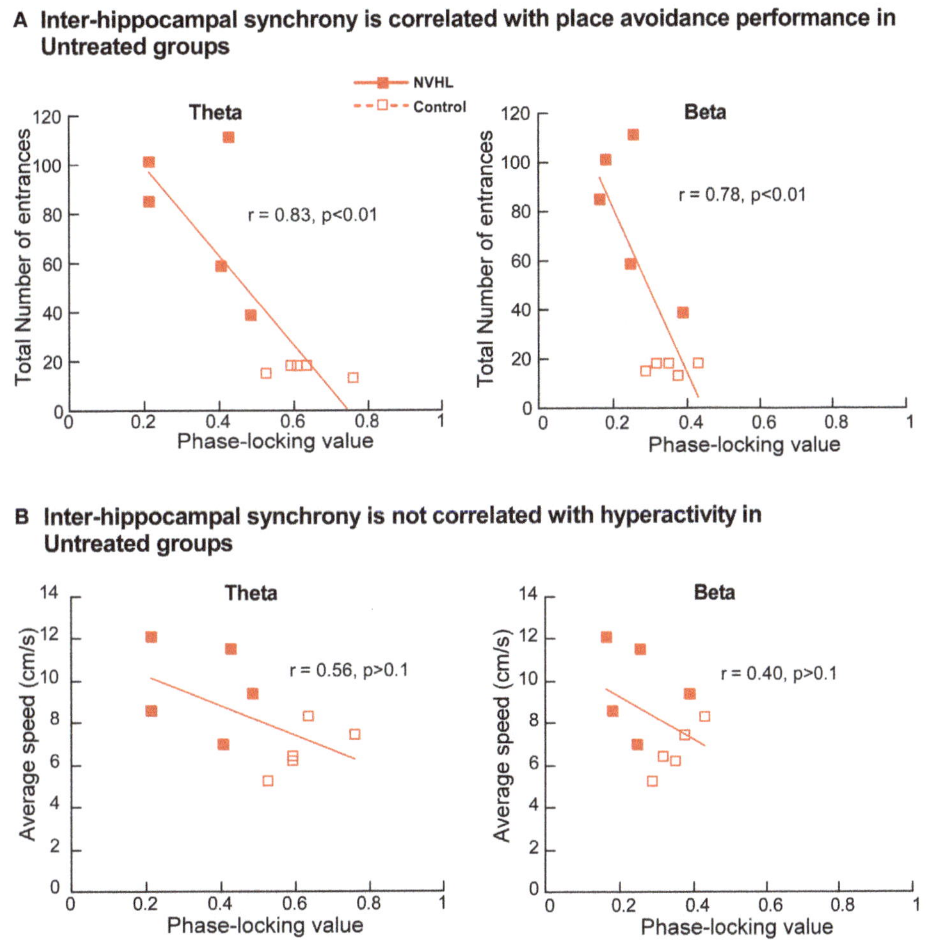

FIGURE 9 | Inter-hippocampal synchrony is correlated with place avoidance performance. **(A)** In the untreated NVHL and control rats, the scatter plot distributions of theta phase-locking values (left) and beta phase-locking values (right) show significant correlation with the total number of errors in the two-frame avoidance task. **(B)** In the untreated NVHL and control rats, theta phase-locking values (left) and beta phase-locking values (right) were not correlated with hyperactivity, measured as running speed during the two-frame avoidance task.

change control synchrony patterns. Because place avoidance behavior in the NVHL group was improved by ethosuximide, we estimated the distance between this group and the others. The distance to the untreated control group was no different than the distance within the NVHL-ethosuximide group, suggesting that the two groups were relatively similar. The complementary estimate of distance, this time to the olanzapine–NVHL group had a different answer. All groups had greater distances to the olanzapine–NVHL group than the distances amongst the group itself, consistent with the synchrony pattern caused by olanzapine being unique, rather than normalizing.

DISCUSSION

SUMMARY

The main finding of this study is that a drug that normalizes aberrant cognition-related neural synchrony in NVHL rats can also attenuate the cognitive control impairment in this schizophrenia-related neurodevelopmental model of mental dysfunction. This work demonstrates that the pattern of abnormal cognition-related neural synchrony is acutely normalized by ethosuximide, and furthermore shows that the synchrony alterations were associated with improved cognitive performance after ethosuximide but not olanzapine, despite both drugs being effective at reducing hyperactive locomotion in the NVHL model. Although olanzapine increased theta and beta synchrony between the two hippocampi, which is correlated with task performance (**Figure 8**), the drug also increased gamma synchrony beyond baseline levels, which may itself be associated with poor place avoidance performance in mutant mice (40, 41). Note that under ethosuximide, and also under olanzapine, the overall neural synchrony pattern in NVHL rats was distinct from the untreated control pattern, but the pattern after ethosuximide was closer to the control pattern than the pattern after olanzapine (**Figure 10D**) and perhaps this is one of the reasons that place avoidance performance was improved by ethosuximide but not olanzapine.

We have used the NVHL model to examine abnormal synchrony and cognitive impairment. Although NVHL rats are not a model of schizophrenia *per se*, these animals are an experimental

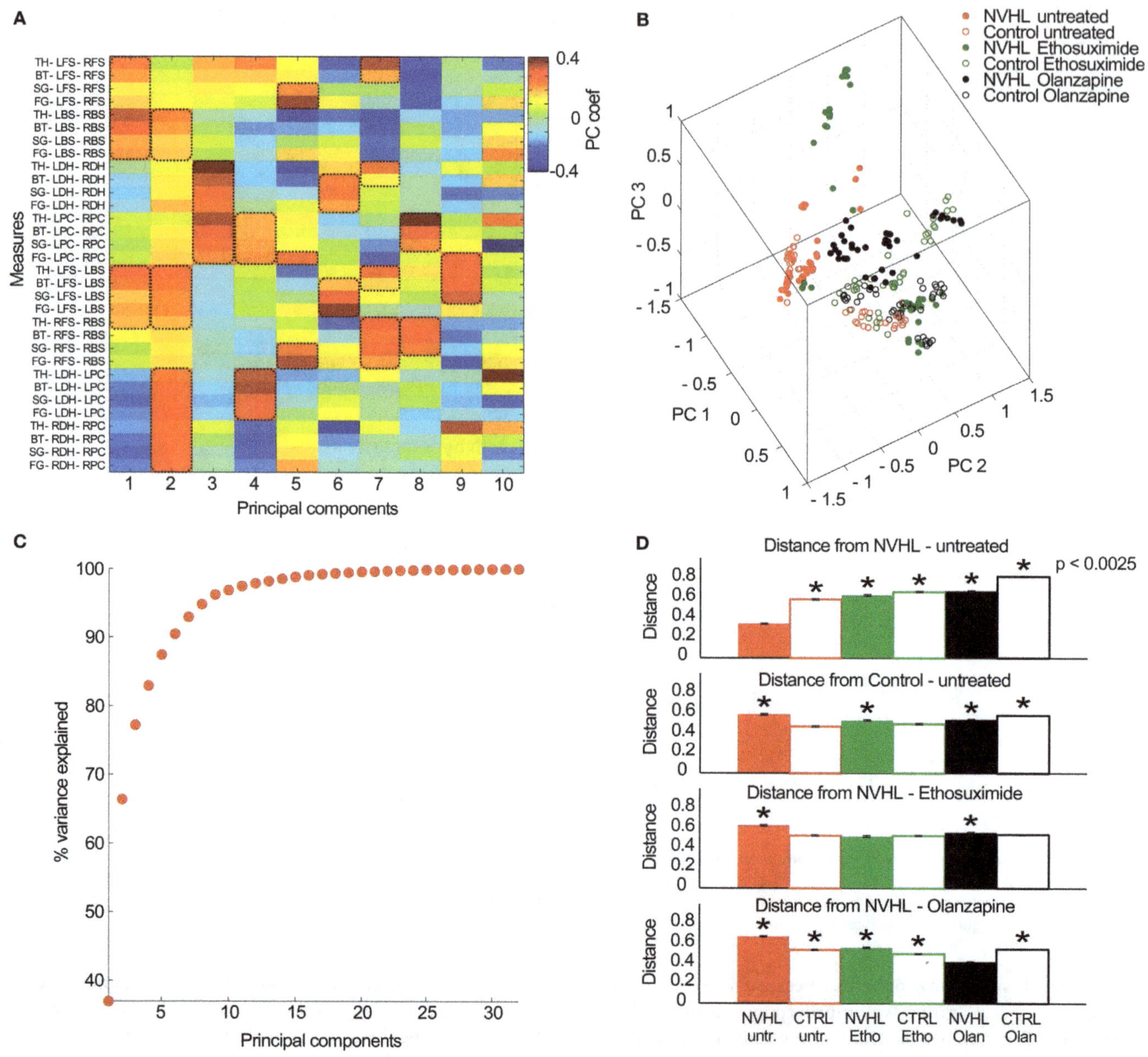

FIGURE 10 | Analysis of the multidimensional pattern of synchrony. **(A)** Thirty-two PLV measures were extracted from the data (8 electrode pairs × 4 frequency bands) and treated as a set of 32-dimensional vectors. PCA analysis was performed on the resulting vector dataset. The first 10 principal components (PC) are shown here (*x*-axis) with the relative contribution of each measurement (*y*-axis) indicated by a color code. The PCs tend to group measures with similar properties. As an example, PC #1 corresponds mostly to frequency band-non-specific phase synchrony between the contralateral cortical electrode pairs as well as ipsilateral cortical electrode pairs, which are measures of global cortical phase synchrony. PC #3 corresponds mostly to frequency band-non-specific phase synchrony between the left and right-hippocampi as well as between the left and right prefrontal cortex, which is an estimate of region-specific inter-hemispheric synchrony. PC #6 corresponds to frequency-specific synchrony in the beta, slow gamma, and fast gamma bands between inter-hemispheric neocortical and hippocampal sites. The key measures of synchrony that contributed to each PC are indicated by the dashed boxes. **(B)** The multidimensional data can be visualized by plotting in the 3-D space of the first three PCs. **(C)** The cumulative probability of the dataset variance is explained by the PCs. The first six principal components explain ~90% of the dataset variance. **(D)** The average Euclidean distance between a pair of vectors estimates their distinctiveness. The distances between all pairs of vectors were computed within a treatment group and between all treatment groups and a specific treatment group to estimate similarity/distinctiveness of the treatment groups. The average distances are given to the untreated NVHL group (top row), to the untreated control group (second row), to the ethosuximide-treated NVHL group (third row), and to the olanzapine-treated NVHL group (bottom row).

model with neural synchrony and related cognitive abnormalities, which allows a prediction of the discoordination hypothesis to be tested. This unifying hypothesis was proposed to account for the schizophrenia syndrome independent of etiology (1, 2, 12, 27, 28). This view acknowledges that schizophrenia may turn out to be heterogeneous and that multiple factors contribute, including genetic alterations, infectious, toxic, and stressful events (42, 43). Whatever the etiology, the discoordination hypothesis asserts that disruption of the physiological synchronization of neural activities produces cognitive abnormalities in schizophrenia, despite otherwise seemingly normal expression of unitary physiological phenomena. The hypothesis is based specifically on the physiological coordination of neural activities, defined as the set of neural processes that control the timing of spike discharge across ensembles of neurons (1, 29, 44, 45). Our group has demonstrated this neural coordination during cognitive control in active place avoidance tasks (46, 47). The current findings support the discoordination hypothesis by demonstrating that correcting the neural synchrony abnormality in NVHL rats can be associated with cognitive improvement, which was the case with ethosuximide but not with olanzapine. Olanzapine did not normalize either neural synchrony or cognitive behavior (**Figures 4**, **5**, and **8**). In further support of the hypothesis, olanzapine caused abnormal neural synchrony in control rats, which seemed to worsen the place avoidance.

SPIKE-WAVE ACTIVITY

A secondary finding in this study is that spike-wave like activity was observed in the epidural cortical EEG of both NVHL and control rats during stillness in the home-cage and only rarely during active place avoidance behavior, consistent with prior observations (32, 34). This observation may have implications for how deficits in NVHL animals are interpreted when those deficits are characterized in tasks during which there is behavioral stillness, like pre-pulse inhibition, inhibitory avoidance, and food-motivated radial-arm mazes. Complex interactions of inhibitory and excitatory systems between the thalamus and cortical structures generate a variety of normal and abnormal rhythmic states including spindle waves and SWDs during absence seizures. Spindle waves are characterized by 1–4 s periods of 6–14 Hz oscillations during normal sleep (48). The characteristic frequency of the SWD is 3–4 Hz in humans (49) and is normally higher (4–12 Hz) in rodents (50, 51). Our analysis of cortical spike-wave activity shows that the features of the spike-wave activity in NVHL and control rats are different (**Figure 2**). The duration of the activity was greater in NVHL rats compared to control rats, further suggesting that this activity in the NVHL rats may be of a different neural origin than it is in control rats. In NVHL rats it may reflect a form of pathological network synchrony and even a sign of epileptiform propensity (52).

Indeed, during several hours of continuous monitoring, we have observed rare, but nonetheless *bona fide* epileptiform discharges and behavioral seizures in NVHL rats (52). The NHVL rats may have increased susceptibility to seizures due to dysregulation of the GABA system (53, 54). There is widespread reduction of GAD67 expression (54, 55), and decreased expression of PV interneurons in the prefrontal cortex and the hippocampus (54) in these rats. There is also increased firing in pyramidal neurons in the NVHL rats. The mPFC pyramidal neurons of NVHL rats respond to stimulation of the ventral tegmental area, the origin of dopamine projections to the PFC, with an increase in firing rates (56) instead of the normal decrease (57), indicating hyperexcitability. It has been shown that NVHL rats developed epileptiform SWDs at a twofold lower dose of pentylenetetrazol (PTZ, a $GABA_A$ antagonist) than sham-operated rats, further evidence that the NVHL rats have increased susceptibility to absence-like seizures (54). Indeed, PD7 injections into ventral hippocampus with kainate, an excitotoxin with a different mechanism of action than ibotenate (58), is used as a model of temporal lobe epilepsy (59). Perturbations of the GABA system, together with the aberrant response reflecting the inability of dopamine to activate interneurons, may result in enhanced cortical excitability and abnormal spike-wave activity in NVHL rats.

ETHOSUXIMIDE TREATMENT

We now discuss the effects of ethosuximide in the contexts of its pharmacological actions, typical use as well as the relevance of the findings with ethosuximide to understanding the cognitive impairments in the NVHL rat model and mental illness such as schizophrenia. To be clear, neither the findings nor the discussion that follows suggest that ethosuximide might be an effective treatment for schizophrenia. Rather, the procognitive and normalizing neural coordination effects of ethosuximide in the NVHL model provides new evidence that attenuating neural synchrony deficits can itself be procognitive.

Ethosuximide is used extensively to treat absence (petit mal) seizures (60–62). The mechanism of action is to block low-threshold Ca^{2+} currents in the T-type Ca^{2+} channels and enhance GABAergic tone (63, 64). We observed that ethosuximide reduced spike-wave activity in NVHL rats, indicating it is effective on abnormal synchrony in NVHL rats during home-cage behaviors (**Figure 3**). The drug also increased inter-hippocampal synchrony in NVHL rats so that neural coordination between the two hippocampi approached normal levels in the theta- and beta-frequency bands. Nonetheless, taken together, after ethosuximide, the overall pattern of neural synchrony in the NVHL rats was modified but the pattern of synchronies was not restored to the pattern of the untreated controls. Indeed, ethosuximide also changed the synchrony pattern in the controls animals too, but these changes were not associated with cognitive disability.

The effectiveness of ethosuximide may be contemplated in relation to the fact that the synchronization of oscillations reflects the temporally precise interaction of neural activities (65). Such coordinated interactions result from an appropriate balance between GABA-mediated inhibition and glutamate-mediated excitation, which may be unbalanced in adult NVHL rats (56). Alterations in one or both of these systems can result in abnormal network synchrony. Schizophrenia has been associated with dysregulation of cortical GABAergic neurotransmission (66) and abnormalities in NMDA-receptor mediated neurotransmission (67). There are significantly decreased levels of GABAergic neuronal markers like parvalbumin mRNA in the prefrontal cortex (68, 69) and in the dorsolateral prefrontal cortex of schizophrenia patients, decreased levels have been reported of glutamic acid decarboxylase (GAD67) mRNA, the GABA-synthesizing enzyme (70, 71). Indeed,

NMDA-receptor hypofunction in schizophrenia (72, 73) is now thought to primarily affect GABA inhibition by reducing GABAergic tone. Thus dysregulation of excitatory and inhibitory neurotransmission contribute to abnormalities in the coordination of neural activities, which according to the hypothesis, is the basis for the impaired cognitive functions that are central to schizophrenia and a logical target for developing cognition promoting therapies. It was recently proposed that aberrant low frequency delta/theta oscillations emerge as a consequence of NMDA-receptor hypofunction (3, 74). The reduced excitation would deinactivate T-type Ca^{2+} channels and exaggerate bursting, especially in thalamic neurons, which may be the origin of the low frequency thalamocortical oscillations that could disrupt cortical function in schizophrenia (75). In this context, given ethosuximide's mechanism of action, it is perhaps not surprising that the drug both normalized neural synchrony and improved cognition in NVHL rats. Ethosuximide reduces excitability primarily by blocking activity-dependent low-threshold Ca^{2+} currents as well as by acting as a partial agonist at the picrotoxin GABA-blocking receptor (64).

In the absence of the forgoing discussion, it may seem surprising to some readers that ethosuximide can improve inter-hippocampal synchrony and place avoidance behavior. Some readers may have assumed that because ethosuximide is antiepileptic it must decrease neural synchrony because epileptiform activity is thought of as excessive synchrony. According to these opinions, ethosuximide would decrease synchrony, not increase it, and thus worsen place avoidance behavior in control as well as NVHL rats. As we have pointed out in the Section "Introduction," epileptiform activity is not simply excessive synchrony, and in the NVHL rat, we have measured the evidence of widespread decreases of synchrony between brain areas, resembling functional disconnection (52). Embedded in this loosening of neural coordination, perhaps by excitation–inhibition uncoupling, we also observed that some brain areas can exhibit relatively increased synchrony. Thus, there are alternative conceptualizations of the ethosuximide effects but they are not supported by the data on the subject in general or on NVHL rats in particular.

Ethosuximide treatment also reduced hyperactivity in NVHL rats, which in animal models, is widely studied as a behavioral analog of the positive symptoms of schizophrenia, although the reduction was not as effective as after olanzapine. Blocking T-type Ca^{2+} channels can produce antipsychotic effects in rats by attenuating the psychomotor effects of both the NMDA antagonist MK-801 and amphetamine, the dopaminergic psychostimulant (76). T-type Ca^{2+} channels are widely expressed in the brain, including areas such as the thalamus, the prefrontal cortex, the hippocampus, and the nucleus accumbens (77), which are regions that have been reported to function abnormally in schizophrenia (74, 78, 79). Interestingly, a number of clinically validated antipsychotics, including haloperidol, pimozide, flunarizine, and clozapine, are potent T-type channel antagonists (76, 80–82). A recent genome-wide study of single-nucleotide polymorphisms (SNP) found that variations in calcium channel genes are associated with schizophrenia as well as a range of major psychiatric disorders (83). These data implicate calcium channels in the pathophysiology of schizophrenia, and while calcium channel abnormality may help to account for why ethosuximide was effective on NVHL rats, it is also possible that ethosuximide was effective because of its fundamental effects on excitation–inhibition balance through the action on otherwise normal calcium channels. Nonetheless, the present work does not imply and we do not propose to use ethosuximide as a treatment for cognitive deficits in schizophrenia. Rather the present findings demonstrate that procognitive effects may be possible if treatments can normalize the coordination of neural activity between cognitive processing centers like the two hippocampi.

OLANZAPINE TREATMENT

Second-generation (atypical) antipsychotic medications, including olanzapine, are effective in treating psychosis, hallucinations, and delusions (84) but ineffective in treating the cognitive impairments that strongly debilitate schizophrenia patients (85). Olanzapine, a thienobenzodiazepine derivative, is classified as a multi-acting receptor-targeted antipsychotic, showing high affinity for dopaminergic, serotonergic, cholinergic, histaminergic, and muscarinic receptors (86, 87). As expected, we observed that olanzapine reduced hyperactivity in NVHL rats to control levels during the place avoidance task, indicating we used an effective antipsychotic dose, at least by traditional measures. The dose was however, ineffective at improving cognitive performance of NVHL rats in the two-frame task. This is of course consistent with the drug's lack of effect on cognitive symptoms in patients.

Olanzapine treatment in NVHL and control rats showed a reversed effect on neural synchrony. Olanzapine increased inter-hippocampal synchrony in NVHL rats to the level of untreated controls in the theta and beta bands and in excess of the control levels in the gamma bands. In contrast, the drug decreased inter-hippocampal synchrony in control rats. The increased synchrony in olanzapine-treated NVHL rats was not associated with improved cognitive performance in the NVHL rats, which would be at odds with the discoordination hypothesis, except that after olanzapine, the gamma synchrony was excessive, indicating that olanzapine changed neural coordination, but as demonstrated with the multidimensional synchrony analysis (**Figure 10**), the synchrony changes did not normalize neural synchrony in NVHL rats. Conversely, but also in support of the discoordination hypothesis, the decreased synchrony in olanzapine-treated control rats was associated with a higher number of errors in the two-frame task when compared to untreated control rats, which is consistent with the observation that the drug changed the neural synchrony pattern in control animals to a pattern that is substantially distinct (**Figures 10B,D**) from the untreated control pattern. It is well documented that antipsychotic drugs cause EEG abnormalities associated with general slowing of background activity, an increase in paroxysmal theta or delta activity and the development of epileptiform discharges (88). In patients on olanzapine, there is an increased diffuse and intermittent slowing of the EEG (89, 90) and an increased high risk of EEG abnormalities such as theta and delta slowing, sharp waves or phase reversal, and/or spike-wave activities (88, 91). Healthy subjects on olanzapine showed an increased power in the theta band and a decrease in the beta band (92). In summary, olanzapine normalized inter-hippocampal synchrony in the theta and beta bands but it also caused abnormal synchrony changes in both the NVHL and control rats that were not associated with improved cognitive performance in the two-frame task.

CONCLUSION

The findings reported here are consistent with the main assertion and prediction of the discoordination hypothesis that abnormal neural synchrony during cognitive effort is associated with impaired cognition and that restoring normal synchrony will promote cognition. As shown here, targeting the pathophysiology of abnormal neural coordination, regardless of the etiology, may be both a rational and effective program for developing a much-needed generation of procognitive treatments for mental illness in general and schizophrenia in particular.

AUTHOR CONTRIBUTIONS

Heekyung Lee collected and analyzed data, Dino Dvorak analyzed data, Heekyung Lee and André A. Fenton wrote the manuscript, and André A. Fenton planned and organized the research.

ACKNOWLEDGMENTS

This work was supported by NIMH grant R01MH084038.

REFERENCES

1. Phillips WA, Silverstein SM. Convergence of biological and psychological perspectives on cognitive coordination in schizophrenia. *Behav Brain Sci* (2003) **26**:65–82. doi:10.1017/S0140525X03000025
2. Uhlhaas PJ, Singer W. Neural synchrony in brain disorders: relevance for cognitive dysfunctions and pathophysiology. *Neuron* (2006) **52**:155–68. doi:10.1016/j.neuron.2006.09.020
3. Lisman JE, Coyle JT, Green RW, Javitt DC, Benes FM, Heckers S, et al. Circuit-based framework for understanding neurotransmitter and risk gene interactions in schizophrenia. *Trends Neurosci* (2008) **31**(5):234–42. doi:10.1016/j.tins.2008.02.005
4. Uhlhaas PJ, Singer W. Abnormal neural oscillations and synchrony in schizophrenia. *Nat Rev Neurosci* (2010) **11**:100–13. doi:10.1038/nrn2774
5. Galderisi S, Mucci A, Volpe U, Boutros N. Evidence-based medicine and electrophysiology in schizophrenia. *Clin EEG Neurosci* (2009) **40**:62–77. doi:10.1177/155005940904000206
6. Schmiedt C, Brand A, Hildebrandt H, Basar-Eroglu C. Event-related theta oscillations during working memory tasks in patients with schizophrenia and healthy controls. *Brain Res Cogn Brain Res* (2005) **25**:936–47. doi:10.1016/j.cogbrainres.2005.09.015
7. Uhlhaas PJ, Linden DE, Singer W, Haenschel C, Lindner M, Maurer K, et al. Dysfunctional long-range coordination of neural activity during Gestalt perception in schizophrenia. *J Neurosci* (2006) **26**:8168–75. doi:10.1523/JNEUROSCI.2002-06.2006
8. Spencer KM, Nestor PG, Perlmutter R, Niznikiewicz MA, Klump MC, Frumin M, et al. Neural synchrony indexes disordered perception and cognition in schizophrenia. *Proc Natl Acad Sci U S A* (2004) **101**:17288–93. doi:10.1073/pnas.0406074101
9. Cho RY, Konecky RO, Carter CS. Impairments in frontal cortical gamma synchrony and cognitive control in schizophrenia. *Proc Natl Acad Sci U S A* (2006) **103**:19878–83. doi:10.1073/pnas.0609440103
10. Sigurdsson T, Stark KL, Karayiorgou M, Gogos JA, Gordon JA. Impaired hippocampal-prefrontal synchrony in a genetic mouse model of schizophrenia. *Nature* (2010) **464**(7289):763–7. doi:10.1038/nature08855
11. Dickerson DD, Wolff AR, Bilkey DK. Abnormal long-range neural synchrony in a maternal immune activation animal model of schizophrenia. *J Neurosci* (2010) **30**(37):12424–31. doi:10.1523/JNEUROSCI.3046-10.2010
12. Lee H, Dvorak D, Kao HY, Duffy AM, Scharfman HE, Fenton AA. Early cognitive experience prevents adult deficits in a neurodevelopmental schizophrenia model. *Neuron* (2012) **75**:714–24. doi:10.1016/j.neuron.2012.06.016
13. Palop JJ, Chin J, Mucke L. A network dysfunction perspective on neurodegenerative diseases. *Nature* (2006) **443**:768–73. doi:10.1038/nature05289
14. Palop JJ, Chin J, Roberson ED, Wang J, Thwin MT, Bien-Ly N, et al. Aberrant excitatory neuronal activity and compensatory remodeling of inhibitory hippocampal circuits in mouse models of Alzheimer's disease. *Neuron* (2007) **55**:697–711. doi:10.1016/j.neuron.2007.07.025
15. Sanchez PE, Zhu L, Verret L, Vossel KA, Orr AG, Cirrito JR, et al. Levetiracetam suppresses neuronal network dysfunction and reverses synaptic and cognitive deficits in an Alzheimer's disease model. *Proc Natl Acad Sci U S A* (2012) **109**:E2895–903. doi:10.1073/pnas.1121081109
16. Lipska BK, Jaskiw GE, Weinberger DR. Postpubertal emergence of hyperresponsiveness to stress and to amphetamine after neonatal excitotoxic hippocampal damage: a potential animal model of schizophrenia. *Neuropsychopharmacology* (1993) **9**:67–75. doi:10.1038/npp.1993.44
17. Lawrie SM, Abukmeil SS. Brain abnormality in schizophrenia. A systematic and quantitative review of volumetric magnetic resonance imaging studies. *Br J Psychiatry* (1998) **172**:110–20. doi:10.1192/bjp.172.2.110
18. Nelson MD, Saykin AJ, Flashman LA, Riordan HJ. Hippocampal volume reduction in schizophrenia as assessed by magnetic resonance imaging: a meta-analytic study. *Arch Gen Psychiatry* (1998) **55**:433–40. doi:10.1001/archpsyc.55.5.433
19. McCarley RW, Wible CG, Frumin M, Hirayasu Y, Levitt JJ, Fischer IA, et al. MRI anatomy of schizophrenia. *Biol Psychiatry* (1999) **45**:1099–119. doi:10.1016/S0006-3223(99)00018-9
20. Wright IC, Rabe-Hesketh S, Woodruff PW, David AS, Murray RM, Bullmore ET. Meta-analysis of regional brain volumes in schizophrenia. *Am J Psychiatry* (2000) **157**:16–25.
21. Goldman MB, Mitchell CP. What is the functional significance of hippocampal pathology in schizophrenia? *Schizophr Bull* (2004) **30**:367–92. doi:10.1093/oxfordjournals.schbul.a007086
22. Harrison PJ. The hippocampus in schizophrenia: a review of the neuropathological evidence and its pathophysiological implications. *Psychopharmacology (Berl)* (2004) **174**:151–62. doi:10.1007/s00213-003-1761-y
23. Jessen F, Scheef L, Germeshausen L, Tawo Y, Kockler M, Kuhn KU, et al. Reduced hippocampal activation during encoding and recognition of words in schizophrenia patients. *Am J Psychiatry* (2003) **160**:1305–12. doi:10.1176/appi.ajp.160.7.1305
24. Luck D, Danion JM, Marrer C, Pham BT, Gounot D, Foucher J. Abnormal medial temporal activity for bound information during working memory maintenance in patients with schizophrenia. *Hippocampus* (2010) **20**:936–48. doi:10.1002/hipo.20689
25. Zierhut K, Bogerts B, Schott B, Fenker D, Walter M, Albrecht D, et al. The role of hippocampus dysfunction in deficient memory encoding and positive symptoms in schizophrenia. *Psychiatry Res* (2010) **183**:187–94. doi:10.1016/j.pscychresns.2010.03.007
26. Erk S, Meyer-Lindenberg A, Schnell K, Opitz Von Boberfeld C, Esslinger C, Kirsch P, et al. Brain function in carriers of a genome-wide supported bipolar disorder variant. *Arch Gen Psychiatry* (2010) **67**:803–11. doi:10.1001/archgenpsychiatry.2010.94
27. Fenton AA. Neural coordination and psychotic disorganization. In: Holscher C, Munk MH, editors. *Information Processing by Neuronal Populations*. London: Cambridge University Press (2008). p. 387–408.
28. Tononi G, Edelman GM. Schizophrenia and the mechanisms of conscious integration. *Brain Res Brain Res Rev* (2000) **31**:391–400. doi:10.1016/S0165-0173(99)00056-9
29. Buzsaki G. Neural syntax: cell assemblies, synapsembles, and readers. *Neuron* (2010) **68**:362–85. doi:10.1016/j.neuron.2010.09.023
30. Dvorak D, Fenton AA. Toward a proper estimation of phase-amplitude coupling in neural oscillations. *J Neurosci Methods* (2014) **225**:42–56. doi:10.1016/j.jneumeth.2014.01.002
31. Lachaux JP, Rodriguez E, Martinerie J, Varela FJ. Measuring phase synchrony in brain signals. *Hum Brain Mapp* (1999) **8**:194–208. doi:10.1002/(SICI)1097-0193(1999)8:4<194::AID-HBM4>3.0.CO;2-C
32. Wiest MC, Nicolelis MA. Behavioral detection of tactile stimuli during 7-12 Hz cortical oscillations in awake rats. *Nat Neurosci* (2003) **6**:913–4. doi:10.1038/nn1107
33. Xanthopoulos P, Rebennack S, Liu CC, Zhang J, Holmes GL, Uthman BM, et al. A novel wavelet based algorithm for spike and wave detection in absence epilepsy. *Bioinformatics and Bioengineering (BIBE) 2010 IEEE International Conference* (2010).

34. Semba K, Szechtman H, Komisaruk BR. Synchrony among rhythmical facial tremor, neocortical 'alpha' waves, and thalamic non-sensory neuronal bursts in intact awake rats. *Brain Res* (1980) **195**:281–98. doi:10.1016/0006-8993(80)90065-7
35. Gomora JC, Daud AN, Weiergraber M, Perez-Reyes E. Block of cloned human T-type calcium channels by succinimide antiepileptic drugs. *Mol Pharmacol* (2001) **60**:1121–32. doi:10.1124/mol.60.5.1121
36. Mitchell KJ, O'Donnell P, Durstewitz D, Fenton AA, Gingrich JA, Gordon JA, et al. A Framework for the Use of Models in Schizophrenia. In: Silverstein SM, Moghaddam B, Wykes T, editors. *Schizophrenia: Evolution and Synthesis*. Cambridge, MA: MIT Press (2013). p. 212–26.
37. Patil ST, Zhang L, Martenyi F, Lowe SL, Jackson KA, Andreev BV, et al. Activation of mGlu2/3 receptors as a new approach to treat schizophrenia: a randomized Phase 2 clinical trial. *Nat Med* (2007) **13**:1102–7. doi:10.1038/nm1007-1264
38. Duncan GE, Moy SS, Lieberman JA, Koller BH. Typical and atypical antipsychotic drug effects on locomotor hyperactivity and deficits in sensorimotor gating in a genetic model of NMDA receptor hypofunction. *Pharmacol Biochem Behav* (2006) **85**:481–91. doi:10.1016/j.pbb.2006.09.017
39. Sun T, Hu G, Li M. Repeated antipsychotic treatment progressively potentiates inhibition on phencyclidine-induced hyperlocomotion, but attenuates inhibition on amphetamine-induced hyperlocomotion: relevance to animal models of antipsychotic drugs. *Eur J Pharmacol* (2009) **602**:334–42. doi:10.1016/j.ejphar.2008.11.036
40. Zhong J, Chuang SC, Bianchi R, Zhao W, Lee H, Fenton AA, et al. BC1 regulation of metabotropic glutamate receptor-mediated neuronal excitability. *J Neurosci* (2009) **29**:9977–86. doi:10.1523/JNEUROSCI.3893-08.2009
41. Zhong J, Chuang SC, Bianchi R, Zhao W, Paul G, Thakkar P, et al. Regulatory BC1 RNA and the fragile X mental retardation protein: convergent functionality in brain. *PLoS One* (2010) **5**:e15509. doi:10.1371/journal.pone.0015509
42. Carpenter WT Jr. How the diagnosis of schizophrenia impeded the advance of knowledge (and what to do about it). In: Silverstein SM, Moghaddam B, Wykes T, editors. *Schizophrenia: Evolution and Synthesis*. Cambridge, MA: MIT Press (2013). p. 49–62.
43. MacDonald AW. What kind of a thing is schizophrenia? Specific causation and general failure models. In: Silverstein SM, Moghaddam B, Wykes T, editors. *Schizophrenia: Evolution and Synthesis*. Cambridge, MA: MIT Press (2013). p. 25–48.
44. Hebb DO. *The Organization of Behavior: A Neuropsychological Theory*. New York: Wiley (1949).
45. Phillips WA, Singer W. In search of common foundations for cortical computation. *Behav Brain Sci* (1997) **20**:657–83. doi:10.1017/S0140525X9700160X
46. Kelemen E, Fenton AA. Dynamic grouping of hippocampal neural activity during cognitive control of two spatial frames. *PLoS Biol* (2010) **8**:e1000403. doi:10.1371/journal.pbio.1000403
47. Kelemen E, Fenton AA. Key features of human episodic recollection in the cross-episode retrieval of rat hippocampus representations of space. *PLoS Biol* (2013) **11**:e1001607. doi:10.1371/journal.pbio.1001607
48. Steriade M, McCormick DA, Sejnowski TJ. Thalamocortical oscillations in the sleeping and aroused brain. *Science* (1993) **262**:679–85. doi:10.1126/science.8235588
49. Panayiotopoulos C. Absence epilepsies. In: Engel J Jr, Pedley TA, editors. *Epilepsy: A Comprehensive Textbook*. Philadelphia: Lippincott-Raven Publishers (1997). p. 2327–46.
50. Buzsaki G, Bickford RG, Ponomareff G, Thal LJ, Mandel R, Gage FH. Nucleus basalis and thalamic control of neocortical activity in the freely moving rat. *J Neurosci* (1988) **8**:4007–26.
51. Hosford DA, Clark S, Cao Z, Wilson WA Jr, Lin FH, Morrisett RA, et al. The role of GABAB receptor activation in absence seizures of lethargic (lh/lh) mice. *Science* (1992) **257**:398–401. doi:10.1126/science.1321503
52. Neymotin SA, Lee H, Fenton AA, Lytton WW. Interictal EEG discoordination in a rat seizure model. *J Clin Neurophysiol* (2010) **27**:438–44. doi:10.1097/WNP.0b013e3181fe059e
53. Endo K, Hori T, Abe S, Asada T. Alterations in GABA(A) receptor expression in neonatal ventral hippocampal lesioned rats: comparison of prepubertal and postpubertal periods. *Synapse* (2007) **61**:357–66. doi:10.1002/syn.20393
54. Francois J, Ferrandon A, Koning E, Angst MJ, Sandner G, Nehlig A. Selective reorganization of GABAergic transmission in neonatal ventral hippocampal-lesioned rats. *Int J Neuropsychopharmacol* (2009) **12**:1097–110. doi:10.1017/S1461145709009985
55. Lipska BK, Lerman DN, Khaing ZZ, Weickert CS, Weinberger DR. Gene expression in dopamine and GABA systems in an animal model of schizophrenia: effects of antipsychotic drugs. *Eur J Neurosci* (2003) **18**:391–402. doi:10.1046/j.1460-9568.2003.02738.x
56. O'Donnell P, Lewis BL, Weinberger DR, Lipska BK. Neonatal hippocampal damage alters electrophysiological properties of prefrontal cortical neurons in adult rats. *Cereb Cortex* (2002) **12**:975–82. doi:10.1093/cercor/12.9.975
57. Lewis BL, O'Donnell P. Ventral tegmental area afferents to the prefrontal cortex maintain membrane potential 'up' states in pyramidal neurons via D(1) dopamine receptors. *Cereb Cortex* (2000) **10**:1168–75. doi:10.1093/cercor/10.12.1168
58. Kohler C, Schwarcz R. Comparison of ibotenate and kainate neurotoxicity in rat brain: a histological study. *Neuroscience* (1983) **8**:819–35. doi:10.1016/0306-4522(83)90013-1
59. Babb TL, Pereira-Leite J, Mathern GW, Pretorius JK. Kainic acid induced hippocampal seizures in rats: comparisons of acute and chronic seizures using intrahippocampal versus systemic injections. *Ital J Neurol Sci* (1995) **16**:39–44. doi:10.1007/BF02229073
60. Zimmerman FT, Burgemeister BB. A new drug for petit mal epilepsy. *Neurology* (1958) **8**:769–75. doi:10.1212/WNL.8.10.769
61. Heathfield KW, Jewesbury EC. Treatment of petit mal with ethosuximide. *Br Med J* (1961) **2**:565–7. doi:10.1136/bmj.2.5251.565
62. Goren MZ, Onat F. Ethosuximide: from bench to bedside. *CNS Drug Rev* (2007) **13**:224–39. doi:10.1111/j.1527-3458.2007.00009.x
63. Coulter DA, Huguenard JR, Prince DA. Specific petit mal anticonvulsants reduce calcium currents in thalamic neurons. *Neurosci Lett* (1989) **98**:74–8. doi:10.1016/0304-3940(89)90376-5
64. Coulter DA, Huguenard JR, Prince DA. Differential effects of petit mal anticonvulsants and convulsants on thalamic neurones: GABA current blockade. *Br J Pharmacol* (1990) **100**:807–13. doi:10.1111/j.1476-5381.1990.tb14095.x
65. Schnitzler A, Gross J. Normal and pathological oscillatory communication in the brain. *Nat Rev Neurosci* (2005) **6**:285–96. doi:10.1038/nrn1650
66. Lewis DA, Hashimoto T, Volk DW. Cortical inhibitory neurons and schizophrenia. *Nat Rev Neurosci* (2005) **6**:312–24. doi:10.1038/nrn1648
67. Moghaddam B. Bringing order to the glutamate chaos in schizophrenia. *Neuron* (2003) **40**:881–4. doi:10.1016/S0896-6273(03)00757-8
68. Beasley CL, Reynolds GP. Parvalbumin-immunoreactive neurons are reduced in the prefrontal cortex of schizophrenics. *Schizophr Res* (1997) **24**:349–55. doi:10.1016/S0920-9964(96)00122-3
69. Woo TU, Miller JL, Lewis DA. Schizophrenia and the parvalbumin-containing class of cortical local circuit neurons. *Am J Psychiatry* (1997) **154**:1013–5.
70. Guidotti A, Auta J, Davis JM, Di-Giorgi-Gerevini V, Dwivedi Y, Grayson DR, et al. Decrease in reelin and glutamic acid decarboxylase67 (GAD67) expression in schizophrenia and bipolar disorder: a postmortem brain study. *Arch Gen Psychiatry* (2000) **57**:1061–9. doi:10.1001/archpsyc.57.11.1061
71. Volk DW, Austin MC, Pierri JN, Sampson AR, Lewis DA. Decreased glutamic acid decarboxylase67 messenger RNA expression in a subset of prefrontal cortical gamma-aminobutyric acid neurons in subjects with schizophrenia. *Arch Gen Psychiatry* (2000) **57**:237–45. doi:10.1001/archpsyc.57.3.237
72. Olney JW, Newcomer JW, Farber NB. NMDA receptor hypofunction model of schizophrenia. *J Psychiatr Res* (1999) **33**:523–33. doi:10.1016/S0022-3956(99)00029-1
73. Javitt DC. Glutamatergic theories of schizophrenia. *Isr J Psychiatry Relat Sci* (2010) **47**:4–16.
74. Lisman JE, Pi HJ, Zhang Y, Otmakhova NA. A thalamo-hippocampal-ventral tegmental area loop may produce the positive feedback that underlies the psychotic break in schizophrenia. *Biol Psychiatry* (2010) **68**:17–24. doi:10.1016/j.biopsych.2010.04.007
75. Llinas RR, Ribary U, Jeanmonod D, Kronberg E, Mitra PP. Thalamocortical dysrhythmia: a neurological and neuropsychiatric syndrome characterized by magnetoencephalography. *Proc Natl Acad Sci U S A* (1999) **96**:15222–7. doi:10.1073/pnas.96.26.15222
76. Uslaner JM, Smith SM, Huszar SL, Pachmerhiwala R, Hinchliffe RM, Vardigan JD, et al. T-type calcium channel antagonism produces antipsychotic-like effects

and reduces stimulant-induced glutamate release in the nucleus accumbens of rats. *Neuropharmacology* (2010) **62**(3):1413–21. doi:10.1016/j.neuropharm.2010.11.015

77. Talley EM, Cribbs LL, Lee JH, Daud A, Perez-Reyes E, Bayliss DA. Differential distribution of three members of a gene family encoding low voltage-activated (T-type) calcium channels. *J Neurosci* (1999) **19**:1895–911.
78. O'Donnell P, Grace AA. Synaptic interactions among excitatory afferents to nucleus accumbens neurons: hippocampal gating of prefrontal cortical input. *J Neurosci* (1995) **15**:3622–39.
79. Grace AA. Gating of information flow within the limbic system and the pathophysiology of schizophrenia. *Brain Res Brain Res Rev* (2000) **31**:330–41. doi:10.1016/S0165-0173(99)00049-1
80. Enyeart JJ, Biagi BA, Mlinar B. Preferential block of T-type calcium channels by neuroleptics in neural crest-derived rat and human C cell lines. *Mol Pharmacol* (1992) **42**:364–72.
81. Santi CM, Cayabyab FS, Sutton KG, McRory JE, Mezeyova J, Hamming KS, et al. Differential inhibition of T-type calcium channels by neuroleptics. *J Neurosci* (2002) **22**:396–403.
82. Choi KH, Rhim H. Inhibition of recombinant Ca(v)3.1 (alpha(1G)) T-type calcium channels by the antipsychotic drug clozapine. *Eur J Pharmacol* (2010) **626**:123–30. doi:10.1016/j.ejphar.2009.09.035
83. Smoller JW, Craddock N, Kendler K, Lee PH, Neale BM, Nurnberger JI, et al. Identification of risk loci with shared effects on five major psychiatric disorders: a genome-wide analysis. *Lancet* (2013) **381**:1371–9. doi:10.1016/S0140-6736(12)62129-1
84. Lieberman JA, Stroup TS, McEvoy JP, Swartz MS, Rosenheck RA, Perkins DO, et al. Effectiveness of antipsychotic drugs in patients with chronic schizophrenia. *N Engl J Med* (2005) **353**:1209–23. doi:10.1056/NEJMoa051688
85. Keefe RS, Bilder RM, Davis SM, Harvey PD, Palmer BW, Gold JM, et al. Neurocognitive effects of antipsychotic medications in patients with chronic schizophrenia in the CATIE trial. *Arch Gen Psychiatry* (2007) **64**:633–47. doi:10.1001/archpsyc.64.6.633
86. Bymaster FP, Calligaro DO, Falcone JF, Marsh RD, Moore NA, Tye NC, et al. Radioreceptor binding profile of the atypical antipsychotic olanzapine. *Neuropsychopharmacology* (1996) **14**:87–96. doi:10.1016/0893-133X(94)00129-N
87. Horacek J, Bubenikova-Valesova V, Kopecek M, Palenicek T, Dockery C, Mohr P, et al. Mechanism of action of atypical antipsychotic drugs and the neurobiology of schizophrenia. *CNS Drugs* (2006) **20**:389–409. doi:10.2165/00023210-200620050-00004
88. Amann BL, Pogarell O, Mergl R, Juckel G, Grunze H, Mulert C, et al. EEG abnormalities associated with antipsychotics: a comparison of quetiapine, olanzapine, haloperidol and healthy subjects. *Hum Psychopharmacol* (2003) **18**:641–6. doi:10.1002/hup.537
89. Pillmann F, Schlote K, Broich K, Marneros A. Electroencephalogram alterations during treatment with olanzapine. *Psychopharmacology (Berl)* (2000) **150**:216–9. doi:10.1007/s002130000426
90. Wichniak A, Szafranski T, Wierzbicka A, Waliniowska E, Jernajczyk W. Electroencephalogram slowing, sleepiness and treatment response in patients with schizophrenia during olanzapine treatment. *J Psychopharmacol* (2006) **20**:80–5. doi:10.1177/0269881105056657
91. Centorrino F, Price BH, Tuttle M, Bahk WM, Hennen J, Albert MJ, et al. EEG abnormalities during treatment with typical and atypical antipsychotics. *Am J Psychiatry* (2002) **159**:109–15. doi:10.1176/appi.ajp.159.1.109
92. Hubl D, Kleinlogel H, Frolich L, Weinandi T, Maurer K, Holstein W, et al. Multi-lead quantitative electroencephalogram profile and cognitive evoked potentials (P300) in healthy subjects after a single dose of olanzapine. *Psychopharmacology (Berl)* (2001) **158**:281–8. doi:10.1007/s002130100861

3

Computational Neuropsychiatry – Schizophrenia as a Cognitive Brain Network Disorder

Maria R. Dauvermann[1]*, Heather C. Whalley[1], André Schmidt[2,3], Graham L. Lee[4], Liana Romaniuk[1], Neil Roberts[5], Eve C. Johnstone[1], Stephen M. Lawrie[1] and Thomas W. J. Moorhead

[1] *Division of Psychiatry, Royal Edinburgh Hospital, University of Edinburgh, Edinburgh, UK*
[2] *Department of Psychiatry, University of Basel, Basel, Switzerland*
[3] *Medical Image Analysis Center, University Hospital Basel, Basel, Switzerland*
[4] *McGovern Institute for Brain Research, Massachusetts Institute of Technology, Cambridge, MA, USA*
[5] *Clinical Research Imaging Centre, QMRI, University of Edinburgh, Edinburgh, UK*

***Correspondence:**
Maria R. Dauvermann, Division of Psychiatry, Royal Edinburgh Hospital, University of Edinburgh, Kennedy Tower, Morningside Park, Edinburgh EH10 5HF, UK
e-mail: m.r.dauvermann@sms.ed.ac.uk, maria.dauvermann@childrens.harvard.edu

Computational modeling of functional brain networks in fMRI data has advanced the understanding of higher cognitive function. It is hypothesized that functional networks mediating higher cognitive processes are disrupted in people with schizophrenia. In this article, we review studies that applied measures of functional and effective connectivity to fMRI data during cognitive tasks, in particular working memory fMRI studies. We provide a conceptual summary of the main findings in fMRI data and their relationship with neurotransmitter systems, which are known to be altered in individuals with schizophrenia. We consider possible developments in computational neuropsychiatry, which are likely to further our understanding of how key functional networks are altered in schizophrenia.

Keywords: computational neuropsychiatry, schizophrenia, fMRI, dynamic causal modeling, cognition, neurotransmitter, dopamine, glutamate

INTRODUCTION

Schizophrenia is a severe psychiatric disorder, which is initially manifested through positive symptoms including delusions, hallucinations, and disorganized thoughts. As the illness progresses negative symptoms such as avolition, alogia, and apathy may occur. Prior to diagnosis of illness, cognitive deficits can occur and illness progression can also be associated with cognitive deficits (1, 2). It is widely established that such cognitive deficits are considered a core symptom of schizophrenia (3) and are associated with reductions in working memory performance. Working memory deficits are one of the main neurocognitive impairments found in subjects with first episode schizophrenia (FES) (4, 5) and in people with established schizophrenia (EST) (6). Similar deficits also occur in individuals at high risk of schizophrenia [HR; Ref. (2)]. Furthermore, recent evidence has been presented, which indicates a relationship between severity of working memory deficits and the severity of negative symptoms (7). The severity of working memory deficits that is evident at the first episode of schizophrenia can predict the quality of life at the established stage of the illness (8, 9).

Two major neurotransmitter circuits have been implicated in clinical and cognitive symptoms in subjects with schizophrenia: these are the dopamine and glutamate neurotransmitter circuits. Evidence has been presented for separate alterations/disruptions of dopamine and glutamate as well as an interactive role between both neurotransmitters[1]. The two main neurobiological hypotheses in schizophrenia are based on the theories of altered dopaminergic transmission ("dopamine hypothesis of schizophrenia") and altered glutamatergic transmission ("glutamate hypothesis of schizophrenia"). It is thought that both dopamine and glutamate modulate the dorsolateral prefrontal cortex (DLPFC) and in schizophrenia alter the performance in cognitive processes such as in working memory (10–13). Such work supports the notion of schizophrenia as a brain disorder. FMRI and positron emission tomography (PET) findings of altered functional activation and functional connectivity (FC) during working memory have been

Abbreviations: AC/ACC, anterior cingulate/anterior cingulate cortex; ARMS, at-risk mental state; BMS, Bayesian model selection; BOLD response, blood-oxygen-level dependent response; D_1 receptor, D_1 subtype of the dopamine receptor; D_2 receptor, D_2 subtype of the dopamine receptor; $D_{2/3}$ receptors, $D_{2/3}$ subtype of the dopamine receptor; DCM, Dynamic Causal Modeling; DMN, default-mode network; DLPFC, dorsolateral prefrontal cortex; EC, effective connectivity; EST, subjects with EST; FC, functional connectivity; FEP, subjects with first episode psychosis; FES, subjects with first episode schizophrenia; GABA, γ-aminobutyric acid; GBC, global-based connectivity; HR, subjects at high risk of schizophrenia; HR+, subjects at high familial risk of schizophrenia with transient psychotic symptoms; HR−, subjects at high familial risk of schizophrenia without transient psychotic symptoms; HRill, subjects at high familial risk of schizophrenia who subsequent to scanning developed schizophrenia; HSCT, Hayling sentence completion task IFG inferior frontal gyrus; MFG, middle frontal gyrus; MRS, magnetic resonance spectroscopy; NMDA, *N*-Methyl-D-aspartate acid; PC, parietal cortex; PET, positron emission tomography; rCBF, regional cerebral blood flow; SPECT, single-photon emission computed tomography; SPL, superior parietal lobe; STG, superior temporal gyrus.

[1] It is noted that other neurotransmitter circuits are interacting with dopaminergic and/or glutamatergic circuits such as serotonin and GABA (24, 29, 149).

reported in people with schizophrenia when they are compared to healthy controls (14, 15). Furthermore, PET studies have presented evidence for indirect markers of altered dopamine transmission, which was correlated with working memory performance (2, 16). Alterations of indirect measures of glutamate concentrations have been reported by proton magnetic resonance spectroscopy (MRS) studies (17).

One subfield within the emerging field of computational neuropsychiatry is based on modeling fMRI networks and the evidence of (i) altered dopaminergic and/or glutamatergic transmission in (ii) cognitive function (i.e., working memory) in people with schizophrenia. Therefore, the objectives are the investigation of impaired cognitive function mediated by large-scale networks in combination with underlying neurobiological circuits such as dopamine and glutamate. Researchers in computational neuropsychiatry examine and model altered cognitive brain function in terms of functionally integrated regions [i.e., effective connectivity (EC)] (18), which may be mediated by genetic factors and neurotransmitter circuits (19–21). Mechanistic responses can be inferred from the computational modeling of cognitive brain function where the localized brain function is monitored through the BOLD response (22). This modeling approach allows computational neuropsychiatry to further our understanding of the neurobiological processes, which underlie altered cognitive brain function in individuals with schizophrenia. Thus, advancing our knowledge of schizophrenia as a cognitive brain network disorder.

In this review, we summarize fMRI findings in verbal/numeric working memory[2] in context of (i) the understanding of schizophrenia as a cognitive brain disorder (from clinical and cognitive neurosciences) and (ii) the understanding of schizophrenia as a cognitive brain network disorder (from computational neuropsychiatry). We discuss these sets of findings in context of the dopamine and the glutamate hypotheses of schizophrenia. We consider two key research questions for the discussion of each set of findings:

(i) To what extent do these sets of findings support the dopamine hypothesis and/or the glutamate hypothesis in subjects with schizophrenia?
(ii) Do the findings from computational neuropsychiatry lead to a better understanding of schizophrenia than that obtained from clinical and cognitive neurosciences?

The review is structured as followed: first, the dopamine and glutamate hypotheses of schizophrenia are summarized (Section Schizophrenia as a Brain Disorder). Second, exemplary findings of verbal/numeric working memory deficits from fMRI studies in subjects with schizophrenia are summarized. These findings are discussed in context of the dopamine hypothesis and the glutamate hypothesis of schizophrenia (Section Schizophrenia as a Cognitive Brain Disorder). Third, we present a brief introduction to computational neuropsychiatry. We provide examples from computational neuropsychiatry and the application to the investigation of cognitive brain large-scale networks in people with schizophrenia[3]. Finally, we consider current methodological limitations of the methods (Section From Computational Neuropsychiatry Towards Schizophrenia as a Cognitive Brain Network Disorder). We outline potential future influences of computational advances in schizophrenia that may shape our understanding of schizophrenia with the aim of developing more effective treatments for the disorder (Section Understanding of Schizophrenia).

SCHIZOPHRENIA AS A BRAIN DISORDER

Neurobiological research into alterations of dopaminergic and/or glutamatergic neurotransmission has paved the way for the understanding of schizophrenia as a disorder of the brain. The dopamine hypothesis posits that dopamine function is altered in schizophrenia and that this dysfunction may be the pathophysiological pathway leading to clinical and cognitive symptoms (23, 24). The glutamate hypothesis proposes that the altered dopaminergic dysfunction may be secondary to aberrant glutamatergic dysregulation, which may contribute to clinical and cognitive symptoms in schizophrenia (25–27).

DOPAMINE HYPOTHESIS OF SCHIZOPHRENIA

The origin of the dopamine hypothesis of schizophrenia is based on the discovery of antipsychotic drugs by Delay et al. (28) in 1952. Carlsson and Lindqvit reported the first findings of an effect of antipsychotic drugs on the metabolism of dopamine (29). The dopamine hypothesis posits that alterations of dopaminergic receptors may underlie the clinical symptoms of schizophrenia (30). Over last three decades, the dopamine hypothesis of schizophrenia has undergone reformulations in light of newly available preclinical and clinical findings. Here, we consider the three main hypotheses: (i) the "dopamine receptor hypothesis," (ii) the "modified dopamine hypothesis of schizophrenia," and (iii) the "dopamine hypothesis: version III."

The dopamine receptor hypothesis goes back to studies reporting antipsychotics affecting the affinity of dopamine receptors (31–33). Further evidence for the hypothesis was presented with increased synaptic monoamine levels during the induction of psychotic symptoms (34). The focus of this hypothesis rests on the excess of dopamine receptors. Thus, the clinical treatment is aimed at blocking the dopamine D_2 subtype of the dopamine receptors (35).

The modified dopamine hypothesis of schizophrenia has been formulated to integrate new findings (36). Preclinical and clinical studies (i.e., post-mortem, metabolite, and dopamine receptor neuroimaging studies) have advanced the understanding of relationships between affinity and occupancy of D_2 and D_1 subtypes of the dopamine receptors and regional specificity (37). Furthermore, it was assumed that findings of altered regional dopaminergic receptor function from preclinical and indirect clinical studies could be linked to clinical symptomatology in schizophrenia (36). The hypothesis suggests that "hypofrontality," as measured with reduced regional cerebral blood flow (rCBF) in the PFC may indicate low dopamine levels in the PFC (36). Findings from preclinical

[2]In this review, we focus on the "2-back" task [verbal "2-back", (104); numeric "2-back", (97)] to review/discuss brain function and PET findings of comparable experimental paradigms, psychological/ cognitive domains/components and activated brain regions.

[3]Exemplary studies on verbal fluency findings are presented.

lesion studies proposed that prefrontal "hypodopaminergia" lead to striatal "hyperdopaminergia" (38, 39). In addition, it is hypothesized that prefrontal "hypodopaminergia" could cause negative symptoms, whereas striatal "hyperdopaminergia" could lead to positive symptoms (36).

The dopamine hypothesis: version III synthesizes published findings on dopamine and its potential role in schizophrenia from the main fields into one unifying hypothesis. The hypothesis aims to provide a framework for findings from developments in clinical research into genetic (risk) factors, environmental risk factors, neurochemical and neuroimaging studies, and preclinical studies, which may be related to increased presynaptic striatal dopaminergic function in schizophrenia (23). The hypothesis is comprised of four components: (i) The interaction of "hits" such as frontotemporal dysfunction, genes, stress, and drugs may lead to striatal dopamine dysregulation (i.e., increased presynaptic dopamine synthesis capacity) and therefore to psychosis. (ii) It is hypothesized that the primary dopaminergic dysfunction is located at the presynaptic dopaminergic level instead of the D_2 receptor level. (iii) The hypothesis assumes that the dopamine dysregulation combined with cultural and societal factors could lead to future clinical diagnosis of "psychosis" rather than schizophrenia. (iv) It is proposed that the dopamine dysfunction could change the perception and judgment of stimuli (possibly through aberrant salience), which could result in cognitive deficits (40, 41).

Recent meta-analyses, which examined markers of striatal dopamine alterations in schizophrenia, reported evidence of different types of elevated dopamine dysfunction. Supporting evidence for the dopamine hypothesis has been shown by increased striatal presynaptic dopaminergic function in medication-free or medication-naïve patients with schizophrenia contrasted to healthy controls (42) and increased striatal dopamine synthesis capacity (43). Contradictory findings have however been reported by Fusar-Poli and Meyer-Lindenberg (44), who found no difference in striatal dopamine active transporter density between patients with schizophrenia and healthy controls.

In summary, while both the dopamine receptor hypothesis and the modified dopamine hypothesis of schizophrenia have their origins in the neurobiological investigation of the mode of action of antipsychotics, the dopamine hypothesis: version III aims at integrating advances in research of schizophrenia into one unifying dopamine hypothesis. The scope of understanding of dopaminergic dysregulation has become more defined, ranging from the whole brain perspective, through the perspective of regional specificity between (DL)PFC and striatum, to the current perspective of elevated presynaptic striatal dopaminergic function. The development of the dopamine hypothesis over the three versions has helped shape the understanding of schizophrenia as a brain disorder.

GLUTAMATE HYPOTHESIS OF SCHIZOPHRENIA

The origin of the glutamate hypothesis of schizophrenia was based on the discovery of psychotomimetic effects of ketamine and phencyclidine, which elicited psychotic symptoms in healthy people. Symptoms such as delusions and hallucinations experienced by healthy individuals were compared to positive symptoms seen in FES (45, 46). The glutamate hypothesis postulates a mechanistic process of altered interacting glutamatergic and/or dopaminergic neurotransmitter circuitries implicated in the pathophysiology of clinical and cognitive symptoms in schizophrenia (47–50). In this review, we consider three models of the glutamate hypothesis with relevance to the investigation of altered working memory function in people with schizophrenia: (i) the "*N*-Methyl-D-aspartate acid (NMDA) receptor hypofunction model" of schizophrenia, (ii) the "acute ketamine model," and (iii) the "dysconnection hypothesis" of schizophrenia.

The NMDA receptor hypofunction model of schizophrenia posits that the subtype of the glutamate receptor is implicated in multiple pathological brain mechanisms of schizophrenia ranging across cellular, chemical, and neuronal levels (51–54). It has been proposed that NMDA receptor hypofunction could underlie the pathophysiology of negative and cognitive symptoms in schizophrenia (29, 51, 55, 56). Clinical trials with agents modulating NMDA receptor in addition to treatment with first-generation antipsychotics (FGA; such as chlorpromazine, haloperidol, perphenazine) and second-generation antipsychotics (SGA; such as clozapine and olanzapine) presented supporting evidence for amelioration of negative and cognitive symptoms (51, 57, 58). Evidence for the involvement of NMDA receptor hypofunction through interactions among different neurotransmitters such as γ-aminobutyric acid (GABAergic) interneurons (51) and dopamine (59, 60) has also been reported.

Evidence for the glutamate hypothesis in humans is based on clinical studies with ketamine in healthy subjects. Results suggest that glutamatergic alterations could explain the pathophysiological mechanisms resulting in positive symptoms predominantly experienced by FES and those with first episode psychosis (FEP) (45, 61). While findings from ketamine injection studies have aided the understanding of glutamatergic signaling in the development of delusions and hallucinations, evidence for altered glutamatergic transmission in negative and cognitive symptoms is scarce. FMRI findings from ketamine studies in healthy subjects propose that altered glutamatergic signaling could be implicated in working memory (12, 45, 62). These findings are in keeping with evidence from glutamatergic animal models, which report aberrant working memory function after the inhibition of glutamatergic receptors (63–66).

The dysconnection hypothesis of schizophrenia posits that altered NMDA receptor-mediated synaptic plasticity may be the underlying pathophysiological mechanism in individuals with schizophrenia (20, 21, 67). The authors propose that altered synaptic plasticity may explain both clinical symptoms and cognitive deficits in people with schizophrenia neurobiologically by altered NMDA receptor neuromodulation. Therefore, the dysconnection hypothesis synthesizes neurobiological findings (i.e., dopamine as one of the main neuromodulators leading to aberrant NMDA receptor function) with clinical and cognitive neuroscientific findings (i.e., cognitive impairment) in individuals with schizophrenia. One of the main objectives of the dysconnection hypothesis is to offer a new approach and therefore new interpretation of neurophysiological and neuroimaging data. This may be used to assist in the understanding of altered cognitive function in people with schizophrenia. For functional neuroimaging data, the biophysical modeling approach of dynamic causal modeling [DCM; Ref.

(18)] has been proposed to infer biophysical processes (namely, NMDA receptor-dependent synaptic plasticity) underlying the blood-oxygen-level-dependent (BOLD) responses. In addition, the authors provide arguments that the development of positive symptoms such as delusions can be explained by a "failure of self-monitoring mechanism" or "corollary discharge" (20). Abnormal EC findings from EEG and fMRI studies across a range of cognitive tasks in subjects with schizophrenia in contrast to healthy controls have been reported (68–70). These lead to a new insight into altered connectivity above those provided by FC studies, which are formulated under different theoretical frameworks, specifically DCM findings enable the inference of biophysical processes underlying neural responses (18, 19, 71).

In summary, the three hypotheses, the NMDA receptor hypofunction model, the acute ketamine model, and the dysconnection hypothesis, have motivated researchers to investigate biophysical circuit processes implicated in glutamatergic and dopaminergic interaction in negative symptoms and cognitive function in schizophrenia. These circuit mechanisms are thought to underlie altered working memory function in schizophrenia. Research on the NMDA receptor hypofunction model has its roots in the pharmacological examination of antipsychotics, the development of new agents, and its effects on clinical and cognitive symptoms in preclinical and clinical research in schizophrenia. The focus of researchers examining the acute ketamine model and the dysconnection hypothesis lies on elucidating proposed neurobiological processes of blockade of NMDA receptor underlying altered cognitive brain function in schizophrenia. The study designs of both versions differ in the investigation of (i) the pharmacological effect of ketamine on altered cognitive brain function and clinical symptomatology in healthy controls (the acute ketamine model) and (ii) altered synaptic plasticity during altered cognitive brain function in subjects with schizophrenia. Despite the different approaches, researchers of both versions of the glutamate hypothesis share the common aim of increasing our insight into schizophrenia by the translation of neurobiological knowledge from basic research to clinical research in schizophrenia. Furthermore, researchers share the common methodological approach of large-scale network analysis of fMRI data. Taken together, development over the three versions of the glutamate hypothesis of schizophrenia have presented promising evidence for shaping the understanding of schizophrenia as a cognitive brain network disorder.

SCHIZOPHRENIA AS A COGNITIVE BRAIN DISORDER

Clinical and cognitive neuroscience studies have applied *in vivo* neuroimaging techniques of fMRI, PET, and single-photon emission computed tomography (SPECT) to assess neurobiological processes that underlie working memory function in people with schizophrenia. Techniques such as PET and SPECT use injections of positron-emitting radionuclide as tracer (for PET) or gamma-emitting radionuclide as tracer (for SPECT) in the living brain. Although these nuclear medical imaging techniques are non-invasive they require the administration of tracers. FMRI provides non-invasive *in vivo* imaging, which measures brain function by means of the BOLD response (72).

In the last two decades, the fields of clinical and cognitive neurosciences merged to provide a multidisciplinary approach to research into schizophrenia. This approach has created the notion of schizophrenia as a cognitive brain disorder (15, 73, 74).

EXAMPLES OF fMRI AND PET STUDIES INVESTIGATING ALTERED WORKING MEMORY FUNCTION IN SUBJECTS WITH SCHIZOPHRENIA

Working memory tasks were initially investigated with fMRI in healthy subjects (75–78). These initial findings led to the use of fMRI as a tool for examining neurobiological markers that could be related to working memory performance. The examination of working memory function was extended to individuals with schizophrenia.

Reported findings of brain function during working memory (among several domains and components of working memory tasks) in healthy controls have led to the understanding that dopamine modulates working memory in healthy controls (79–81). This evidence of dopaminergic involvement in working memory was extended by the findings of altered dopaminergic modulation in schizophrenia (74, 82). Subsequently, converging findings were reported that regions such as DLPFC, anterior cingulate cortex (ACC), and parietal cortex (PC) are activated in working memory in both healthy controls and in subjects with schizophrenia (83–86). However, in those with schizophrenia, these regions exhibit increased or reduced functional activations and FC between prefrontal and parietal regions as well as between prefrontal and temporal regions in contrast to healthy controls. Alterations in FC occur at all stages of the illness (87, 88): (i) in HR subjects (89); (ii) in FES and FEP (90), and (iii) in subjects with EST (91).

Systematic reviews and meta-analyses of working memory fMRI studies in people with schizophrenia do not report consistent findings (92–95). Some studies report increased activation of the DLPFC, commonly referred to as "hyperfrontality," however, others report decreased activation or "hypofrontality." This picture of differing functional activation in terms of the direction, extent, and/or pattern of BOLD responses was attributed to the variation of domains and components of working memory tasks (92–95). Also it was considered that methodological factors in the applied analyses would contribute to these variations in functional activation (93, 95, 96). In addition, differences in medication could contribute to variation in the reported functional activation between studies.

Here, we review exemplary fMRI studies using the numeric or verbal "N-back" task in subjects with EST and healthy controls, which reported functional activation and FC findings (**Table 1**). The reviewed studies present group differences between subjects with schizophrenia and healthy controls. In functional activation studies, evidence was reported for increased activation in DLPFC, PFC, ventral PFC, medial frontal gyrus, and AC during high working memory load in subjects with EST (89, 97–101). However, reduced activation in prefrontal regions, such as ventral PFC, DLPFC, AC, and parietal regions was found during high working memory load in subjects with EST (97, 98, 102). One study in FES found a reduction of activation in inferior frontal gyrus (IFG), superior frontal gyrus, and AC during high working memory load (103). We note three factors, which contributed to difficulties in comparing the findings across the reviewed studies: (i) missing information of phase of schizophrenia (100), (ii)

Table 1 | Understanding of schizophrenia as a cognitive brain disorder – I summary of main findings in verbal/numeric working memory.

Study	Subjects – phase of schizophrenia: HC – HR, FES, EST	Medication	Experimental paradigm	Functional connectivity method; seed regions/ROIs/VOIs; seed regions/ ROIs/VOIs; definition; sphere size	Main finding(s)
fMRI STUDIES – FA					
(97)	18 HC; 13 EST[a]	Not reported	Numeric "2-back"	N/A	↑ With increasing WM load in right DLPFC, left PFC, left AC; ↓ with increasing WM load includ. right AC, right PC, left vPFC
(102)	16 HC; 17 EST	17 EST, stable injectable FGA for 2 months	Verbal "2-back"	N/A	Main effect of group: ↑ subgenual AC gyrus; group × WM load interaction for high WM load: ↓ in right DLPFC
(98)	14 HC; 14 Patients[b] subdivided into HP: 8 HC, 7 patients; LP: 6 HC, 7 patients	14 Patients, 476.3 (291.7)[c]; 7 Patients, 556.0 (157.0)[c]; 6 Patients, 237.7 (96.4)[c]	Numeric "2-back"	N/A	↑ and ↓ for high WM load in different subdivisions of the right and left DLPFC in 14 patients; bilateral prefrontal areas of ↑ and ↓ for high WM load in HP patients; bilateral prefrontal areas of ↓ for high WM load in LP patients
(99)	22 HC; 14 EST	Not reported	Verbal "2-back"	N/A	↑ For high WM load in right medial FG; ↑ for hits during for high WM load in right medial FG
fMRI STUDIES – FC					
(100)	26 HC; 15 Patients[b], subdivided into HP: 14 HC, 8 patients; LP: 12 HC, 7 patients	15 Patients, 501 (337.0)[c]	Numeric "2-back"	Seed-based cross-correlation; seed regions: right dPFC and left vPFC; functional ROIs 10 mm sphere size	↑ FA with increasing WM load in bilateral vPFC in 15 patients; ↑ FC between left vPFC and left SPL in 15 patients; ↓ FC between right dPFC and bilateral IPL in 15 patients
(89)	153 HC; 78 EST[b]	75 EST, FGA, and SGA; 3 EST, data missing	Numeric "2-back"	Seed-based cross-correlation[d]; Seed regions: right DLPFC; functional ROIs 6 mm sphere size	↑ FA for high WM load in right DLPFC; ↓ FC between right DLPFC and bilateral HF; ↓ FC between right DLPFC and right IPL
(103)	28 HC; 30 FES[a]	Not reported	Numeric "2-back"	Seed-based cross-correlation; seed regions: left gyrus rectus, left IFG, left SFG, left AC, right PHG, right amygdala; functional ROIs sphere size not reported	↑ FA for high WM load in left gyrus rectus, left IFG, left SFG, left AC, right PHG, right amygdala; ↓ FC between medial FG and right precuneus; between medial FG and left OFG; between medial frontal gyrus and right precentral gyrus
(101)	28 HC; 28 EST[a,b]	24 EST, 294.45 (316.36)[c]	Numeric "2-back"	ROI-to-ROI FC; ROIs: bilateral DLPFC, vlPFC, putamen, caudate nuclei, IPL; functional ROIs sphere size not reported	↑ FA for high WM load in bilateral putamen, left DLPFC, OFC, cuneus, and PC; ↓ FC between left putamen and right vlPFC; ↓ FC between left putamen and left vlPFC; between right IPL and right vlPFC

↑ Increased in subjects with schizophrenia in contrast to HC.

↓ Decreased in subjects with schizophrenia in contrast to HC.

AC, anterior cingulate; DLPFC, dorsolateral prefrontal cortex; dPFC, dorsal prefrontal cortex; EST, subjects with established schizophrenia; FA, functional activation; FC, Functional connectivity; FES, subjects with first episode schizophrenia; FG, frontal gyrus; FGA, First-generation antipsychotics; HC, healthy controls; HF, hippocampal formation; HP, high-performers; HR, subjects at high risk of schizophrenia; IFG, inferior frontal gyrus; IPL, inferior parietal lobe; LP, low-performers; OFG, orbitofrontal gyrus; PC, posterior cingulate; PHG, parahippocampal gyrus; ROI, region of interest; SGA, second-generation antipsychotics; SFG, superior frontal gyrus; SPL, superior parietal lobule; vPFC, ventral prefrontal cortex; vlPFC, ventrolateral PFC; WM, working memory.

[a] *Patients with different schizophrenia subtypes, such as paranoid subtype, schizoaffective subtype, undifferentiated subtype.*

[b] *Phase of illness, illness onset, and illness duration not reported. Phase of illness based on symptoms scores.*

[c] *Chlorpromazine equivalents in milligrams per day.*

[d] *Seed-based connectivity only reported here.*

heterogeneous groups of subjects with EST (97, 101, 103), and (iii) limited information on antipsychotic treatment (89, 97–101, 103). Fundamentally, none of the functional activation findings was interpreted in context of the dopamine or glutamate hypothesis. The lack of a clear understanding in terms of neural activation and pathophysiological mechanism suggests there is a need for studies examining wider prefrontal circuitry underlying working memory deficits in schizophrenia (93, 95).

Functional connectivity studies applied voxel-based seed approaches to the BOLD response (89, 100, 103), with the exception of one study, which applied an ROI-to-ROI approach (101). Despite equivalent methodological approaches, the FC findings are not entirely comparable due to the use of different seed locations. Findings of reduced connectivity involving subregions of the PFC were found in FES and EST. Reduced FC findings in subjects with schizophrenia and EST were reported in the majority of studies: (i) Reduced prefrontal–parietal[4] FC in subjects with schizophrenia (100); (ii) Reduced prefrontal–hippocampal, prefrontal–striatal, and within-PFC FC in EST (89); and (iii) Reduced parieto-prefrontal FC and between putamen and ventrolateral PFC in EST (101). Further evidence for reduced FC between medial frontal gyrus and putamen was found in FES (103). In contrast to most studies that report reduced FC in the early and late phases of the illness, increased FC between the ventral PFC and posterior PC was shown in subjects with schizophrenia (100). The findings of both reduced and increased FC between subregions of the PFC and the posterior PC may be related to variations in behavioral response to task load for subjects with schizophrenia (100). Similar difficulties in comparing the FC findings among the studies are present as in the comparison of the functional activation studies due to unclear and missing information regarding the illness phase, diagnosis, and medication treatment. Similarly, no reference is made to the dopamine or glutamate hypothesis in interpreting the FC findings.

In summary, findings presented by FC studies during the "N-back" task have paved the way for the understanding of large-scale functional networks in working memory. Furthermore, the insight of brain alterations in subjects with schizophrenia has advanced with FC from individually activated regions to connectivity between brain regions. The perspective of circuit-based neurobiology and cognitive brain function opens the doors for translational research from preclinical and clinical research in schizophrenia. However, FC is limited as the connection assessments are based upon regional correlations and this approach does not allow inferences of directions or causality between connected regions (18).

Positron emission tomography and SPECT imaging in schizophrenia research are used to investigate indirect markers of dopamine measures such as D2/3 receptors, presynaptic dopaminergic function, dopamine synthesis capacity, dopamine release, and dopamine transporters. Three [H215O] PET studies consistently reported reduced rCBF in DLPFC and PC in verbal/numeric "2-back" in subjects with EST in contrast to healthy controls (104–106). Reduced prefrontal–hippocampal FC findings in subjects with schizophrenia in contrast to healthy controls (105, 106) confirmed the hypothesis of reduced functional connections in working memory. Correlational PET studies provided support for dopaminergic alterations and measures of the "2-back" task in subjects with schizophrenia (2, 16).

In summary, fMRI and PET studies in the field of clinical and cognitive neurosciences have been used to investigate brain function during working memory in people with schizophrenia (**Figure 1**). Both fMRI and PET findings have advanced the understanding of altered working memory performance and brain function in subjects with schizophrenia. This has led to better insight into the interaction between altered working memory function and experimental/clinical factors (such as cognitive domains of working memory function, performance level, phases of illness, clinical symptomatology, and effects of antipsychotic medication) in individuals with schizophrenia.

EXAMPLES OF fMRI STUDIES INVESTIGATING ALTERED SPATIAL WORKING MEMORY FUNCTION – GLUTAMATE HYPOTHESIS OF SCHIZOPHRENIA

The role of the DLPFC in working memory deficits has been associated with glutamatergic alterations and more specifically in dopamine–glutamate interactions (10, 50, 51). Furthermore, it has been reported that ketamine, a NMDA receptor antagonist, can induce psychosis-like symptoms in healthy subjects (45). Here, we briefly summarize the main functional activation and FC findings of fMRI studies on the spatial "N-back" task in the context of the glutamate hypothesis of schizophrenia (**Table 2**).

Anticevic et al. (12) presented ketamine-induced reduced functional activation in task-activated regions (such as the DLPFC and the precuneus) and task-deactivated regions of the default-mode network (DMN). In addition, the combination of a spiking local-circuit model of performance during the spatial "N-back" task and the functional activation findings revealed that the modulation of

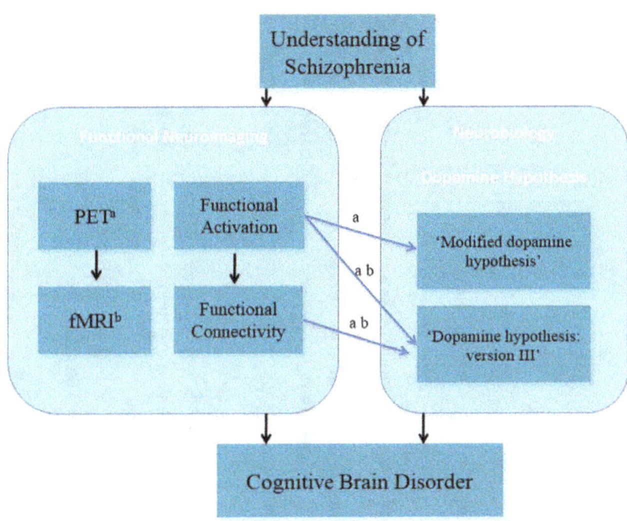

FIGURE 1 | Understanding of schizophrenia as a cognitive brain disorder – verbal/numeric "N-back" task. [a]fMRI; [b]PET, positron emission tomography.

[4]Reduced FC between the dorsal PFC and posterior PC.

Table 2 | Schizophrenia as a cognitive brain disorder II – summary of main findings in spatial working memory.

Study	Subjects HC	Medication/ketamine injection	Experimental paradigm	Functional connectivity method Seed regions/ROIs Seed regions/ROIs definition Sphere size	Computational modeling	Main finding(s)
fMRI + KETAMINE STUDIES						
(12)	19 HC	One saline injection; initial ketamine bolus 0.23 mg/kg for I min; subsequent ketamine bolus 0.58 mg/kg for 1 h	Spatial "2-back" and "4-back"	Seed-based cross-correlation Seeds: FP–DMN pair; CO–DMN pair; anatomical ROIs 15 mm sphere size	Modeling of the acute ketamine effect of local and long-range E–I connections Spiking E and I cell local-circuit models: task-activated module and task-deactivated module	Ketamine attenuated task-activated regions (i.e., DLPFC and precuneus) Ketamine attenuated task-deactivated regions overlapping the DMN; ↓ E–I conductance led to attenuation in task-activated regions; modulation of task-activated FC between FP–DMN networks during delay of WM
(62)	22 HC	One saline injection; one initial ketamine bolus 0.23 mg/kg for 1 min; one subsequent ketamine bolus 0.58 mg/kg for 1 h	Spatial "2-back" and "4-back"	(1) Seed-based cross-correlation; seed regions: bilateral MFG, IFG, SFG, and Heschl's gyrus; anatomical ROIs 10 mm sphere size (2) Global-based connectivity; see details as in (1)	N/A	Ketamine effect using (1): ↓ FC between right DLPFC and MFG, IFG, frontal OC, insula, medial FG; angular gyrus; ketamine effect using (2): ↓ FC within left DLPFC

↓ Reduced.

CO, cingulo-occipital; DLPFC, dorsolateral prefrontal cortex; DMN, default-mode network; E cells, excitatory cells; FC, functional connectivity; FG, frontal gyrus; FP, fronto-parietal; HC, healthy controls; I cells, inhibitory cells; IFG, inferior frontal gyrus; MFG, middle frontal gyrus; NMDA, N-Methyl-d-aspartate acid; OC, orbital cortex; ROI, region of interest; SFG, superior frontal gyrus; WM, working memory.

ketamine alters the association between the task-activated and the task-deactivated networks. Finally, it was shown that ketamine modulates FC between the fronto-parietal and DMN networks. In a recent study, Driesen et al. (62) provided further support for ketamine-induced reduced prefrontal FC during the spatial "N-back" task. Two FC approaches with the same seed regions were employed, seed-based FC and global-based connectivity (GBC), which revealed both decreased FC within the DLPFC. The seed-based analysis resulted in reduced FC between DLPFC and middle frontal gyrus [MFG, IFG, and insula (among other regions) under ketamine in contrast to saline]. The GBC analysis showed decreased FC of the DLPFC under ketamine.

In summary, these studies on altered spatial working memory function inform on the glutamate hypothesis, through the acute ketamine model (**Figure 2**). In this, they have advanced the understanding of NMDA receptor-modulated brain function in healthy subjects.

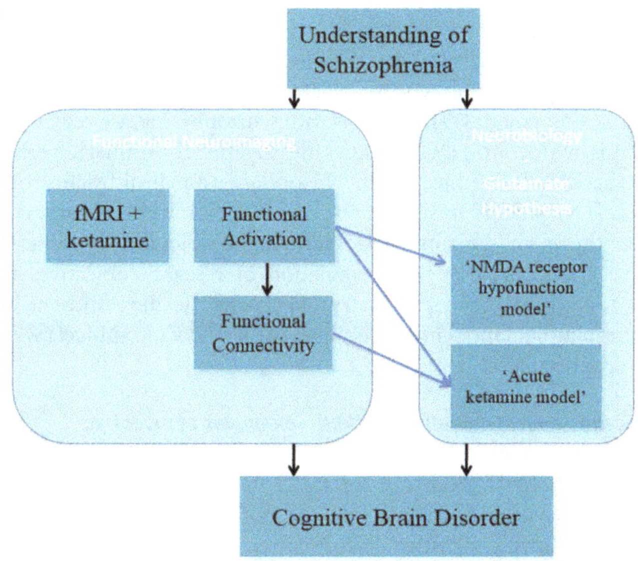

FIGURE 2 | Understanding of schizophrenia as a cognitive brain disorder – spatial "N-back" task.

FROM COMPUTATIONAL NEUROPSYCHIATRY TOWARD SCHIZOPHRENIA AS A COGNITIVE BRAIN NETWORK DISORDER

Clinical and cognitive neurosciences have advanced the understanding of altered working memory function in subjects with schizophrenia. FMRI studies in working memory among other neuroimaging and electrophysiological techniques, have reported on functional activation and FC findings in subjects with schizophrenia. Both findings of functional activation and FC revealed methodological, cognitive, and clinical factors related to our understanding of altered working memory function in patients with schizophrenia. In particular, FC findings mark the beginning of the notion of "disconnection" and "dysconnection" (20, 21, 67, 107) in working with people with schizophrenia. FC is defined as the statistical association or dependency among two or more anatomically distinct time-series (107). FC findings cannot be interpreted in terms of causal effects between connected regions and thus, does not allow for a mechanistic inference of the BOLD responses.

The modeling of functional large-scale networks[5] during working memory function in schizophrenia could provide mechanistic explanations for altered brain function in individuals with schizophrenia. The advantage of modeling functional large-scale networks in terms of EC over FC is that inferences can be drawn on mechanistic processes, which are not directly observable in the BOLD response.

COMPUTATIONAL NEUROSCIENCE AND COMPUTATIONAL NEUROPSYCHIATRY

Marr proposes a theoretical framework for computational research on the brain on three levels (1976). At the first level, researchers should aim to gain knowledge of the high-level computations of the brain such as working memory ("computational level"). At the next level, the testing of the brain's methods and algorithms for the high-level working memory function is led by hypotheses derived from the acquired knowledge and testing how appropriate an algorithm such as Bayesian inference is for modeling the working memory brain function ("algorithmic level"). Finally, when an algorithm is found, which is valid and more likely than alternative algorithms to predict known brain function/behavior, then the investigation of the biological implementation can be pursued ("physical level").

Computational neuropsychiatry is an emerging field within computational neuroscience. Computational neuropsychiatry aims to provide an explanatory bridge between altered cognitive function and neurobiological mechanisms associated with the development of mental illness (108, 109, Huys, unreferred preprint). Computational neuropsychiatry in humans has been defined by outlining a set of components, which include biophysical modeling and computational modeling (109). Different types of computational models at different neural levels are used dependent on the study hypothesis (108, Huys, unreferred preprint).

COMPUTATIONAL NEUROPSYCHIATRY AND MODELING OF FUNCTIONAL LARGE-SCALE NETWORKS IN SUBJECTS WITH SCHIZOPHRENIA

Connectionist and neural network models in working memory/cognitive control in subjects with schizophrenia have added to our understanding of both the brain function and the neurobiological mechanism underlying working memory (74, 76). The strength of these models is based on the translational link between human brain function (i.e., functional activation) and preclinical neurobiological evidence (namely, dopaminergic modulation) during working memory.

Following on from the work of Cohen and Braver, evidence for the understanding of schizophrenia as a cognitive network disorder has been presented by both preclinical studies (8, 10, 110–113) and human FC studies in working memory (89, 100, 101, 103). Recent studies examining biophysical mechanisms underlying

[5]As one subfield within computational psychiatry.

altered functional large-scale networks aim to bridge the gap between the human functional network used in working memory and the preclinical neurobiological processes. Examples of such computational neuropsychiatric studies, including EC during working memory in subjects with schizophrenia, are reviewed. In this, we focus on DCM studies investigating the numeric/verbal "N-back" task in subjects with schizophrenia and healthy controls. This is considered in the context of the dopamine and glutamate hypotheses of schizophrenia. Both neurobiological hypotheses have contributed to the formulation of research objectives in computational neuropsychiatry (114) and the development of computational modeling techniques of fMRI data in subjects with schizophrenia (20).

Dynamic causal modeling for fMRI – examples of modeling functional large-scale networks

Dynamic causal modeling for fMRI has been introduced as a method to provide insight into the notion of "functional integration" during cognitive performance. "Functional integration" has been advanced from the historic notion of "functional specialization" (115), which is defined by context-dependent interactions among different brain regions (18, 116–118).

Dynamic causal modeling has been described as a biophysical modeling of neuronal dynamic processes (18, 19)[6], which can be used as a method for the computation of synaptic plasticity from fMRI task-based studies (20, 21). Together biophysical modeling and Bayesian inference analysis form the framework for DCM (71, 117, 118). Thus, DCM is a modeling approach, which combines defined network models (i.e., hypotheses) with Bayesian inversion methods (19, 117). Specifically, DCM assesses inter-regional EC through assessment of experimentally induced changes (18) and therefore allows for mechanistic inferences from neuronal function.

Bilinear DCM infers dynamics at the neuronal level by translating modeled neuronal responses into predicted BOLD measurements (18). Non-linear DCM for fMRI (71, 119) is an advanced approach for increasing the biological plausibility of DCMs by the means of modeling "gain modulation" (i.e., non-linear modulation of neuronal connections) (19, 117, 118). In non-linear DCM, the modulation of connection strengths by experimental inputs is supplemented by direct modulation of neural activity in one or more network regions (18, 119). The computations for gating in neural networks use the multiplicative computation of non-linear modulation (120, 121). Accordingly, non-linear DCM can be used for inferring that the strength of a connection is modulated by activity of other neuronal populations (119, 122).

Findings of altered effective connectivity during working memory in subjects with schizophrenia. The first DCM studies in healthy controls described large-scale networks in working memory and a similar task [continuous performance test; (123–125)]. A recent study in healthy controls built the linkage between EC results and underlying dopaminergic modulation of large-scale networks comprising of the DLPFC and PC during verbal memory performance (126).

To date four DCM studies have examined the verbal/numeric "N-back" task in subjects with schizophrenia using bilinear DCM (127–130) (**Table 3**). These provide novel insights into reduced task-dependent EC and increased task-independent EC measures through modeling large-scale networks in schizophrenia.

In the first study, increased fronto-temporal intrinsic connectivity was found to be associated with increased functional activation of the superior temporal gyrus (STG) during the numeric "N-back" task in the subjects at the prodromal and at the acutely psychotic stage of schizophrenia in contrast to the healthy controls. This suggests a potential marker for vulnerability to the disorder (127). Furthermore, progressively decreased intrinsic connectivity between the STG and the MFG in subjects at-risk mental state (ARMS) and FES subjects in contrast to the healthy controls was reported. This finding suggested that functional activation may resemble increased task-independent EC between the PFC and the STG. However, the results of the study are not comparable to other DCM studies because (i) only one model was examined and (ii) the biological plausibility of the EC measures is not clearly accessible. No reference to the dopamine or glutamate hypotheses was made.

The second study investigated the working memory-dependent modulatory effect for the prefrontal–parietal connectivity in subjects with EST and healthy subjects during the numeric "N-back" task (128). The large-scale networks included the right DLPFC, the PC, and the visual cortex with bidirectional connection between all regions. The main finding was decreased task-dependent EC from the DLPFC to the PC in the subjects with EST. Thus, this finding could resemble evidence for the glutamate hypothesis of schizophrenia, specifically the NMDA receptor hypofunction model and the dysconnection hypothesis.

The third study examined possible vulnerability markers for psychosis from the verbal "N-back" task in ARMS subjects, FES subjects, and healthy subjects (129). This study examined reduced task-dependent EC measures as well as relationships between connectivity parameters and antipsychotic medication received by subjects. In this study, EC in interhemispheric large-scale networks between the bilateral superior parietal lobes (SPL) and the bilateral MFG was assessed. This study reported novel findings of progressively decreased working memory and induced modulation of connectivity between the MFG and the SPL (from healthy subjects to ARMS). Additionally, further decreased EC of modulatory effects were observed in non-medicated subjects with FEP contrasted to healthy controls. Evidence for amelioration of reduced EC between the MFG and the SPL in subjects with FES, who received SGA medication, could reflect alterations of dopaminergic regulation of NMDA receptor-dependent synaptic plasticity of fronto-parietal connections. However, this interpretation is limited by the lack of a control group of FES who are treated with different types of antipsychotic medication. These findings across different subpopulations of schizophrenia together with the effect of antipsychotic medication may reflect support for the NMDA receptor hypofunction model and the dysconnection hypothesis.

[6]We consider DCM as the generative model approach as introduced in the seminal article by Friston et al. (18).

Table 3 | Schizophrenia as a cognitive brain network disorder II – summary of main findings in verbal/numeric working memory – neuroimaging and biophysical modeling.

Study	Subjects – phase of schizophrenia; HC – HR, FES/FEP, EST	Medication	Experimental paradigm	Networks – model space; number of models; regions	DCM settings – DCM version; sphere size; inference technique(s)	Main finding(s)
(127)	13 HC; 16 HR[a]; 10 FES	HR, not medicated; 7 FES, risperidone or quetiapine, 3 FES, not medicated	Numeric "2-back"	1 Left hemispheric model; STG, SMA, MFG, INS, PPC	DCM in SPM5; Sphere sizes not reported; BMS not performed	Progressively ↑ IC of the prefrontal–temporal connection in HR and FES
(128)	42 HC; 41 EST	35 EST, FGA; 5 EST, SGA; 1 EST, not medicated	Numeric "2-back"	48 Intrahemispheric models; 3 model families; DLPFC, PC, VC	DCM10 in SPM8; 4 mm spheres; random-effects BMS[e,f]; BMA	↓ EC (effect of task-modulation) from DLPFC to PC
(129)	20 HC; 17 HR[a]; 21 FEP	HR, not medicated; 7 FEP, completely antipsychotic naïve; 6 FEP, antipsychotic naïve at the time of scanning; 8 FEP, SGA	Verbal "2-back"	12 Intrahemispheric models; bilateral SPL, bilateral MFG	DCM10 in SPM8; 12 mm spheres; random-effects BMS[e]; BMA	Progressively ↓ EC (effect of task-modulation) between MFG and SPL in HC, HR, and FES. Ameliorated EC correlated with antipsychotic treatment.
(130)	15 HC; 14 FES[b]; 19 FES[c]	FES[b], 254.76 (192.09)[d]; FES[c], 325.88 (185.19)[d]	Verbal "2-back"	5 Left hemispheric models; medial PFC, PCC	DCM version not reported; SPM8; 6 mm spheres; BMS[e]; BMA	↑ IC from PCC to medial PFC in both FES[e] and FES[f]

↑Increased in subjects with schizophrenia in contrast to HC.

↓Decreased in subjects with schizophrenia in contrast to HC.

BMA, Bayesian model averaging; BMS, Bayesian model selection; DLPFC, dorsolateral prefrontal cortex; EC, effective connectivity; EST, subjects with established schizophrenia; FES, subjects with first episode schizophrenia; FEP, subjects with first episode psychosis; FGA, first-generation antipsychotics; HC, healthy controls; HR, subjects at high risk of schizophrenia; IC, intrinsic connectivity; IFG, inferior frontal gyrus; INS, insula; MFG, middle frontal gyrus; PC, parietal cortex; PCC, posterior parietal cortex; PFC, prefrontal cortex; SGA, second-generation antipsychotics; SMA, supramarginal area; SPL, superior parietal lobe; STG, superior temporal gyrus; VC, visual cortex.

[a]Subjects at high clinical risk of schizophrenia.

[b]With high suicidal risk.

[c]With low suicidal risk.

[d]Chlorpromazine equivalents in mg/day.

[e]BMS at the group-level.

[f]BMS at the model family level.

In the fourth study, Zhang et al. (130) explored EC measures in terms of possible neurobiological markers in groups of subjects with schizophrenia with high or low suicide risk and contrasted these with healthy controls during the verbal "N-back" task. The large-scale networks were defined by unidirectional and bidirectional connections between the two regions of the medial PFC and PC as well as working memory effects on these regions. This pilot study presented novel findings in subjects with schizophrenia at suicidal risk in terms of increased intrinsic connectivity from the PC to the MFG in both groups with FES (in comparison to healthy controls). This finding was interpreted as a possible association to schizophrenia, in which increased intrinsic connectivity from the MFG to the PC in the subjects with high risk of suicide could reflect vulnerability of suicide. However, the results are not directly comparable to the other DCM studies because of the study population, which focused on the issue of suicide. The findings were also not interpreted in context of the dopamine or glutamate hypotheses.

We highlight main experimental and methodological limitations in the four DCM studies, which impede the comparability of findings (please see **Table 3** for details). The main experimental limitation focuses on the discrepancies between the different patient subpopulations. Two studies analyzed working memory fMRI data of subjects with ARMS and FES in comparison to healthy controls (127, 129), whereas one study modeled scans from subjects with EST (128). Zhang et al. (130) reported findings of a unique patient population of FES with high and low suicidal risk. In terms of methodological issues, one limitation lies in different definitions of model spaces for the large-scale networks, despite equivalence in the experimental tasks. Another limitation is that the reviewed DCM studies employed deterministic DCM for the comparison of the models. Deterministic models can predict processes perfectly if all inputs are known (131). However, at this early stage of employing biophysical modeling approaches to human brain function, we do not have a full understanding of the brain responses to working memory. Future studies may employ stochastic DCM as an extension (117, 118, 132). A further limitation is that different DCM versions were applied across the four studies, which impede the comparability of the findings. The priors are differently defined in the used DCM versions, which give rise to a variation in model evidence between the studies (117). Thus, it is possible that discrepancies in EC findings could be due to the prior definition and may not be solely due to differences in performance, brain function, or clinical aspects of subjects with schizophrenia. Lastly, a general limitation of DCM for fMRI is that maximally 10 regions within a large-scale network can be modeled. This simplification results in difficulties of biophysical modeling of tasks, which are likely to encompass more than ten regions. Furthermore, not only the definition of different regions and different numbers of regions but also different modulatory inputs result in further extensions to the model space. Such model spaces are difficult to validate and analyze.

The four DCM studies presented evidence for increased task-dependent EC and increased task-independent EC findings during verbal/numeric working memory in subjects with schizophrenia. We discuss these EC findings in context of (i) the dopamine and glutamate hypothesis and (ii) FC findings during verbal/numeric working memory in subjects with schizophrenia.

The four studies modeled large-scale networks during the "N-back" task in subjects with schizophrenia. However, only two out of these four studies consider their DCM results in the light of biophysical processes (128, 129). The findings of reduced EC (namely, the effect of task-modulation) of the prefrontal–parietal connection in subjects with schizophrenia in contrast to healthy controls were interpreted biophysically and linked to the NMDA receptor hypofunction model and the dysconnection hypothesis (128, 129). Both studies reported reduced EC findings of the prefrontal–parietal connection during working memory, however, these findings need to be considered carefully due to different experimental designs (i.e., patient subpopulations, antipsychotic medication treatment of FGA and SGA) and methodological implementation (i.e., model space, DCM settings, and inference techniques).

Three of the DCM studies reported altered EC findings of the prefrontal–parietal and parieto-prefrontal connections during the "N-back" task in subjects with schizophrenia in contrast to healthy controls. Deserno et al. (128) and Schmidt et al. (129) presented reduced EC (effect of task-modulation) of the prefrontal–parietal connection in subjects with schizophrenia in contrast to healthy controls, whereas Zhang et al. (130) found increased EC (intrinsic connectivity) of the parietal–prefrontal connection. The reduced task-dependent EC findings are in keeping with reduced FC findings of these connections, although increased FC between a different prefrontal subregion and the PC was reported (100).

The study by Crossley et al. (127) reported increased EC (intrinsic connectivity) of the prefrontal–temporal connection in subjects at HR and FES (in contrast to healthy controls). Reduced FC of the prefrontal–temporal connection during the "N-back" task in subjects with schizophrenia has been previously reported in PET studies (105, 106). However, the regions within the PFC and temporal region differ between the studies.

Findings of altered effective connectivity during verbal fluency in subjects with schizophrenia. Here, we discuss bilinear and non-linear DCM studies, which have assessed large-scale networks during verbal fluency [namely, the Hayling sentence completion task (HSCT)] in subjects with schizophrenia and healthy controls (**Table 4**). One bilinear DCM study in healthy controls investigated the task-dependent modulation of response initiation and response suppression in EC between left hemispheric temporal and prefrontal regions (133). The main finding was a difference in connection strength of the modulatory effect in response initiation and response suppression.

Two clinical bilinear DCM studies have investigated EC measures during the HSCT in HR subjects and healthy controls: (i) Subjects at high clinical risk of schizophrenia [ARMS; Ref. (134)] and (ii) subjects at high familial risk of schizophrenia (135). Allen et al. (134) investigated increased fronto-temporal EC (intrinsic connectivity) as a potential measure of vulnerability of developing schizophrenia. Two main findings were reported: firstly, no significant effect of task-dependent modulation on the fronto-temporal connection between ARMS subjects and healthy controls was revealed. Secondly, ARMS subjects displayed increased intrinsic connectivity between the ACC and the MTG in comparison to healthy controls. Furthermore, the Bayesian model selection (BMS) approach revealed that the same network was equally likely

Table 4 | Schizophrenia as a cognitive brain network disorder II – summary of main findings in verbal fluency – neuroimaging and biophysical modeling.

Study	Subjects – phase of schizophrenia; HC – HR, FES/FEP, EST	Medication	Experimental paradigm	Networks – model space; number of models; regions	DCM settings – DCM version; sphere size; inference technique(s)	Main finding(s)
(134)	15 HC; 15 HR[a]	2 HR risperidone and quetiapine[c]	HCST	14 Left hemispheric models; MFG, ACC, MTG	DCM in SPM5; 12 mm spheres; random-effects BMS4	↑ IC between ACC and MTG; same winning model in both groups
(135)	19 HC; 26 HR[b] – 20 HR+, 4 HRill	Not medicated	HCST	8 Left hemispheric models; 3 model families; IPS, IFG, ACC, MTG, MD thalamus	DCM8 in SPM8; 8 mm spheres (IPS, DLPFC, MTG); 6 mm spheres (ACC, MD thalamus); Random-effects BMS[d,e]; BMA	Progressively ↓ connection strength with non-linear modulation of the thalamo-cortical connection in HR+ and HRill in contrast to HC

↑ Increased in subjects with schizophrenia in contrast to HC.

↓ Decreased in subjects with schizophrenia in contrast to HC.

ACC, anterior cingulate cortex; ARMS, subjects with at-risk mental state; BMA, Bayesian model averaging; BMS, Bayesian model selection; EC, effective connectivity; FEP, subjects with first episode psychosis; FES, subjects with first episode schizophrenia; HC, healthy controls; HR–, subjects at high familial risk of schizophrenia without transient psychotic symptoms; HR+, subjects at high familial risk of schizophrenia with transient psychotic symptoms; HRill, subjects at familial risk of schizophrenia who subsequent to the scanning developed schizophrenia; HSCT, Hayling sentence completion task; IC, intrinsic connectivity; IFG, inferior frontal gyrus; IPS, intraparietal sulcus; MD mediodorsal; MFG, middle frontal gyrus; MTG, middle temporal gyrus;

[a] *Subjects at high clinical risk of schizophrenia.*

[b] *Subjects at high familial risk of schizophrenia.*

[c] *At the time of scanning.*

[d] *BMS at the group-level.*

[e] *BMS at the model family level.*

to explain the given HSCT fMRI data in both the ARMS subjects and the healthy controls. No reference to the glutamate hypothesis was made.

Dauvermann et al. (135) modeled EC measures in a similar version of the HSCT that was used by Allen et al. (134). This study was conducted in subjects at high familial risk of schizophrenia and healthy subjects. The results reported by Allen et al. (134) of a similar large-scale network in both HR subjects and healthy controls was replicated[7]. This finding was also confirmed by Dauvermann et al. (135), when the group of HR subjects was subdivided into high risk subjects without transient psychotic symptoms (referred to as HR−), high risk subjects with transient psychotic symptoms (referred to as HR+) and high risk subjects who subsequent to scanning developed schizophrenia [referred to as HRill; please see Ref. (136, 137)]. Comparability between these two studies is limited due to differences in the model space. The model space in Dauvermann et al. (135) includes the IPS and the mediodorsal thalamus, which are not incorporated in the model space by Allen et al. (134). In addition, endogenous connections and task-dependent modulations were accordingly changed [Ref. (135); **Table 4**]. There was no reference to the glutamate hypothesis of schizophrenia.

Limitations of bilinear DCM have been addressed through the development of non-linear DCM for fMRI (119). This method was applied in the genetic high risk study reported by Dauvermann et al. (135). The progress from the bilinear DCM to the non-linear DCM as reported by Dauvermann is based on the biophysical modeling of connection strength with non-linear modulation during the HSCT response. The authors show that relative to healthy controls there is reduced connection strength with non-linear modulation of the thalamo-cortical connection during the HSCT in HR+ subjects and a further reduction in this connection strength in HRill subjects (135). The authors suggest that reduced gain control may underlie the reduced strength in the thalamo-cortical connection. Furthermore, the findings of reduced connection strength with non-linear modulation of the thalamo-cortical connection could reflect altered glutamatergic neurotransmission, which may underlie a disruption of synaptic plasticity in this thalamo-cortical connection [Ref. (135); **Table 4**]. Thus, the findings were interpreted in context of the NMDA receptor hypofunction model and the dysconnection hypothesis.

Summary of studies modeling functional large-scale networks – dynamic causal modeling for fMRI

Evidence from brain function in working memory in subjects with schizophrenia at the level of functional large-scale networks (i.e., clinical and cognitive neurosciences) and neurobiological mechanisms in working memory in animal models of schizophrenia (preclinical neurobiological research) in combination with computational neuroscientific approaches has informed and enabled research in computational neuropsychiatry.

Exemplary DCM studies in subjects with schizophrenia have reported both increased and reduced EC findings during cognition in subjects with schizophrenia in contrast to healthy controls. These studies applied DCM as a biophysical modeling approach to functional large-scale networks, which enabled the interpretation of EC findings on the basis of the glutamate hypothesis of schizophrenia, namely the NMDA receptor hypofunction model and the dysconnection hypothesis (128, 129, 135). We emphasize that the findings support not only the glutamate hypothesis but also the dopamine hypothesis. Dopamine is a neuromodulator that may crucially affect glutamate-induced synaptic plasticity. Synaptic plasticity may be involved in a regulation of dopamine synthesis and release via other neurotransmitter systems. Specifically for non-linear effects, it has been shown that dopamine acts as a neuromodulator mediating postsynaptic gain (74, 138).

In a recent study, it has been reported that the combination of the DCM analysis of numerical "N-back" task in EST (128) and generative embedding resulted in the dissection of three subgroups of EST based on the mechanistically inferred DCM findings (139). This exemplary study showed that DCM can be applied as a generative model of large-scale networks in individuals with schizophrenia. In summary, DCM is a promising approach for modeling synaptic plasticity; nevertheless in its current form it cannot reflect the full complexity in the processing required for the implementation of tasks such as working memory (**Figure 3**).

UNDERSTANDING OF SCHIZOPHRENIA IN DEVELOPMENT

Our understanding of schizophrenia is in continuous development and with more preclinical and clinical findings being published this understanding will advance further. A critical aspect of this understanding is the facilitation of multidisciplinary approach between preclinical and clinical research in schizophrenia.

The original understanding of schizophrenia as a brain disorder stems from observational clinical work, which led onto preclinical

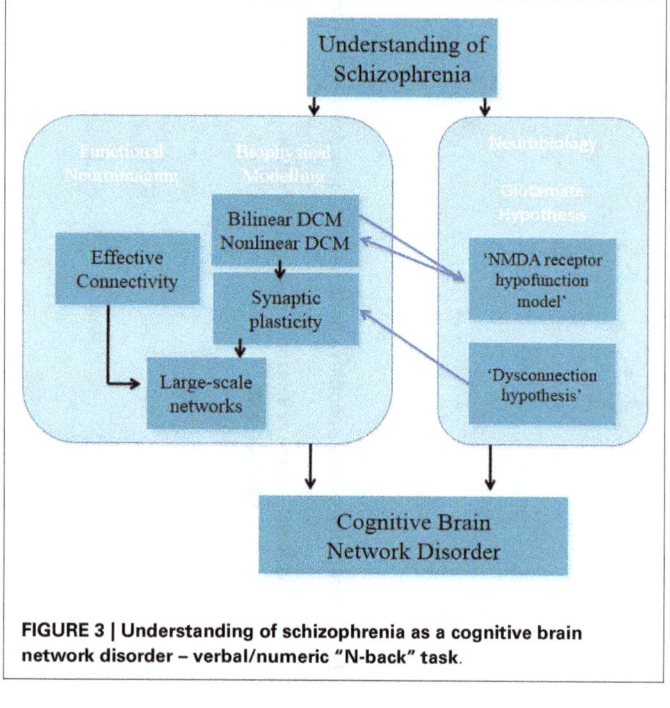

FIGURE 3 | Understanding of schizophrenia as a cognitive brain network disorder – verbal/numeric "N-back" task.

---

[7] It is noted, however, that the large-scale networks differed slightly from the previous study.

investigation. Over time, the knowledge of alterations of cellular, chemical, and molecular mechanisms has increased: (i) findings of dopaminergic and glutamatergic modulation of working memory (and clinical features) in animal models of schizophrenia contributed to form the understanding of schizophrenia as a cognitive brain disorder; (ii) findings of neurotransmitter circuit systems, mainly dopaminergic and glutamatergic systems, were found to modulate working memory in animal models of schizophrenia in combination with computational studies (140), which plays a role in shaping the understanding of schizophrenia as a cognitive network disorder.

Understanding of schizophrenia has not only been shaped by preclinical research but also by clinical research in subjects with schizophrenia, which has been and continues to be illuminated by preclinical neurobiological and computational work. The field of clinical and cognitive neurosciences has contributed to forming our understanding of schizophrenia as a cognitive brain disorder. Importantly, the multidisciplinary field of computational neuropsychiatry (preclinical neurobiology, clinical and cognitive neurosciences, and computational psychiatry) has allowed for progress in our understanding of schizophrenia as a cognitive brain network disorder.

SCHIZOPHRENIA AS COGNITIVE BRAIN NETWORK DISORDER

The use of computational neuropsychiatric research in developing our understanding of schizophrenia as a cognitive brain network disorder is at an early stage. Here, we focused on FC and EC studies (DCM studies) during the verbal/numeric "N-back" task in subjects with schizophrenia and healthy controls. We discuss these FC and EC findings in context of two key research questions. Consideration of these questions was seen as a means to inform future schizophrenia research in the fields of clinical and cognitive neurosciences and/or computational neuropsychiatry:

To what extent do these sets of findings support the dopamine hypothesis and/or the glutamate hypothesis in subjects with schizophrenia?

Studies reported both increased and reduced FC during the "N-back" task in subjects with schizophrenia in contrast to healthy controls. These findings have introduced the notion of human large-scale networks underlying brain function during working memory. The FC correlational analyses do not allow for the inference of directions or weights of in functional connections. Thus, from FC findings it is not practical to draw inferences on neurobiological causal processing.

Studies, which applied DCM as a biophysical modeling approach to functional large-scale networks, showed that reduced EC findings could be interpreted in context of the NMDA receptor hypofunction model and the dysconnection hypothesis.

In summary, FC findings cannot be interpreted in context of the dopamine or glutamate hypothesis. For EC findings, the computational neuropsychiatric approach of modeling large-scale networks requires biophysically plausible networks, which are hypothesis-driven from neurobiological and cognitive neuroscience in subjects with schizophrenia. EC findings have been interpreted in the context of the glutamate hypothesis and the dopamine hypothesis.

Do the findings from computational neuropsychiatry lead to a gain in understanding of schizophrenia in comparison to the findings from clinical and cognitive neurosciences?

Functional connectivity findings from cognitive and clinical neuroscience have contributed to the understanding of schizophrenia as a cognitive brain disorder. The analysis of altered working memory at the level of large-scale networks has advanced our knowledge of cognitive function in humans. However, it is not wholly understood what altered FC during cognition neurobiologically means in schizophrenia. EC findings from computational neuropsychiatry, here specifically modeling functional large-scale networks with DCM, have shown indications of linkage between clinical network-based working memory (large-scale networks) and preclinical neurotransmitter modulation of cognitive function. Altered synaptic plasticity during working memory can be interpreted with dopaminergic and glutamatergic mechanisms. We emphasize that the interpretation of altered neurotransmitter circuits should be considered carefully because the DCM method is likely to underestimate the processing complexity in neurobiological circuits. Nonetheless, a strength of DCM lies in interpretation of altered synaptic plasticity based on the inference of mechanistic information.

The consideration of schizophrenia as a cognitive brain network disorder from computational neuropsychiatry offers a holistic view of schizophrenia. Computational neuropsychiatry seeks to bridge the gap between neurobiology and cognitive and clinical neurosciences in subjects with schizophrenia. It is hoped that this research will enhance our understanding of schizophrenia, clinical treatment, and improve outcome in people with schizophrenia.

FUTURE OUTLOOK AND OPEN QUESTIONS

The reviewed findings in biophysical modeling of functional large-scale networks are promising. In order to reach the objective of predicting and improving clinical treatment in subjects with schizophrenia, longitudinal study designs, and the combination of subfields within computational neuropsychiatry should be pursued.

We consider computational neuropsychiatric research areas for the combination of biophysical modeling of functional large-scale networks and other computational (neuro)psychiatric approaches, which are of clinical relevance for subjects with schizophrenia, for example:

- Neurotransmitter systems
- Behavior
- Clinical symptoms
- Effects of antipsychotic medication
- Clinical outcome.

We suggest specific study designs, which may increase our understanding for developing clinical treatment for subjects with schizophrenia:

(i) Combination of biophysical modeling of functional large-scale networks with computation, for example:
  (a) Brain function and brain circuit model (12);
  (b) Brain function and behavior (141);
  (c) Brain function and effect of antipsychotic medication:

(ii) Combination of biophysical modeling of functional large-scale networks with multimodal neuroimaging study designs, for example:
   (a) FMRI and EEG/magnetoencephalography study designs;
   (b) FMRI and transcranial magnetic stimulation study designs (142);
   (c) FMRI and MRS study designs;
   (d) FMRI and PET study designs;
(iii) Combination of biophysical modeling of functional large-scale networks and computational modeling for the investigation of clinical (sub)groups, for example:
   (a) Associative learning (143, 144);
   (b) Machine learning approach (139, 145);
   (c) Reinforcement learning (109).

Findings of modeling functional large-scale networks contribute to shaping the understanding of schizophrenia as a cognitive brain network disorder. The combination of computational neuropsychiatric areas may bring researchers closer to the common long-term objectives of developing a diagnostic tool for schizophrenia along with the development of more effective treatments.

ACKNOWLEDGMENTS

We acknowledge Vincent Valton for his help. Maria R. Dauvermann and Thomas W. J. Moorhead are supported by Dr Mortimer and Theresa Sackler Foundation. Heather C. Whalley is supported by Royal Society Dorothy Hodgkin Fellowship.

REFERENCES

1. MacDonald AW, Schulz SC. What we know: findings that every theory of schizophrenia should explain. *Schizophr Bull* (2009) **35**:493–508. doi:10.1093/schbul/sbp017
2. Fusar-Poli P, Howes OD, Allen P, Broome M, Valli I, Asselin MC, et al. Abnormal frontostriatal interactions in people with prodromal signs of psychosis: a multimodal imaging study. *Arch Gen Psychiatry* (2010) **67**(7):683–91. doi:10.1001/archgenpsychiatry.2010.77
3. Gold JM. Cognitive deficits as treatment targets in Schizophrenia. *Schizophr Res* (2004) **72**(1):21–8. doi:10.1016/j.schres.2004.09.008
4. Seidman LJ, Giuliano AJ, Meyer EC, Addington J, Cadenhead KS, Cannon TD, et al. Neuropsychology of the prodrome to psychosis in the NAPLS consortium: relationship to family history and conversion to psychosis. *Arch Gen Psychiatry* (2010) **67**:578–88. doi:10.1001/archgenpsychiatry.2010.66
5. Kim HS, Shin NY, Jang JH, Kim E, Shim G, Park HY, et al. Social cognition and neurocognition as predictors of conversion to psychosis in individuals at ultra-high risk. *Schizophr Res* (2011) **130**:170–5. doi:10.1016/j.schres.2011.04.023
6. Genevsky A, Garrett CT, Alexander PP, Vinogradov S. Cognitive training in schizophrenia: a neuroscience-based approach. *Dialogues Clin Neurosci* (2010) **12**(3):416–21.
7. Bora E, Murray RM. Meta-analysis of cognitive deficits in ultra-high risk to psychosis and first-episode psychosis: do the cognitive deficits progress over, or after the onset of psychosis? *Schizophr Bull* (2013). doi:10.1093/schbul/sbt085
8. Seshadri S, Zeledon M, Sawa A. Synapse-specific contributions in the cortical pathology of schizophrenia. *Neurobiol Dis* (2013) **53**:26–35. doi:10.1016/j.nbd.2013.01.009
9. Kukla M, Davis LW, Lysaker PH. Cognitive behavioral therapy and work outcomes: correlates of treatment engagement and full and partial success in schizophrenia. *Behav Cogn Psychother* (2013). doi:10.1017/S1352465813000428
10. Tanaka S. Dopaminergic control of working memory and its relevance to schizophrenia: a circuit dynamics perspective. *Neuroscience* (2006) **139**:153–71. doi:10.1016/j.neuroscience.2005.08.070
11. Tan HY, Callicott JH, Weinberger DR. Dysfunctional and compensatory prefrontal cortical systems, genes and the pathogenesis of schizophrenia. *Cereb Cortex* (2007) **17**:i171–81. doi:10.1093/cercor/bhm069
12. Anticevic A, Gancsos M, Murray JD, Repovs G, Driesen NR, Ennis DJ, et al. NMDA receptor function in large-scale anticorrelated neural systems with implications for cognition and schizophrenia. *Proc Natl Acad Sci U S A* (2012) **109**:16720–5. doi:10.1073/pnas.1208494109
13. Volk DW, Lewis DA. Prefrontal cortical circuits in schizophrenia. *Curr Top Behav Neurosci* (2010) **4**:485–508. doi:10.1007/7854_2010_44
14. Kim JJ, Kwon JS, Park HJ, Youn DH, Kang MS, Kim MS, et al. Functional disconnection between the prefrontal and parietal cortices during working memory processing in schizophrenia: a [15(O)]H20 PET study. *Am J Psychiatry* (2003) **160**(5):919–23. doi:10.1176/appi.ajp.160.5.919
15. Honey GD, Fletcher PC. Investigating principles of human brain function underlying working memory: what insights from schizophrenia? *Neuroscience* (2006) **139**:59–71. doi:10.1016/j.neuroscience.2005.05.036
16. Abi-Dargham A, Mawlawi O, Lombardo I, Gil R, Martinez D, Huang Y, et al. Prefrontal dopamine D1 receptors and working memory in schizophrenia. *J Neurosci* (2002) **22**(9):3708–19.
17. Poels EM, Kegeles LS, Kantrowitz JT, Javitt DC, Lieberman JA, Abi-Dargham A, et al. Glutamatergic abnormalities in schizophrenia: a review of proton MRS findings. *Schizophr Res* (2014) **152**(2–3):325–32. doi:10.1016/j.schres.2013.12.013
18. Friston KJ, Harrison L, Penny W. Dynamic causal modelling. *Neuroimage* (2003) **19**:1273–302. doi:10.1016/S1053-8119(03)00202-7
19. Friston KJ, Dolan RJ. Computational and dynamic models in neuroimaging. *Neuroimage* (2010) **52**:752–65. doi:10.1016/j.neuroimage.2009.12.068
20. Stephan KE, Friston KJ, Frith CD. Dysconnection in schizophrenia: from abnormal synaptic plasticity to failures of self-monitoring. *Schizophr Bull* (2009) **35**:509–27. doi:10.1093/schbul/sbn176
21. Stephan KE, Baldeweg T, Friston KJ. Synaptic plasticity and dysconnection in schizophrenia. *Biol Psychiatry* (2006) **59**:929–39. doi:10.1016/j.biopsych.2005.10.005
22. Stephan KE, Mathys C. Computational approaches to psychiatry. *Curr Opin Neurobiol* (2014) **25**:85–92. doi:10.1016/j.conb.2013.12.007
23. Howes OD, Kapur S. The dopamine hypothesis of schizophrenia: version III – the final common pathway. *Schizophr Bull* (2009) **35**:549–62. doi:10.1093/schbul/sbp006
24. Qi Z, Miller GW, Voit EO. Computational modeling of synaptic neurotransmission as a tool for assessing dopamine hypotheses of schizophrenia. *Pharmacopsychiatry* (2010) **43**(Suppl 1):S50–60. doi:10.1055/s-0030-1248317
25. Coyle JT. NMDA receptor and schizophrenia: a brief history. *Schizophr Bull* (2012) **38**(5):920–6. doi:10.1093/schbul/sbs076
26. Coyle JT, Basu A, Benneyworth M, Balu D, Konopaske G. Glutamatergic synaptic dysregulation in schizophrenia: therapeutic implications. *Handb Exp Pharmacol* (2012) **2012**:267–95. doi:10.1007/978-3-642-25758-2_10
27. Kantrowitz JT, Javitt DC. *N*-methyl-D-aspartate (NMDA) receptor dysfunction or dysregulation: the final common pathway on the road to schizophrenia? *Brain Res Bull* (2010) **83**:108–21. doi:10.1016/j.brainresbull.2010.04.006
28. Delay J, Deniker P, Harl JM. Therapeutic use in psychiatry of phenothiazine of central elective action (4560 RP). *Ann Med Psychol (Paris)* (1952) **110**(2):112–7.
29. Carlsson A. Does dopamine have a role in schizophrenia? *Biol Psychiatry* (1978) **13**(1):3–21.
30. Emilien G, Maloteaux JM, Geurts M, Owen MJ. Dopamine receptors and schizophrenia: contribution of molecular genetics and clinical neuropsychology. *Int J Neuropsychpharmacol* (1999) **2**(3):197–227. doi:10.1017/S1461145799001479
31. Seeman P, Lee T. Antipsychotic drugs: direct correlation between clinical potency and presynaptic action on dopamine neurons. *Science* (1975) **188**:1217–9. doi:10.1126/science.1145194
32. Creese I, Burt DR, Snyder SH. Dopamine receptor binding predicts clinical and pharmacological potencies of antischizophrenic drugs. *Science* (1976) **192**:481–3. doi:10.1126/science.3854
33. Seeman P, Lee T, Chau-Wong M, Wong K. Antipsychotic drug doses and neuroleptic/dopamine receptors. *Nature* (1976) **261**:77–9. doi:10.1038/261717a0
34. Lieberman AN, Goldstein M, Gopinathan G, Nophytides A. D-1 and D-2 agonists in Parkinson's disease. *Can J Neurol Sci* (1987) **14**(3 Suppl):466–73.
35. Snyder SH. The dopamine hypothesis of schizophrenia: focus on the dopamine receptor. *Am J Psychiatry* (1976) **133**(2):197–202.

36. Davis KL, Kahn RS, Ko G, Davidson M. Dopamine in schizophrenia: a review and reconceptualization. *Am J Psychiatry* (1991) **148**:1474–86.
37. Kapur S, Seeman P. Does fast dissociation from the dopamine D(2) receptor explain the action of atypical antipsychotics? A new hypothesis. *Am J Psychiatry* (2001) **158**:360–9. doi:10.1176/appi.ajp.158.3.360
38. Pycock CJ, Kerwin RW, Carter CJ. Effect of lesion of cortical dopamine terminals on subcortical dopamine receptors in rats. *Nature* (1980) **286**:74–6. doi:10.1038/286074a0
39. Scatton B, Worms P, Lloyd KG, Bartholini G. Cortical modulation of striatal function. *Brain Res* (1982) **232**(2):331–43. doi:10.1016/0006-8993(82)90277-3
40. Heinz A. Dopaminergic dysfunction in alcoholism and schizophrenia – psychopathological and behavioral correlates. *Eur Psychiatry* (2002) **17**(1):9–16. doi:10.1016/S0924-9338(02)00628-4
41. Kapur S. Psychosis as a state of aberrant salience: a framework linking biology, phenomenology, and pharmacology in schizophrenia. *Am J Psychiatry* (2003) **160**(1):13–23. doi:10.1176/appi.ajp.160.1.13
42. Howes OD, Kambeitz J, Kim E, Stahl D, Slifstein M, Abi-Dargham A, et al. The nature of dopamine dysfunction in schizophrenia and what this means for treatment. *Arch Gen Psychiatry* (2012) **69**(8):776–86. doi:10.1001/archgenpsychiatry.2012.169
43. Fusar-Poli P, Meyer-Lindenberg A. Striatal presynaptic dopamine in schizophrenia, part I: meta-analysis of dopamine active transporter (DAT) density. *Schizophr Bull* (2013) **39**(1):22–32. doi:10.1093/schbul/sbr111
44. Fusar-Poli P, Meyer-Lindenberg A. Striatal presynaptic dopamine in schizophrenia, part II: meta-analysis of [(18)F/(11)C]-DOPA PET studies. *Schizophr Bull* (2013) **39**(1):33–42. doi:10.1093/schbul/sbr180
45. Krystal JH, Karper LP, Seibyl JP, Freeman GK, Delaney R, Bremner JD, et al. Subanesthetic effects of the noncompetitive NMDA antagonist, ketamine, in humans. Psychotomimetic, perceptual, cognitive, and neuroendocrine responses. *Arch Gen Psychiatry* (1994) **51**(3):199–214. doi:10.1001/archpsyc.1994.03950030035004
46. Abi-Saab WM, D'Souza DC, Moghaddam B, Krystal JH. The NMDA antagonist model for schizophrenia: promise and pitfalls. *Pharmacopsychiatry* (1998) **31**(Suppl 2):104–9. doi:10.1055/s-2007-979354
47. Luby E, Cohen B, Rosenbaum G, Gottlieb J, Kelley J. Study of a new schizophrenomimetic drugs. *AMA Arch Neurol Psychiatry* (1959) **81**:363–9. doi:10.1001/archneurpsyc.1959.02340150095011
48. Carlsson A, Waters N, Waters S, Carlsson ML. Network interactions in schizophrenia – therapeutic implications. *Brain Res Brain Res Rev* (2000) **31**(2–3):342–9. doi:10.1016/S0165-0173(99)00050-8
49. Farber NB, Kim SH, Dikranian K, Jiang XP, Heinkel C. Receptor mechanisms and circuitry underlying NMDA antagonist neurotoxicity. *Mol Psychiatry* (2002) **7**:32–43. doi:10.1038/sj.mp.4000912
50. Javitt DC. Glutamate and schizophrenia: phencyclidine, *N*-methyl-D-aspartate receptors, and dopamine-glutamate interactions. *Int Rev Neurobiol* (2007) **78**:69–108. doi:10.1016/S0074-7742(06)78003-5
51. Coyle JT. Glutamate and schizophrenia: beyond the dopamine hypothesis. *Cell Mol Neurobiol* (2006) **26**:365–84. doi:10.1007/s10571-006-9062-8
52. Coyle JT, Balu D, Benneyworth M, Basu A, Roseman A. Beyond the dopamine receptor: novel therapeutic targets for treating schizophrenia. *Dialogues Clin Neurosci* (2010) **12**(3):359–82.
53. Moghaddam B, Krystal JH. Capturing the angel in "angel dust": twenty years of translational neuroscience studies of NMDA receptor antagonists in animals and humans. *Schizophr Bull* (2012) **38**:942–9. doi:10.1093/schbul/sbs075
54. Javitt DC, Zukin SR, Heresco-Levy U, Umbricht D. Has an angel shown the way? Etiological and therapeutic implications of the PCP/NMDA model of schizophrenia. *Schizophr Bull* (2012) **38**:958–66. doi:10.1093/schbul/sbs069
55. Javitt DC. Glutamatergic theories of schizophrenia. *Isr J Psychiatry Relat Sci* (2010) **47**(1):4–16.
56. Goff DC, Coyle JT. The emerging role of glutamate in the pathophysiology and treatment of schizophrenia. *Am J Psychiatry* (2001) **158**:1367–77. doi:10.1176/appi.ajp.158.9.1367
57. Heresco-Levy U, Ermilov M, Shimoni J, Shapira B, Silipo G, Javitt DC. Placebo-controlled trial of D-cycloserine added to conventional neuroleptics, olanzapine, or risperidone in schizophrenia. *Am J Psychiatry* (2002) **159**(3):480–2. doi:10.1176/appi.ajp.159.3.480
58. Lane HY, Chang YC, Liu YC, Chiu CC, Tsai GE. Sarcosine or D-serine add-on treatment for acute exacerbation of schizophrenia: a randomized, double-blind, placebo-controlled study. *Arch Gen Psychiatry* (2005) **62**(11):1196–204. doi:10.1001/archpsyc.62.11.1196
59. Tzschentke TM. Pharmacology and behavioral pharmacology of the mesocortical dopamine system. *Prog Neurobiol* (2001) **63**(3):241–320. doi:10.1016/S0301-0082(00)00033-2
60. Sesack SR, Carr DB. Selective prefrontal cortex inputs to dopamine cells: implications for schizophrenia. *Physiol Behav* (2002) **77**(4–5):513–7. doi:10.1016/S0031-9384(02)00931-9
61. Krystal JH, D'Souza DC, Karper LP, Bennett A, Abi-Dargham A, Abi-Saab D, et al. Interactive effects of subanesthetic ketamine and haloperidol in healthy humans. *Psychopharmacology* (1999) **145**(2):193–204. doi:10.1007/s002130051049
62. Driesen NR, McCarthy G, Bhagwagar Z, Bloch MH, Calhoun VD, D'Souza DC, et al. The impact of NMDA receptor blockade on human working memory-related prefrontal function and connectivity. *Neuropsychopharmacology* (2013) **38**(13):2613–22. doi:10.1038/npp.2013.170
63. Moghaddam B, Adams B, Verma A, Daly D. Activation of glutamatergic neurotransmission by ketamine: a novel step in the pathway from NMDA receptor blockade to dopaminergic and cognitive disruptions associated with the prefrontal cortex. *J Neurosci* (1997) **17**:2921–7.
64. Timofeeva OA, Levin ED. Glutamate and nicotinic receptor interactions in working memory: importance for the cognitive impairment of schizophrenia. *Neuroscience* (2011) **195**:21–36. doi:10.1016/j.neuroscience.2011.08.038
65. Fitzgerald PJ. The NMDA receptor may participate in widespread suppression of circuit level neural activity, in addition to a similarly prominent role in circuit level activation. *Behav Brain Res* (2012) **230**:291–8. doi:10.1016/j.bbr.2012.01.057
66. Arnsten AF, Wang MJ, Paspalas CD. Neuromodulation of thought: flexibilities and vulnerabilities in prefrontal cortical network synapses. *Neuron* (2012) **76**:223–39. doi:10.1016/j.neuron.2012.08.038
67. Stephan KE, Penny WD, Daunizeau J, Moran RJ, Friston KJ. Bayesian model selection for group studies. *Neuroimage* (2009) **46**:1004–17. doi:10.1016/j.neuroimage.2009.03.025
68. Dima D, Roiser JP, Dietrich DE, Bonnemann C, Lanfermann H, Emrich HM, et al. Understanding why patients with schizophrenia do not perceive the hollow-mask illusion using dynamic causal modelling. *Neuroimage* (2009) **46**(4):1180–6. doi:10.1016/j.neuroimage.2009.03.033
69. Dima D, Dietrich DE, Dillo W, Emrich HM. Impaired top-down processes in schizophrenia: a DCM study of ERPs. *Neuroimage* (2010) **52**(3):824–32. doi:10.1016/j.neuroimage.2009.12.086
70. Wagner G, Koch K, Schachtzabel C, Schultz CC, Gaser C, Reichenbach JR, et al. Structural basis of the fronto-thalamic dysconnectivity in schizophrenia: a combined DCM-VBM study. *Neuroimage Clin* (2013) **3**:95–105. doi:10.1016/j.nicl.2013.07.010
71. Stephan KE, Friston KJ. Analyzing effective connectivity with fMRI. *Wiley Interdiscip Rev Cogn Sci* (2010) **1**:446–59. doi:10.1002/wcs.58
72. Ogawa S, Lee TM, Kay AR, Tank DW. Brain magnetic resonance imaging with contrast dependent on blood oxygenation. *Proc Natl Acad Sci U S A* (1990) **87**:9868–72. doi:10.1073/pnas.87.24.9868
73. Cohen JD, Servan-Schreiber D. A theory of dopamine function and its role in cognitive deficits in schizophrenia. *Schizophr Bull* (1993) **19**:85–104. doi:10.1093/schbul/19.1.85
74. Braver TS, Barch DM, Cohen JD. Cognition and control in schizophrenia: a computational model of dopamine and prefrontal function. *Biol Psychiatry* (1999) **46**:312–28. doi:10.1016/S0006-3223(99)00116-X
75. Cohen JD, Servan-Schreiber D. Context, cortex, and dopamine: a connectionist approach to behavior and biology in schizophrenia. *Psychol Rev* (1992) **99**:45–77. doi:10.1037/0033-295X.99.1.45
76. Cohen JD, Braver TS, O'Reilly RC. A computational approach to prefrontal cortex, cognitive control and schizophrenia: recent developments and current challenges. *Philos Trans R Soc Lond B Biol Sci* (1996) **351**:1515–27. doi:10.1098/rstb.1996.0138
77. Smith EE, Jonides J. Storage and executive processes in the frontal lobes. *Science* (1999) **283**:1657–61. doi:10.1126/science.283.5408.1657

78. Collette F, Van der Linden M. Brain imaging of the central executive component of working memory. *Neurosci Biobehav Rev* (2002) **26**:105–25. doi:10.1016/S0149-7634(01)00063-X
79. Braver TS, Cohen JD, Nystrom LE, Jonides J, Smith EE, Noll DC. A parametric study of prefrontal cortex involvement in human working memory. *Neuroimage* (1997) **5**:49–62. doi:10.1006/nimg.1996.0247
80. Cohen JD, Braver TS, Brown JW. Computational perspectives on dopamine function in prefrontal cortex. *Curr Opin Neurobiol* (2002) **12**:223–9. doi:10.1016/S0959-4388(02)00314-8
81. Cools R, Gibbs SE, Miyakawa A, Jagust W, D'Esposito M. Working memory capacity predicts dopamine synthesis capacity in the human striatum. *J Neurosci* (2008) **28**(5):1208–12. doi:10.1523/JNEUROSCI.4475-07.2008
82. Hazy TE, Frank MJ, O'Reilly RC. Banishing the homunculus: making working memory work. *Neuroscience* (2006) **139**:105–18. doi:10.1016/j.neuroscience.2005.04.067
83. Cole MW, Schneider W. The cognitive control network: integrated cortical regions with dissociable functions. *Neuroimage* (2007) **37**:343–60. doi:10.1016/j.neuroimage.2007.03.071
84. Lenartowicz A, McIntosh AR. The role of anterior cingulate cortex in working memory is shaped by functional connectivity. *J Cogn Neurosci* (2005) **17**(7):1026–42. doi:10.1162/0898929054475127
85. Woodward TS, Cairo TA, Ruff CC, Takane Y, Hunter MA, Ngan ET. Functional connectivity reveals load dependent neural systems underlying encoding and maintenance in verbal working memory. *Neuroscience* (2006) **139**:317–25. doi:10.1016/j.neuroscience.2005.05.043
86. Gazzaley A, Nobre AC. Top-down modulation: bridging selective attention and working memory. *Trends Cogn Sci* (2012) **16**:129–35. doi:10.1016/j.tics.2011.11.014
87. Broome MR, Matthiasson P, Fusar-Poli P, Woolley JB, Johns LC, Tabraham P, et al. Neural correlates of executive function and working memory in the 'at-risk mental state'. *Br J Psychiatry* (2009) **194**:25–33. doi:10.1192/bjp.bp.107.046789
88. Liemburg EJ, Knegtering H, Klein HC, Kortekaas R, Aleman A. Antipsychotic medication and prefrontal cortex activation: a review of neuroimaging findings. *Eur Neuropsychopharmacol* (2012) **22**:387–400. doi:10.1016/j.euroneuro.2011.12.008
89. Rasetti R, Sambataro F, Chen Q, Callicott JH, Mattay VS, Weinberger DR. Altered cortical network dynamics: a potential intermediate phenotype for schizophrenia and association with ZNF804A. *Arch Gen Psychiatry* (2011) **68**:1207–17. doi:10.1001/archgenpsychiatry.2011.103
90. Barch DM, Carter CS, Braver TS, Sabb FW, MacDonald A III, Noll DC, et al. Selective deficits in prefrontal cortex function in medication-naive patients with schizophrenia. *Arch Gen Psychiatry* (2001) **58**:280–8. doi:10.1001/archpsyc.58.3.280
91. Potkin SG, Turner JA, Brown GG, McCarthy G, Greve DN, Glover GH, et al. Working memory and DLPFC inefficiency in schizophrenia: the FBIRN study. *Schizophr Bull* (2009) **35**:19–31. doi:10.1093/schbul/sbn162
92. Brown GG, Thompson WK. Functional brain imaging in schizophrenia: selected results and methods. *Curr Top Behav Neurosci* (2010) **4**:181–214. doi:10.1007/7854_2010_54
93. Manoach DS. Prefrontal cortex dysfunction during working memory performance in schizophrenia: reconciling discrepant findings. *Schizophr Res* (2003) **60**:285–98. doi:10.1016/S0920-9964(02)00294-3
94. Wager TD, Smith EE. Neuroimaging studies of working memory: a meta-analysis. *Cogn Affect Behav Neurosci* (2003) **3**:255–74. doi:10.3758/CABN.3.4.255
95. Glahn DC, Ragland JD, Abramoff A, Barrett J, Laird AR, Bearden CE, et al. Beyond hypofrontality: a quantitative meta-analysis of functional neuroimaging studies of working memory in schizophrenia. *Hum Brain Mapp* (2005) **25**(1):60–9. doi:10.1002/hbm.20138
96. van Snellenberg JX, Torres IJ, Thornton AE. Functional neuroimaging of working memory in schizophrenia: task performance as a moderating variable. *Neuropsychology* (2006) **20**(5):497–510. doi:10.1037/0894-4105.20.5.497
97. Callicott JH, Bertolino A, Mattay VS, Langheim FJ, Duyn J, Coppola R, et al. Physiological dysfunction of the dorsolateral prefrontal cortex in schizophrenia revisited. *Cereb Cortex* (2000) **10**:1078–92. doi:10.1093/cercor/10.11.1078
98. Callicott JH, Mattay VS, Verchinski BA, Marenco S, Egan MF, Weinberger DR. Complexity of prefrontal cortical dysfunction in schizophrenia: more than up or down. *Am J Psychiatry* (2003) **160**:2209–15. doi:10.1176/appi.ajp.160.12.2209
99. Thermenos HW, Goldstein JM, Buka SL, Poldrack RA, Koch JK, Tsuang MT, et al. The effect of working memory performance on functional MRI in schizophrenia. *Schizophr Res* (2005) **74**(2–3):19–94. doi:10.1016/j.schres.2004.07.021
100. Tan HY, Sust S, Buckholtz JW, Mattay VS, Meyer-Lindenberg A, Egan MF, et al. Dysfunctional prefrontal regional specialization and compensation in schizophrenia. *Am J Psychiatry* (2006) **163**(11):1969–77. doi:10.1176/appi.ajp.163.11.1969
101. Quidé Y, Morris RW, Shepherd AM, Rowland JE, Green MJ. Task-related fronto-striatal functional connectivity during working memory performance in schizophrenia. *Schiozphr Res* (2013) **150**(2–3):468–75. doi:10.1016/j.schres.2013.08.009
102. Perlstein WM, Carter CS, Noll DC, Cohen JD. Relation of prefrontal cortex dysfunction to working memory and symptoms in schizophrenia. *Am J Psychiatry* (2001) **158**(7):1105–13. doi:10.1176/appi.ajp.158.7.1105
103. Guerrero-Pedraza A, McKenna PJ, Gomar JJ, Sarró S, Salvador R, Amann B, et al. First-episode psychosis is characterized by failure of deactivation but not by hypo- or hyperfrontality. *Psychol Med* (2012) **42**(1):73–84. doi:10.1017/S0033291711001073
104. Carter CS, Perlstein W, Ganguli R, Brar J, Mintun M, Cohen JD. Functional hypofrontality and working memory dysfunction in schizophrenia. *Am J Psychiatry* (1998) **155**(9):1285–7.
105. Meyer-Lindenberg A, Poline JB, Kohn PD, Holt JL, Egan MF, Weinberger DR, et al. Evidence for abnormal cortical functional connectivity during working memory in schizophrenia. *Am J Psychiatry* (2001) **158**(11):1809–17. doi:10.1176/appi.ajp.158.11.1809
106. Meyer-Lindenberg AS, Olsen RK, Kohn PD, Brown T, Egan MF, Weinberger DR, et al. Regionally specific disturbance of dorsolateral prefrontal-hippocampal functional connectivity in schizophrenia. *Arch Gen Psychiatry* (2005) **62**(4):379–86. doi:10.1001/archpsyc.62.4.379
107. Friston KJ, Frith CD. Schizophrenia: a disconnection syndrome? *Clin Neurosci* (1995) **3**(2):89–97.
108. Huys QJ, Moutoussis M, Williams J. Are computational models of any use to psychiatry? *Neural Netw* (2011) **24**:544–51. doi:10.1016/j.neunet.2011.03.001
109. Montague PR, Dolan RJ, Friston KJ, Dayan P. Computational psychiatry. *Trends Cogn Sci* (2012) **16**:72–80. doi:10.1016/j.tics.2011.11.018
110. Lewis DA, Moghaddam B. Cognitive dysfunction in schizophrenia: convergence of gamma-aminobutyric acid and glutamate alterations. *Arch Neurol* (2006) **63**:1372–6. doi:10.1001/archneur.63.10.1372
111. Lewis DA, Gonzalez-Burgos G. Neuroplasticity of neocortical circuits in schizophrenia. *Neuropsychopharmacology* (2008) **33**:141–65. doi:10.1038/sj.npp.1301563
112. Gonzalez-Burgos G, Hashimoto T, Lewis DA. Alterations of cortical GABA neurons and network oscillations in schizophrenia. *Curr Psychiatry Rep* (2010) **12**:335–44. doi:10.1007/s11920-010-0124-8
113. Volk DW, Eggan SM, Lewis DA. Alterations in metabotropic glutamate receptor 1 alpha and regulator of G protein signaling 4 in the prefrontal cortex in schizophrenia. *Am J Psychiatry* (2010) **167**:1489–98. doi:10.1176/appi.ajp.2010.10030318
114. Schwartz TL, Sachdeva S, Stahl SM. Glutamate neurocircuitry: theoretical underpinnings in schizophrenia. *Front Pharmacol* (2012) **3**:195. doi:10.3389/fphar.2012.00195
115. Friston K. Beyond phrenology: what can neuroimaging tell us about distributed circuitry? *Annu Rev Neurosci* (2002) **25**:221–50. doi:10.1146/annurev.neuro.25.112701.142846
116. McIntosh AR. Towards a network theory of cognition. *Neural Netw* (2000) **13**:861–70. doi:10.1016/S0893-6080(00)00059-9
117. Daunizeau J, David O, Stephan KE. Dynamic causal modelling: a critical review of the biophysical and statistical foundations. *Neuroimage* (2011) **58**:312–22. doi:10.1016/j.neuroimage.2009.11.062
118. Daunizeau J, Preuschoff K, Friston KJ, Stephan KE. Optimizing experimental d esign for comparing models of brain function. *PLoS Comput Biol* (2011) **7**:e1002280. doi:10.1371/journal.pcbi.1002280
119. Stephan KE, Kasper L, Harrison LM, Daunizeau J, den Ouden HE, Breakspear M, et al. Nonlinear dynamic causal models for fMRI. *Neuroimage* (2008) **42**:649–62. doi:10.1016/j.neuroimage.2008.04.262

120. Salinas E, Sejnowski TJ. Gain modulation in the central nervous system: where behavior, neurophysiology, and computation meet. *Neuroscientist* (2001) **7**:430–40. doi:10.1177/107385840100700512
121. Volman V, Levine H, Sejnowski TJ. Shunting inhibition controls the gain modulation mediated by asynchronous neurotransmitter release in early development. *PLoS Comput Biol* (2010) **6**:e1000973. doi:10.1371/journal.pcbi.1000973
122. Stephan KE, Harrison LM, Kiebel SJ, David O, Penny WD, Friston KJ. Dynamic causal models of neural system dynamics: current state and future extensions. *J Biosci* (2007) **32**:129–44. doi:10.1007/s12038-007-0012-5
123. Tana MG, Montin E, Cerutti S, Bianchi AM. Exploring cortical attentional system by using fMRI during a continuous performance test. *Comput Intell Neurosci* (2010) **2010**:329213. doi:10.1155/2010/329213
124. Wang L, Liu X, Guise KG, Knight RT, Ghajar J, Fan J. Effective connectivity of the fronto-parietal network during attentional control. *J Cogn Neurosci* (2010) **22**:543–53. doi:10.1162/jocn.2009.21210
125. Brazdil M, Mikl M, Marecek R, Krupa P, Rektor I. Effective connectivity in target stimulus processing: a dynamic causal modeling study of visual oddball task. *Neuroimage* (2007) **35**:827–35. doi:10.1016/j.neuroimage.2006.12.020
126. Tan HY, Chen AG, Kolachana B, Apud JA, Mattay VS, Callicott JH, et al. Effective connectivity of AKT1-mediated dopaminergic working memory networks and pharmacogenetics of anti-dopaminergic treatment. *Brain* (2012) **135**:1436–45. doi:10.1093/brain/aws068
127. Crossley NA, Mechelli A, Fusar-Poli P, Broome MR, Matthiasson P, Johns LC, et al. Superior temporal lobe dysfunction and frontotemporal dysconnectivity in subjects at risk of psychosis and in first-episode psychosis. *Hum Brain Mapp* (2009) **30**:4129–37. doi:10.1002/hbm.20834
128. Deserno L, Sterzer P, Wustenberg T, Heinz A, Schlagenhauf F. Reduced prefrontal-parietal effective connectivity and working memory deficits in schizophrenia. *J Neurosci* (2012) **32**:12–20. doi:10.1523/JNEUROSCI.3405-11.2012
129. Schmidt A, Smieskova R, Aston J, Simon A, Allen P, Fusar-Poli P, et al. Brain connectivity abnormalities predating the onset of psychosis: correlation with the effect of medication. *JAMA Psychiatry* (2013) **70**(9):903–12. doi:10.1001/jamapsychiatry.2013.117
130. Zhang H, Wei X, Tao H, Mwansisya TE, Pu W, He Z, et al. Opposite effective connectivity in the posterior cingulate and medial prefrontal cortex between first-episode schizophrenic patients with suicide risk and healthy controls. *PLoS One* (2013) **8**:e63477. doi:10.1371/journal.pone.0063477
131. Dayan P, Abbot LF. *Theoretical Neuroscience: Computational and Mathematical Modeling of Neural Systems.* Cambridge, MA: The MIT Press (2000).
132. Li B, Daunizeau J, Stephan KE, Penny W, Hu D, Friston K. Generalised filtering and stochastic DCM for fMRI. *Neuroimage* (2011) **58**:442–57. doi:10.1016/j.neuroimage.2011.01.085
133. Allen P, Mechelli A, Stephan KE, Day F, Dalton J, Williams S, et al. Fronto-temporal interactions during overt verbal initiation and suppression. *J Cogn Neurosci* (2008) **20**:1656–69. doi:10.1162/jocn.2008.20107
134. Allen P, Stephan KE, Mechelli A, Day F, Ward N, Dalton J, et al. Cingulate activity and fronto-temporal connectivity in people with prodromal signs of psychosis. *Neuroimage* (2010) **49**:947–55. doi:10.1016/j.neuroimage.2009.08.038
135. Dauvermann MR, Whalley HC, Romaniuk L, Valton V, Owens DG, Johnstone EC, et al. The application of nonlinear dynamic causal modelling for fMRI in subjects at high genetic risk of schizophrenia. *Neuroimage* (2013) **73**:16–29. doi:10.1016/j.neuroimage.2013.01.063
136. Whalley HC, Simonotto E, Flett S, Marshall I, Ebmeier KP, Owens DG, et al. FMRI correlates of state and trait effects in subjects at genetically enhanced risk of schizophrenia. *Brain* (2004) **127**:478–90. doi:10.1093/brain/awh070
137. Whalley HC, Simonotto E, Marshall I, Owens DG, Goddard NH, Johnstone EC, et al. Functional disconnectivity in subjects at high genetic risk of schizophrenia. *Brain* (2005) **128**:2097–108. doi:10.1093/brain/awh556
138. Friston KJ, Shiner T, FitzGerald T, Galea JM, Adams R, Brown H, et al. Dopamine, affordance and active inference. *PLoS Comput Biol* (2012) **8**(1):e1002327. doi:10.1371/journal.pcbi.1002327
139. Brodersen KJ, Deserno L, Schlagenhauf F, Lin Z, Penny WD, Buhmann JM, et al. Dissecting psychiatric spectrum disorders. *Neuroimage Clin* (2013) **4**:98–111. doi:10.1016/j.nicl.2013.11.002
140. Durstewitz D, Seamans JK. The computational role of dopamine D1 receptors in working memory. *Neural Netw* (2002) **15**(4–6):561–72. doi:10.1016/S0893-6080(02)00049-7
141. Murray JD, Anticevic A, Gancsos M, Ichinose M, Corlett PR, Krystal JH, et al. Linking microcircuit dysfunction to cognitive impairment: effects of disinhibition associated with schizophrenia in a cortical working memory model. *Cereb Cortex* (2012) **24**(4):859–72. doi:10.1093/cercor/bhs370
142. D'Ardenne K, Eshel N, Luka J, Lenartowicz A, Nystrom LE, Cohen JD. Role of prefrontal cortex and the midbrain dopamine system in working memory updating. *Proc Natl Acad Sci U S A* (2012) **109**:19900–9. doi:10.1073/pnas.1116727109
143. den Ouden HE, Friston KJ, Daw ND, McIntosh AR, Stephan KE. A dual role for prediction error in associative learning. *Cereb Cortex* (2009) **19**(5):1175–85. doi:10.1093/cercor/bhn161
144. den Ouden HE, Daunizeau J, Roiser J, Friston KJ, Stephan KE. Striatal prediction error modulates cortical coupling. *J Neurosci* (2010) **30**(9):3210–9. doi:10.1523/JNEUROSCI.4458-09.2010
145. Brodersen KH, Schofield TM, Leff AP, Ong CS, Lomakina EI, Buhmann JM, et al. Generative embedding for model-based classification of fMRI data. *PLoS Comput Biol* (2011) **7**(6):e1002079. doi:10.1371/journal.pcbi.1002079
146. Stephan KE, Penny WD, Moran RJ, den Ouden HE, Daunizeau J, Friston KJ. Ten simple rules for dynamic causal modeling. *Neuroimage* (2010) **49**(4):3099–109. doi:10.1016/j.neuroimage.2009.11.015
147. Penny WD, Stephan KE, Mechelli A, Friston KJ. Comparing dynamic causal models. *Neuroimage* (2004) **22**(3):1157–72. doi:10.1016/j.neuroimage.2004.03.026
148. Penny WD, Stephan KE, Daunizeau J, Rosa MJ, Friston KJ, Schofield TM, et al. Comparing families of dynamic causal models. *PLoS Comput Biol* (2010) **6**(3):e1000709. doi:10.1371/journal.pcbi.1000709
149. Lisman JE, Coyle JT, Green RW, Javitt DC, Benes FM, Heckers S, et al. Circuit-based framework for understanding neurotransmitter and risk gene interactions in schizophrenia. *Trends Neurosci* (2008) **31**:234–42. doi:10.1016/j.tins.2008.02.005

APPENDIX

DYNAMIC CAUSAL MODELING

Dynamic causal modeling is general framework for model-based assessment of competing theories about neuronal circuits (18, 146). In particular, DCM is a generic Bayesian system identification technique, which allows for inference on "hidden" neurophysiological mechanisms that generated observed measures, such as blood-oxygen-level-dependent signal in functional magnetic resonance imaging (fMRI) or evoked responses measured with electroencephalography (EEG). The principle idea thereby is to formulate a simplified model of neuronal population responses (z) and combine this with a modality-specific forward model (λ) such that one can predict the measurement (y) that would arise from any particular neuronal circuit (18).

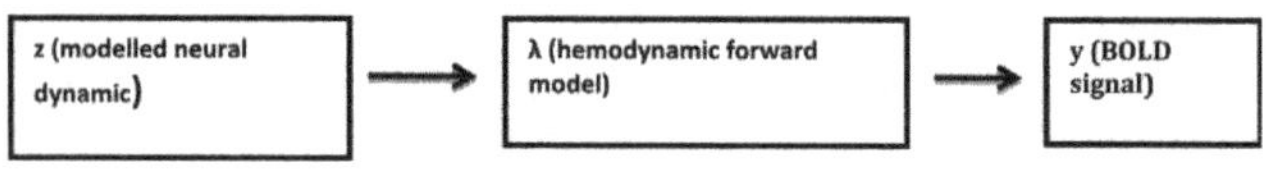

In DCM for fMRI, the dynamics of the neural states underlying regional BOLD response are modeled by a bilinear differential equation that describes how the neural states (x) change over time (t) as a function of endogenous inter-regional connections (matrix A), modulatory effects on these connections (matrix B), and direct (driving) inputs (matrix C) (Eq. A1) (18, 122). The endogenous connections represent coupling strengths in the absence of input u_j to the system, whereas the modulatory effects represent task-specific alterations in this connectivity.

$$f(x, u) = \frac{dx}{xt} = \left(A + \sum_{i=1}^{m} uB^{(j)}\right) x + Cu \qquad \text{(A1)}$$

The bilinear state equation has subsequently been extended by a non-linear term, where the modulation of connection strengths by experimental inputs is supplemented by direct modulation with neural activity in one or more regions (119). In other words, non-linear DCMs allow addressing how the connection between two neuronal units is gated by activity in other units. This is of particular interest as gating processes represent a key mechanism for many neurobiological processes and thus increasing the biological realism of non-linear compared to bilinear DCMs. To this end, compared with the bilinear state equation, the new term in the non-linear equations are the D matrices (Eq. A2), which encode how the n regions gate connections in the system.

$$f(x, u) = \frac{dx}{dt} = \left(A + \sum_{i=1}^{m} uB^{(j)} + \sum_{j=1}^{n} x_j D^{(j)}\right) x + Cu \qquad \text{(A2)}$$

BAYESIAN MODEL SELECTION AND BAYESIAN MODEL AVERAGING

Bayesian model selection is an essential procedure of DCM studies as it can be used to test competing hypotheses (different DCMs) about the neural mechanisms generating the data. BMS rests on comparing the evidence of a predefined set of models (the model space). The model evidence is the probability of observing the empirical data, given a model, and represents a principled measure of model quality, derived from probability theory (147, 148). Concretely, it represents the mean predicted data under random sampling from the model's priors or, alternatively, a principled measure of the balance between model fit and model complexity. A random-effects BMS approach has been suggested for group studies, which is capable of quantifying the degree of heterogeneity in a population while being extremely robust to potential outliers (20, 67). The probability that one model is more likely than any other model, given the group data, can be expressed by the exceedance probability (φ_k) of each model:

$$\exists k \in \{1 \ldots k\}, \forall j \in \{1 \ldots k | j \neq k\}:$$
$$\varphi_k = p(r_k > r_j | y; a)$$

After inference on the most likely network architecture underlying a specific neural process, one can compare the parameter estimates of the most likely model obtained from BMS (winning model) for between-group inferences. However, statistical comparison of model parameter estimates across groups is only valid if those estimates stem from the same model. Given that different models may be found to be optimal across groups, Bayesian model averaging (BMA) has been recommended as standard approach for clinical DCM studies (146). BMA averages posterior parameter estimates over models, weighted by the posterior model probabilities (148). Thus, models with a low posterior probability contribute little to the estimation of the marginal posterior. In brief, BMS and BMA are central components of DCM studies to infer on neural mechanisms at the neural system level and on specific model parameters across groups, respectively (146).

In non-linear DCM analysis, the connection strengths between selected nodes are assessed for activity-dependent modulation of the reciprocal neuronal projections by the introduction of gating mechanisms. Non-linear DCM is applied to the models identified as winning models from the application of bilinear state equation. The bilinear model and the non-linear models differ only in the introduction of gating mechanisms such as a parametric response in the tested functional task. Such gating mechanisms are applied to nodal connections, which are expected to explain the variation in subject response to the functional task. The appropriate placement of the gating input is assessed through the application of model space partitioning and family inference. The exceedance probabilities of the models are compared and the non-linear models, which provide higher exceedance probabilities than the bilinear models are identified as winning models.

4

Effects of Nicotine on the Neurophysiological and Behavioral Effects of Ketamine in Humans

Daniel H. Mathalon[1,2]*, Kyung-Heup Ahn[3,4,5], Edward B. Perry Jr.[3,4,5], Hyun-Sang Cho[3,6], Brian J. Roach[2], Rebecca K. Blais[3], Savita Bhakta[3], Mohini Ranganathan[3], Judith M. Ford[1,2] and Deepak Cyril D'Souza[3,4,5]

[1] Department of Psychiatry, University of California San Francisco, San Francisco, CA, USA
[2] Mental Health Service (116D), San Francisco VA Medical Center, San Francisco, CA, USA
[3] Department of Psychiatry, Yale University School of Medicine, New Haven, CT, USA
[4] Schizophrenia Biological Research Center (116A), VA Connecticut Healthcare System, West Haven, CT, USA
[5] Abraham Ribicoff Research Facilities, Connecticut Mental Health Center, New Haven, CT, USA
[6] Department of Psychiatry, Yonsei University College of Medicine, Seoul, South Korea

***Correspondence:**
Daniel H. Mathalon, Mental Health Service (116D), San Francisco VA Medical Center, 4150 Clement Street, San Francisco, CA 94121, USA
e-mail: daniel.mathalon@ucsf.edu

Background: *N*-methyl-D-aspartate (NMDA) receptor hypofunction has been implicated in the pathophysiology of schizophrenia and its associated neurocognitive impairments. The high rate of cigarette smoking in schizophrenia raises questions about how nicotine modulates putative NMDA receptor hypofunction in the illness. Accordingly, we examined the modulatory effects of brain nicotinic acetylcholine receptor (nAChR) stimulation on NMDA receptor hypofunction by examining the interactive effects of nicotine, a nAChR agonist, and ketamine, a non-competitive NMDA receptor antagonist, on behavioral and neurophysiological measures in healthy human volunteers.

Methods: From an initial sample of 17 subjects (age range 18–55 years), 8 subjects successfully completed 4 test sessions, each separated by at least 3 days, during which they received ketamine or placebo and two injections of nicotine or placebo in a double-blind, counterbalanced manner. Schizophrenia-like effects Positive and Negative Syndrome Scale, perceptual alterations Clinician Administered Dissociative Symptoms Scale, subjective effects Visual Analog Scale and auditory event-related brain potentials (mismatch negativity, MMN; P300) were assessed during each test session.

Results: Consistent with existing studies, ketamine induced transient schizophrenia-like behavioral effects. P300 was reduced and delayed by ketamine regardless of whether it was elicited by a target (P3b) or novel (P3a) stimulus, while nicotine only reduced the amplitude of P3a. Nicotine did not rescue P300 from the effects of ketamine; the interactions of ketamine and nicotine were not significant. While nicotine significantly reduced MMN amplitude, ketamine did not.

Conclusion: Nicotine failed to modulate ketamine-induced neurophysiological and behavioral effects in this preliminary study. Interestingly, ketamine reduced P3b amplitude and nicotine reduced P3a amplitude, suggesting independent roles of NMDA receptor and nAChR in the generation of P3b and P3a, respectively.

Keywords: schizophrenia, nicotine, ketamine, *N*-methyl-D-aspartate receptor, nicotinic acetylcholine receptor, event-related potential, mismatch negativity, P300

INTRODUCTION

Several lines of evidence support a glutamatergic hypothesis of schizophrenia involving *N*-methyl-D-aspartate (NMDA) receptor hypofunction (1–7). Studies with the NMDA receptor antagonist, ketamine, in healthy human subjects have been a cornerstone of the glutamatergic hypothesis of schizophrenia, producing clinical symptoms and cognitive impairments similar to those observed in schizophrenia (4, 5, 7–13). Nicotine has been shown to have cognitive enhancing effects in some (14–16), although not all (17, 18), studies. It has been suggested that the high rate of cigarette smoking in schizophrenia patients may reflect their efforts to use nicotine to "self-medicate" (19–21). In the present, exploratory study, we examined the interactive effects of ketamine and nicotine in healthy volunteers in order to determine whether impairments in brain function mediated by NMDA receptor hypofunction can be ameliorated by nicotine.

PARALLEL EFFECTS OF KETAMINE AND SCHIZOPHRENIA ON CLINICAL, COGNITIVE, AND NEUROPHYSIOLOGICAL FUNCTION

When administered at subanesthetic doses, ketamine produces an array of transient effects in healthy humans that resemble the positive and negative symptoms and cognitive deficits of schizophrenia (4, 7–13, 22–26). Ketamine has also been shown to produce some of the event-related brain potential (ERP) abnormalities observed in schizophrenia including reductions of two ERP components associated with controlled and automatic processing of deviant stimuli, P300 and mismatch negativity (MMN), as described below.

P300 is a positive voltage ERP component occurring about 300 ms following infrequent deviant stimuli interspersed among frequent "standard" stimuli, typically elicited in auditory or visual "oddball" tasks (27). P300 has been posited to reflect allocation of attentional resources (28–30), stimulus categorization (31), and contextual updating of working memory (32). Multiple brain regions have been implicated as neural generators of the P300, including the temporo-parietal junction and prefrontal cortex (33, 34). P300 comprises two subcomponents, the P3b and P3a that are differentially present depending on task conditions (27, 35–38). The P3b is primarily elicited by infrequent target stimuli, reflects top-down allocation of attention, and has a parietal scalp maximum (27, 36, 37). The P3a is primarily elicited by an infrequent non-target distractor or novel stimuli in an oddball sequence, reflects bottom-up orienting of attention, and has a fronto-central scalp maximum (27, 38–41).

P300 amplitude reduction, particularly auditory P3b, is one of the most widely replicated brain abnormalities observed in patients with schizophrenia (42, 43), although it is also reduced in a number of other psychiatric and neurological disorders (44, 45). Furthermore, several studies have shown that ketamine reduces P300 amplitude in healthy volunteers (46–51), consistent with the possibility that NMDA receptor hypofunction contributes to P300 amplitude reduction in schizophrenia. Interestingly, in the Knott et al. (47) study, the reduction of P300 amplitude by ketamine was only evident in the subgroup of non-smokers, consistent with a possible protective effect of nicotine.

Mismatch negativity is a negative ERP component elicited automatically by infrequent deviant auditory stimuli randomly interspersed among frequent "standard" stimuli (52, 53). MMN has been widely interpreted to reflect auditory sensory echoic memory because the detection of deviance requires an online representation of what has recently been "standard" in the auditory stream (52). More recently, interpretations of the MMN have emphasized its reflection of both short-term (seconds) and long-term (minutes to hours) synaptic plasticity in the service of auditory sensory/perceptual learning since the amplitude of the MMN to a deviant stimulus increases as a function of the number of repetitions of the preceding standard stimulus (54, 55). From this perspective, memory traces of the recent auditory past code predictions of future auditory events, with the MMN signaling a prediction error, when the auditory expectancy is violated by a deviant stimulus (54–56). Auditory deviance along a number of dimensions elicits MMN, including pitch, duration, intensity, and location, among others (52, 57). MMN generators have been localized to the auditory cortex and to the frontal lobes (52). MMN is considered to be largely pre-attentive (52), and it is typically elicited while subjects perform a distractor task.

Mismatch negativity has been shown to be reduced in schizophrenia, particularly the duration-deviant MMN (58–60). Moreover, MMN abnormalities, relative to P300 abnormalities, appear to be more specific to schizophrenia (61, 62). Non-competitive NMDA receptor antagonism by phencyclidine (PCP) and ketamine has been shown to reduce MMN in non-human primates (63, 64) and healthy volunteers (26, 46, 65–68), respectively. However, some studies failed to find an effect of ketamine on MMN (50) or showed the effect to depend on the type of auditory deviance or the underlying cortical source examined (65, 67). Recently, Knott and colleagues (66) reported that reduction of MMN with ketamine was only seen in people with a predisposition to experience auditory hallucinations and delusions. Moreover, this effect was blocked when these subjects were chewing nicotine gum, consistent with a possible protective effect of nicotine (66).

EFFECTS OF NICOTINE ON NEUROCOGNITIVE AND NEUROPHYSIOLOGICAL FUNCTION

Nicotine has been shown to enhance cognitive functions including attention, episodic memory, and working memory in humans in some (14–16, 69, 70), but not all (17, 18), studies. The effects of nicotine administration or smoking on neurophysiological measures related to processing of deviant stimuli have been examined in a number of studies (71, 72). In experienced tobacco users, cigarette smoking or nicotine administration has been shown to increase P300 amplitude (73–75), especially in non-smokers (47), and/or to reduce P300 latency (74, 76, 77). However, some studies have failed to show such effects (78–81) or have found effects on visual, but not auditory, P300 (77). In addition, some studies (75, 82, 83), but not others (84), have shown reduced P300 amplitudes in chronic smokers, suggesting a distinction between the effects of acute and chronic exposure to nicotine. Indeed, Knott and colleagues reported that the enhancement of P300 produced by nicotine administration was only evident in non-smokers (47).

Regarding MMN, some studies have reported that nicotine or nicotinic agonists increase MMN amplitude (85–88) or shorten MMN latency (86, 89, 90), whereas others have failed to show such amplitude increases (89–91) or latency reductions (66, 88, 91) with nicotine administration.

NICOTINE AND SCHIZOPHRENIA

There is a high prevalence of cigarette smoking among patients with schizophrenia (92–95). This may reflect an effort by schizophrenia patients to "self-medicate" clinical symptoms and a number of neurocognitive impairments including deficits in attention and memory (19) and deficient sensory gating (96). Thus, there is significant interest in developing nicotinic acetylcholine receptor (nAChR) agonists to target the neurocognitive symptoms of schizophrenia. Indeed, an alpha7 nicotinic agonist, 3-[(2,4-dimethoxy) benzylidene] Anabaseine (DMXAB) has been shown to produce significant improvements in cognitive function and P50 sensory gating in patients with schizophrenia (97).

Several studies have examined the effects of nicotine administration on MMN in patients with schizophrenia. Regarding MMN amplitude, a study of schizophrenic smokers showed that nicotine increases the amplitude and the latency of duration-deviant MMN, but shows no effect on frequency-deviant MMN (98). An earlier study from the same group examined the effects of nicotine on a mixed sample of smoking and non-smoking schizophrenia patients with high levels of auditory hallucinations and found no effects on MMN amplitudes in response to duration, frequency, and intensity deviants, although the latency of the intensity-deviant MMN was shortened by nicotine (99). Another study of non-smoking schizophrenia patients failed to show any effect of nicotine on a frequency-deviant MMN (90).

NICOTINIC RECEPTOR MODULATION OF GLUTAMATERGIC NEUROTRANSMISSION

One possible mechanism by which nAChR agonists might enhance neurocognitive and neurophysiological function is facilitating glutamatergic neurotransmission via presynaptic nAChR (100) or via GABA interneurons (101, 102). Nicotine or nAChR agonists have been shown to facilitate glutamatergic transmission in rat prefrontal cortex (103, 104) and hippocampus (105). Specifically relevant to this study, nicotine attenuates or reverses memory and attentional deficits induced by the NMDA receptor antagonist MK-801 (dizocilpine) in rats (106, 107). Moreover, dizocilpine blocked nicotinic enhancement of memory consolidation in mice (108). Knott et al. (47) examined the effects of nicotine and a sub-perceptual dose of ketamine on P300 in men and women, smokers and non-smokers. In non-smokers, ketamine reduced P300, an effect that did not interact with nicotine. However, in the third assessment block, following the drug infusion, nicotine increased P300 amplitude on its own but further reduced P300 when combined with ketamine. In a subsequent study, Knott and colleagues (66) found that ketamine reduces the amplitude of MMN in healthy individuals with a high propensity toward hallucinatory experiences and/or delusional thinking, an effect that was blocked by nicotine. Similar effects were not evident in individuals with a low propensity toward these psychotic symptoms.

THE RATIONALE AND HYPOTHESES FOR CURRENT STUDY

It is difficult to isolate and study the NMDA receptor hypofunction and its consequences in schizophrenia. The ketamine paradigm in healthy subjects offers a pharmacological model for investigating nicotine's effect on putative NMDA receptor hypofunction in schizophrenia. Specifically, this study examined the effects of nAChR activation on NMDA receptor hypofunction by investigating the interactions of ketamine, a non-competitive NMDA receptor antagonist, and nicotine, a nAChR agonist, when administered to healthy volunteers in a placebo-controlled study over four test days. The neurophysiological outcome measures, chosen based on their established sensitivity to schizophrenia, consisted of: (1) two variants of the auditory P300, the P3b elicited by target stimuli and the P3a elicited by novel distractor stimuli, and (2) the MMN elicited automatically by a duration-deviant auditory stimulus. The primary and secondary hypotheses were that nicotine would attenuate the neurophysiological abnormalities and schizophrenia-like clinical symptoms induced by ketamine, respectively.

MATERIALS AND METHODS

RESEARCH PARTICIPANTS

The study was approved by the Institutional Review Boards of VA Connecticut Healthcare System (West Haven, CT, USA) and Yale University School of Medicine (New Haven, CT, USA). Subjects were recruited via public advertisements and were paid for their study participation. Written informed consent was obtained from all subjects. Smokers who were not interested in quitting and lifetime non-smokers who had tried nicotine in the past were both invited to participate. Subjects were medically healthy by physical examination, history, electrocardiography, and laboratory testing. They had no history of a DSM-IV Axis-I disorder (other than nicotine dependence), major current or recent (<6 weeks) life stressors, and first-degree relative with a history of psychosis. Screening procedures included the Structured Clinical Interview for DSM-IV, Non-Patient Edition (109), selected sub-tests from the Wechsler Adult Intelligence Scale (Information, Vocabulary, Block Design, Picture Completion) to provide an estimate of general level of cognitive ability (110), and the Fagerström Test for Nicotine Dependence (111) to measure the severity of nicotine dependence in smokers. Subjects were instructed to refrain from consuming psychoactive substances from 1 week prior to testing through completion of the study. An outside informant identified by the subject was interviewed to corroborate information provided by potential subjects. Urine toxicology testing was performed at screening and on the morning of each test day to rule out recent illicit substance use. Subjects were instructed to fast overnight and abstain from smoking after 11:00 p.m. prior to arrival for each test day. They were excluded if breath carbon monoxide levels were higher than 10 ppm.

Seventeen subjects participated in at least one test day. Eight of the 17 subjects scheduled for four test days did not complete testing: 3 of 5 (60%) non-smokers and 5 of 12 (42%) smokers. The reasons for discontinuation were mostly related to adverse effects of ketamine or nicotine ($n = 6$). Adverse events and study discontinuations were reported to the VA Connecticut Human Studies Subcommittee. As with all of our prior ketamine studies, clinical follow-ups indicated that all adverse events associated with acute ketamine administration resolved spontaneously without any late appearing or persistent adverse effects. There were no significant differences in age, sex, education, smoking status, or Fagerström Nicotine Dependence scores between study completers and non-completers. Only nine subjects completed all four test days. Demographic data for these nine completers are presented in **Table 1**. Of the nine completers (five men, four women), one woman was excluded from the ERP analyses because she was too somnolent and impaired to perform the oddball task or the MMN distractor task during the Ketamine Alone test day. In addition, one man was dropped from the ERP MMN analysis because of technical problems running the MMN paradigm during his Nicotine Alone test day.

Table 1 | Demographic data for study completers ($N = 9$).

Variable	Number of subjects
Gender (male/female)	5/4
Smoking status (smoker/non-smoker)	7/2
	Mean (SD)
Age (years)	29.8 (7.9)
Education (years)	16.8 (3.0)
Fagerström nicotine dependence score	1.78 (2.28)

TEST DAYS

Across the four test days, subjects received ketamine and nicotine in a double-blind, randomized, 2 × 2 crossover design. On each test day, subjects received ketamine (a bolus of 0.26 mg/kg over 1 min, followed by maintenance infusion at 0.65 mg/kg/h × 2 h) or placebo (normal saline). Fifteen minutes after the ketamine bolus, subjects received an intravenous infusion of nicotine (1.0 μg/kg/min × 10 min) or placebo followed by another nicotine or placebo injection 70 min later. The reason for two spaced nicotine injections was to attempt to minimize the possibility of desensitization that is known to occur with nicotine exposure. The dose of nicotine administered with each infusion (1.0 μg/kg/min × 10 min) = 0.7 mg in a 70-kg individual. A regular cigarette contains about 1.2–1.4 mg nicotine and an average of 0.88 mg of nicotine is delivered to a smoker from each cigarette. The timing of procedures is detailed in **Table 2**. Behavioral ratings were obtained at baseline and repeated periodically after the administration of ketamine and nicotine, but ERP data were collected only once per test day. Plasma ketamine and nicotine levels were measured after each infusion to rule out any pharmacokinetic interactions.

Table 2 | Study procedures.

Time (minutes)	Procedure
−110	IV lines and EEG leads placed, PANSS, CADSS, VAS, VS, plasma cotinine level, breath carbon monoxide, urine toxicology, training for AX-CPT
−20	Ketamine or placebo bolus plus infusion
−19	VS, PANSS, CADSS, VAS
−5	VS
0	Nicotine or placebo
+3	VS
+5	AX-CPT, ERP recording for MMN, periodic VS
+35	Plasma ketamine and nicotine levels, VS, PANSS, CADSS, VAS
+58	VS
+60	Nicotine or placebo
+63	VS
+65	ERP recording for P300, periodic VS
+98	Plasma ketamine and nicotine levels
+100	VS
+110	PANSS, CADSS, VAS, VS
+180	PANSS, CADSS, VAS, VS
+240	VS, discharge

PANSS, Positive and Negative Syndrome Scale; CADSS, Clinician Administered Dissociative Symptoms Scale; VAS, Visual Analog Scale; VS, vital signs; MMN, mismatch negativity; AX-CPT, AX-Continuous Performance Test.

BEHAVIORAL MEASURES

The schizophrenia-like clinical symptoms induced by ketamine were assessed using the Positive and Negative Syndrome Scale (PANSS) (112). Perceptual alterations were assessed using the Clinician Administered Dissociative Symptoms Scale (CADSS) (113). The following subjective states were rated by participants using 100-mm Visual Analog Scales (VASs) (10): Talkative, Happy, Drowsy, Tense, Dad, Calm, Depressed, Anxious, Energetic, Fearful, Mellow, High, Angry, Mania, Irritable, Tired, Hungry, and Craving.

ANALYSIS OF NICOTINE AND KETAMINE LEVELS

Plasma ketamine and norketamine were assayed using the identical method as described in detail elsewhere (114). Plasma nicotine concentrations were assayed using reversed-phase high-performance liquid chromatography (HPLC) based on a modification of a previously described method (115, 116). The nicotine assay involved HPLC/MS operated in the APCI/SIM mode using deuterated nicotine as an internal standard. After addition of the internal standard the plasma is deproteinized with sulfosalicylic acid and the supernatant made alkaline and extracted with heptane methylene chloride 85:15. This solvent is then dried down via vacuum centrifuge. The residue is redissolved in ethanol and an aliquot is injected into the HPLC. The HPLC column (Nova Pak C18 30 cm × 3.9 mm, 4 μm) is run in the isocratic mode using methanol acetonitrile ammonium formate (pH 4.0) 32.5:42.5:35.0 as mobile phase. The standard curve encompassing a range of 1–200 ng/ml was linear with negligible intercept. Plasma controls containing 4, 40, and 80 ng/ml nicotine in six consecutive runs demonstrated an inter-assay relative standard deviation RSD of 8.6, 7.4, and 8.3%, respectively.

ERP MEASURES

Electroencephalography (EEG) data were recorded using a 23-channel Physiometrix electrode cap. The cap included one ground electrode placed on the forehead (FPz), and the mean of freely placed bilateral earlobe electrodes served as the reference channel. Vertical and horizontal electro-oculograms (VEOGs and HEOGs) were recorded and used to correct EEG data for eye blink and eye-movement artifacts. Electrode impedances were maintained at <5 kΩ. The data were recorded using Neuroscan Synamps amplifiers, which were calibrated prior to each session. Data were acquired using a 0.05–100-Hz band pass filter, and the sampling rate was 1000 Hz.

P300 was elicited during an auditory oddball target detection task. Three types of stimuli were delivered through Etymotic ER-3A insert earphones: (1) standard tones: 500 Hz pure tones (rise/fall 5 ms; 50 ms duration), (2) target tones: 1000 Hz pure tones (rise/fall 5 ms; 50 ms duration), and (3) novel distractor sounds, selected from a corpus of novel sounds (average duration of 250 ms) developed by Friedman et al. (117). All auditory stimuli were presented at an identical sound pressure level (~80 dB SPL C scale). The task was presented in three blocks. Each block comprised of 150 pseudo-randomized stimuli (80% standards, 10% targets, 10% novel distractors) presented with a stimulus onset asynchrony (SOA) of 1250 ms. Subjects were instructed to press a response button with the index finger of their dominant hand each time a target tone occurred, giving equal emphasis to speed and accuracy.

For the MMN paradigm, subjects were presented with a pseudorandom sequence of standard tones (90% probability;

633 Hz; 5 ms rise/fall time; 50 ms duration) and duration-deviant tones (10% probability; 633 Hz, 5 ms rise/fall time, 100 ms duration) presented at 80 dB SPL, with a 510-ms SOA. A long duration-deviant MMN paradigm was chosen because of some evidence that it may more sensitive to the effect of schizophrenia than other types of MMN (58, 60, 61). The MMN paradigm was presented in two blocks, with each block comprising 783 standard tones and 87 deviant tones. These tones were presented binaurally through earphone inserts, while subjects performed a visual AX-Continuous Performance Task (AX-CPT) (118). Because several of the behavioral performance files from this task were irretrievably corrupted resulting in many subjects with missing behavioral performance data, the AX-CPT performance data were not analyzed in the current study. Thus, the AX-CPT essentially served as the distractor task during MMN recording.

ERP DATA PROCESSING

As the MMN and P300 measures generally achieve their maximum amplitudes along the midline and do not typically show hemispheric lateralization, EEG data from the midline fronto-central sites (Fz, Cz) and fronto-central-parietal sites (Fz, Cz, Pz) were analyzed for the MMN and P300 components, respectively. The processing pipeline for the P300 elicited during the three-stimulus auditory oddball task involved the following steps: continuous data were separated into 1000 ms epochs time-locked to stimulus onset, with a 100-ms pre-stimulus baseline. VEOG and HEOG data were used to correct EEG for eye-movements and blinks with a regression-based algorithm (119). After baseline correction, epochs containing artifacts (voltages exceeding ±100 µV) were rejected. P300 was identified as the most positive peak in a 235- to 400-ms time window following stimulus onset; however, because target P3b and novelty P3a have different topographies, different rules were used for identifying their peaks. The target P3b peak was first identified at Pz, then a 50-ms window (±25 ms) surrounding this peak's latency was used to identify target P3b peaks at other sites. Novelty P3a showed more scalp variability in peak latency than target P3b, particularly at frontal sites, leading us to adopt a more flexible peak identification approach. Novelty P3a peaks were first identified at all central and parietal sites. From the range of peak latencies obtained at central sites (C3, Cz, C4), minimum and maximum latencies were identified. By subtracting 50 ms from the minimum and adding 50 ms to the maximum, the search window for identification of P3a peaks at frontal sites was defined. Somewhat early latency cut-off (400 ms) for auditory P300s was chosen to avoid picking the second late positive component, which peaked around 550 ms (see **Figure 1**). Peak amplitudes and latencies for target P3b and novelty P3a were extracted from electrodes Fz, Cz, and Pz for statistical analyses.

The same eye-movement correction and artifact rejection criteria used in the P300 data processing pipeline were applied to the MMN standard and deviant trials, but these data were segmented into 550 ms epochs and baseline corrected using the 50-ms

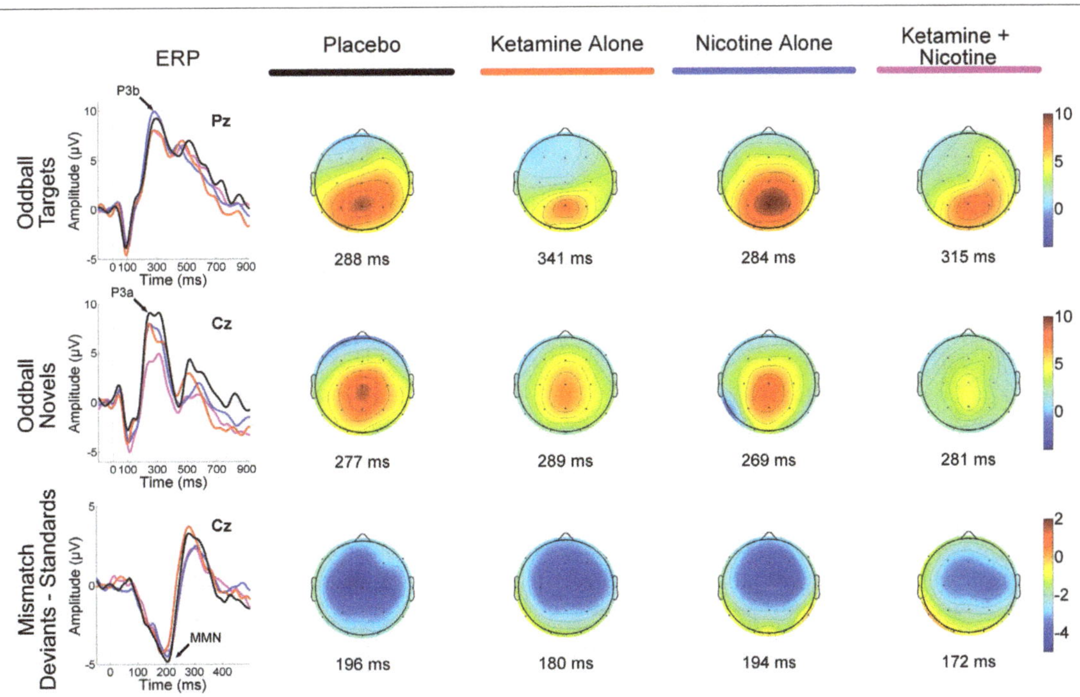

FIGURE 1 | Event-related brain potential grand average waveforms (left) and corresponding topographic maps (right) are shown for placebo (black), ketamine alone (red), nicotine alone (blue), and ketamine + nicotine (magenta) days. ERPs, overlaid for each test day, are shown to oddball targets at Pz (top row), to oddball novels at Cz (middle row), and to difference waveforms (deviants-standards) at Cz. The oddball target elicited a P3b, the oddball novel elicited a P3a, and the deviant elicited a MMN, with each peak denoted by an arrow on the ERP waveforms. Amplitude in microvolts is on the *y*-axis, and latency in milliseconds is on the *x*-axis. Stimulus onset is at 0 ms. Negativity is plotted down. Scalp topography maps are shown for each test day for each stimulus, at the peak latency for P3b (top), P3a (middle), and MMN (bottom). Hot colors indicate positive voltage and cool colors, negative voltage.

preceding tone onset. Standard and deviant trials remaining after artifact rejection were averaged separately, and the resulting ERP for the standard was subtracted from the deviant to create a difference wave. MMN was identified as the most negative peak between 90 and 270 ms post-tone onset in the difference wave at electrodes Fz and Cz. Peak amplitudes and latencies were extracted for statistical analyses.

STATISTICAL ANALYSES

Behavioral data

Initially, behavioral data were examined descriptively using means, standard deviations, and graphs. Each measure was tested for normality using Kolmogorov-Smirnov test statistics and normal probability plots. All PANSS, CADSS, and VAS measures were highly skewed. Thus, these non-normal behavioral data were first ranked and then fitted using a mixed-effects model with an unstructured variance-covariance matrix and *p*-values adjusted for Analysis of Variance (ANOVA)-type statistics (ATS). In these models, Ketamine (active vs. placebo), Nicotine (active vs. placebo), and Time (−110, −19, +35, +110, and +180 min) were included as within-subjects explanatory factors, while Subject was the clustering factor. Time reflected the time point, in minutes, relative to Time 0 when the first intravenous infusion of active-nicotine or placebo-nicotine was initiated (see **Table 2**). All two- and three-way interactions were modeled. Significant interactions were followed by appropriate *post hoc* tests and graphical displays to interpret the effects. All results were considered statistically significant at $p < 0.05$. Bonferroni correction was applied within but not across domains. Thus, for example, a cut-off alpha level of $0.05/2 = 0.025$ was used to declare effects significant for the two CADSS ratings (Subject- and Clinician-Rated).

ERP data

For the ERP data, which were collected once per test day, repeated-measures ANOVAs were conducted with Ketamine (active vs. placebo) and Nicotine (active vs. placebo) as within-subjects factors. The ANOVA models assessing P300 amplitudes and latencies included two additional within-subjects factors: Deviant Type (target vs. novel) and Lead (Fz vs. Cz vs. Pz). The ANOVA model for MMN amplitude and latency included one additional within-subjects factor: Lead (Fz vs. Cz). Analyses proceeded in a hierarchical fashion, with higher order interactions being parsed by examining lower order simple main effects and interactions. Ultimately, condition comparisons were tested with single degree of freedom contrasts.

RESULTS

BEHAVIORAL DATA

Ketamine produced significant increases in PANSS Total, CADSS Subject-Rated and Clinician-Rated Perceptual Alterations, and VAS subjective "High" ratings (see **Figure 2**). All Ketamine main effects and Ketamine × Time interactions were significant at $p < 0.0001$ (**Table 3**). *Post hoc* analyses showed significant effects of Ketamine at time points −19, +35, and +110 (all $p < 0.05$) for each of these measures. There were no significant main effects of Nicotine. Nor were there any significant Ketamine × Nicotine

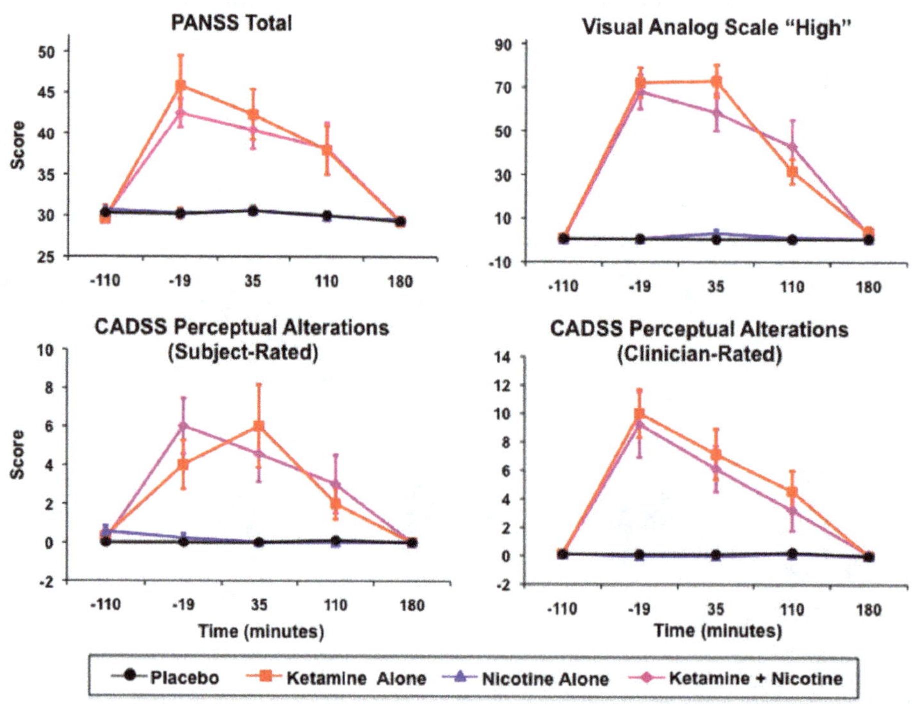

FIGURE 2 | Mean and standard errors are plotted for Positive and Negative Syndrome Scale (PANSS) total scores (upper left), Visual Analog Scale of subjective states (upper right), subject-rate (lower-left) and clinician-rated (lower-right) perceptual alterations using the Clinician Administered Dissociative Symptoms Scale (CADSS). For each plot, values for each of the four test days are overlaid, for Placebo (black), Ketamine Alone (red), Nicotine Alone (blue), and Ketamine + Nicotine (magenta) days.

Table 3 | Analysis of clinical scales.

Effect	Positive and Negative Syndrome Scale				Visual Analog Scale				CADSS perceptual alterations							
	Total score				"High"				Subject-rated				Clinician-rated			
	Num *df*	ATS	*p*-Value	Direction of effect	Num *df*	ATS	*p*-Value	Direction of effect	Num *df*	ATS	*p*-Value	Direction of effect	Num *df*	ATS	*p*-Value	Direction of effect
Nicotine (nicotine vs. placebo-nicotine)	1	0.36	0.551		1	0.59	0.441		1	0.96	0.327		1	0.20	0.655	
Ketamine (ketamine vs. placebo-ketamine)	1	24.60	**<0.0001**	Ketamine > placebo	1	77.01	**<0.0001**	Ketamine > placebo	1	23.39	**<0.0001**	Ketamine > placebo	1	43.32	**<0.0001**	Ketamine > placebo
Time (−110 vs. −19 vs. 35 vs. 110 vs. 180 min)	2.58	21.50	**<0.0001**	(−19, 35, 110) > (−110, 180)	3.39	29.94	**<0.0001**	(−19, 35, 110) > (−110, 180)	2.66	9.32	**<0.0001**	(−19, 35, 110) > (−110, 180)	2.46	19.98	**<0.0001**	(−19, 35, 110) > (−110, 180)
Nicotine × ketamine	1	0.020	0.892		1	0.190	0.660		1	0.050	0.829		1	0.100	0.751	
Nicotine × time	2.72	0.18	0.892		3.47	0.31	0.847		3.11	1.10	0.349		3.42	0.65	0.601	
Ketamine × time	3.12	22.12	**<0.0001**		3.09	22.97	**<0.0001**		3.15	16.39	**<0.0001**		2.72	23.10	**<0.0001**	
Ketamine effect at −110 min	*1*	*2.99*	*0.084*		*1*	*0.00*	*0.953*		*1*	*0.18*	*0.672*		*1*	*0.00*	*1.000*	
Ketamine effect at −19 min	*1*	*38.06*	***<0.0001***	*Ketamine > placebo*	*1*	*96.57*	***<0.0001***	*Ketamine > placebo*	*1*	*27.32*	***<0.0001***	*Ketamine > placebo*	*1*	*142.70*	***<0.0001***	*Ketamine > placebo*
Ketamine effect at 35 min	*1*	*41.12*	***<0.0001***	*Ketamine > placebo*	*1*	*75.97*	***<0.0001***	*Ketamine > placebo*	*1*	*33.83*	***<0.0001***	*Ketamine > placebo*	*1*	*51.34*	***<0.0001***	*Ketamine > placebo*
Ketamine effect at 110 min	*1*	*26.90*	***<0.0001***	*Ketamine > placebo*	*1*	*29.44*	***<0.0001***	*Ketamine > placebo*	*1*	*12.09*	***0.0005***	*Ketamine > placebo*	*1*	*15.17*	***<0.0001***	*Ketamine > placebo*
Ketamine effect at 180 min	*1*	*0.57*	*0.449*		*1*	*3.40*	*0.065*		*1*	*0.00*	*1.000*		*1*	*0.34*	*0.559*	
Nicotine × ketamine × time	2.67	0.04	0.983		3.34	1.00	0.399		3.05	1.34	0.258		3.49	1.00	0.399	

Results are based on a non-parametric mixed-effects model of ranked data with an unstructured variance-covariance matrix and p-values adjusted for ANOVA-type statistics (ATS). Follow-up test results are shown in italics. Significant p-values are shown in bold. Num df, numerator degrees of freedom.

or Ketamine × Nicotine × Time interactions for any of these outcome measures.

P300 AMPLITUDE

Event-related brain potential overlays showing P300 waves and topographic maps are shown in **Figure 1**, P300 peak amplitude and latency means are presented in **Table 4** and histograms showing the effects of the drug conditions on P3b and P3a are shown in **Figure 3**. Results of the Ketamine × Nicotine × Deviant Type × Lead repeated-measures ANOVA for P300 amplitude and latency are presented in **Table 5**.

In terms of main effects, only the effect of Lead was significant, with contrasts indicating equivalent P300 amplitudes at Pz and Cz that were both larger than P300 amplitude at Fz. In terms of two-way interactions, there were significant Ketamine × Lead ($p = 0.02$) and Deviant Type × Lead ($p = 0.001$) effects, with a trend ($p = 0.057$) toward a Deviant Type × Nicotine effect. The Ketamine × Lead effect was parsed by examining the main effects of Ketamine separately for each of the three midline leads, with results showing ketamine to significantly reduce P300 amplitude at electrode Cz ($p = 0.046$), but not at Fz ($p = 0.384$) or Pz ($p = 0.11$). This ketamine-induced reduction of midline vertex P300 amplitude did not significantly depend on Deviant Type ($p = 0.389$). The Deviant Type × Lead effect was parsed by examining lead effects separately for targets and novels, both of which were significant. These Lead effects reflected the typical midline scalp topographies of target P3b amplitude (i.e., Fz < Cz < Pz) and novelty P3a amplitude (i.e., Fz < Cz = Pz). The Deviant Type × Nicotine trend was parsed by examining the main effect of Nicotine for each Deviant Type separately. Nicotine significantly reduced the amplitude of novelty P3a ($p = 0.02$) but not target P3b ($p = 0.737$). No other main effects or interactions were significant.

Table 4 | Means and standard errors for auditory oddball P300 amplitude and latency across the four test sessions.

Condition	Deviant type	Lead	P300 peak			
			Amplitude (μV)		Latency (ms)	
			Mean	SE	Mean	SE
Placebo	Target P3b	Fz	4.232	0.961	283.625	12.659
		Cz	8.423	1.213	274.125	9.003
		Pz	10.981	0.713	288.500	10.544
	Novelty P3a	Fz	7.049	1.052	313.125	17.845
		Cz	11.409	0.727	277.000	12.694
		Pz	11.036	0.727	296.625	14.493
Ketamine alone	Target P3b	Fz	3.043	1.639	338.125	20.994
		Cz	5.490	2.337	333.750	21.874
		Pz	9.744	1.300	341.500	19.991
	Novelty P3a	Fz	7.356	0.935	311.125	15.725
		Cz	9.973	1.480	289.000	17.537
		Pz	8.882	0.886	311.375	13.950
Nicotine alone	Target P3b	Fz	4.698	1.120	292.375	7.426
		Cz	8.792	1.671	280.375	9.653
		Pz	10.990	1.695	284.000	7.778
	Novelty P3a	Fz	6.163	0.870	300.375	14.645
		Cz	9.142	1.471	269.125	9.875
		Pz	8.208	1.331	284.250	13.080
Ketamine + nicotine	Target P3b	Fz	4.126	0.719	311.625	21.304
		Cz	6.741	0.736	306.250	21.445
		Pz	9.790	1.119	315.000	20.376
	Novelty P3a	Fz	5.189	0.614	311.875	10.419
		Cz	6.364	1.108	280.500	13.340
		Pz	5.916	1.185	298.625	13.143

P300 LATENCY

There was a significant main effect of Ketamine ($p = 0.043$) indicating that ketamine delayed P300 latency by 25.44 ms relative to placebo (**Tables 4** and **5**). There was also a significant main effect of Lead ($p = 0.018$) indicating that P300's peak latency was significantly shorter at Cz than at Pz and Fz. No other main effects or interactions were significant (see **Table 5**).

MISMATCH NEGATIVITY AMPLITUDE

Event-related brain potential overlays showing MMN difference waves and topographic maps are shown in **Figure 1**, MMN peak amplitude and latency means are presented in **Table 6**, and histograms showing the effects of the drug conditions on MMN are shown in **Figure 4**. The ANOVA results for MMN amplitude are presented in **Table 7**. None of the main effects were significant, but there were significant Nicotine × Ketamine and Nicotine × Ketamine × Lead interactions. The Nicotine × Ketamine × Lead three-way interaction was parsed by examining the Nicotine × Ketamine effect separately for Fz and Cz. The Nicotine × Ketamine effect was significant at Cz

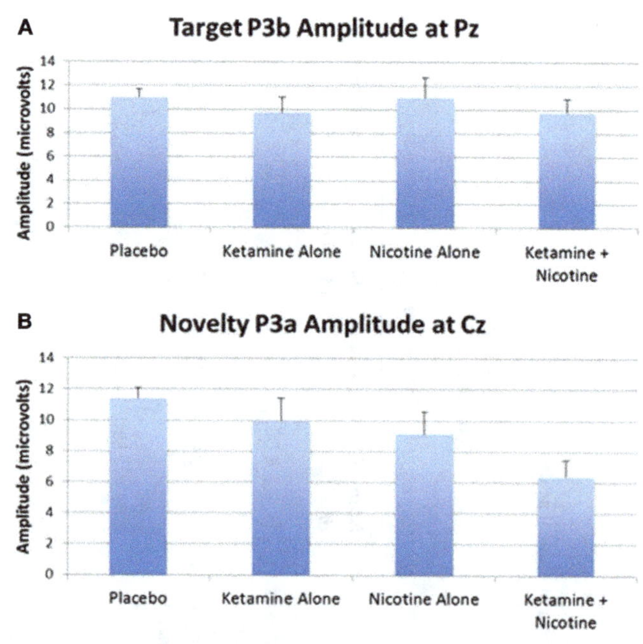

FIGURE 3 | Mean P300 amplitude across four test days. (A) Mean target P3b amplitude for each test day. **(B)** Mean novelty P3a amplitude for each test day. Error bars indicate standard errors.

Table 5 | Analysis of variance (ANOVA) of P300 peak amplitudes and latencies.

Effect	P300 peak amplitude				P300 peak latency		
	df	*F*	*p*-Value	Direction of effect	*F*	*p*-Value	Direction of effect
Deviant type (target vs. novel)	1.7	1.33	0.287		2.72	0.143	
Nicotine (nicotine vs. placebo-nicotine)	1.7	0.85	0.388		1.12	0.325	
Ketamine (ketamine vs. placebo-ketamine)	1.7	3.64	0.098		6.09	**0.043**	Ketamine > placebo
Lead (Fz vs. Cz vs. Pz)	2.6	61.71	**<0.001**	Fz < Cz = Pz	8.52	**0.018**	Cz < Fz = Pz
Deviant type × ketamine	1.7	0.001	0.982		2.21	0.181	
Deviant type × nicotine	1.7	5.20	0.057		0.01	0.912	
Nicotine effect for targets	*1.7*	*0.12*	*0.737*				
Nicotine effect for novels	*1.7*	*9.06*	**0.020**	*Nicotine < placebo*			
Deviant type × lead	2.6	26.95	**0.001**		4.59	0.062	
Lead effect for targets	*2.6*	*53.08*	**<0.001**	*Fz < Cz < Pz*			
Lead effect for novels	*1.7*	*17.69*	**0.001**	*Fz < Cz = Pz*			
Nicotine × ketamine	1.7	0.02	0.900		0.87	0.381	
Nicotine × lead	2.6	0.82	0.486		1.40	0.317	
Ketamine × lead	2.6	8.04	**0.020**		0.34	0.723	
Ketamine effect at Fz	*1.7*	*0.86*	*0.384*				
Ketamine effect at Cz	*1.7*	*5.87*	**0.046**	*Ketamine < placebo*			
Ketamine effect at Pz	*1.7*	*3.34*	*0.110*				
Deviant type × ketamine × lead	2.6	1.11	0.389		0.07	0.932	
Deviant type × nicotine × lead	2.6	2.01	0.215		0.00	1.000	
Deviant type × nicotine × ketamine	1.7	1.02	0.346		0.79	0.405	
Nicotine × ketamine × lead	2.6	0.04	0.958		0.33	0.729	
Deviant type × nicotine × ketamine × lead	2.6	3.16	0.116		0.21	0.818	

ANOVA results are based on mutlivariate assumptions for repeated-measures, and all F-tests are based on Wilks' Lambda. Follow-up ANOVA results are shown in italics. Significant p-values are shown in bold.

Table 6 | Means and standard errors for mismatch negativity amplitude and latency across the four test sessions.

Condition	Lead	MMN peak			
		Amplitude (μV)		Latency (ms)	
		Mean	SE	Mean	SE
Placebo	Fz	−4.591	0.687	196.286	8.216
	Cz	−4.905	0.604	196.143	7.802
Ketamine alone	Fz	−4.216	0.949	179.429	11.487
	Cz	−4.286	1.083	180.143	11.531
Nicotine alone	Fz	−4.270	0.763	201.143	7.561
	Cz	−4.239	0.873	194.143	11.754
Ketamine + nicotine	Fz	−3.890	1.012	177.571	10.040
	Cz	−4.411	1.152	172.000	11.103

($p = 0.015$) but not at Fz ($p = 0.347$). The Nicotine × Ketamine effect at Cz and the overall Nicotine × Ketamine two-way interaction (averaged over leads) were parsed by examining the main effect of each drug condition separately for the active and placebo days of the other drug condition. Nicotine Alone produced a trend level reduction of MMN amplitude relative to Placebo ($p = 0.058$ for Cz; $p = 0.084$ for average of Fz and Cz), but this Nicotine effect was not evident when Nicotine + Ketamine was compared to Ketamine Alone. In contrast, Ketamine did not significantly affect MMN amplitude when administered alone or along with Nicotine. No other interaction effects were significant.

MISMATCH NEGATIVITY LATENCY

Analysis of variance results for MMN latency are presented in **Table 7**. There was a significant main effect of ketamine ($p = 0.025$) indicating that ketamine shortened MMN latency by 19.64 ms relative to placebo. No other main effects or interactions were significant.

PLASMA DRUG LEVELS

Mean plasma levels for ketamine, norketamine, dehydroketamine, and nicotine are presented in **Table 8**. There were no significant differences in levels of plasma ketamine, norketamine, or dehydroketamine levels between the ketamine alone condition and the ketamine–nicotine condition. In addition, there were no significant differences in plasma nicotine levels between the nicotine alone condition and the ketamine–nicotine condition.

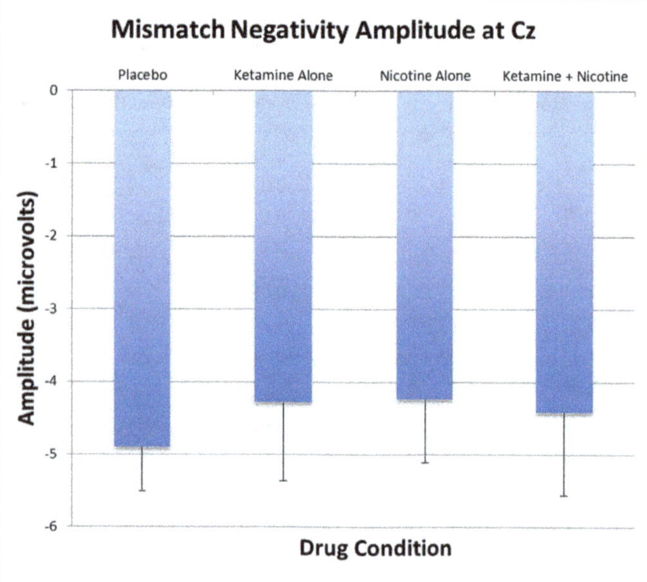

FIGURE 4 | Mean and standard errors for MMN amplitudes recorded at Cz are plotted for the four test days.

DISCUSSION

The principal findings of the current study are the differential effects of ketamine and nicotine on MMN and P300, and their interactive effects on MMN.

EFFECTS OF KETAMINE

Consistent with previous studies (4, 5, 7–13, 120), ketamine induced transient schizophrenia-like behavioral effects in healthy subjects. In terms of the electrophysiological measures, ketamine decreased the amplitude and delayed the latency of P300, regardless of whether P300 was elicited by a target or novel stimulus. The decrease in amplitude is consistent with the other ERP studies showing ketamine to reduce P300 amplitude at parietal leads (46–51), although we did not observe the previously reported increase in novelty P3a at frontal leads with ketamine (51). Our results are also consistent with a prior study showing ketamine to decrease the amplitude of the late positive potential in a working memory task (9). These results provide evidence that glutamatergic neurotransmission at NMDA receptors contribute to P300 generation, both in response to infrequent target stimuli (P3b) and infrequent novel stimuli (P3a). Moreover, inasmuch as P300 amplitude reduction and latency delay are well established in schizophrenia (42, 43, 121, 122), our findings are consistent with the NMDA receptor hypofunction model of schizophrenia (1–3, 5, 6, 123, 124) and its possible role in mediating P300 deficits.

The current study did not find ketamine to significantly reduce MMN amplitude. This conflicts with a number of previous studies (26, 46, 65–68), but is consistent with some studies that either failed to show a ketamine effect on MMN (50) or showed the ketamine-induced MMN reduction to be limited to a subset of task conditions or cortical source locations (26, 65, 67), or to a subgroup of subjects (66). The discrepant results across these studies may be due to differences in the dosage and dosing schedule of ketamine. For example, the study with the most robust effects (26) used a high dose of ketamine (0.9 mg/kg), while the study with a non-significant result (50) used a relatively low dose (0.3 mg/kg). Heekeren and colleagues (65) also demonstrated dose-dependent changes in MMN amplitude using two different doses of ketamine (0.1–0.15 and 0.15–0.20 mg/kg). The absence of a significant ketamine effect on MMN in our study may also have been related to the relatively small size of our subject sample, resulting in limited power to detect an effect. For the ketamine vs. placebo effect on MMN amplitude during the placebo-nicotine day, the effect size (Cohen's d) was estimated to be -0.43. This effect size, which appears to be smaller than the effects reported in prior studies showing ketamine to reduce MMN, would reach significance ($p < 0.05$) with a sample of about 25 subjects. This underscores the limited power in our current study, and points to an effect of ketamine on MMN that may emerge with moderate sample sizes.

However, it is noteworthy that our sample size was sufficiently large to detect robust psychotomimetic effects of ketamine, as well as significant ketamine-induced reductions and delays in the P300 ERP component. Thus, consistent with the report of Oranje and colleagues (50), the P300 ERP component appears to be more sensitive to the effects of NMDA receptor blockade than the MMN component. In terms of MMN latency, ketamine reduced MMN latency by about 19 ms. This effect has not been previously reported to our knowledge, and therefore should be regarded as preliminary pending replication in future studies.

EFFECTS OF NICOTINE

To our knowledge, this is the first study to show nicotine to reduce the novelty P300 (P3a) in humans. This unexpected finding appears to conflict with the plethora of evidence showing nicotine to enhance cognitive functions, including attention (14–16). It is possible to construe the novelty P3a reduction by nicotine as a reflection of enhanced focus on the target detection task and reduced susceptibility to distraction by non-target distractors. However, such an interpretation is not consistent with other evidence showing P3a reduction in patients with schizophrenia (43, 121, 125–128) and patients with frontal lobe lesions (129–131), two conditions known to be associated with attentional impairments and increased distractibility. Thus, nicotine's reduction of the P3a response to novel distractors is unlikely to be a reflection of its cognitive enhancing effects.

We did not observe significant effects of nicotine on target P300 (P3b), inconsistent with some prior reports showing nicotine to increase P300 amplitude (47, 73, 74) and decrease P300 latency (75, 77) in smokers. However, our results are consistent with other studies reporting no effects of nicotine on P300 (76, 78–80). Our study was relatively unique in its use of the intravenous route for nicotine administration, which may partially account for inconsistencies between our results and some prior studies. More generally, inconsistencies among studies may also be related to differences in the type of nicotinic agonist and dosage used, differences in sensory modality of the oddball task used to elicit the P300, and different representations of smokers and non-smokers in the study samples.

The differential effects of nicotine on P3a and P3b in our study is consistent with other evidence that the neuroanatomical (33)

Table 7 | Analysis of variance (ANOVA) of MMN peak amplitudes and latencies.

Effect	df	MMN peak amplitude			MMN peak latency		
		F	p-Value	Direction of effect	F	p-Value	Direction of effect
Nicotine (active-nicotine vs. placebo-nicotine)	1.6	2.04	0.203		0.03	0.875	
Ketamine (active ketamine vs. placebo-ketamine)	1.6	0.20	0.668		8.77	**0.025**	Ketamine < placebo
Lead (Fz vs. Cz)	1.6	1.27	0.302		0.27	0.624	
Nicotine × ketamine	1.6	7.04	**0.038**		0.11	0.756	
Nicotine effect during placebo-ketamine	*1.6*	*4.27*	*0.084*	*Nicotine < placebo*			
Nicotine effect during active ketamine	*1.6*	*0.26*	*0.629*				
Ketamine effect during placebo-nicotine	*1.6*	*1.28*	*0.301*				
Ketamine effect during active-nicotine	*1.6*	*0.47*	*0.519*				
Nicotine × lead	1.6	0.01	0.914		1.81	0.227	
Ketamine × lead	1.6	0.26	0.627		0.04	0.854	
Nicotine × ketamine × lead	1.6	9.50	**0.022**		0.00	0.972	
Nicotine × ketamine at Fz	*1.6*	*1.04*	*0.347*				
Nicotine × ketamine at Cz	*1.6*	*11.38*	***0.015***				
Nicotine effect during placebo-ketamine	*1.6*	*5.48*	*0.058*	*Nicotine < placebo*			
Nicotine effect during active ketamine	*1.6*	*0.003*	*0.960*	*Nicotine ≥ placebo*			
Ketamine effect during placebo-nicotine	*1.6*	*1.40*	*0.281*	*Ketamine ≤ placebo*			
Ketamine effect during active-nicotine	*1.6*	*2.94*	*0.137*	*Ketamine ≥ placebo*			

ANOVA results are based on mutlivariate assumptions for repeated-measures, and all F-tests are based on Wilks' Lambda. Follow-up ANOVA results are shown in italics. Significant p-values are shown in bold.

Table 8 | Plasma ketamine, norketamine, dehydroketamine and nicotine levels.

Blood level (ng/ml)	Time	Placebo	Ketamine alone	Nicotine alone	Ketamine + nicotine
Ketamine	+35		174.91 (59.92)		171.22 (62.21)
	+98		222.40 (57.55)		229.78 (64.52)
Norketamine	+35		70.82 (32.61)		73.78 (40.92)
	+98		147.20 (52.21)		138.67 (45.92)
Dehydroketamine	+35		16.09 (9.86)		17.78 (9.04)
	+98		42.20 (19.77)		42.33 (23.52)
Nicotine	+35			6.92 (3.23)	10.18 (4.31)
	+98			6.65 (2.63)	12.93 (7.01)

Ketamine levels were assayed only on the days that subjects received ketamine (ketamine alone and ketamine + nicotine) and nicotine was assayed only on the days that subjects received nicotine (nicotine alone and nicotine + ketamine).

and neurochemical (71) underpinnings of P3a and P3b are at least partially dissociable. Polich and Criado (71) proposed dopaminergic/frontal processes for P3a generation and locus coeruleus-mediated noradrenergic/parietal processes for P3b generation. Evidence for this includes demonstrations that chronic abuse of different street drugs are associated with differential effects on P3a and P3b amplitudes (71). Nonetheless, roles for nicotinic cholinergic neurotransmission, as well as glutamatergic neurotransmission, have not figured prominently in prior neurochemical models of P300 generation.

Nicotine alone produced a trend level reduction of MMN amplitude, but this effect was not evident when comparing the Nicotine + Ketamine condition to Ketamine alone. These results conflict with some prior studies showing nicotine or nicotinic agonists to enhance MMN amplitude in response to duration (85), frequency (86, 87), or inter-stimulus interval (88) deviants in healthy volunteers, and similarly failed to corroborate studies showing nicotine to enhance duration-deviant MMN amplitude in schizophrenia patients (98). One possible reason for the discrepancy between our findings and those reported previously is that our study used an intravenous route of nicotine administration whereas prior studies used either gum (85, 88, 98) or a transdermal patch (87). While differences in the pharmacokinetics and pharmacodynamics between intravenous vs. gum and transdermal routes of administration have not been systematically studied', it is likely that time to onset of action and peak levels achieved would differ between these modes of nicotine delivery, and such differences could account for variability in the effects of nicotine on

MMN. At the same time, it should be noted that a number of studies using gum (47, 99) or transdermal patches (89, 90) failed to demonstrate an enhancement of MMN amplitude by nicotine. Moreover, the fact that our study focused on duration-deviant MMN, in part because of evidence that it is more sensitive to schizophrenia than other types of MMN (58, 60, 61) cannot be the reason we failed to observe enhancement by nicotine, since at least two prior studies have shown the amplitude of the duration-deviant MMN to be increased by nicotine [Ref. (85, 98); but, see Ref. (99)].

COMBINED EFFECT OF KETAMINE AND NICOTINE

Discordant with the study hypothesis, nicotine did not improve either the behavioral or neurophysiological abnormalities induced by ketamine. Of the many drugs tested in the ketamine model, few have been shown to reduce the schizophrenia-like behavioral and cognitive effects of ketamine in healthy human subjects. Lamotrigine, but not haloperidol or lorazepam, has been shown to reduce some of the behavioral and cognitive symptoms induced by ketamine in healthy volunteers (132–134). With previous findings from animal and human studies documenting cognitive enhancing effects of nicotine in humans (135–138) and animals (139, 140), including animal data showing nicotine to ameliorate NMDA-antagonist induced cognitive deficits (106, 107) or NMDA-antagonists to block cognitive enhancing effects of nicotine (108), it was surprising that nicotine did not show any tendency to reverse ketamine's psychotomimetic or cognitive ERP effects. Inconsistencies among studies may be due to differences in nicotine dose, rate, and route of nicotine administration, and the smoking status of the subjects tested. Importantly, our results are consistent with other studies showing that nicotine did not block ketamine's deleterious effects on P300 (47) or on neurocognitive test performance (141) in humans, suggesting that any pro-cognitive effects of nicotine may not be able to overcome the impairments produced by NMDA receptor blockade. However, our results were not consistent with a prior study that showed nicotine to prevent ketamine's reduction on MMN amplitude, an effect that was only observed in the subgroup of healthy volunteers with a high propensity to have hallucinatory experiences (66). However, this prior study used a substantially lower dose of ketamine than used in the current study, and nicotine was administered with chewing gum rather than the intravenous route employed here.

LIMITATIONS

The main limitations of the current study include the small sample size, the high dropout rate, the heterogeneous smoking status of our sample, and the use of only one dose of nicotine. Future studies aimed at elucidating the effects of nicotine on patients with schizophrenia by using pharmacological models of psychosis in healthy volunteers must consider the fact that the large majority of schizophrenia patients are significantly dependent on nicotine. Accordingly, for studies about nAChR function to be relevant to schizophrenia, heavy smokers need to be included in the subject sample. However, the inclusion of nicotine-dependent heavy smokers in such studies raises the question of when to schedule the nicotine challenge relative to the timing of their last cigarette. Studying smokers who have been asked to abstain from smoking for several hours or more prior to study onset would mean studying them in a nicotine-withdrawal state. On the other hand, studying smokers who have smoked recently and are in a nicotine-satiated state may obscure the effects of intravenous nicotine. Further complicating this issue, studying non-smokers would result in high dropout routes because nicotine is generally unpleasant to non-smokers. Moreover, data from non-smokers may not generalize to schizophrenia patients, most of whom are heavy smokers.

In conclusion, the results of this study suggest that activation of nACH receptors does not influence ketamine's psychotomimetic effects or physiological effects on MMN and P300 in healthy human volunteers. However, ketamine and nicotine appear to have independent effects on P3a, P3b, and MMN suggesting differential effects of nACH and NMDA receptor systems on these ERP components. Moreover, this is the first study to report a significant reduction in P3a amplitude by nicotine.

ACKNOWLEDGMENTS

The authors also thank Angelina Genovese, R.N.C., M.B.A.; Elizabeth O'Donnell, R.N.; Brenda Breault, R.N., B.S.N.; Sonah Yoo, R.Ph.; Robert Sturwold, R.Ph.; and Willie Ford of the Neurobiological Studies Unit at the VA Connecticut Healthcare System, West Haven Campus for their central contributions to the success of this project. The authors also acknowledge the contributions of John Krystal, MD for his role in providing the impetus in conducting the study. The Department of Veterans Affairs Schizophrenia Biological Research Center and a NARSAD Young Investigator Award to Hyun-Sang Cho supported this study.

REFERENCES

1. Coyle JT, Tsai G, Goff D. Converging evidence of NMDA receptor hypofunction in the pathophysiology of schizophrenia. *Ann N Y Acad Sci* (2003) **1003**:318–27. doi:10.1196/annals.1300.020
2. Javitt DC, Zukin SR. Recent advances in the phencyclidine model of schizophrenia. *Am J Psychiatry* (1991) **148**:1301–8.
3. Javitt DC, Zukin SR, Heresco-Levy U, Umbricht D. Has an angel shown the way? Etiological and therapeutic implications of the PCP/NMDA model of schizophrenia. *Schizophr Bull* (2012) **38**:958–66. doi:10.1093/schbul/sbs069
4. Krystal JH, Anand A, Moghaddam B. Effects of NMDA receptor antagonists: implications for the pathophysiology of schizophrenia. *Arch Gen Psychiatry* (2002) **59**:663–4. doi:10.1001/archpsyc.59.7.663
5. Krystal JH, D'Souza DC, Mathalon D, Perry E, Belger A, Hoffman R. NMDA receptor antagonist effects, cortical glutamatergic function, and schizophrenia: toward a paradigm shift in medication development. *Psychopharmacology (Berl)* (2003) **169**:215–33. doi:10.1007/s00213-003-1582-z
6. Moghaddam B, Javitt D. From revolution to evolution: the glutamate hypothesis of schizophrenia and its implication for treatment. *Neuropsychopharmacology* (2012) **37**:4–15. doi:10.1038/npp.2011.181
7. Moghaddam B, Krystal JH. Capturing the angel in "angel dust": twenty years of translational neuroscience studies of NMDA receptor antagonists in animals and humans. *Schizophr Bull* (2012) **38**:942–9. doi:10.1093/schbul/sbs075
8. Adler CM, Goldberg TE, Malhotra AK, Pickar D, Breier A. Effects of ketamine on thought disorder, working memory, and semantic memory in healthy volunteers. *Biol Psychiatry* (1998) **43**:811–6. doi:10.1016/S0006-3223(97)00556-8
9. Ahn KH, Youn T, Cho SS, Ha TH, Ha KS, Kim MS, et al. N-methyl-D-aspartate receptor in working memory impairments in schizophrenia: event-related potential study of late stage of working memory process. *Prog Neuropsychopharmacol Biol Psychiatry* (2003) **27**:993–9. doi:10.1016/S0278-5846(03)00159-3
10. Krystal JH, Karper LP, Seibyl JP, Freeman GK, Delaney R, Bremner JD, et al. Subanesthetic effects of the noncompetitive NMDA antagonist, ketamine,

in humans. Psychotomimetic, perceptual, cognitive, and neuroendocrine responses. *Arch Gen Psychiatry* (1994) **51**:199–214. doi:10.1001/archpsyc.1994.03950030035004

11. Lahti AC, Weiler MA, Tamara Michaelidis BA, Parwani A, Tamminga CA. Effects of ketamine in normal and schizophrenic volunteers. *Neuropsychopharmacology* (2001) **25**:455–67. doi:10.1016/S0893-133X(01)00243-3
12. Malhotra AK, Pinals DA, Weingartner H, Sirocco K, Missar CD, Pickar D, et al. NMDA receptor function and human cognition: the effects of ketamine in healthy volunteers. *Neuropsychopharmacology* (1996) **14**:301–7. doi:10.1016/0893-133X(95)00137-3
13. Morgan CJ, Mofeez A, Brandner B, Bromley L, Curran HV. Acute effects of ketamine on memory systems and psychotic symptoms in healthy volunteers. *Neuropsychopharmacology* (2004) **29**:208–18. doi:10.1038/sj.npp.1300342
14. Newhouse PA, Potter A, Singh A. Effects of nicotinic stimulation on cognitive performance. *Curr Opin Pharmacol* (2004) **4**:36–46. doi:10.1016/j.coph.2003.11.001
15. Rezvani AH, Levin ED. Cognitive effects of nicotine. *Biol Psychiatry* (2001) **49**:258–67. doi:10.1016/S0006-3223(00)01094-5
16. Swan GE, Lessov-Schlaggar CN. The effects of tobacco smoke and nicotine on cognition and the brain. *Neuropsychol Rev* (2007) **17**:259–73. doi:10.1007/s11065-007-9035-9
17. Park S, Knopick C, McGurk S, Meltzer HY. Nicotine impairs spatial working memory while leaving spatial attention intact. *Neuropsychopharmacology* (2000) **22**:200–9. doi:10.1016/S0893-133X(99)00098-6
18. Sakurai Y, Kanazawa I. Acute effects of cigarettes in non-deprived smokers on memory, calculation and executive functions. *Hum Psychopharmacol* (2002) **17**:369–73. doi:10.1002/hup.424
19. George TP, Vessicchio JC, Termine A, Sahady DM, Head CA, Pepper WT, et al. Effects of smoking abstinence on visuospatial working memory function in schizophrenia. *Neuropsychopharmacology* (2002) **26**:75–85. doi:10.1016/S0893-133X(01)00296-2
20. Kumari V, Postma P. Nicotine use in schizophrenia: the self medication hypotheses. *Neurosci Biobehav Rev* (2005) **29**:1021–34. doi:10.1016/j.neubiorev.2005.02.006
21. Sacco KA, Bannon KL, George TP. Nicotinic receptor mechanisms and cognition in normal states and neuropsychiatric disorders. *J Psychopharmacol* (2004) **18**:457–74. doi:10.1177/0269881104047273
22. Hetem LA, Danion JM, Diemunsch P, Brandt C. Effect of a subanesthetic dose of ketamine on memory and conscious awareness in healthy volunteers. *Psychopharmacology (Berl)* (2000) **152**:283–8. doi:10.1007/s002130000511
23. Honey RA, Turner DC, Honey GD, Sharar SR, Kumaran D, Pomarol-Clotet E, et al. Subdissociative dose ketamine produces a deficit in manipulation but not maintenance of the contents of working memory. *Neuropsychopharmacology* (2003) **28**:2037–44. doi:10.1038/sj.npp.1300272
24. Krystal JH, Bennett A, Abi-Saab D, Belger A, Karper LP, D'Souza DC, et al. Dissociation of ketamine effects on rule acquisition and rule implementation: possible relevance to NMDA receptor contributions to executive cognitive functions. *Biol Psychiatry* (2000) **47**:137–43. doi:10.1016/S0006-3223(99)00097-9
25. Rowland LM, Astur RS, Jung RE, Bustillo JR, Lauriello J, Yeo RA. Selective cognitive impairments associated with NMDA receptor blockade in humans. *Neuropsychopharmacology* (2005) **30**:633–9. doi:10.1038/sj.npp.1300642
26. Umbricht D, Schmid L, Koller R, Vollenweider FX, Hell D, Javitt DC. Ketamine-induced deficits in auditory and visual context-dependent processing in healthy volunteers: implications for models of cognitive deficits in schizophrenia. *Arch Gen Psychiatry* (2000) **57**:1139–47. doi:10.1001/archpsyc.57.12.1139
27. Polich J. Updating P300: an integrative theory of P3a and P3b. *Clin Neurophysiol* (2007) **118**:2128–48. doi:10.1016/j.clinph.2007.04.019
28. Isreal JB, Chesney GL, Wickens CD, Donchin E. P300 and tracking difficulty: evidence for multiple resources in dual-task performance. *Psychophysiology* (1980) **17**:259–73. doi:10.1111/j.1469-8986.1980.tb00146.x
29. Kramer AF, Strayer DL. Assessing the development of automatic processing: an application of dual-task and event-related brain potential methodologies. *Biol Psychol* (1988) **26**:231–67. doi:10.1016/0301-0511(88)90022-1
30. Ravden D, Polich J. Habituation of P300 from visual stimuli. *Int J Psychophysiol* (1998) **30**:359–65. doi:10.1016/S0167-8760(98)00039-7
31. Johnson R Jr, Donchin E. P300 and stimulus categorization: two plus one is not so different from one plus one. *Psychophysiology* (1980) **17**:167–78. doi:10.1111/j.1469-8986.1980.tb00131.x
32. Donchin E, Coles M. Is the P300 component a manifestation of context updating? (Commentary on Verleger's critique of the context updating model). *Behav Brain Sci* (1988) **11**:357–74. doi:10.1017/S0140525X00058027
33. Halgren E, Marinkovic K, Chauvel P. Generators of the late cognitive potentials in auditory and visual oddball tasks. *Electroencephalogr Clin Neurophysiol* (1998) **106**:156–64. doi:10.1016/S0013-4694(97)00119-3
34. Smith ME, Halgren E, Sokolik M, Baudena P, Musolino A, Liegeois-Chauvel C, et al. The intracranial topography of the P3 event-related potential elicited during auditory oddball. *Electroencephalogr Clin Neurophysiol* (1990) **76**:235–48. doi:10.1016/0013-4694(90)90018-F
35. Dien J, Spencer KM, Donchin E. Parsing the late positive complex: mental chronometry and the ERP components that inhabit the neighborhood of the P300. *Psychophysiology* (2004) **41**:665–78. doi:10.1111/j.1469-8986.2004.00193.x
36. Polich J, Kok A. Cognitive and biological determinants of P300: an integrative review. *Biol Psychol* (1995) **41**:103–46. doi:10.1016/0301-0511(95)05130-9
37. Spencer KM, Dien J, Donchin E. Spatiotemporal analysis of the late ERP responses to deviant stimuli. *Psychophysiology* (2001) **38**:343–58. doi:10.1111/1469-8986.3820343
38. Squires NK, Squires KC, Hillyard SA. Two varieties of long-latency positive waves evoked by unpredictable auditory stimuli in man. *Electroencephalogr Clin Neuropysiol* (1975) **38**:387–401. doi:10.1016/0013-4694(75)90263-1
39. Comerchero MD, Polich J. P3a, perceptual distinctiveness, and stimulus modality. *Brain Res Cogn Brain Res* (1998) **7**:41–8. doi:10.1016/S0926-6410(98)00009-3
40. Courchesne E, Hillyard S, Galambos R. Stimulus novelty, task relevance and the visual evoked potential in man. *Electroencephalogr Clin Neurophysiol* (1975) **39**:131–43. doi:10.1016/0013-4694(75)90003-6
41. Goldstein A, Spencer KM, Donchin E. The influence of stimulus deviance and novelty on the P300 and novelty P3. *Psychophysiology* (2002) **39**:781–90. doi:10.1111/1469-8986.3960781
42. Bramon E, Rabe-Hesketh S, Sham P, Murray RM, Frangou S. Meta-analysis of the P300 and P50 waveforms in schizophrenia. *Schizophr Res* (2004) **70**:315–29. doi:10.1016/j.schres.2004.01.004
43. Jeon YW, Polich J. Meta-analysis of P300 and schizophrenia: patients, paradigms, and practical implications. *Psychophysiology* (2003) **40**:684–701. doi:10.1111/1469-8986.00070
44. Charles G, Hansenne M. P 300 slow potential. Clinical interest in 3 mental diseases and neurobiology: a review. *Encephale* (1992) 18:225-236.
45. Hansenne M. The p300 cognitive event-related potential. II. Individual variability and clinical application in psychopathology. *Neurophysiol Clin* (2000) **30**:211–31. doi:10.1016/S0987-7053(00)00224-0
46. Gunduz-Bruce H, Reinhart RM, Roach BJ, Gueorguieva R, Oliver S, D'Souza DC, et al. Glutamatergic modulation of auditory information processing in the human brain. *Biol Psychiatry* (2012) **71**:969–77. doi:10.1016/j.biopsych.2011.09.031
47. Knott V, Millar AM, McIntosh JF, Shah DK, Fisher DJ, Blais CM, et al. Separate and combined effects of low dose ketamine and nicotine on behavioural and neural correlates of sustained attention. *Biol Psychol* (2011) **88**:83–93. doi:10.1016/j.biopsycho.2011.06.012
48. Musso F, Brinkmeyer J, Ecker D, London MK, Thieme G, Warbrick T, et al. Ketamine effects on brain function – simultaneous fMRI/EEG during a visual oddball task. *Neuroimage* (2011) **58**:508–25. doi:10.1016/j.neuroimage.2011.06.045
49. Oranje B, Gispen-de Wied CC, Westenberg HG, Kemner C, Verbaten MN, Kahn RS. Haloperidol counteracts the ketamine-induced disruption of processing negativity, but not that of the P300 amplitude. *Int J Neuropsychopharmacol* (2009) **12**:823–32. doi:10.1017/S1461145708009814
50. Oranje B, van Berckel BN, Kemner C, van Ree JM, Kahn RS, Verbaten MN. The effects of a sub-anaesthetic dose of ketamine on human selective attention. *Neuropsychopharmacology* (2000) **22**:293–302. doi:10.1016/S0893-133X(99)00118-9
51. Watson TD, Petrakis IL, Edgecombe J, Perrino A, Krystal JH, Mathalon DH. Modulation of the cortical processing of novel and target stimuli by drugs affecting glutamate and GABA neurotransmission. *Int J Neuropsychopharmacol* (2009) **12**:357–70. doi:10.1017/S1461145708009334
52. Naatanen R, Alho K. Mismatch negativity – a unique measure of sensory processing in audition. *Int J Neurosci* (1995) **80**:317–37. doi:10.3109/00207459508986107

53. Naatanen R, Gaillard AW, Mantysalo S. Early selective-attention effect on evoked potential reinterpreted. *Acta Psychol (Amst)* (1978) **42**:313–29. doi:10.1016/0001-6918(78)90006-9
54. Stephan KE, Baldeweg T, Friston KJ. Synaptic plasticity and dysconnection in schizophrenia. *Biol Psychiatry* (2006) **59**:929–39. doi:10.1016/j.biopsych.2005.10.005
55. Stephan KE, Friston KJ, Frith CD. Dysconnection in schizophrenia: from abnormal synaptic plasticity to failures of self-monitoring. *Schizophr Bull* (2009) **35**:509–27. doi:10.1093/schbul/sbn176
56. Garrido MI, Kilner JM, Stephan KE, Friston KJ. The mismatch negativity: a review of underlying mechanisms. *Neurophysiol Clin* (2009) **120**:453–63. doi:10.1016/j.clinph.2008.11.029
57. Naatanen R, Pakarinen S, Rinne T, Takegata R. The mismatch negativity (MMN): towards the optimal paradigm. *Clin Neurophysiol* (2004) **115**:140–4. doi:10.1016/j.clinph.2003.04.001
58. Michie PT. What has MMN revealed about the auditory system in schizophrenia? *Int J Psychophysiol* (2001) **42**:177–94. doi:10.1016/S0167-8760(01)00166-0
59. Todd J, Michie PT, Schall U, Karayanidis F, Yabe H, Naatanen R. Deviant matters: duration, frequency, and intensity deviants reveal different patterns of mismatch negativity reduction in early and late schizophrenia. *Biol Psychiatry* (2008) **63**:58–64. doi:10.1016/j.biopsych.2007.02.016
60. Umbricht D, Krljes S. Mismatch negativity in schizophrenia: a meta-analysis. *Schizophr Res* (2005) **76**:1–23. doi:10.1016/j.schres.2004.12.002
61. Naatanen R, Kahkonen S. Central auditory dysfunction in schizophrenia as revealed by the mismatch negativity (MMN) and its magnetic equivalent MMNm: a review. *Int J Neuropsychopharmacol* (2009) **12**:125–35. doi:10.1017/S1461145708009322
62. Umbricht D, Koller R, Schmid L, Skrabo A, Grubel C, Huber T, et al. How specific are deficits in mismatch negativity generation to schizophrenia? *Biol Psychiatry* (2003) **53**:1120–31. doi:10.1016/S0006-3223(02)01642-6
63. Javitt DC, Steinschneider M, Schroeder CE, Arezzo JC. Role of cortical N-methyl-D-aspartate receptors in auditory sensory memory and mismatch negativity generation: implications for schizophrenia. *Proc Natl Acad Sci U S A* (1996) **93**:11962–7. doi:10.1073/pnas.93.21.11962
64. Javitt DC, Steinschneider M, Schroeder CE, Vaughan HG Jr, Arezzo JC. Detection of stimulus deviance within primate primary auditory cortex: intracortical mechanisms of mismatch negativity (MMN) generation. *Brain Res* (1994) **667**:192–200. doi:10.1016/0006-8993(94)91496-6
65. Heekeren K, Daumann J, Neukirch A, Stock C, Kawohl W, Norra C, et al. Mismatch negativity generation in the human 5HT2A agonist and NMDA antagonist model of psychosis. *Psychopharmacology (Berl)* (2008) **199**:77–88. doi:10.1007/s00213-008-1129-4
66. Knott V, Shah D, Millar A, McIntosh J, Fisher D, Blais C, et al. Nicotine, auditory sensory memory, and sustained attention in a human ketamine model of schizophrenia: moderating influence of a hallucinatory trait. *Front Pharmacol* (2012) **3**:172. doi:10.3389/fphar.2012.00172
67. Kreitschmann-Andermahr I, Rosburg T, Demme U, Gaser E, Nowak H, Sauer H. Effect of ketamine on the neuromagnetic mismatch field in healthy humans. *Brain Res Cogn Brain Res* (2001) **12**:109–16. doi:10.1016/S0926-6410(01)00043-X
68. Schmidt A, Bachmann R, Kometer M, Csomor PA, Stephan KE, Seifritz E, et al. Mismatch negativity encoding of prediction errors predicts S-ketamine-induced cognitive impairments. *Neuropsychopharmacology* (2012) **37**:865–75. doi:10.1038/npp.2011.261
69. Froeliger B, Gilbert DG, McClernon FJ. Effects of nicotine on novelty detection and memory recognition performance: double-blind, placebo-controlled studies of smokers and nonsmokers. *Psychopharmacology (Berl)* (2009) **205**:625–33. doi:10.1007/s00213-009-1571-y
70. Pineda JA, Herrera C, Kang C, Sandler A. Effects of cigarette smoking and 12-h abstention on working memory during a serial-probe recognition task. *Psychopharmacology (Berl)* (1998) **139**:311–21. doi:10.1007/s002130050722
71. Polich J, Criado JR. Neuropsychology and neuropharmacology of P3a and P3b. *Int J Psychophysiol* (2006) **60**:172–85. doi:10.1016/j.ijpsycho.2005.12.012
72. Pritchard W, Sokhadze E, Houlihan M. Effects of nicotine and smoking on event-related potentials: a review. *Nicotine Tob Res* (2004) **6**:961–84. doi:10.1080/14622200412331324848
73. Houlihan ME, Pritchard WS, Robinson JH. Effects of smoking/nicotine on performance and event-related potentials during a short-term memory scanning task. *Psychopharmacology (Berl)* (2001) **156**:388–96. doi:10.1007/s002130100751
74. Knott V, Bosman M, Mahoney C, Ilivitsky V, Quirt K. Transdermal nicotine: single dose effects on mood, EEG, performance, and event-related potentials. *Pharmacol Biochem Behav* (1999) **63**:253–61. doi:10.1016/S0091-3057(99)00006-4
75. Kodama E, Morita K, Kinoshita S, Miyahira A, Nakamura J, Maeda H. Inhibitory effect of smoking on event-related potentials in schizophrenic patients: comparison with healthy subjects. *Prog Neuropsychopharmacol Biol Psychiatry* (1998) **22**:1275–88. doi:10.1016/S0278-5846(98)00082-7
76. Edwards JA, Wesnes K, Warburton DM, Gale A. Evidence of more rapid stimulus evaluation following cigarette smoking. *Addict Behav* (1985) **10**:113–26. doi:10.1016/0306-4603(85)90017-6
77. Houlihan ME, Pritchard WS, Robinson JH. Faster P300 latency after smoking in visual but not auditory oddball tasks. *Psychopharmacology (Berl)* (1996) **123**:231–8. doi:10.1007/BF02246577
78. Knott V, McIntosh J, Millar A, Fisher D, Villeneuve C, Ilivitsky V, et al. Nicotine and smoker status moderate brain electric and mood activation induced by ketamine, an N-methyl-D-aspartate (NMDA) receptor antagonist. *Pharmacol Biochem Behav* (2006) **85**:228–42. doi:10.1016/j.pbb.2006.08.005
79. Lindgren M, Molander L, Verbaan C, Lunell E, Rosen I. Electroencephalographic effects of intravenous nicotine – a dose-response study. *Psychopharmacology (Berl)* (1999) **145**:342–50. doi:10.1007/s002130051067
80. Lindgren M, Stenberg G, Rosen I. Effects of nicotine in a bimodal attention task. *Neuropsychobiology* (1998) **38**:42–9. doi:10.1159/000026515
81. Michel C, Hasenfratz M, Nil R, Battig K. Cardiovascular, electrocortical, and behavioral effects of nicotine chewing gum. *Klin Wochenschr* (1988) **66**(Suppl 11):72–9.
82. Anokhin AP, Vedeniapin AB, Sirevaag EJ, Bauer LO, O'Connor SJ, Kuperman S, et al. The P300 brain potential is reduced in smokers. *Psychopharmacology (Berl)* (2000) **149**:409–13. doi:10.1007/s002130000387
83. Neuhaus A, Bajbouj M, Kienast T, Kalus P, von Haebler D, Winterer G, et al. Persistent dysfunctional frontal lobe activation in former smokers. *Psychopharmacology (Berl)* (2006) **186**:191–200. doi:10.1007/s00213-006-0366-7
84. Ascioglu M, Dolu N, Golgeli A, Suer C, Ozesmi C. Effects of cigarette smoking on cognitive processing. *Int J Neurosci* (2004) **114**:381–90. doi:10.1080/00207450490270668
85. Baldeweg T, Wong D, Stephan KE. Nicotinic modulation of human auditory sensory memory: evidence from mismatch negativity potentials. *Int J Psychophysiol* (2006) **59**:49–58. doi:10.1016/j.ijpsycho.2005.07.014
86. Dunbar G, Boeijinga PH, Demazieres A, Cisterni C, Kuchibhatla R, Wesnes K, et al. Effects of TC-1734 (AZD3480), a selective neuronal nicotinic receptor agonist, on cognitive performance and the EEG of young healthy male volunteers. *Psychopharmacology* (2007) **191**:919–29. doi:10.1007/s00213-006-0675-x
87. Harkrider AW, Hedrick MS. Acute effect of nicotine on auditory gating in smokers and non-smokers. *Hear Res* (2005) **202**:114–28. doi:10.1016/j.heares.2004.11.009
88. Martin LF, Davalos DB, Kisley MA. Nicotine enhances automatic temporal processing as measured by the mismatch negativity waveform. *Nicotine Tob Res* (2009) **11**:698–706. doi:10.1093/ntr/ntp052
89. Inami R, Kirino E, Inoue R, Arai H. Transdermal nicotine administration enhances automatic auditory processing reflected by mismatch negativity. *Pharmacol Biochem Behav* (2005) **80**:453–61. doi:10.1016/j.pbb.2005.01.001
90. Inami R, Kirino E, Inoue R, Suzuki T, Arai H. Nicotine effects on mismatch negativity in nonsmoking schizophrenic patients. *Neuropsychobiology* (2007) **56**:64–72. doi:10.1159/000111536
91. Knott V, Heenan A, Shah D, Bolton K, Fisher D, Villeneuve C. Electrophysiological evidence of nicotine's distracter-filtering properties in non-smokers. *J Psychopharmacol* (2011) **25**:239–48. doi:10.1177/0269881109348158
92. Dalack GW, Healy DJ, Meador-Woodruff JH. Nicotine dependence in schizophrenia: clinical phenomena and laboratory findings. *Am J Psychiatry* (1998) **155**:1490–501.
93. de Leon J, Diaz FJ. A meta-analysis of worldwide studies demonstrates an association between schizophrenia and tobacco smoking behaviors. *Schizophr Res* (2005) **76**:135–57. doi:10.1016/j.schres.2005.02.010

94. Hughes JR, Hatsukami DK, Mitchell JE, Dahlgren LA. Prevalence of smoking among psychiatric outpatients. *Am J Psychiatry* (1986) **143**:993–7.
95. Ziedonis DM, George TP. Schizophrenia and nicotine use: report of a pilot smoking cessation program and review of neurobiological and clinical issues. *Schizophr Bull* (1997) **23**:247–54. doi:10.1093/schbul/23.2.247
96. Adler LE, Hoffer LD, Wiser A, Freedman R. Normalization of auditory physiology by cigarette smoking in schizophrenic patients. *Am J Psychiatry* (1993) **150**:1856–61.
97. Olincy A, Harris JG, Johnson LL, Pender V, Kongs S, Allensworth D, et al. Proof-of-concept trial of an alpha7 nicotinic agonist in schizophrenia. *Arch Gen Psychiatry* (2006) **63**:630–8. doi:10.1001/archpsyc.63.6.630
98. Dulude L, Labelle A, Knott VJ. Acute nicotine alteration of sensory memory impairment in smokers with schizophrenia. *J Clin Psychopharmacol* (2010) **30**:541–8. doi:10.1097/JCP.0b013e3181f0c9c6
99. Fisher DJ, Grant B, Smith DM, Borracci G, Labelle A, Knott VJ. Nicotine and the hallucinating brain: effects on mismatch negativity (MMN) in schizophrenia. *Psychiatry Res* (2012) **196**:181–7. doi:10.1016/j.psychres.2012.01.026
100. McGehee DS, Heath MJ, Gelber S, Devay P, Role LW. Nicotine enhancement of fast excitatory synaptic transmission in CNS by presynaptic receptors. *Science* (1995) **269**:1692–6. doi:10.1126/science.7569895
101. Alkondon M, Pereira EF, Eisenberg HM, Albuquerque EX. Nicotinic receptor activation in human cerebral cortical interneurons: a mechanism for inhibition and disinhibition of neuronal networks. *J Neurosci* (2000) **20**:66–75.
102. Ji D, Dani JA. Inhibition and disinhibition of pyramidal neurons by activation of nicotinic receptors on hippocampal interneurons. *J Neurophysiol* (2000) **83**:2682–90.
103. Gioanni Y, Rougeot C, Clarke PB, Lepouse C, Thierry AM, Vidal C. Nicotinic receptors in the rat prefrontal cortex: increase in glutamate release and facilitation of mediodorsal thalamo-cortical transmission. *Eur J Neurosci* (1999) **11**:18–30. doi:10.1046/j.1460-9568.1999.00403.x
104. Lambe EK, Picciotto MR, Aghajanian GK. Nicotine induces glutamate release from thalamocortical terminals in prefrontal cortex. *Neuropsychopharmacology* (2003) **28**:216–25. doi:10.1038/sj.npp.1300032
105. Radcliffe KA, Fisher JL, Gray R, Dani JA. Nicotinic modulation of glutamate and GABA synaptic transmission of hippocampal neurons. *Ann N Y Acad Sci* (1999) **868**:591–610. doi:10.1111/j.1749-6632.1999.tb11332.x
106. Levin ED, Bettegowda C, Weaver T, Christopher NC. Nicotine-dizocilpine interactions and working and reference memory performance of rats in the radial-arm maze. *Pharmacol Biochem Behav* (1998) **61**:335–40. doi:10.1016/S0091-3057(98)00109-9
107. Rezvani AH, Levin ED. Nicotinic-glutamatergic interactions and attentional performance on an operant visual signal detection task in female rats. *Eur J Pharmacol* (2003) **465**:83–90. doi:10.1016/S0014-2999(03)01439-0
108. Ciamei A, Aversano M, Cestari V, Castellano C. Effects of MK-801 and nicotine combinations on memory consolidation in CD1 mice. *Psychopharmacology (Berl)* (2001) **154**:126–30. doi:10.1007/s002130000584
109. Spitzer RL, Williams JB, Gibbon M, First MB. *Structured Clinical Interview for DSM-III-R – Non-Patient Edition (SCID-NP, Version 1.0 with Supplement for DSM-IV).* Washington, DC: American Psychiatric Press (1990).
110. Wechsler D. *Manual for the Wechsler Adult Intelligence Scale.* New York: Psychological Corporation (1955). 110 p.
111. Heatherton T, Kozlowski L, Frecker R, Fagerstrom K. The Fagerstrom test for nicotine dependence: a revision of the Fagerstrom tolerance questionnaire. *Br J Addict* (1991) **86**:1119–27. doi:10.1111/j.1360-0443.1991.tb01879.x
112. Kay S, Fiszbein A, Opler L. The Positive and Negative Syndrome Scale (PANSS) for schizophrenia. *Schizophr Bull* (1987) **13**:261–76. doi:10.1093/schbul/13.2.261
113. Bremner JD, Krystal JH, Putnam FW, Southwick SM, Marmar C, Charney DS, et al. Measurement of dissociative states with the Clinician-Administered Dissociative States Scale (CADSS). *J Trauma Stress* (1998) **11**:125–36. doi:10.1023/A:1024465317902
114. Krystal JH, Perry EB Jr, Gueorguieva R, Belger A, Madonick SH, Abi-Dargham A, et al. Comparative and interactive human psychopharmacologic effects of ketamine and amphetamine: implications for glutamatergic and dopaminergic model psychoses and cognitive function. *Arch Gen Psychiatry* (2005) **62**:985–94. doi:10.1001/archpsyc.62.9.985
115. Hariharan M, VanNoord T, Greden JF. A high-performance liquid-chromatographic method for routine simultaneous determination of nicotine and cotinine in plasma. *Clin Chem* (1988) **34**:724–9.
116. Staley JK, Krishnan-Sarin S, Cosgrove KP, Krantzler E, Frohlich E, Perry E, et al. Human tobacco smokers in early abstinence have higher levels of beta2* nicotinic acetylcholine receptors than nonsmokers. *J Neurosci* (2006) **26**:8707–14. doi:10.1523/JNEUROSCI.0546-06.2006
117. Friedman D, Simpson G, Hamberger M. Age-related changes in scalp topography to novel and target stimuli. *Psychophysiology* (1993) **30**:383–96. doi:10.1111/j.1469-8986.1993.tb02060.x
118. Cohen JD, Barch DM, Carter C, Servan-Schreiber D. Context-processing deficits in schizophrenia: converging evidence from three theoretically motivated cognitive tasks. *J Abnorm Psychol* (1999) **108**:120–33. doi:10.1037/0021-843X.108.1.120
119. Gratton G, Coles MG, Donchin E. A new method for off-line removal of ocular artifact. *Electroencephalogr Clin Neurophysiol* (1983) **55**:468–84. doi:10.1016/0013-4694(83)90135-9
120. Cho HS, Perry EB, Gunduz-Bruce H, D'Souza DC. The ketamine paradigm in humans: relevance to psychotic disorders. In: Heresco-Levy U, Daniel C, Javitt DC, editors. *Glutamate in Neuropsychiatric Disorders Trivandrum.* Kerala, India: Research Signpost (2008). p. 99–131.
121. Mathalon DH, Ford JM, Pfefferbaum A. Trait and state aspects of P300 amplitude reduction in schizophrenia: a retrospective longitudinal study. *Biol Psychiatry* (2000) **47**:434–49. doi:10.1016/S0006-3223(99)00277-2
122. Mathalon DH, Ford JM, Rosenbloom M, Pfefferbaum A. P300 reduction and prolongation with illness duration in schizophrenia. *Biol Psychiatry* (2000) **47**:413–27. doi:10.1016/S0006-3223(99)00151-1
123. Abi-Saab WM, D'Souza DC, Moghaddam B, Krystal JH. The NMDA antagonist model for schizophrenia: promise and pitfalls. *Pharmacopsychiatry* (1998) **31**(Suppl 2):104–9. doi:10.1055/s-2007-979354
124. Coyle JT. NMDA receptor and schizophrenia: a brief history. *Schizophr Bull* (2012) **38**:920–6. doi:10.1093/schbul/sbs076
125. Alain C, Bernstein LJ, Cortese F, Yu H, Zipursky RB. Deficits in automatically detecting changes in conjunction of auditory features in patients with schizophrenia. *Psychophysiology* (2002) **39**:599–606. doi:10.1111/1469-8986.3950599
126. Devrim-Ucok M, Keskin-Ergen HY, Ucok A. Novelty P3 and P3b in first-episode schizophrenia and chronic schizophrenia. *Prog Neuropsychopharmacol Biol Psychiatry* (2006) **30**:1426–34. doi:10.1016/j.pnpbp.2006.05.019
127. Grillon C, Courchesne E, Ameli R, Geyer MA, Braff DL. Increased distractibility in schizophrenic patients. Electrophysiologic and behavioral evidence. *Arch Gen Psychiatry* (1990) **47**:171–9. doi:10.1001/archpsyc.1990.01810140071010
128. Merrin EL, Floyd TC. P300 responses to novel auditory stimuli in hospitalized schizophrenic patients. *Biol Psychiatry* (1994) **36**:527–42. doi:10.1016/0006-3223(94)90617-3
129. Daffner KR, Mesulam MM, Holcomb PJ, Calvo V, Acar D, Chabrerie A, et al. Disruption of attention to novel events after frontal lobe injury in humans. *J Neurol Neurosurg Psychiatry* (2000) **68**:18–24. doi:10.1136/jnnp.68.1.18
130. Daffner KR, Mesulam MM, Scinto LF, Acar D, Calvo V, Faust R, et al. The central role of the prefrontal cortex in directing attention to novel events. *Brain* (2000) **123**(Pt 5):927–39. doi:10.1093/brain/123.5.927
131. Woods DL, Knight RT. Electrophysiologic evidence of increased distractibility after dorsolateral prefrontal lesions. *Neurology* (1986) **36**:212–6. doi:10.1212/WNL.36.2.212
132. Anand A, Charney DS, Oren DA, Berman RM, Hu XS, Cappiello A, et al. Attenuation of the neuropsychiatric effects of ketamine with lamotrigine: support for hyperglutamatergic effects of N-methyl-D-aspartate receptor antagonists. *Arch Gen Psychiatry* (2000) **57**:270–6. doi:10.1001/archpsyc.57.3.270
133. Krystal JH, D'Souza DC, Karper LP, Bennett A, Abi-Dargham A, Abi-Saab D, et al. Interactive effects of subanesthetic ketamine and haloperidol in healthy humans. *Psychopharmacology (Berl)* (1999) **145**:193–204. doi:10.1007/s002130051049
134. Krystal JH, Karper LP, Bennett A, D'Souza DC, Abi-Dargham A, Morrissey K, et al. Interactive effects of subanesthetic ketamine and subhypnotic lorazepam in humans. *Psychopharmacology (Berl)* (1998) **135**:213–29. doi:10.1007/s002130050503
135. Ernst M, Heishman SJ, Spurgeon L, London ED. Smoking history and nicotine effects on cognitive performance. *Neuropsychopharmacology* (2001) **25**:313–9. doi:10.1016/S0893-133X(01)00257-3

136. Lawrence NS, Ross TJ, Stein EA. Cognitive mechanisms of nicotine on visual attention. *Neuron* (2002) **36**:539–48. doi:10.1016/S0896-6273(02)01004-8
137. Mancuso G, Andres P, Ansseau M, Tirelli E. Effects of nicotine administered via a transdermal delivery system on vigilance: a repeated measure study. *Psychopharmacology (Berl)* (1999) **142**:18–23. doi:10.1007/s002130050857
138. McClernon FJ, Gilbert DG, Radtke R. Effects of transdermal nicotine on lateralized identification and memory interference. *Hum Psychopharmacol* (2003) **18**:339–43. doi:10.1002/hup.488
139. Arendash GW, Sanberg PR, Sengstock GJ. Nicotine enhances the learning and memory of aged rats. *Pharmacol Biochem Behav* (1995) **52**:517–23. doi:10.1016/0091-3057(95)00119-H
140. Levin ED, Simon BB. Nicotinic acetylcholine involvement in cognitive function in animals. *Psychopharmacology (Berl)* (1998) **138**:217–30. doi:10.1007/s002130050667
141. D'Souza DC, Ahn K, Bhakta S, Elander J, Singh N, Nadim H, et al. Nicotine fails to attenuate ketamine-induced cognitive deficits and negative and positive symptoms in humans: implications for schizophrenia. *Biol Psychiatry* (2012) **72**:785–94. doi:10.1016/j.biopsych.2012.05.009

5

Magnetic Resonance Imaging in Studying Schizophrenia, Negative Symptoms and the Glutamate System

***Oliver Gruber*[1]*, *Antonella Chadha Santuccione*[2] *and Helmut Aach*[2]**

[1] *Center for Translational Research in Systems Neuroscience and Psychiatry, Clinic for Psychiatry and Psychotherapy, University Medical Center Göttingen, Göttingen, Germany*

[2] *Medical Affairs – Psychiatry, Roche Pharma AG, Grenzach-Wyhlen, Germany*

Correspondence:
Oliver Gruber, Clinic for Psychiatry and Psychotherapy, University Medical Center Göttingen, Von-Siebold-Str. 5, Göttingen 37075, Germany
e-mail: ogruber@gwdg.de

Schizophrenia is characterized by positive, negative, and cognitive symptoms. While positive symptoms occur periodically during psychotic exacerbations, negative and cognitive symptoms often emerge before the first psychotic episode and persist with low functional outcome and poor prognosis. This review article outlines the importance of modern functional magnetic resonance imaging techniques for developing a stratified therapy of schizophrenic disorders. Functional neuroimaging evidence on the neural correlates of positive and particularly negative symptoms and cognitive deficits in schizophrenic disorders is briefly reviewed. Acute dysregulation of dopaminergic neurotransmission is crucially involved in the occurrence of psychotic symptoms. However, increasing evidence also implicates glutamatergic pathomechanisms, in particular *N*-methyl-D-aspartate (NMDA) receptor dysfunction in the pathogenesis of schizophrenia and in the appearance of negative symptoms and cognitive dysfunctions. In line with this notion, several gene variants affecting the NMDA receptor's pathway have been reported to increase susceptibility for schizophrenia, and have been investigated using the imaging genetics approach. In recent years, several attempts have been made to develop medications modulating the glutamatergic pathway with modest evidences for efficacy. The most successful approaches were those that aimed at influencing this pathway using compounds that enhance NMDA receptor function. More recently, the selective glycine reuptake inhibitor bitopertin has been shown to improve NMDA receptor hypofunction by increasing glycine concentrations in the synaptic cleft. Further research is required to test whether pharmacological agents with effects on the glutamatergic system can help to improve the treatment of negative symptoms in schizophrenic disorders.

Keywords: schizophrenia, glutamate, negative symptoms, cognitive deficits, neuroimaging biomarkers, stratified therapy

Neuroimaging techniques have been developed as important tools to investigate brain dysfunctions that underlie psychiatric disorders. In particular, modern functional magnetic resonance imaging (fMRI) holds the promise to provide neurofunctional biomarkers for improved diagnosis, prognosis, and optimized treatment of mental disorders [e.g., Ref. (1–4)]. In this brief, not exhaustive review, we will exemplify this translational neuroimaging research by focusing on schizophrenia and current challenges to advancing therapeutic approaches for this heterogeneous diagnostic category. First, the importance of negative symptoms and cognitive deficits for successful treatment of schizophrenic disorders will be highlighted, and an overview will be given on the neural correlates of these symptom domains as revealed by fMRI studies. Second, neuroimaging studies of glutamate levels and genetic risk factors pointing to an important role of glutamate–dopamine interactions in the pathophysiology of schizophrenic disorders will be briefly reviewed and will be related to recent findings of pharmacological and animal studies. In the final part of this review, we will present current approaches to develop therapeutic strategies that target the glutamatergic pathway in schizophrenic disorders.

"PSYCHOPATHOPHYSIOLOGY" OF SCHIZOPHRENIC DISORDERS AND THE IMPORTANCE OF NEGATIVE SYMPTOMS AND COGNITIVE DEFICITS

In traditional psychiatry, mental disorders are diagnosed and classified on the basis of more or less specific psychopathological symptoms in the course of the disorder. Numerous recent findings from modern systems neuroscience and molecular neuroscience strongly suggest that diagnoses made on the basis of psychopathological criteria do not represent "natural disease entities" in the sense of diseases with uniform pathogenesis and pathology [see Ref. (1, 3–8)]. Therefore, schizophrenia represents a group of mental disorders that share more or less characteristic psychopathological symptoms, such as verbal hallucinations, delusions, and formal thought disorders.

During the last two decades, modern brain imaging techniques have allowed for the first time scientific investigations into the neural correlates of different symptom dimensions that characterize schizophrenic disorders. These studies of pathophysiological processes that underlie different psychopathological symptoms and syndromes (an approach that may be termed "psychopathophysiology") are briefly reviewed in the following.

Positive symptoms of schizophrenic disorders such as verbal hallucinations ("hearing voices") and delusional symptoms are certainly the most impressive characteristics of schizophrenic disorders. Nevertheless, much evidence has been provided that negative symptoms and cognitive disturbances are more strongly associated with the long-term functional outcome of patients suffering from schizophrenia than positive symptoms (9–14). Cognitive deficits are even present at first episode and remain relatively constant over the course of illness (15–17). In contrast to the dopamine model of schizophrenia, glutamatergic theories of schizophrenia account for negative symptoms and cognitive dysfunction as well, and may therefore lead to new treatment approaches specifically targeting the unmet medical need to improve negative symptomatology and cognitive deficits (18).

NEURAL CORRELATES OF POSITIVE SYMPTOMS IN SCHIZOPHRENIC DISORDERS

The positive symptoms of schizophrenic disorders particularly include auditory–verbal hallucinations ("hearing voices") and delusional symptoms like paranoia. As regards auditory–verbal hallucinations, a number of functional brain imaging studies have been performed in the past. Overall, findings of these studies appear quite heterogeneous. However, a finding that has been replicated several times is overactivation of the superior temporal gyrus during experimental phases in which the patients exhibited the symptom of hearing voices [e.g., Ref. (19–21)]. In most of these studies, this activation of auditory association cortices was associated with additional activations in other brain regions. For instance, some of these studies also reported an increased brain activity in Broca's area, the anterior cingulate cortex, the hippocampus, and the amygdala [e.g., Ref. (20)]. Some of these findings have also been confirmed on the meta-analytical level. Jardri et al. (22) confirmed that phases of "hearing voices" are associated with increased activity in Broca's area, anterior insula, precentral gyrus, frontal opercular cortex, middle and superior temporal gyrus, inferior parietal lobule as well as in hippocampus and parahippocampal gyrus. It has to be noted, however, that patients suffering from this kind of intermittently occurring auditory–verbal hallucinations are probably not representative for most types of schizophrenic disorders in which the hallucinations persist for longer time periods. A second meta-analysis by Kühn and Gallinat (23) came to the conclusion that a current psychopathological state of experiencing auditory–verbal hallucinations may be associated with abnormal activation of brain regions that are also involved in speech production (e.g., Broca's area), whereas a subgroup of schizophrenic patients that exhibits the symptom of auditory–verbal hallucinations (in comparison to a subgroup without "life-time diagnosis" of auditory–verbal hallucinations) may be particularly characterized by abnormal brain activation in areas involved in speech processing and, more generally, the processing of auditory stimuli. In another, qualitative and quantitative review, Goghari et al. (24) showed an association between positive symptoms, in particular ideas of persecution, with the activity in medial prefrontal cortex, amygdala, hippocampus, and parahippocampal gyrus.

NEURAL CORRELATES OF NEGATIVE SYMPTOMS IN SCHIZOPHRENIC DISORDERS

Negative symptoms of schizophrenic disorders are usually defined as symptoms representing a qualitative and/or quantitative reduction of mental capacities or qualities of experience. This class of symptoms is relatively heterogeneous and traditionally includes the five "A"s, which are affective flattening, apathy (reduced drive), anhedonia, asociality (social withdrawal), and alogia (impoverishment of thought) [e.g., Ref. (25)]. Early studies on the structural correlates of negative symptoms in schizophrenic disorders have shown gray matter reduction in temporal, medial frontal, insular, and hippocampal regions [e.g., Ref. (26)]. On the other hand, evidence on brain structural correlates of negative symptoms is very heterogeneous as there are also several studies that failed to find any correlation of brain volumes to negative symptoms in schizophrenia [e.g., Ref. (27–30)].

The development of functional neuroimaging techniques like PET and fMRI led to an increasing number of studies on the neurofunctional correlates of negative symptoms. Several studies have shown a reduced activation of the prefrontal cortex in schizophrenic patients with negative symptoms (25, 31–33). This principal finding of "hypofrontality" associated with negative symptoms has been confirmed by later studies though for different subregions of the prefrontal cortex. For example, in a study using memory retrieval tasks, Heckers et al. (34) found a significantly reduced recruitment of left frontal cortex (Brodmann area 44/9) in schizophrenic patients with deficit syndrome (i.e., patients with negative symptoms as primary and enduring features) as compared to both schizophrenic patients without deficit syndrome and healthy controls. Using auditory working memory tasks (*n*-back tasks), Menon et al. (35) found an inverse correlation of negative symptoms with activation in the frontal opercular cortex and in the right DLPFC. In contrast to that, another experiment using the *n*-back task (36) reported a correlation of activation deficits in the DLPFC with disorganization symptoms rather than with negative symptoms.

A number of functional neuroimaging studies have also reported associations of negative symptoms with activation in other brain regions including temporal cortices and the ventral striatum. For instance, Tamminga et al. (37) found both limbic system abnormalities and neocortical alterations associated with the deficit syndrome. A later series of studies have demonstrated a significant correlation of activation in temporal cortices with negative symptoms (38–40). Using the monetary incentive delay task, which activates the reward system, Juckel et al. (41) found a correlation of diminished ventral striatal activation with negative symptoms in schizophrenic patients. In another study by Simon et al. (42), a ventral striatal activation during reward anticipation was negatively correlated with symptoms of apathy, while activation during receipt of reward was negatively correlated with severity of depressive symptoms. Finally, in a recent systematic review and meta-analysis of 25 fMRI studies on schizophrenic symptomatology, Goghari and colleagues (24) have confirmed a relationship of negative symptoms with the functioning of the ventrolateral prefrontal cortex and the ventral striatum.

NEURAL CORRELATES OF COGNITIVE DYSFUNCTIONS IN SCHIZOPHRENIC DISORDERS

Traditionally, psychiatric diagnosis of schizophrenic disorders is based on psychopathological, particularly positive and negative symptoms. Over the last few decades, the advent of modern experimental neuropsychological and functional neuroimaging techniques has switched the focus of interest toward brain dysfunctions in the domains of cognitive, emotional, and motivational processes that are highly prevalent in schizophrenic disorders. Especially cognitive deficits are of major interest as they have been proposed to represent core deficits of schizophrenic disorders [e.g., Ref. (43, 44)]. These core cognitive deficits of schizophrenic disorders include deficits in working memory, executive functions, episodic memory, and social cognitions.

Deficits in working memory in schizophrenic disorders have been found to be associated with dysfunctions of prefrontal cortices, especially of the dorsolateral prefrontal cortex, of the deep fronto-opercular cortex, and of the anterior cingulate cortex [e.g., Ref. (45–50)]. In the last few years, there have also been several reports of a disturbed connectivity between these prefrontal areas and the medial temporal lobe, particularly the hippocampus [e.g., Ref. (51, 52)].

Executive function is a construct that encompasses a variety of sub-functions [see for example Ref. (53, 54)], among them selective attention, background monitoring of the environment for potentially significant sensory events [e.g., Ref. (55)], and the adaptation of behavior to changing environmental conditions [e.g., Ref. (56–60)]. Patients with schizophrenic disorders exhibit multiple dysfunctions in these areas of executive control mechanisms that are associated with reduced activity in the posterior frontal medial cortex and the inferior frontal junction area (IFJA; a cortical subregion at the intersection of the precentral sulcus and the inferior frontal sulcus) (61, 62) as well as with abnormally increased activations in brain stem nuclei and the ventral striatum (63).

Episodic memory deficits in schizophrenic disorders have been found to be associated firstly with dysfunction of the extended hippocampal formation (including the hippocampus proper and the surrounding medial temporal structures) [e.g., Ref. (64)], and secondly with dysfunctions of prefrontal cognitive control mechanisms that are involved in encoding and retrieval processes (65).

Disturbed social cognitions in schizophrenic disorders include particularly impaired recognition of facial emotional expressions and reduced theory-of-mind capacities. Neuroimaging studies have revealed that deficits in these domains of social cognitions are associated, firstly, with reduced activation in the amygdala and the fusiform gyrus (66) and, secondly, with reduced activity in the fronto-median cortex, in the temporo-parietal junction cortex, and the amygdala–hippocampus complex [e.g., Ref. (67)]. Disturbed functional coupling between prefrontal areas and the amygdala has also been reported as a correlate of impaired emotional regulation mechanisms (68).

Taken together, neuroimaging studies on the neural correlates of different (positive, negative, cognitive) symptom domains in schizophrenic disorders suggest the involvement of different lateral and medial prefrontal, temporal (particularly including hippocampus and amygdala), and subcortical (in particular ventral striatum as part of the dopaminergic reward system) brain regions in the occurrence of these symptoms.

PATHOGENESIS, PATHOPHYSIOLOGY, AND TREATMENT OF SCHIZOPHRENIC DISORDERS: THE ROLE OF GLUTAMATE–DOPAMINE INTERACTIONS

It is well-established that acute dysregulation of dopaminergic (and glutamatergic) neurotransmission is crucially involved in the occurrence of psychotic symptoms, whereas more chronic cellular neuropathology may be responsible for the development of cognitive deficits and negative symptoms (69). In more recent years, classical elements of the dopamine hypothesis such as the overactive mesolimbic dopamine system and a reduced mesocortical dopamine turnover are considered rather as a "final common pathway" (70), i.e., as the expression of upstream pathophysiological changes. In particular, it is postulated that *N*-methyl-D-aspartate (NMDA) receptor dysfunction may lead to dopaminergic dysregulation in schizophrenic disorders through a complex interaction between glutamatergic and dopaminergic, but also GABA-ergic mechanisms. Schwartz and co-workers (71), for example, explain both positive and negative symptoms of schizophrenia with dysfunctions of NMDA-glutamatergic synapses. Via effects on various complex circuits including GABA-ergic interneurons, these dysfunctions ultimately result both in hyperfunction of the mesolimbic dopamine system leading to positive symptoms, and also in hypofunction of the mesocortical dopamine system associated with negative symptoms and cognitive dysfunctions (**Figure 1**). Such pathomechanisms in functional interactions between prefrontal cortices and brain stem nuclei, in particular the ventral tegmental area (VTA), the striatum, and the thalamus, may be influenced by predisposing and/or protective genetic variants that exert effects on the glutamatergic synapse. Thus, the glutamatergic hypothesis is also compatible with our knowledge about the effects of susceptibility genes of schizophrenia (see below).

Modern pharmacological and animal research approaches are increasingly focusing on the interactions between the dopaminergic and glutamatergic system, especially within fronto-striato-thalamo-frontal loops and in the interactions between frontal cortex, hippocampus, nucleus accumbens, and VTA. Within and between these brain regions, the dopamine and the glutamate system interact in a very complex way, and dysfunctions in these interactions are a central pathomechanistic explanation for the development of schizophrenic disorders [e.g., Ref. (73, 74)]. Particularly, the hippocampus plays a major role in regulating the dopaminergic reward system. Animal studies have shown that increased activity of the ventral hippocampus (subiculum) leads to increased dopamine turnover in the ventral striatum (nucleus accumbens) (75, 76). Other recent findings suggest that this glutamatergically mediated effect of the subiculum on the nucleus accumbens further leads to increased GABA-ergic projection onto the ventral pallidum with reduced tonic activity of the pallidum and consecutive disinhibition of dopamine neurons in the VTA (77). In this way, hyperactivity of the ventral hippocampus observed in schizophrenic disorders could lead to overstimulation and hyperactivity of dopaminergic VTA neurons which may account for various symptoms, in particular for delusional

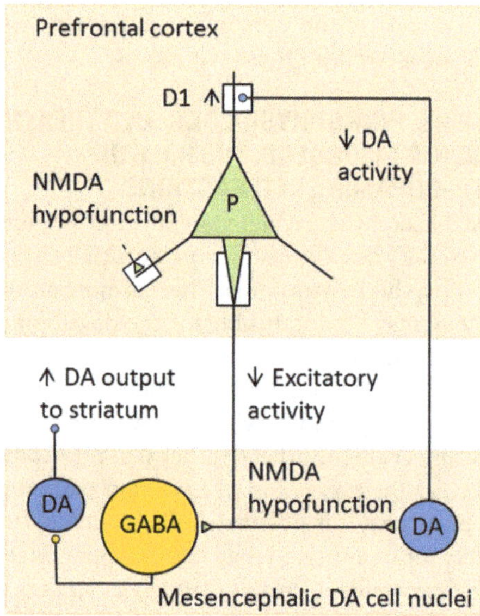

FIGURE 1 | Example for consequences of NMDA receptor hypofunction in glutamatergic–dopaminergic circuits. Hypofunction of NMDA receptors mediating excitatory inputs to prefrontal pyramidal cells in schizophrenia leads to decreased activity in cortical excitatory projections to mesencephalic DA cell nuclei. This results in decreased activity of DA neurons projecting to the DLPFC and increased activity of DA cells projecting to the striatum, as a consequence of decreased stimulation of GABA interneurons. Reduced DA levels in DLPFC lead to compensatory, but functionally insufficient, upregulation of D1 receptors [adapted from Lewis and Gonzalez-Burgos (72)].

phenomena. Further support for this theory is provided by studies using the MAM animal model of schizophrenia which have shown that the relevant pathophysiological changes such as VTA hyperactivity and increased response to amphetamines are no longer present after inactivation of the subiculum. This indicates that the subiculum is necessary to induce hyperdopaminergic states in this animal model (78).

The pathophysiological role of glutamatergic disbalances has also been investigated *in vivo* in patients with schizophrenia, for example using magnetic resonance spectroscopy (MRS). In very recent publications (79, 80), findings of such glutamatergic proton magnetic resonance spectroscopic imaging studies have been nicely reviewed, particularly with respect to their implications for drug discovery. Overall, neuroimaging studies support the current glutamate model of schizophrenia by suggesting a hypofunction of the NMDA receptor. In particular, proton magnetic resonance spectroscopic (1H-MRS) studies have provided evidence for altered levels of glutamate and glutamine in the medial prefrontal cortex and in the basal ganglia in early-stage, drug-naïve, or drug-free schizophrenia patients.

Some studies with unmedicated patients with schizophrenia have reported elevated glutamatergic levels in the medial prefrontal cortex as compared to healthy controls (81–84). More precisely, a recent meta-analysis by Marsman and colleagues (79) indicated that it is glutamine which is increased in the frontal cortex in schizophrenic patients, whereas glutamate is reduced. Such an elevated glutamine/glutamate ration may result from either a deficiency in glutaminase, which converts glutamine into glutamate, or from NMDA receptor hypofunction which has also been shown to increase glutamine levels and decrease glutamate levels (79). Further, glutamate levels in the medial prefrontal cortex have been found to be associated with negative symptoms and worse global functioning and to be decreased in remitted patients as compared to non-remitted patients (85). Consistent with that, most studies comparing medicated patients with healthy control subjects reported unchanged glutamate levels in the medial prefrontal cortex (81, 86–92). The meta-analysis by Marsman and colleagues (79) provided additional support for a progressive decrease of frontal glutamate and glutamine in patients with schizophrenia possibly indicating a progressive loss of synaptic activity. Finally, particularly in first episodes schizophrenic patients, increased glutamatergic levels have also been reported in the basal ganglia (93–95), and they appear to decrease to normal levels during antipsychotic treatment with risperidone (94).

Over the last 10–15 years, numerous potential susceptibility genes of schizophrenia have been identified, among them COMT, dysbindin-1, neuregulin-1, RGS4, GRM3, and DISC1. Many of these candidate genes have been shown to influence dopaminergic and/or glutamatergic neurotransmission, and effects on neuroplastic processes and particularly on synaptogenesis have also been reported. Imaging genetics is still a relatively novel approach that, however, has already made substantial contributions to our knowledge about genetic effects on brain structure and function. Early studies, for example, demonstrated the influence of variants in the COMT gene on working memory-related prefrontal activation (96) and on the functional interplay between dopamine synthesis in the midbrain and prefrontal function (97). Although the evidence for an association between the COMT gene and schizophrenia is not unequivocal, these findings nevertheless have high biological plausibility insofar as the influence of the COMT gene on the dopaminergic tone in the prefrontal cortex has been convincingly demonstrated (98). Further studies on the COMT genotype have shown more complex haplotype effects on prefrontal cerebral activations (99) and on gene–gene interactions between COMT and other genes such as RGS4, G72, DISC1, and GRM3 (49, 100, 101). Especially the latter finding is consistent with a role of glutamate–dopamine interactions in the pathophysiology and pathogenesis of schizophrenic disorders.

The number of genome-wide association studies between gene variants and diseases has markedly increased over the last few years due to the availability of modern chips. This has also inspired imaging genetics studies as genome-wide confirmed risk variants have also been investigated for their effects on brain structure and function. Two examples of this are the zinc finger protein 804A (ZNF804A), the function of which has not yet been more closely characterized, but which showed a genome-wide significant association with schizophrenia and also with bipolar disorder (102), as well as the CACNA1C gene, which was first discovered as a risk gene for bipolar disorder, but later also for schizophrenia (103). Studies on the ZNF804A polymorphism have shown an effect on the connectivity between the prefrontal cortex and the hippocampus (104–106). Effects of the CACNA1C gene have been reported with regard to activation of the hippocampus and the subgenual

ACC (107) as well as activation of the amygdala during reward and fear recognition paradigms (108, 109).

Taken together, the studies summarized here support the important pathophysiological role of glutamate in schizophrenia and encourage further development of therapeutic strategies that target the glutamatergic pathway in schizophrenia.

THERAPEUTIC STRATEGIES TARGETING THE GLUTAMATERGIC PATHWAY IN SCHIZOPHRENIA

A valid treatment for positive symptoms, based on the use of antipsychotic agents and their main capacity to modulate the dopaminergic system, is currently available for schizophrenia. However, antipsychotics are less effective in reducing negative symptoms or in ameliorating cognitive dysfunctions (110–112). Based on the novel findings that the glutamatergic system plays an important role in the pathogenesis of schizophrenia, several attempts have been made to identify drugs which, by modulating this system, could improve negative symptoms and cognitive dysfunction (113). Pharmacological targets are different types of glutamate receptors, which interact in a complex not yet fully understood way within glutamatergic synapses. These receptors include both ionotropic receptors [NMDA, α-amino-3-hydroxy-5-methyl-4-isoxazolepropionic acid (AMPA), and kainate receptors] and metabotropic glutamate receptors (mGluRs) [reviewed in Ref. (114)]. AMPA and kainate receptors are fast gating by glutamate binding and permeable for Na^+ and K^+ ions, whereas NMDA receptors exhibit a slow gating kinetic and need a predepolarization of the neuronal membrane for activation by glutamate binding. This predepolarization occurs when vicinal AMPA receptors are frequently activated and leads to the release of a blocking Mg^{2+} ion from the NMDA receptor. Activated NMDA receptor channels are not ion specific and pass Ca^{2+}, Na^+, and K^+ ions, which leads not only to further depolarization but also intracellular processes making the synapse more sensible for signals from upstream and sending stronger signals downstream. This so-called long-term potentiation (LTP) provides the basis for synaptic and dendritic proliferation or pruning, learning, and memory (115).

Metabotropic glutamate receptors are G protein-coupled receptors influencing intracellular metabolic processes and are present on presynaptic and postsynaptic neurons as well as on glial cells near glutamatergic synapses. Currently, eight mGlu receptors are known of which the mGlu 2/3 receptors are investigated as targets for schizophrenia therapy, because they regulate presynaptic glutamate secretion.

After successful completion of preclinical trial programs of pharmacodynamic activity and safety, potential compounds are investigated in escalating clinical study programs. Phase 1 studies are open label, single to multiple dose trials with healthy volunteers, exploring pharmacokinetic and first safety characteristics. Phase 2 studies are explorative or proof-of-concept studies that are usually controlled and blinded with small to medium numbers of patients, and designed for dosis finding and first in patient proof of safety and efficacy. Phase 3 studies are large scale, double blinded controlled studies to confirm safety and efficacy. Some of the following described trial results are not yet published in peer-reviewed journals, and we had to quote congress presentations or company statements.

COMPOUNDS ENHANCING NMDA RECEPTOR FUNCTION

Since the activation of the NMDA receptor also requires glycine as a co-agonist, the glycine binding site at the NMDA receptor is regarded as a promising pharmacological target to enhance its activity, thereby minimizing the risk of excitotoxicity that is associated with direct overactivation of the glutamate binding site (116). A first review of clinical trials published until 2003 with agonists of the glycine binding site of the NMDA receptor including glycine, D-cycloserine, and D-serine reported moderate effect sizes for glycine and D-serine on negative symptoms, but no effect of D-cycloserine (117). It included 358 small randomized trials with 6–51 participants and a maximum duration of 12 weeks. Up to now, the amount of data has grown confirming these early results. In almost all trials, the compounds were used as adjunctive treatment to regular antipsychotic therapy, and generally no effect was reported in patients taking clozapine.

Several clinical trials have been conducted using glycine, a substance that is endogenously produced and that can act as a co-agonist of NMDA receptors binding at the glycine modulatory site. The results of these studies suggest that glycine can significantly improve symptoms of schizophrenia (118), including negative symptoms, although there are also negative and equivocal studies (119).

D-Cycloserine is a selective co-agonist of NMDA receptors containing the NR2C subunit, and these receptors are involved in fear conditioning and memory consolidation (120). When used as a single dosis in rodents, D-cycloserine led to enhanced memory consolidation of novel information (120). In an exploratory clinical trial, once weekly dosing of D-cycloserine augmentation over 8 weeks did not improve cognitive symptoms but reduced negative symptoms and delusion severity in stable schizophrenic patients medicated with a range of different antipsychotics excluding clozapine (121).

D-Serine, another agonist of the glycine modulatory site within the NMDA receptor, has been shown in clinical trials to be capable of ameliorating several symptom domains in schizophrenia (122–124).

GLYCINE TRANSPORTER-1 INHIBITORS

Sarcosine is a potent natural glycine transporter-1 inhibitor (GlyT-1) (125). The inhibition of this transporter leads to increased levels of glycin in the synapsis and consequently enhanced NMDA receptor activation, which may represent a possible treatment mechanism for schizophrenic disorders in which a hypofunction of NMDA receptors is present (126). As recently shown, sarcosine may reduce negative symptoms in acutely ill schizophrenia patients receiving atypical antipsychotics, being more effective than the NMDA/glycine site agonist D-serine (125).

A meta-analysis including all abovementioned molecules found that, overall, the NMDA-enhancers were effective against most symptom domains of schizophrenia. Glycine, D-serine, and sarcosine significantly improved multiple symptom domains, whereas no symptom domain was improved by D-cycloserine. Furthermore, glycine, D-serine, and sarcosine were found to be superior to D-cycloserine in improving overall psychopathology [Ref. (118); see **Figure 2**]. However, these compounds have individual disadvantages to be developed to drugs licensed for long-term

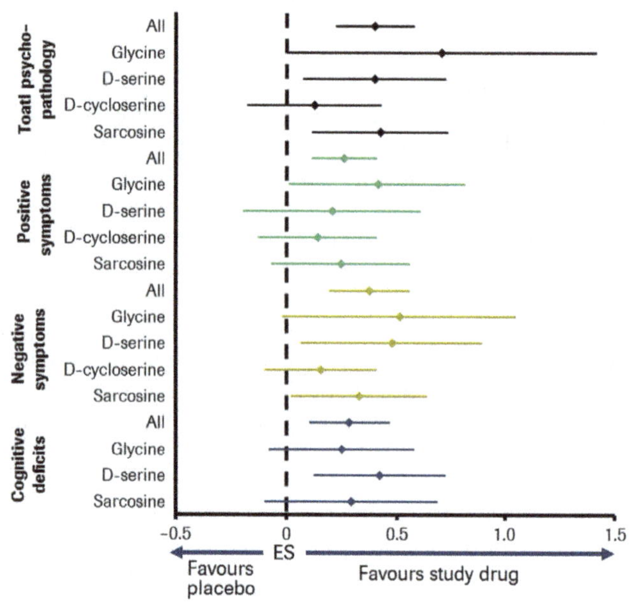

FIGURE 2 | Meta-analysis of double-blind, placebo-controlled studies of small-molecule NMDA receptor enhancers in patients with schizophrenia. Sample size: 26 studies comprising about 800 patients. Effect size (ES) for glycine, d-serine, d-cycloserine, sarcosine, and all in different symptom domains of schizophrenia [adapted from Tsai and Lin (118)].

use. Glycine is fast metabolized and passes the blood–brain barrier poorly. So it has to be applied with daily doses up to 60 g. Although D-serine is substantially metabolized, daily doses of 30–120 mg/kg were effective. But there is concern about nephrotoxicity at higher doses, although no significant adverse events have yet been observed at doses of $\leq$4 g/day (127). According to Sreekumar et al. (128), sarcosine might play a role in aggravating prostate cancer progression.

Bitopertin is a GlyT-1 inhibitor that increases levels of the glycine neurotransmitter by inhibiting its reuptake from the synaptic cleft. Preclinical evidence showed that this molecule is capable of ameliorating the symptoms of schizophrenia in animal models (129, 130). These preclinical findings encouraged a double blinded placebo-controlled phase IIb clinical trial which showed that adjunctive treatment with bitopertin in stable patients with predominant negative symptoms was capable of ameliorating negative symptoms and improving general clinical status (131). Currently, several phase III studies are underway with the hope that bitopertin may help in the treatment of currently unsatisfyingly responding stages of schizophrenia.

A major goal for future research combining psychopharmacology and modern functional neuroimaging techniques would be to understand how these molecules modulate the activity of pathophysiologically relevant neural structures as outlined above. Such studies could, for example, provide important information on whether these pharmacological agents can be successfully used to treat patient subgroups that are characterized by specific symptoms of schizophrenia.

AMPA RECEPTOR MODULATORS

As described above, the fast trafficking of AMPA receptors in the synaptic cleft has an impact on NMDA receptor-mediated LTP and depression. These intracellular mechanisms influence synaptic strength and therefore constitute the basis of learning and memory (132). Therefore, modulation of AMPA activity could lead to amelioration of cognitive dysfunction in schizophrenia. To this aim and based on preclinical evidences, two molecules have been used in schizophrenia clinical trials: piracetam (133) and CX516 (121, 134).

Piracetam augmentation of haloperidol was capable of improving psychotic symptoms in schizophrenia, but had no effect on PANSS (133). Because only 30 patients (all receiving haloperidol) completed the placebo-controlled trial, more scientific evidence is needed to support such an effect. Trials with CX156 led to controversial results. In a small study, CX156 improved cognitive functions and negative symptoms in schizophrenic patients when compared to patients treated with clozapine (134). However, a larger study was unable to show any effect of CX516 on cognition or negative symptoms when compared to controls (135). Taken together, there is only little evidence about these molecules and their therapeutic effect.

mGlu RECEPTOR MODULATORS

In contrast to the concept of improving symptoms of schizophrenia with ampakines, a line of evidence points to an overactivation of AMPA synapses in the prefrontal cortex downstream of NMDA receptor hypofunction (136). NMDA receptor blockade on GABA-ergic interneurons reduces inhibition of pyramidal cells and leads to excessive glutamate release in AMPA receptor synapses in the prefrontal cortex (137). Metabolic glutamate receptors 2 and 3 (mGlu 2/3) facilitate a feedback regulation of synaptic glutamate release (138). Consequently, mGlu 2/3 enhancing agents were developed to delimit pathologically enhanced glutamate release. In schizophrenia, clinical trials were conducted with the mGluR2/3 agonist, pomaglumetad methionil (LY2140023) and the mGlu2 positive allosteric modulator, ADX71149.

Pomaglumetad methionil was investigated as monotherapy in three clinical trials. At first, a phase 2 proof-of-concept trial showed significant improvement of positive and negative symptoms versus placebo (139). In a following phase 2 dose ranging trial, all of the four investigated dosing groups did not differ from placebo (140), which was also the case for a phase 2 trial comparing pomaglumetad methionil to olanzapine and a placebo group. In this trial, both active treatment groups did not separate regarding efficacy and safety parameters from the placebo group (141).

After demonstrating an augmentation of the efficacy of atypical antipsychotics in preclinical trials, a phase 1 study was conducted to prove the safety of the combination of pomaglumetad methionil with four different second generation antipsychotics in healthy subjects (142). A following placebo-controlled phase 2 study tested the substance as adjunctive to standard of care in patients with prominent negative symptoms of schizophrenia. This trial did not indicate a significantly greater reduction of negative symptoms or an improvement of secondary efficacy endpoints over placebo (143). Based on these results, a phase 3 study started in the meantime was stopped.

The mGluR2 selective positive allosteric modulator ADX71149 is co-developed by Addex Therapeutics (144) and Johnson & Johnson, who code it JNJ40411813. Results of a randomized placebo-controlled phase 2 study evaluating the safety, tolerability, and exploratory efficacy of the compound given in two different doses as adjunctive to an ongoing antipsychotic medication were reported at the 2013 annual meeting of the American Psychiatric Society. The study population comprised three groups: patients with residual negative symptoms, patients with residual positive symptoms, and patients with insufficient response to clozapine treatment. Tolerability results suggest that dose titration may be beneficial. An efficacy signal seen in the negative symptoms subgroup treated with the lower dose suggests this population warrants further evaluation in a formal proof-of-concept study (144, 145).

CONCLUSION AND FUTURE PERSPECTIVES

In this brief review article, we have summarized recent findings from genetic, animal, and functional neuroimaging studies that together point to an important role of glutamate–dopamine interactions within cortico-striato-thalamo-cortical (CSTC) loops, which are modulated by hippocampal and amygdala inputs, in the pathophysiology of schizophrenic disorders. These findings provide the empirical basis for the development of novel treatment approaches for schizophrenic disorders that target glutamatergic mechanisms. The new findings from animal studies may also inspire analogous clinical neuroimaging investigations of neurofunctional interactions within CSTC loops as well as of the dynamic effects of mediotemporal structures such as hippocampus and amygdala on these CSTC loops in the human brain. Here, the development of valid animal model-supported experimental paradigms is of major importance as it may allow for the targeted *in vivo* investigation of these pathomechanisms involved in the pathophysiology of schizophrenic disorders [e.g., Ref. (4)]. Such targeted investigations may enable a future stratification of the heterogeneous group of schizophrenic disorders into pathophysiologically more homogenous "natural disease entities" (146). Moreover, the development of neurofunctional MRI biomarkers for sub-classification of patient groups and prediction of individual treatment responses may generally play an important role in a future individualized medicine in psychiatry [e.g., Ref. (4)].

ACKNOWLEDGMENTS

This publication was supported by a grant of the Roche Pharma AG, Germany.

REFERENCES

1. Insel TR, Wang PS. Rethinking mental illness. *JAMA* (2010) **303**(19):1970–1. doi:10.1001/jama.2010.555
2. Meyer-Lindenberg A. From maps to mechanisms through neuroimaging of schizophrenia. *Nature* (2010) **468**(7321):194–202. doi:10.1038/nature09569
3. Gruber O, Falkai P. Von der Identifizierung neurofunktioneller Systeme zur Individualisierung der Therapie schizophrener Störungen. *Nervenarzt* (2009) **80**:12–8. doi:10.1007/s00115-008-2615-y
4. Gruber O. Hirnbildgebungsmarker. *Nervenarzt* (2011) **82**:1404–13. doi:10.1007/s00115-011-3347-y
5. Insel TR, Cuthbert BN. Endophenotypes: bridging genomic complexity and disorder heterogeneity. *Biol Psychiatry* (2009) **66**(11):988–9. doi:10.1016/j.biopsych.2009.10.008
6. Insel T, Cuthbert B, Garvey M, Heinssen R, Pine DS, Quinn K, et al. Research domain criteria (RDoC): toward a new classification framework for research on mental disorders. *Am J Psychiatry* (2010) **167**(7):748–51. doi:10.1176/appi.ajp.2010.09091379
7. Insel TR. Rethinking schizophrenia. *Nature* (2010) **468**(7321):187–93. doi:10.1038/nature09552
8. Gruber O, Gruber E, Falkai P. Neural correlates of working memory deficits in schizophrenic patients. Ways to establish neurocognitive endophenotypes of psychiatric disorders. *Radiologe* (2005) **45**(2):153–60.
9. Green MF. What are the functional consequences of neurocognitive deficits in schizophrenia? *Am J Psychiatry* (1996) **153**:321–30.
10. Green MF, Kern RS, Braff DL, Mintz J. Neurocognitive deficits and functional outcome in schizophrenia: are we measuring the "right stuff"? *Schizophr Bull* (2000) **26**:119–36. doi:10.1093/oxfordjournals.schbul.a033430
11. Green MF, Kern RS, Heaton RK. Longitudinal studies of cognition and functional outcome in schizophrenia: implications for MATRICS. *Schizophr Res* (2004) **72**:41–51. doi:10.1016/j.schres.2004.09.009
12. Kurtz MM, Moberg PJ, Ragland JD, Gur RC, Gur RE. Symptoms versus neurocognitive test performance as predictors of psychosocial status in schizophrenia: a 1- and 4-year prospective study. *Schizophr Bull* (2005) **31**:167–74. doi:10.1093/schbul/sbi004
13. Fenton WS, McGlashan TH. Antecedents, symptom progression, and long-term outcome of the deficit syndrome in schizophrenia. *Am J Psychiatry* (1994) **151**:351–6.
14. Kirkpatrick B, Buchanan RW, Ross DE, Carpenter WT Jr. A separate disease within the syndrome of schizophrenia. *Arch Gen Psychiatry* (2001) **58**:165–71. doi:10.1001/archpsyc.58.2.165
15. Kantrowitz JT, Javitt DC. Thinking glutamatergically: changing concepts of schizophrenia based upon changing neurochemical models. *Clin Schizophr Relat Psychoses* (2010) **4**:189–200. doi:10.3371/CSRP.4.3.6
16. Woodberry KA, Giuliano AJ, Seidman LJ. Premorbid IQ in schizophrenia: a meta-analytic review. *Am J Psychiatry* (2008) **165**:579–87. doi:10.1176/appi.ajp.2008.07081242
17. Bilder RM, Goldman RS, Robinson D, Reiter G, Bell L, Bates JA, et al. Neuropsychology of first-episode schizophrenia: initial characterization and clinical correlates. *Am J Psychiatry* (2000) **157**:549–59. doi:10.1176/appi.ajp.157.4.549
18. Moghaddam B, Javitt D. From revolution to evolution: the glutamate hypothesis of schizophrenia and its implication for treatment. *Neuropsychopharmacology* (2012) **37**:4–15. doi:10.1038/npp.2011.181
19. Suzuki M, Yuasa S, Minabe Y, Murata M, Kurachi M. Left superior temporal blood flow increases in schizophrenic and schizophreniform patients with auditory hallucination: a longitudinal case study using 123I-IMP SPECT. *Eur Arch Psychiatry Clin Neurosci* (1993) **242**(5):257–61. doi:10.1007/BF02190383
20. Dierks T, Linden DE, Jandl M, Formisano E, Goebel R, Lanfermann H, et al. Activation of Heschl's gyrus during auditory hallucinations. *Neuron* (1999) **22**(3):615–21. doi:10.1016/S0896-6273(00)80715-1
21. Lennox BR, Park SBG, Medley I, Morris PG, Jones PB. The functional anatomy of auditory hallucinations in schizophrenia. *Psychiatry Res* (2000) **100**:13–20. doi:10.1016/S0925-4927(00)00068-8
22. Jardri R, Pouchet A, Pins D, Thomas P. Cortical activations during auditory verbal hallucinations in schizophrenia: a coordinate-based meta-analysis. *Am J Psychiatry* (2011) **168**:73–81. doi:10.1176/appi.ajp.2010.09101522
23. Kühn S, Gallinat J. Quantitative meta-analysis on state and trait aspects of auditory verbal hallucinations in schizophrenia. *Schizophr Bull* (2012) **38**:779–86. doi:10.1093/schbul/sbq152
24. Goghari VM, Sponheim SR, MacDonald AW. The functional neuroanatomy of symptom dimensions in schizophrenia: a qualitative and quantitative review of a persistent question. *Neurosci Biobehav Rev* (2010) **34**:468–86. doi:10.1016/j.neubiorev.2009.09.004
25. Andreasen NC, Olsen S. Negative vs positive schizophrenia. Definition and validation. *Arch Gen Psychiatry* (1982) **39**:789–94. doi:10.1001/archpsyc.1982.04290070025006
26. Turetsky B, Cowell PE, Gur RC, Grossman RI, Shtasel DL, Gur RE. Frontal and temporal lobe brain volumes in schizophrenia. Relationship to symptoms and clinical subtype. *Arch Gen Psychiatry* (1995) **52**:1061–70. doi:10.1001/archpsyc.1995.03950240079013
27. Bogerts B, Lieberman JA, Ashtari M, Bilder RM, Degreef G, Lerner G, et al. Hippocampus-amygdala volumes and psychopathology in chronic schizophrenia. *Biol Psychiatry* (1993) **33**:236–46. doi:10.1016/0006-3223(93)90289-P

28. Buchanan RW, Breier A, Kirkpatrick B, Elkashef A, Munson RC, Gellad F, et al. Structural abnormalities in deficit and nondeficit schizophrenia. *Am J Psychiatry* (1993) **150**:59–65.
29. Gur RE, Cowell P, Turetsky BI, Gallacher F, Cannon T, Bilker W, et al. A follow-up magnetic resonance imaging study of schizophrenia. Relationship of neuroanatomical changes to clinical and neurobehavioral measures. *Arch Gen Psychiatry* (1998) **55**:145–52. doi:10.1001/archpsyc.55.2.145
30. Gur RE, Turetsky BI, Bilker WB, Gur RC. Reduced gray matter volume in schizophrenia. *Arch Gen Psychiatry* (1999) **56**:905–11. doi:10.1001/archpsyc.56.10.905
31. Schröder J, Buchsbaum MS, Siegel BV, Geider FJ, Niethammer R. Structural and functional correlates of subsyndromes in chronic schizophrenia. *Psychopathology* (1995) **28**:38–45. doi:10.1159/000284898
32. Schröder J, Buchsbaum MS, Siegel BV, Geider FJ, Lohr J, Tang C, et al. Cerebral metabolic activity correlates of subsyndromes in chronic schizophrenia. *Schizophr Res* (1996) **19**:41–53. doi:10.1016/0920-9964(95)00043-7
33. Potkin SG, Alva G, Fleming K, Anand R, Keator D, Carreon D, et al. A PET study of the pathophysiology of negative symptoms in schizophrenia. *Am J Psychiatry* (2002) **159**:227–37. doi:10.1176/appi.ajp.159.2.227
34. Heckers S, Goff D, Schacter DL, Savage CR, Fischman AJ, Alpert NM, et al. Functional imaging of memory retrieval in deficit vs nondeficit schizophrenia. *Arch Gen Psychiatry* (1999) **56**:1117–23. doi:10.1001/archpsyc.56.12.1117
35. Menon V, Anagnoson RT, Mathalon DH, Glover GH, Pfefferbaum A. Functional neuroanatomy of auditory working memory in schizophrenia: relation to positive and negative symptoms. *Neuroimage* (2001) **13**:433–46. doi:10.1006/nimg.2000.0699
36. Perlstein WM, Carter CS, Noll DC, Cohen JD. Relation of prefrontal cortex dysfunction to working memory and symptoms in schizophrenia. *Am J Psychiatry* (2001) **158**:1105–13. doi:10.1176/appi.ajp.158.7.1105
37. Tamminga CA, Thaker GK, Buchanan R, Kirkpatrick B, Alphs LD, Chase TN, et al. Limbic system abnormalities identified in schizophrenia using positron emission tomography with fluorodeoxyglucose and neocortical alterations with deficit syndrome. *Arch Gen Psychiatry* (1992) **49**:522–30. doi:10.1001/archpsyc.1992.01820070016003
38. Ebmeier KP, Blackwood DH, Murray C, Souza V, Walker M, Dougall N, et al. Single-photon emission computed tomography with 99mTc-exametazime in unmedicated schizophrenic patients. *Biol Psychiatry* (1993) **33**:487–95. doi:10.1016/0006-3223(93)90002-U
39. Kawasaki Y, Maeda Y, Sakai N, Higashima M, Yamaguchi N, Koshino Y, et al. Regional cerebral blood flow in patients with schizophrenia: relevance to symptom structures. *Psychiatry Res* (1996) **67**:49–58. doi:10.1016/0925-4927(96)02685-6
40. Min SK, An SK, Jon DI, Lee JD. Positive and negative symptoms and regional cerebral perfusion in antipsychotic-naive schizophrenic patients: a high-resolution SPECT study. *Psychiatry Res* (1999) **90**:159–68. doi:10.1016/S0925-4927(99)00014-1
41. Juckel G, Schlagenhauf F, Koslowski M, Wustenberg T, Villringer A, Knutson B, et al. Dysfunction of ventral striatal reward prediction in schizophrenia. *Neuroimage* (2006) **29**:409–16. doi:10.1016/j.neuroimage.2005.07.051
42. Simon JJ, Biller A, Walther S, Roesch-Ely D, Stippich C, Weisbrod M, et al. Neural correlates of reward processing in schizophrenia – relationship to apathy and depression. *Schizophr Res* (2010) **118**:154–61. doi:10.1016/j.schres.2009.11.007
43. Elvevag B, Goldberg TE. Cognitive impairment in schizophrenia is the core of the disorder. *Crit Rev Neurobiol* (2000) **14**(1):1–21. doi:10.1615/CritRevNeurobiol.v14.i1.10
44. Silver H, Feldman P, Bilker W, Gur RC. Working memory deficit as a core neuropsychological dysfunction in schizophrenia. *American Journal of Psychiatry* (2003) **160**(10):1809–16. doi:10.1176/appi.ajp.160.10.1809
45. Weinberger DR, Berman KF, Suddath R, Torrey EF. Evidence of dysfunction of a prefrontal-limbic network in schizophrenia: a magnetic resonance imaging and regional cerebral blood flow study of discordant monozygotic twins. *Am J Psychiatry* (1992) **149**(7):890–7.
46. Callicott JH, Bertolino A, Mattay VS, Langheim FJ, Duyn J, Coppola R, et al. Physiological dysfunction of the dorsolateral prefrontal cortex in schizophrenia revisited. *Cereb Cortex* (2000) **10**(11):1078–92. doi:10.1093/cercor/10.11.1078
47. Manoach DS, Gollub RL, Benson ES, Searl MM, Goff DC, Halpern E, et al. Schizophrenic subjects show aberrant fMRI activation of dorsolateral prefrontal cortex and basal ganglia during working memory performance. *Biol Psychiatry* (2000) **48**(2):99–109. doi:10.1016/S0006-3223(00)00227-4
48. Perlstein WM, Dixit NK, Carter CS, Noll DC, Cohen JD. Prefrontal cortex dysfunction mediates deficits in working memory and prepotent responding in schizophrenia. *Biol Psychiatry* (2003) **53**(1):25–38. doi:10.1016/S0006-3223(02)01675-X
49. Tan H-Y, Chen Q, Sust S, Buckholtz JW, Meyers JD, Egan MF, et al. Epistasis between catechol-O-methyltransferase and type II metabotropic glutamate receptor 3 genes on working memory brain function. *Proc Natl Acad Sci U S A* (2007) **104**:12536–41. doi:10.1073/pnas.0610125104
50. Henseler I, Falkai P, Gruber O. A systematic fMRI investigation of the brain systems subserving different working memory components in schizophrenia. *Eur J Neurosci* (2009) **30**:693–702. doi:10.1111/j.1460-9568.2009.06850.x
51. Meyer-Lindenberg A, Olsen R, Kohn P. Regionally specific disturbance of dorsolateral prefrontal-hippocampal functional connectivity in schizophrenia. *Arch Gen Psychiatry* (2005) **62**:379–86. doi:10.1001/archpsyc.62.4.379
52. Henseler I, Falkai P, Gruber O. Disturbed functional connectivity within brain networks subserving domain-specific subcomponents of working memory in schizophrenia: relation to performance and clinical symptoms. *J Psychiatr Res* (2010) **44**:364–72. doi:10.1016/j.jpsychires.2009.09.003
53. Smith EE, Jonides J. Storage and executive processes in the frontal lobes. *Science* (1999) **283**(5408):1657–61. doi:10.1126/science.283.5408.1657
54. Gruber O, Goschke T. Executive control emerging from dynamic interactions between brain systems mediating language, working memory and attentional processes. *Acta Psychol (Amst).* (2004) **115**(2-3):105–21. doi:10.1016/j.actpsy.2003.12.003
55. Gruber O, Melcher T, Diekhof EK, Karch S, Falkai P, Goschke T. Brain mechanisms associated with background monitoring of the environment for potentially significant sensory events. *Brain Cogn* (2009) **69**:559–64. doi:10.1016/j.bandc.2008.11.008
56. Montague PR, Berns GS. Neural economics and the biological substrates of valuation. *Neuron* (2002) **36**(2):265–84. doi:10.1016/S0896-6273(02)00974-1
57. Cools R, Clark L, Owen AM, Robbins TW. Defining the neural mechanisms of probabilistic reversal learning using event-related functional magnetic resonance imaging. *J Neurosci* (2002) **22**(11):4563–7.
58. Kringelbach ML, Rolls ET. Neural correlates of rapid reversal learning in a simple model of human social interaction. *Neuroimage* (2003) **20**(2):1371–83. doi:10.1016/S1053-8119(03)00393-8
59. O'Doherty J, Winston J, Critchley H, Perrett D, Burt DM, Dolan RJ. Beauty in a smile: the role of medial orbitofrontal cortex in facial attractiveness. *Neuropsychologia* (2003) **41**(2):147–55. doi:10.1016/S0028-3932(02)00145-8
60. Gruber O, Diekhof EK, Kirchenbauer L, Goschke T. A neural system for evaluating the behavioural relevance of salient events outside the current focus of attention. *Brain Res* (2010) **1351**:212–21. doi:10.1016/j.brainres.2010.06.056
61. Minzenberg MJ, Laird AR, Thelen S, Carter CS, Glahn DC. Meta-analysis of 41 functional neuroimaging studies of executive function in schizophrenia. *Arch Gen Psychiatry* (2009) **66**:811–22. doi:10.1001/archgenpsychiatry.2009.91
62. Krabbendam L, O'Daly O, Morley LA, van Os J, Murray RM, Shergill SS. Using the Stroop task to investigate the neural correlates of symptom change in schizophrenia. *Br J Psychiatry* (2009) **194**:373–4. doi:10.1192/bjp.bp.108.055459
63. Murray GK, Corlett PR, Clark L, Pessiglione M, Blackwell AD, Honey G, et al. Substantia nigra/ventral tegmental reward prediction error disruption in psychosis. *Mol Psychiatry* (2008) **13**:267–76. doi:10.1038/sj.mp.4002058
64. Achim AM, Lepage M. Episodic memory-related activation in schizophrenia: meta-analysis. *Br J Psychiatry* (2005) **187**:500–9. doi:10.1192/bjp.187.6.500
65. Lesh TA, Niendam TA, Minzenberg MJ, Carter CS. Cognitive control deficits in schizophrenia: mechanisms and meaning. *Neuropsychopharmacology* (2011) **36**:316–38. doi:10.1038/npp.2010.156
66. Li H, Chan RCK, McAlonan GM, Gong Q. Facial emotion processing in schizophrenia: a meta-analysis of functional neuroimaging data. *Schizophr Bull* (2010) **36**:1029–39. doi:10.1093/schbul/sbn190
67. Brunet-Gouet E, Decety J. Social brain dysfunctions in schizophrenia: a review of neuroimaging studies. *Psychiatry Res* (2006) **148**:75–92. doi:10.1016/j.pscychresns.2006.05.001
68. Rasetti R, Mattay VS, Wiedholz LM, Kolachana BS, Hariri AR, Callicott JH, et al. Evidence that altered amygdala activity in schizophrenia is related to clinical state and not genetic risk. *Am J Psychiatry* (2009) **166**:216–25. doi:10.1176/appi.ajp.2008.08020261

69. Straub RE, Weinberger DR. Schizophrenia genes – famine to feast. *Biol Psychiatry* (2006) **60**:81–3. doi:10.1016/j.biopsych.2006.002
70. Howes OD, Kapur S. The dopamine hypothesis of schizophrenia: version III–the final common pathway. *Schizophr Bull* (2009) **35**(3):549–62. doi:10.1093/schbul/sbp006
71. Schwartz TL, Sachdeva S, Stahl SM. Glutamate neurocircuitry: theoretical underpinnings in schizophrenia. *Front Pharmacol* (2012) **3**:195. doi:10.3389/fphar.2012.00195
72. Lewis DA, Gonzalez-Burgos G. Pathophysiologically based treatment interventions in schizophrenia. *Nat Med* (2006) **12**:1016–22. doi:10.1038/nm1478
73. O'Donnell P, Grace AA. Dysfunctions in multiple interrelated systems as the neurobiological bases of schizophrenic symptom clusters. *Schizophr Bull* (1998) **24**(2):267–83. doi:10.1093/oxfordjournals.schbul.a033325
74. Tost H, Meyer-Lindenberg A. Dopamine-glutamate interactions: a neural convergence mechanism of common schizophrenia risk variants. *Biol Psychiatry* (2011) **69**(10):912–3. doi:10.1016/j.biopsych.2011.03.013
75. Blaha CD, Yang CR, Floresco SB, Barr AM, Phillips AG. Stimulation of the ventral subiculum of the hippocampus evokes glutamate receptor-mediated changes in dopamine efflux in the rat nucleus accumbens. *Eur J Neurosci* (1997) **9**:902–11. doi:10.1111/j.1460-9568.1997.tb01441.x
76. Legault M, Wise RA. Injections of N-methyl-D-aspartate into the ventral hippocampus increase extracellular dopamine in the ventral tegmental area and nucleus accumbens. *Synapse* (1999) **31**:241–9. doi:10.1002/(SICI)1098-2396(19990315)31:4<241::AID-SYN1>3.0.CO;2-#
77. Lodge DJ, Grace AA. Gestational methylazoxymethanol acetate administration alters proteomic and metabolomic markers of hippocampal glutamatergic transmission. *Neuropsychopharmacology* (2012) **37**:319–20. doi:10.1038/npp.2011.255
78. Lodge DJ, Grace AA. Aberrant hippocampal activity underlies the dopamine dysregulation in an animal model of schizophrenia. *J Neurosci* (2007) **27**:11424–30. doi:10.1523/JNEUROSCI.2847-07.2007
79. Marsman A, van den Heuvel MP, Klomp DWJ, Kahn RS, Luijten PR, Hulshoff Pol HE. Glutamate in schizophrenia: a focused review and meta-analysis of ^{1}H-MRS studies. *Schizophr Bull* (2013) **39**(1):120–9. doi:10.1093/schbul/sbr069
80. Poels EMP, Kegeles LS, Kantrowitz JT, Slifstein M, Javitt DC, Lieberman JA, et al. Imaging glutamate in schizophrenia: review of findings and implications for drug discovery. *Mol Psychiatry* (2013) **19**(1):20–9. doi:10.1038/mp.2013.136
81. Kegeles LS, Mao X, Stanford AD, Girgis R, Ojeil N, Xu X, et al. Elevated prefrontal cortex γ-aminobutyric acid and glutamate-glutamine levels in schizophrenia measured in vivo with proton magnetic resonance spectroscopy. *Arch Gen Psychiatry* (2012) **69**:449–59. doi:10.1001/archgenpsychiatry.2011.1519
82. Theberge J, Bartha R, Drost DJ, Menon RS, Malla A, Takhar J, et al. Glutamate and glutamine measured with 4.0 T proton MRS in never-treated patients with schizophrenia and healthy volunteers. *Am J Psychiatry* (2002) **159**:1944–6. doi:10.1176/appi.ajp.159.11.1944
83. Bartha R, Williamson PC, Drost DJ, Malla A, Carr TJ, Cortese L, et al. Measurement of glutamate and glutamine in the medial prefrontal cortex of never-treated schizophrenic patients and healthy controls by proton magnetic resonance spectroscopy. *Arch Gen Psychiatry* (1997) **54**:959–65. doi:10.1001/archpsyc.1997.01830220085012
84. Théberge J, Williamson KE, Aoyama N, Drost DJ, Manchanda R, Malla AK, et al. Longitudinal grey-matter and glutamatergic losses in first-episode schizophrenia. *Br J Psychiatry* (2007) **191**:325–34. doi:10.1192/bjp.bp.106.033670
85. Egerton A, Brugger S, Raffin M, Barker GJ, Lythgoe DJ, McGuire PK, et al. Anterior cingulate glutamate levels related to clinical status following treatment in first-episode schizophrenia. *Neuropsychopharmacology* (2012) **37**:2515–21. doi:10.1038/npp.2012.113
86. Ohrmann P, Kugel H, Bauer J, Siegmund A, Kölkebeck K, Suslow T, et al. Learning potential on the WCST in schizophrenia is related to the neuronal integrity of the anterior cingulate cortex as measured by proton magnetic resonance spectroscopy. *Schizophr Res* (2008) **106**:156–63. doi:10.1016/j.schres.2008.08.005
87. Bustillo JR, Chen H, Gasparovic C, Mullins P, Caprihan A, Qualls C, et al. Glutamate as a marker of cognitive function in schizophrenia: a proton spectroscopic imaging study at 4 Tesla. *Biol Psychiatry* (2011) **69**:19–27. doi:10.1016/j.biopsych.2010.08.024
88. Ongür D, Jensen JE, Prescot AP, Stork C, Lundy M, Cohen BM, et al. Abnormal glutamatergic neurotransmission and neuronal-glial interactions in acute mania. *Biol Psychiatry* (2008) **64**:718–26. doi:10.1016/j.biopsych.2008.05.014
89. Wood SJ, Yücel M, Wellard RM, Harrison BJ, Clarke K, Fornito A, et al. Evidence for neuronal dysfunction in the anterior cingulate of patients with schizophrenia: a proton magnetic resonance spectroscopy study at 3 T. *Schizophr Res* (2007) **94**:328–31. doi:10.1016/j.schres.2007.05.008
90. Kraguljac NV, Reid MA, White DM, den Hollander J, Lahti AC. Regional decoupling of N-acetyl-aspartate and glutamate in schizophrenia. *Neuropsychopharmacology* (2012) **37**:2635–42. doi:10.1038/npp.2012.126
91. Bustillo JR, Rowland LM, Mullins P, Jung R, Chen H, Qualls C, et al. 1H-MRS at 4 Tesla in minimally treated early schizophrenia. *Mol Psychiatry* (2010) **15**:629–36. doi:10.1038/mp.2009.121
92. Reid MA, Stoeckel LE, White DM, Avsar KB, Bolding MS, Akella NS, et al. Assessments of function and biochemistry of the anterior cingulate cortex in schizophrenia. *Biol Psychiatry* (2010) **68**:625–33. doi:10.1016/j.biopsych.2010.04.013
93. de la Fuente-Sandoval C, León-Ortiz P, Favila R, Stephano S, Mamo D, Ramírez-Bermúdez J, et al. Higher levels of glutamate in the associative-striatum of subjects with prodromal symptoms of schizophrenia and patients with first-episode psychosis. *Neuropsychopharmacology* (2011) **36**:1781–91. doi:10.1038/npp.2011.65
94. de la Fuente-Sandoval C, León-Ortiz P, Azcárraga M, Stephano S, Favila R, Díaz-Galvis L, et al. Glutamate levels in the associative striatum before and after 4 weeks of antipsychotic treatment in first-episode psychosis: a longitudinal proton magnetic resonance spectroscopy study. *JAMA Psychiatry* (2013) **70**:1057–66. doi:10.1001/jamapsychiatry.2013.289
95. Goto N, Yoshimura R, Kakeda S, Nishimura J, Moriya J, Hayashi K, et al. Six-month treatment with atypical antipsychotic drugs decreased frontal-lobe levels of glutamate plus glutamine in early-stage first-episode schizophrenia. *Neuropsychiatr Dis Treat* (2012) **8**:119–22. doi:10.2147/NDT.S25582
96. Egan MF, Goldberg TE, Kolachana BS, Callicott JH, Mazzanti CM, Straub RE, et al. Effect of COMT Val(108/158) Met genotype on frontal lobe function and risk for schizophrenia. *Proc Natl Acad Sci U S A* (2001) **98**:6917–22. doi:10.1073/pnas.111134598
97. Meyer-Lindenberg A, Kohn PD, Kolachana B, Kippenhan S, McInerney-Leo A, Nussbaum R, et al. Midbrain dopamine and prefrontal function in humans: interaction and modulation by COMT genotype. *Nat Neurosci* (2005) **8**:594–6. doi:10.1038/nn1438
98. Meyer-Lindenberg A, Weinberger DR. Intermediate phenotypes and genetic mechanisms of psychiatric disorders. *Nat Rev Neurosci* (2006) **7**:818–27. doi:10.1038/nrn1993
99. Meyer-Lindenberg A, Nichols T, Callicott JH, Ding J, Kolachana B, Buckholtz J, et al. Impact of complex genetic variation in COMT on human brain function. *Mol Psychiatry* (2006) **11**:867–77. doi:10.1038/sj.mp.4001860
100. Nixon DC, Prust MJ, Sambataro F, Tan H-Y, Mattay VS, Weinberger DR, et al. Interactive effects of DAOA (G72) and catechol-O-methyltransferase on neurophysiology in prefrontal cortex. *Biol Psychiatry* (2011) **69**:1006–8. doi:10.1016/j.biopsych.2010.10.031
101. Nicodemus KK, Kolachana BS, Vakkalanka R, Straub RE, Giegling I, Egan MF, et al. Evidence for statistical epistasis between catechol-O-methyltransferase (COMT) and polymorphisms in RGS4, G72 (DAOA), GRM3, and DISC1: influence on risk of schizophrenia. *Hum Genet* (2007) **120**:889–906. doi:10.1007/s00439-006-0257-3
102. O'Donovan MC, Craddock N, Norton N, Williams H, Peirce T, Moskvina V, et al. Identification of loci associated with schizophrenia by genome-wide association and follow-up. *Nat Genet* (2008) **40**:1053–5. doi:10.1038/ng.201
103. Ferreira MAR, O'Donovan MC, Meng YA, Jones IR, Ruderfer DM, Jones L, et al. Collaborative genome-wide association analysis supports a role for ANK3 and CACNA1C in bipolar disorder. *Nat Genet* (2008) **40**:1056–8. doi:10.1038/ng.209
104. Esslinger C, Walter H, Kirsch P, Erk S, Schnell K, Arnold C, et al. Neural mechanisms of a genome-wide supported psychosis variant. *Science* (2009) **324**:605. doi:10.1126/science.1167768
105. Paulus FM, Krach S, Bedenbender J, Pyka M, Sommer J, Krug A, et al. Partial support for ZNF804A genotype-dependent alterations in prefrontal connectivity. *Hum Brain Mapp* (2013) **34**:304–13. doi:10.1002/hbm.21434
106. Rasetti R, Sambataro F, Chen Q, Callicott JH, Mattay VS, Weinberger DR. Altered cortical network dynamics a potential intermediate phenotype for schizophrenia and association with ZNF804A RID E-3426-2010. *Arch Gen Psychiatry* (2011) **68**:1207–17. doi:10.1001/archgenpsychiatry.2011.103

107. Erk S, Meyer-Lindenberg A, Schnell K, Opitz von Boberfeld C, Esslinger C, Kirsch P, et al. Brain function in carriers of a genome-wide supported bipolar disorder variant. *Arch Gen Psychiatry* (2010) **67**:803–11. doi:10.1001/archgenpsychiatry.2010.94
108. Bigos KL, Mattay VS, Callicott JH, Straub RE, Vakkalanka R, Kolachana B, et al. Genetic variation in CACNA1C affects brain circuitries related to mental illness. *Arch Gen Psychiatry* (2010) **67**:939–45. doi:10.1001/archgenpsychiatry.2010.96
109. Wessa M, Linke J, Witt SH, Nieratschker V, Esslinger C, Kirsch P, et al. The CACNA1C risk variant for bipolar disorder influences limbic activity. *Mol Psychiatry* (2010) **15**:1126–7. doi:10.1038/mp.2009.103
110. Tandon R, Nasrallah HA, Keshavan MS. Schizophrenia, "just the facts" 5. Treatment and prevention. Past, present, and future. *Schizophr Res* (2010) **122**:1–23. doi:10.1016/j.schres.2010.05.025
111. Leucht S, Corves C, Arbter D, Engel RR, Li C, Davis JM. Second-generation versus first-generation antipsychotic drugs for schizophrenia: a meta-analysis. *Lancet* (2009) **373**:31–41. doi:10.1016/S0140-6736(08)61764-X
112. Hill SK, Bishop JR, Palumbo D, Sweeney JA. Effect of second-generation antipsychotics on cognition: current issues and future challenges. *Expert Rev Neurother* (2010) **10**:43–57. doi:10.1586/ern.09.143
113. Hashimoto K, Malchow B, Falkai P, Schmitt A. Glutamate modulators as potential therapeutic drugs in schizophrenia and affective disorders. *Eur Arch Psychiatry Clin Neurosci* (2013) **263**(5):367–77. doi:10.1007/s00406-013-0399-y
114. Traynelis SF, Wollmuth LP, McBain CJ, Menniti FS, Vance KM, Ogden KK, et al. Glutamate receptor ion channels: structure, regulation, and function. *Pharmacol Rev* (2010) **62**:405–96. doi:10.1124/pr.109.002451
115. Shepherd JD, Huganir RL. The cell biology of synaptic plasticity: AMPA receptor trafficking. *Annu Rev Cell Dev Biol* (2007) **23**:613–43. doi:10.1146/annurev.cellbio.23.090506.123516
116. Johnson JW, Ascher P. Glycine potentiates the NMDA response in cultured mouse brain neurons. *Nature* (1987) **325**:529–31. doi:10.1038/325529a0
117. Tuominen HJ, Tiihonen J, Wahlbeck K. Glutamatergic drugs for schizophrenia. *Cochrane Database Syst Rev* (2006) (2):CD003730. doi:10.1002/14651858.CD003730.pub2
118. Tsai GE, Lin P-Y. Strategies to enhance N-methyl-D-aspartate receptor-mediated neurotransmission in schizophrenia, a critical review and meta-analysis. *Curr Pharm Des* (2010) **16**:522–37. doi:10.2174/138161210790361452
119. Buchanan RW, Javitt DC, Marder SR, Schooler NR, Gold JM, McMahon RP, et al. The cognitive and negative symptoms in schizophrenia trial (CONSIST): the efficacy of glutamatergic agents for negative symptoms and cognitive impairments. *Am J Psychiatry* (2007) **164**:1593–602. doi:10.1176/appi.ajp.2007.06081358
120. Goff DC. D-cycloserine: an evolving role in learning and neuroplasticity in schizophrenia. *Schizophr Bull* (2012) **38**:936–41. doi:10.1093/schbul/sbs012
121. Goff DC, Cather C, Gottlieb JD, Evins AE, Walsh J, Raeke L, et al. Once-weekly D-cycloserine effects on negative symptoms and cognition in schizophrenia: an exploratory study. *Schizophr Res* (2008) **106**:320–7. doi:10.1016/j.schres.2008.08.012
122. Tsai G, Yang P, Chung LC, Lange N, Coyle JT. D-serine added to antipsychotics for the treatment of schizophrenia. *Biol Psychiatry* (1998) **44**:1081–9. doi:10.1016/S0006-3223(98)00279-0
123. Heresco-Levy U, Javitt DC, Ebstein R, Vass A, Lichtenberg P, Bar G, et al. D-serine efficacy as add-on pharmacotherapy to risperidone and olanzapine for treatment-refractory schizophrenia. *Biol Psychiatry* (2005) **57**:577–85. doi:10.1016/j.biopsych.2004.12.037
124. Kantrowitz JT, Malhotra AK, Cornblatt B, Silipo G, Balla A, Suckow RF, et al. High dose D-serine in the treatment of schizophrenia. *Schizophr Res* (2010) **121**:125–30. doi:10.1016/j.schres.2010.05.012
125. Lane H-Y, Lin C-H, Huang Y-J, Liao C-H, Chang Y-C, Tsai GE. A randomized, double-blind, placebo-controlled comparison study of sarcosine (N-methylglycine) and D-serine add-on treatment for schizophrenia. *Int J Neuropsychopharmacol* (2010) **13**:451–60. doi:10.1017/S1461145709990939
126. Javitt DC. Glycine transport inhibitors in the treatment of schizophrenia. *Handb Exp Pharmacol* (2012) **213**:367–99. doi:10.1007/978-3-642-25758-2_12
127. Javitt DC, Zukin SR, Heresco-levy U, Umbricht D. Has an angel shown the way? Etiological and therapeutic implications of the PCP/NMDA model of schizophrenia. *Schizophr Bull* (2012) **38**:958–66. doi:10.1093/schbul/sbs069
128. Sreekumar A, Poisson LM, Rajendiran TM, Khan AP, Cao Q, Yu J, et al. Metabolomic profiles delineate potential role for sarcosine in prostate cancer progression. *Nature* (2012) **12**(457):910–4. doi:10.1038/nature07762
129. Pinard E, Alanine A, Alberati D, Bender M, Borroni E, Bourdeaux P, et al. Selective GlyT1 inhibitors: discovery of [4-(3-fluoro-5-trifluoromethylpyridin-2-yl)piperazin-1-yl][5-methanesulfonyl-2-((S)-2,2,2-trifluoro-1-methylethoxy)phenyl]methanone (RG1678), a promising novel medicine to treat schizophrenia. *J Med Chem* (2010) **53**:4603–14. doi:10.1021/jm100210p
130. Alberati D, Moreau J-L, Lengyel J, Hauser N, Mory R, Borroni E, et al. Glycine reuptake inhibitor RG1678: a pharmacologic characterization of an investigational agent for the treatment of schizophrenia. *Neuropharmacology* (2012) **62**:1152–61. doi:10.1016/j.neuropharm.2011.11.008
131. Roche Global Web Site. *Phase II Study with First-in-Class Investigational Drug Demonstrates Improvement in Negative Symptoms in Patients with Schizophrenia.* (2010). Available from: http://www.roche.com/investors/ir_update/inv-update-2010-12-06b.htm
132. Bliss TV, Collingridge GL. A synaptic model of memory: long-term potentiation in the hippocampus. *Nature* (1993) **361**:31–9. doi:10.1038/361031a0
133. Noorbala AA, Akhondzadeh S, Davari-Ashtiani R, Amini-Nooshabadi H. Piracetam in the treatment of schizophrenia: implications for the glutamate hypothesis of schizophrenia. *J Clin Pharm Ther* (1999) **24**:369–74. doi:10.1046/j.1365-2710.1999.00238.x
134. Goff DC, Leahy L, Berman I, Posever T, Herz L, Leon AC, et al. A placebo-controlled pilot study of the ampakine CX516 added to clozapine in schizophrenia. *J Clin Psychopharmacol* (2001) **21**:484–7. doi:10.1097/00004714-200110000-00005
135. Goff DC, Lamberti JS, Leon AC, Green MF, Miller AL, Patel J, et al. A placebo-controlled add-on trial of the ampakine CX516, for cognitive deficits in schizophrenia. *Neuropsychopharmacology* (2008) **33**:465–72. doi:10.1038/sj.npp.1301444
136. Moghaddam B, Adams B, Verma A, Daly D. Activation of glutamatergic neurotransmission by ketamine: a novel step in the pathway from NMDA receptor blockade to dopaminergic and cognitive disruptions associated with the prefrontal cortex. *J Neurosci* (1997) **17**(8):2921–7.
137. Coyle JT, Basu A, Benneyworth M, Balu D, Konopaske G. Glutamatergic synaptic dysregulation in schizophrenia: therapeutic implications. *Handb Exp Pharmacol* (2012) **213**:267–95. doi:10.1007/978-3-642-25758-2_10
138. Niswender CM, Conn PJ. Metabotropic glutamate receptors: physiology, pharmacology, and disease. *Annu Rev Pharmacol Toxicol* (2010) **50**:295–322. doi:10.1146/annurev.pharmtox.011008.145533
139. Patil ST, Zhang L, Martenyi F, Lowe SL, Jackson KA, Andreev BV, et al. Activation of mGlu2/3 receptors as a new approach to treat schizophrenia: a randomized Phase 2 clinical trial. *Nat Med* (2007) **13**(9):1102–7. doi:10.1038/nm1007-1264
140. Kinon BJ, Zhang L, Millen BA, Osuntokun OO, Williams JE, Kollack-Walker S, et al. A multicenter, inpatient, phase 2, double-blind, placebo-controlled dose-ranging study of LY2140023 monohydrate in patients with DSM-IV schizophrenia. *J Clin Psychopharmacol* (2011) **31**(3):349–55. doi:10.1097/JCP.0b013e318218dcd5
141. Adams DH, Kinon BJ, Baygani S, Millen BA, Velona I, Kollack-Walker S, et al. A long-term, phase 2, multicenter, randomized, open-label, comparative safety study of pomaglumetad methionil (LY2140023 monohydrate) versus atypical antipsychotic standard of care in patients with schizophrenia. *BMC Psychiatry* (2013) **13**(1):143. doi:10.1186/1471-244X-13-143
142. Stauffer VL, Ayan-Oshodi M, Wondmagegnehu ET, Witcher J, Shen T, Yuen ESM, et al. A phase 1B study investigating the potential interaction between LY2140023 and second generation antipsychotics in subjects with schizophrenia or schizoaffective disorder. *Schizophr Res* (2012) **136**:S169–70. doi:10.1016/S0920-9964(12)70533-9
143. Stauffer VL, Millen BA, Andersen S, Kinon BJ, Lagrandeur L, Lindenmayer JP, et al. Pomaglumetad methionil: no significant difference as an adjunctive treatment for patients with prominent negative symptoms of schizophrenia compared to placebo. *Schizophr Res* (2013) **150**:434–41. doi:10.1016/j.schres.2013.08.020
144. Addex Therapeutics. *Addex Reports Top-line Data from a Successful Phase 2a Clinical Study with ADX71149 in Schizophrenia Patients.* Addex Therapeutics Press Release (2012). Available from: http://www.addextherapeutics.com/about/about-addex/

145. Kent JM, Anghelescu IG, Kezic I, Daly E, Ceusters M, De Smedt H, et al. Safety, tolerability and potential therapeutic efficacy of a novel glutamate modulator as adjunctive treatment in patients with schizophrenia. *APA 2013 Annual Meeting*. San Francisco (2013).
146. Kraepelin E. *Psychiatrie – Ein Lehrbuch für Studierende und Ärzte*. 5th ed. Leipzig: Barth (1896).

6

Reinforcement Learning and Dopamine in Schizophrenia: Dimensions of Symptoms or Specific Features of a Disease Group?

Lorenz Deserno[1,2]*, Rebecca Boehme[2], Andreas Heinz[2] and Florian Schlagenhauf[1,2]

[1] Max Planck Institute for Human Cognitive and Brain Sciences, Leipzig, Germany
[2] Department of Psychiatry and Psychotherapy, Charité – Universitätsmedizin Berlin, Berlin, Germany

Correspondence:
Lorenz Deserno, Department of Psychiatry and Psychotherapy, Charité – Universitätsmedizin Berlin, Campus Mitte, Charitéplatz 1, 10117 Berlin, Germany
e-mail: lorenz.deserno@charite.de

Abnormalities in reinforcement learning are a key finding in schizophrenia and have been proposed to be linked to elevated levels of dopamine neurotransmission. Behavioral deficits in reinforcement learning and their neural correlates may contribute to the formation of clinical characteristics of schizophrenia. The ability to form predictions about future outcomes is fundamental for environmental interactions and depends on neuronal teaching signals, like reward prediction errors. While aberrant prediction errors, that encode non-salient events as surprising, have been proposed to contribute to the formation of positive symptoms, a failure to build neural representations of decision values may result in negative symptoms. Here, we review behavioral and neuroimaging research in schizophrenia and focus on studies that implemented reinforcement learning models. In addition, we discuss studies that combined reinforcement learning with measures of dopamine. Thereby, we suggest how reinforcement learning abnormalities in schizophrenia may contribute to the formation of psychotic symptoms and may interact with cognitive deficits. These ideas point toward an interplay of more rigid versus flexible control over reinforcement learning. Pronounced deficits in the flexible or model-based domain may allow for a detailed characterization of well-established cognitive deficits in schizophrenia patients based on computational models of learning. Finally, we propose a framework based on the potentially crucial contribution of dopamine to dysfunctional reinforcement learning on the level of neural networks. Future research may strongly benefit from computational modeling but also requires further methodological improvement for clinical group studies. These research tools may help to improve our understanding of disease-specific mechanisms and may help to identify clinically relevant subgroups of the heterogeneous entity schizophrenia.

Keywords: schizophrenia, dopamine, computational modeling, reinforcement learning, aberrant salience, prediction error, fMRI, PET imaging

INTRODUCTION AND OUTLINE

The "dopamine-hypothesis" of schizophrenia was initially built upon the observation that dopamine receptor antagonists, such as haloperidol, attenuate psychotic symptoms (1). Evidence showing that elevated dopamine levels are indeed involved in the pathophysiology of psychotic symptoms and schizophrenia is primarily derived from neurochemical studies using positron-emission-tomography (PET) with radioactive ligands targeting the brain's dopamine system. Such studies clearly indicate elevated levels of presynaptic dopamine function (2, 3) with particularly strong evidence from meta-analyses for elevated dopamine synthesis capacity (4, 5). A hallmark of dopamine research was the observation that phasic releases of dopaminergic neurons code a temporal-difference prediction error, which was later shown to be causally involved in learning (6–8). This ability to form predictions about future outcomes is fundamental for interactions with the environment and depends on neuronal representations of such teaching signals. Behavioral impairments in reinforcement learning are a key finding in schizophrenia patients and have been proposed to be closely linked to reports of elevated presynaptic dopamine neurotransmission. Influential theoretical work suggests that dysfunctional reinforcement learning may contribute to the formation of the prominent clinical characteristics of schizophrenia patients, namely positive and negative symptoms (9–11). Furthermore, prediction errors are involved in learning-related changes in synaptic plasticity (12), and aberrant plasticity has been suggested as a potential common biological mechanism characterizing the schizophrenia spectrum (13, 14).

Embedded in this context, the central attempt of this article is to review studies on reinforcement learning in schizophrenia and to disentangle dimensions of symptom formation and potential disease-specific mechanisms in the existing literature. The primary focus of this article is to provide an up-to-date overview of the existing literature with the aim to review existing evidence for two influential theories. Therefore, we only include a brief introduction (see Reinforcement Learning in Schizophrenia: Theoretical Considerations) to these hypotheses and refer to the original publications for more detailed theoretical descriptions. The empirical studies reviewed here comprise behavioral and functional neuroimaging studies [restricted to functional magnetic resonance imaging (fMRI) and PET] in patients suffering from schizophrenia. In the first part, we start with studies on reward anticipation and processing based on pre-learned contingencies. Subsequently, we focus on studies that directly examine learning over time with a focus on studies that implemented reinforcement learning models. Finally, we summarize studies that combined experimental perturbations of the brain's dopamine system, such as pharmacological challenges and molecular imaging (PET), with measures of reinforcement learning.

FEEDBACK ANTICIPATION AND PROCESSING

A series of studies used the monetary incentive delay task (MID), a paradigm invented by Knutson and colleagues [(15), see also Ref. (16)]. The initial study demonstrated that participants speed up motor responses to obtain rewards and that anticipation as well as delivery of rewards evoke ventral striatal activation. The first application of this task in schizophrenia patients was carried out by Juckel and colleagues: they found reduced ventral striatal activation in unmedicated patients (17). This finding was subsequently replicated in a larger cohort of drug-naïve, first-episode patients (18, 19). In the study by Juckel et al. (17), it was demonstrated that blunting of anticipatory ventral striatal activation elicited by monetary reward reflected the individual degree of negative symptoms (17). This association was also present in patients treated with typical or first generation antipsychotics (FGAs, or "typical" antipsychotics), who showed reduced ventral striatal activation during reward anticipation, while patients treated with atypical or second generation antipsychotics (SGAs, or "atypical" antipsychotics) showed intact activation during anticipation of monetary reward in the same region (20, 21). This effect of SGAs was recently replicated in a larger cohort of patients (22). In line with these results, further studies applying the MID task in chronic schizophrenia patients medicated predominantly with SGAs did not find reduced ventral striatal anticipation of monetary reward in the patient group, as a whole (23–25). Two studies replicated the association of reward anticipation with negative symptoms (25) and apathy (24), while two other studies reported a correlation of ventral striatal activation during reward anticipation with positive symptoms (18, 19).

Although the static MID task is thought to mirror aspects of animal experiments studying reinforcement learning in the dopaminergic system [e.g., Ref. (6)], the gross time scale of fMRI compared to neurophysiological studies needs to be taken into account (26). Nevertheless, it has been demonstrated that ventral striatal activation during reward anticipation is indeed modulated by dopamine: a positive correlation between the anticipatory activation in core dopamine areas and reward-induced dopamine release was observed via competition of endogenous dopamine with a PET D2/3-receptor radioligand (27). In a study by Knutson et al. (28), diminished ventral striatal reward anticipation was reported when comparing healthy participants receiving amphetamine (resulting in a massive release of dopamine) to placebo (28). The latter study coincides with the results reported above in schizophrenia patients during reward anticipation and the well-established finding of elevated presynaptic dopamine function in schizophrenia using PET with FDOPA and similar tracers [for meta-analyses see: Ref. (4, 5)]. Based on this, it appears conceivable that event-related responses to reward-indicating cues disappear in the noise of elevated dopaminergic activity observed in schizophrenia patients and that this may ultimately contribute to a failure of salience attribution to environmentally relevant stimuli (9, 10, 29). Interestingly, Esslinger et al. (18) implemented the MID task in combination with another task possibly reflecting salience and showed in an exploratory correlation analysis that more pronounced ventral striatal hypoactivation during reward anticipation was associated with more salience attribution to neutral stimuli (18). In line with this, a recent study using emotional picture stimuli demonstrated that schizophrenia patients rate neutral pictures as more salient (30). These results provide some rather indirect support for the idea of aberrant salience in schizophrenia, which we will briefly introduce in the following section.

In contrast to reward anticipation, fewer studies used the MID task to examine the delivery of monetary outcome. One study (31) found that violations of outcome expectancies triggered abnormal neural responses in unmedicated patients: While medial-prefrontal activation was exaggerated when an expected-reward was omitted, ventral striatum (VS) displayed reduced activation for successful versus unsuccessful loss avoidance. The degree of delusion severity was found to be associated with activation in medial-prefrontal cortex (PFC) for successful versus unsuccessful loss avoidance. Moreover, functional connectivity between VS and medial PFC was reduced in patients. In a similar vein, Waltz et al. (25) found reduced activation in the medial PFC and lateral PFC when comparing win versus loss trials in schizophrenia patients medicated with SGAs. Activation to reward delivery in lateral PFC was negatively correlated with the degree of positive and negative symptoms (25). Another study (23) tested high and low rewards together with high and low punishments against neutral events and found significant activation in lateral PFC of healthy controls, most likely reflecting salience. This activation pattern was diminished in patients treated with SGAs. Interestingly, a recent study showed exaggerated activation in dorsolateral PFC elicited by neutral outcomes in unmedicated patients (19).

Two studies examined classical conditioning that actually took place outside the MRI scanner (32, 33). These designs might be thought of as extensions to studies using the MID task: Contingencies were pre-learned before scanning, but allow one to distinguish between expected-rewards, unexpected-rewards (presumably mirroring positive prediction errors), and unexpected omissions of rewards (presumably mirroring negative prediction errors; (32)). Juice was used as a primary reinforcer in 18 medicated patients (32). Attenuated neural responses in dopaminergic core areas (midbrain and striatum) to expected and unexpected-reward deliveries were observed, while activation in reward omission trials was largely intact. Morris et al. (33) completed this approach in a full 2 × 2 design, thereby enabling an orthogonalization of the factors "rewards" and "surprise" as well as the interaction of both factors, which is assumed to mirror prediction-error-related brain activation. In 21 schizophrenia patients medicated with SGAs, this revealed a disrupted differentiation between expected and unexpected events in a way that ventral striatal activation is not coding prediction errors: while response to expected events in right VS was exaggerated, response to unexpected outcomes in left VS was found to be blunted (33).

In summary, fMRI studies in reward processing using the MID task have so far provided important insights into the neural processes underlying outcome anticipation and delivery in schizophrenia. In particular, the finding of reduced ventral striatal activation during outcome anticipation was consistently replicated across three studies involving a total of 68 unmedicated patients. An association of anticipatory ventral striatal activation with negative symptoms was reported in five studies involving 10 unmedicated patients and 52 medicated patients. Antipsychotic medication remains a crucial issue since these drugs specifically block those striatal D2-receptors that are (among others) activated by potentially prediction-error-associated dopamine release [e.g., Ref. (34, 35)] and moreover affect presynaptic dopamine synthesis (36, 37). Therefore, assessing unmedicated patients is key to understanding dopamine dysfunction in schizophrenia and to avoiding confounds by medication effects, which also appear to differ depending on FGAs versus SGAs (20, 21). Furthermore, one important limitation of the studies discussed thus far is the fact that all reward contingencies are pre-learned (i.e., before participants enter the MRI scanner and perform the task). Anticipatory brain activation during the MID task is likely to capture some aspects of reinforcement learning in particular with respect to cue- or action-related value signals. Some kind of value quantification is usually the main outcome variable of reinforcement learning models. It is important to note that these functions evolve over time, which is also a fundamental principle of brain signals. This points out an important limitation of the MID studies which may therefore provide a rather coarse proxy of value-related brain activation and consequently emphasizes the necessity to study learning over the course of time. Thus, studying the temporal dynamics underlying the actual learning process may provide more insights into symptom- and disease-specific processes associated with schizophrenia. In contrast to studies which used the MID task or similar designs, all studies discussed in Section "Behavioral Studies of Reinforcement Learning in Schizophrenia" refer to experimental paradigms that investigate learning on a trial-by-trial basis. Detailed computational modeling of such temporal dynamics may be particularly helpful to elucidate dysfunctional processes in patients and to improve characterization of a heterogeneous disease entity that is so far still based on symptoms (38–41).

REINFORCEMENT LEARNING IN SCHIZOPHRENIA: THEORETICAL CONSIDERATIONS

Reinforcement learning represents a promising, theory-driven tool (42) which aims to quantify learning on a trial-by-trial basis and has so far been implemented in a limited number of clinical group studies [e.g., Ref. (43), **Table 1**]. Although there are several different variants of models, most of them separate two main contributors to the learning process and both of them change on trial-by-trial (**Box 1**): first, the delivered outcome which refers to the time point when prediction errors arise. This teaching signal is thought to be crucially involved in driving any learning process. Second, the values of environmental cues or actions which are learned via this teaching signal. Concepts of motivational or incentive salience are closely linked with values of actions or environmental cues (44) that can be acquired during prediction-error-driven trial-and-error learning. Differences in the perceived properties of feedback stimuli *per se* (e.g., shifts in hedonic experience or salience) may also influence the elicitation of prediction errors and thus potentially corrupt learning processes. Based on these two main time points, we will proceed with a brief summary of two influential hypotheses with respect to the potential contribution of reinforcement learning to symptom dimensions and disease-specific features in schizophrenia.

We begin with the "aberrant salience" hypothesis: schizophrenia patients may attribute salience to otherwise neutral environmental stimuli, and those stimuli may ultimately appear meaningful and evoke delusional mood in patients (9, 10). This process has been described as closely linked to a dysregulation of the dopamine system where both chaotic dopamine firing (45) and elevated baseline dopamine levels (46, 47) have been proposed to be involved. Whether this process actually reflects reinforcement learning in the same way as it was theoretically and mechanistically defined for healthy people (42) remains an open and exciting question. If this is the case, then neutral events should elicit prediction errors which may consequently train values for the associated cues or actions, and these values may finally exceed incentive values associated with rewarding or otherwise reinforcing events. In other words, patients are assumed to attribute importance to stimuli ignored by healthy volunteers and thereby learn something else. The degree of this alteration should be related to positive symptom levels, in particular delusions. It is important to note, that a prerequisite for the latter idea is that misattributed salience to certain neutral events remains stable over a period of time. Alternatively, it may also be possible that the process of misattributing salience is fluctuating permanently, resulting in a random pattern (a state where "everything is salient") that would formally result in no learning at all and might therefore be harder to quantify. It is also conceivable that aberrant aspects of reinforcement learning have not yet been formulated correctly. Here, the role of unsigned prediction errors, as a valence-unspecific salience signal, might be of interest and could possibly be integrated in models of reinforcement learning (48–50).

The second hypothesis focuses on a deficit in the representation of learned values (11). This hypothesis posits that prediction errors are not adequately used to learn values even though hedonic experience itself remains mainly intact. This concept relates closely to the idea that reward feedback is not adequately transformed into motivational drive for goal-directed behavior (51) and has been proposed as a potential mechanism for the origin of negative symptoms (11). In general, a failure to learn any value may also be based on a reduction of hedonic experience, in which case no prediction errors are elicited and therefore no values can be learned; based on studies reviewed in the next section, this appears to be unlikely in schizophrenia patients. On the other hand, a deficit in using monetary and primary rewards for motivated behavior would appear similar to what was proposed in the incentive-sensitization theory of addiction disorders, which assumes a shift from non-drug rewards to drug-related rewards (44). In schizophrenia, such a shift may predominantly concern neutral stimuli and therefore result in aberrant learning as pointed out in the aberrant salience hypothesis.

Table 1 | Studies in schizophrenia patients using a computational model approach.

Reference	Paradigm	Methods	Model	Main findings
Strauss et al. (89)	Temporal utility integration task	51 Medicated schizophrenia and schizoaffective patients, behavioral data only	RT-based RW	Impaired go, intact nogo learning in patients, correlation with negative symptom level
Gold et al. (64)	Instrumental probabilistic reward-approach versus punishment avoidance learning	47 Medicated schizophrenia and schizoaffective patients, behavioral data only	Actor-critic Q-learning hybrid of these two	High negative symptoms patients fail to represent and learn from reward value properly, loss avoidance is preserved
Murray et al. (43)	Instrumental reward learning	13 First-episode patients, 8 on SGAss, later diagnosed: 1 bipolar, 1 psychosis, 11 schizophrenia, fMRI	Q-learning	Impaired differentiation between neutral and reward predicting stimuli, attenuated activity for reward predicting stimulus, trend-wise augmented for neutral stimulus, reduced RPE activity in midbrain and VS
Koch et al. (103)	Instrumental gambling task	19 Medicated (except 1) schizophrenia patients, fMRI	TD	Impaired behavioral performance, reduced dorsolateral PFC and cingulate gyrus probability related activity, reduced RPE response in PFC, putamen, hippocampus and insula
Gradin et al. (106)	Instrumental probabilistic reward learning	15 Medicated schizophrenia patients, fMRI	SARSA-TD	Less rewards achieved, reduced RPE related activity in striatum, thalamus, amygdala-hippocampal complex, and insula, reduced encoding of expected value in amygdala-hippocampal complex and parahippocampal gyrus, correlation with positive symptoms
Romaniuk et al. (93)	Aversive classical conditioning	20 Medicated schizophrenia patients, fMRI	TD	No difference in RT, difference in skin conductance, impaired amygdala activation during conditioning, impaired midbrain activation during learning, inappropriate activation of nucleus accumbens in response to neutral cues
Schlagenhauf et al. (77)	Instrumental reversal learning task	24 Unmedicated schizophrenic patients, fMRI	RW, double-update, Hidden–Markov	Deficit in reversal learning, relation to positive symptoms, VS learning signals are reduced independent of task insight in contrast to prefrontal activation

RW, Rescorla–Wagner-model; TD, temporal-difference model; SARSA, state action response state action; RPE, reward prediction error; VS, ventral striatum; RT, reaction time.

As indicated, the two hypotheses are only partially independent. It is possible that both mentioned mechanisms exist in parallel and converge in producing a behavioral deficit but diverge in their differential contribution to symptom formation. In the following, we will review studies that aimed to test these hypotheses. Thereby, we try to build a coherent picture of how reinforcement learning may contribute to the formation of psychotic symptoms and if this appears to be dimensional or categorical. Finally, we endeavor to interpret previous studies with regard to their disease specificity by summarizing and discussing those studies that examined learning over time. We start with behavioral studies followed by a section on imaging studies. We also mention if studies implemented models of reinforcement learning and how parameters underlying these models were inferred.

BEHAVIORAL STUDIES OF REINFORCEMENT LEARNING IN SCHIZOPHRENIA

Behavioral deficits in associative learning, particularly in instrumental tasks where feedback is used to guide behavior, are frequently replicated in schizophrenia patients. So far, only seven studies have implemented models of reinforcement learning (see **Table 1**), and although reinforcement learning modeling quantifies the observed behavior, only two of these studies were purely behavioral; the other five studies also collected fMRI data and regressed model-derived learning time-series (e.g., prediction errors) against imaging data. Studies on classical conditioning are reported in the subsequent section, because all the clinical studies conducted so far have assessed classical conditioning effects via physiological measures. In the following we will summarize studies that used instrumental tasks. We will also describe modeling studies in detail, because this approach represents a powerful tool to provide a more fine-grained understanding of learning mechanisms and psychopathology (40, 41, 52, 53).

Based on the direct involvement of dopamine in both reinforcement learning and the neurobiology of schizophrenia, more systematic experimental examinations of alterations in reinforcement learning have been reported in the last decade. With regard to aberrant salience and the described ideas about aberrant learning,

Box 1 | Reinforcement learning models.

A prediction error is defined as the difference between a delivered reward R and an expected value, here denoted as Q. t and a denote indices that refer to time and the value associated with a chosen action, respectively.

$$\delta_{Qa,t} = R_t - Q_{a,t} \quad (1)$$

In model-free learning, this error signal can be used to update values:

$$Q_{a,t+1} = Q_{a,t} + \alpha\delta_{Qa,t} \quad (2)$$

Here, α represent a learning rate, which weighs the influence of $\delta_{Qa,t}$ on $Q_{a,t+1}$ with natural boundaries between 0 and 1. For examples of clinical studies using this algorithm, please compare Murray et al. (43) or Schlagenhauf et al. (77). Equation 2 refers to environments, in which each time point or trial t consists of one stage, e.g., one action, which results in feedback delivery. This can be extended to sequential decision tasks, where each trial consists of multiple numbers of stages and for example only the final stage is associated with feedback delivery. For an extension of the Eqs 1 and 2 for sequential decisions, please compare the work by Daw et al. (80) or Glascher et al. (79).

Still referring to model-free learning, we can define δ and the update equation differently, as for example in actor-critic models. The same error signal, generated by the critic, updates values of the critic and the actor:

$$\delta_{C,s,t} = R_t - C_{s,t} \quad (3)$$

$$C_{s,t+1} = C_{s,t} + \alpha_s\delta_{Cs,t} \quad (4)$$

Notably, the critic Eqs 5 and 6 neglects the specific action that was chosen in trial t. The actor learns specific action values via the same error signal $\delta_{Cs,t}$:

$$A_{s,a,t+1} = A_{s,a,t} + \alpha_s\delta_{Cs,t} \quad (5)$$

This approach was applied in one clinical study (64).

So far, all presented models are examples for model-free learning. Subsequently, we present one example, which touches the ground of model-based learning. Depending on task structure, it is possible to implement certain aspects of the environment. For instance, in an environment with two choice options prediction errors may also be used to update values of unchosen actions ua; this can be done by an additional extension of Eq. 2:

$$Q_{ua,t+1} = Q_{ua,t} - \alpha\delta_{Qa,t} \quad (6)$$

Equation 8 represents a full double-update learner (77), while it is also possible to weigh the influence of the double-update by adding another free parameter:

$$Q_{ua,t+1} = Q_{ua,t} - \kappa\alpha\delta_{Qa,t} \quad (7)$$

Here, we use chosen prediction errors to update unchosen values. Based on the task design, it may be possible to use unchosen prediction errors (143). An elegant approach is to mix values learned by two different algorithms. This can be achieved by introducing a weighing parameter, for example as in Eq. 7. Please note that the contribution of additional free parameters (e.g., different learning rates for rewards and punishments in Eq. 2 or different learning rates for the critic and the actor in Eqs 4 and 5) needs to be quantified and that this is ultimately a question answered by model selection procedures [e.g., Ref. (115)].

For all the described models, learned values need to be transformed into choice probabilities to generate behavior. One commonly used approach is the softmax equation, which can be written as:

$$p(a, t) = \frac{\exp(\beta \times Q_{a,t})}{\sum_{a'} \exp(\beta \times Q_{a',t})} \quad (8)$$

Here, all models refer to instrumental tasks. Most of the equations are applicable in similar forms to classical conditioning. For detailed reading, we refer to the scholarly book by Sutton and Barto (42).

so far only one experiment has been developed which specifically tests changes in adaptive (speeding up of reaction times for relevant cues) and aberrant salience (speeding up for irrelevant cues). This work by Roiser et al. (54) showed reduced adaptive salience in schizophrenia patients mostly medicated with SGAs but no general group difference in reaction time measures of aberrant salience. Within patients only, the individual degree of delusions was positively correlated with explicit measures of aberrant salience (54). Furthermore, using the same task, it was demonstrated that unmedicated people with an at-risk mental state for psychosis exhibit greater measures of aberrant salience, and this bias was correlated with their severity of delusion-like symptoms (55). Imaging results from this multimodal study (55) are reported in the next section of this article. These findings point toward the expected direction but rather support a dimensional perspective on positive symptoms, in particular delusions, in a way that the presence of aberrant learning may fluctuate with changes in clinical symptoms. Nevertheless, the findings require further validation in unmedicated patients, since antipsychotic medication directly affects dopamine neurotransmission and primarily attenuates positive symptoms. Other evidence for aberrant learning primarily comes from classical conditioning during fMRI and is reported in the next section on fMRI studies.

Studies from Gold and colleagues have contributed an important body of work to the field. These studies provide evidence for the second hypothesis that postulates a deficit in value representation (11). With regard to hedonic experience, they demonstrated that stable-medicated, chronic patients do not differ in ratings on affective picture material nor do they differ in terms of speeded motor responses to repeat or to endure viewing of these pictures. It was observed that patients respond slightly faster to repeat viewing of neutral pictures (56). These results are in line with behavioral ratings in other studies using similar affective pictures (30, 57, 58).

Together, these findings indicate that schizophrenia patients are surprisingly unimpaired in short hedonic experiences. It is important to ask how these experiences are used to learn values that may guide behavior. Studies showed that delay discounting is altered in schizophrenia in such a way that immediate rewards are preferred over larger rewards in the future and with the degree of this difference being associated with working memory deficits (59–62). A study by Heerey et al. (63) found that in two separate tasks stable-medicated, chronic patients show intact reward sensitivity but impaired weighing of potential outcomes in a decision making task: only potential losses were weighed less by patients (63). Again, the ability to use potential outcomes to guide behavior was correlated with working memory function in patients.

Hypothetically, this deficit may be based on a shift from a goal-directed to a more inflexible learning system. Even in relatively simple tasks learning speed may increase based on additional use of a goal-directed system that accurately maps separate stimulus values to their potential outcome consequences, which may then be used for appropriate action selection. Models of reinforcement learning do not map perfectly on this distinction. Instead, several agents that update values based on prediction errors can be summarized as model-free controllers of learning and decision processes, because they neglect the contribution of additional environmental features (task structure) to the learning process (compare **Box 1**). Nevertheless, the kind of teaching signal used to update values can even be varied within the group of model-free agents. Formally, one class includes model-free Q-learning algorithms, where each possible action becomes associated with a single value and these specific values are used to compute a prediction error. In contrast, a more rigid model-free system may learn values based on teaching signals that convey information about rewarded or punished states (e.g., a pair of stimuli) as, for example, formulated in actor-critic learning (42). This appears to be accompanied by slower learning compared to the more precise mapping of one Q-value to each stimulus associated with a certain value. Gold et al. (64) approached this question by applying a task that requires learning from rewards in one condition and the avoidance of punishment in another condition in a sample of 47 stable-medicated, chronic patients. Patients were split into two subgroups with high and low levels of negative symptoms, respectively. Only patients with high levels of negative symptoms were shown to be selectively impaired in the reward-approach condition but demonstrated intact loss avoidance learning. This dissociation was also confirmed in a post-acquisition transfer test (64). A deficit in reward-based learning, but not in the avoidance of punishment, which was associated with negative symptoms, was also found in two other independent studies, both in patients treated with antipsychotic medication (65, 66). In the study by Gold et al. (64), an actor-critic model, a Q-learner, and a hybrid of these two models were fitted to the observed data and parameters were inferred using maximum-likelihood estimation. Based on model selection, data of the high-negative-symptom group was better explained by the actor-critic model, while healthy participants and the low-negative-symptom group of patients were better explained by the Q-learner. Such a deficit in value-based learning may also be closely connected to a deficit in cost computation of effortful behavior (67). The impact of this shift to a more rigid and rather imprecise learning system may depend on task demands and may in some rare cases be advantageous – if tasks require participants to behave rigid and at low levels of exploration (68). Again, it is important to note that most of the summarized studies were conducted in stable-medicated, rather chronic patients. The important question as to what extent these findings generalize remains to be examined.

The deficit of using outcomes to guide behavior may exacerbate when patients are confronted with situations where they are required to adapt their behavior flexibly. This can be examined in tasks like the Wisconsin Card Sorting Task or reversal learning. Indeed, a deficit in such tasks has been reported repeatedly in chronic, medicated states of schizophrenia (69–73). Studies in medication-free, first-episode patients indicate that such impairments are already present at the beginning of the disease and are stable over time (for at least 6 years), independent of general IQ effects (74, 75). Two recent studies demonstrate that the deficit in rapid behavioral adaptation is most likely due to an increased tendency to switch in schizophrenia patients (76, 77). A study by Schlagenhauf et al. (77) implemented detailed computational modeling of learning – ranging from standard Rescorla–Wagner-Models to Double-Update-Models (**Box 1**) and finally belief-based Hidden–Markov-Models (78) – to the data of 24 unmedicated patients. While the used Rescorla–Wagner-Models clearly provide a model-free account of reinforcement learning, the Double-Update- and the Hidden–Markov-Models can both be regarded as a model-based account of reinforcement learning because both incorporate important aspects of the experimental environment of the given task but in different ways: the Double-Update-Model simply integrates the dichotomy of the two choice options in the reversal learning task by updating each action value with the same prediction error but in different directions; the Hidden–Markov-Model approaches this differently by updating the probability of being in one of the two states and thereby actually building an internal model of the task's states (in the following, this is referred to as the participant's belief about the visited trial being informative about the state or not). Maximum-a-posteriori estimates of model parameters were inferred using random-effects Bayesian techniques complemented by model selection at the population and at the individual level. Random-effects parameters refer to individual parameter estimates per participant in contrast to fixed-effects parameters, which assume one set of parameters for a population. Note that random-effects fitting of models and model selection are crucially important to compare how models map to learning processes across groups and to compare parameters between groups. Also, individual model comparison is important because the meaning of underlying parameters remains unclear if the probability that a participant's data is given by the inferred parameters (the likelihood) is around chance (please also compare Section "Methodological Remarks"). Based on these methods, it was demonstrated that the belief-based model explained the observed data best. This is in line with another study on reversal learning in healthy participants (78). Modeling results revealed increased switching in patients due to false beliefs with respect to feedback-conveyed information about the state of the task, which are based on reversals of reward contingencies (77). The study by Schlagenhauf et al. (77) was conducted in 24 unmedicated patients, of whom a substantial number was not able to apply the belief-based strategy. In these patients ($n = 11$), the reversal learning deficit was more pronounced. This was best explained by the actual presence of their positive symptoms, which is a remarkable contrast to several studies examining stable-medicated, chronic patients with attenuated positive symptoms. This subgroup of patients was additionally characterized by the model in terms of reduced reward sensitivity and showed a relatively better (although still poor) fit by the simple, model-free Rescorla–Wagner algorithm. Parameters of the models were used to generate regressors for the analysis of fMRI data and the results are discussed in the subsequent section.

There is convincing support that deficits in flexible behavioral adaptation and reversal learning, in particular, are important features of schizophrenia patients with an increased tendency to switch as a potential specific mechanism (76, 77). This is in line with an important assumption concerning the hypothesis of a deficit in value representation: an impaired functioning of the so-called rapid learning system that is assumed to rely on prefrontal and orbitofrontal brain structures deeply involved in cognitive functions such as working memory, which allows for flexible adaptation of decisions (47). This system is thought to interact with a more rigid learning system supposedly implemented in the basal ganglia pathways. As already mentioned above, these complementary learning systems may also be associated with the distinction of model-free and model-based controllers of learning, where the latter is implicated in using an internal model of the environment to optimize choice behavior (79, 80). It appears plausible that potential deficits in the model-based domain may be closely linked to well-established findings of impaired cognitive control with most evidence from measures of working memory and cognitive processing speed. Model-based learning relies on precise mapping of the environment and uses this map for forward planning of decisions. This process requires individuals to keep online values of multiple stimuli to allow for flexible decision making.

There is indeed evidence that working memory capacity limits the ability to learn multiple stimulus values to guide decisions and the degree of model-based behavior (81, 82), while, at the same time, possibly directing patients toward more inflexible aspects of learning, which themselves may be affected or spared in schizophrenia. There is additional evidence that patients learn reward contingencies, but that they may need more time depending on task demands (68, 83, 84). Interestingly, in a post-acquisition test-phase, Waltz et al. (83) observed that medicated patients learned to avoid previously punished stimuli, while preference for the previously rewarded cues was weakened compared to controls. In a next step, Waltz et al. (85) studied stable-medicated, chronic patients with an established go-nogo learning task (86). During the training phase, patients showed an overall go-bias but no gradual adaptation to the more frequently rewarded stimuli, while the gradual adaptation to negative outcomes appeared to be intact (85). In line with deficits in reversal learning, rapid trial-to-trial adjustments were impaired in patients. This analysis was compared with predictions from a neurocomputational model of dopamine-induced basal ganglia-cortex interactions proposed by Frank et al. (87): high levels of presynaptic dopamine accompanied by alterations in D1-receptor density may specifically impair go-pathways which are proposed to facilitate reward-approach rather than punishment avoidance (47). This idea is also supported by recent optogenetic animal research (88). In accordance, it was also demonstrated that patients are less able to speed up responses to approach reward and show reduced exploration. Both effects were most pronounced in a subgroup of high-level negative symptoms (89).

In this section, we summarized results from studies on behavioral impairments during performance of instrumental tasks and only three studies, to date, have implemented reinforcement learning modeling to the observed behavioral data (64, 77, 89). Two of those studies demonstrated the ability to identify subgroups of the heterogeneous clinical entity referred to as schizophrenia. Further studies with similar experiments are needed across different disease states (e.g., first-episode) and medication states (in particular unmedicated patients as well as different medications to rule out the possibility that alterations in learning mechanisms are secondary to medication effects). This may be a potentially helpful route toward an identification of patient subgroups based on generative computational models of behavior and neural mechanisms. Recent methodological progress shows improved classification accuracy and allows for clustering within patients based on parameters of generative models of brain connectivity (90, 91), and this may also apply to generative models of behavior.

FUNCTIONAL IMAGING STUDIES OF REINFORCEMENT LEARNING IN SCHIZOPHRENIA

This section will summarize studies that collected fMRI data during reinforcement learning to examine neural substrates of the behavioral alterations discussed in the previous section of this article. First, we summarize studies that examined classical conditioning. This process of associative learning has not been discussed in the previous section because classical conditioning paradigms do not usually require an instrumental response. Nevertheless, physiological responses reflect associative changes in stimulus contingencies, namely the unconditioned and the conditioned stimuli

(US and CS). Second, we report studies that investigated instrumental conditioning during fMRI. In both parts, we explicitly describe the application of reinforcement learning models, how parameters underlying these models were inferred, and how these measures were further applied to the imaging data.

CLASSICAL CONDITIONING

Jensen et al. (92) studied aversive classical conditioning in 13 medicated patients. Their analysis focused on the onset of CS associated with a neutral or an aversive event. In patients, they found elevated left ventral striatal activation to CS preceding neutral events compared to CS preceding aversive events (92). This aberrant attribution of salience was confirmed in skin conductance measures and post-learning self-reports. In a slightly different aversive conditioning paradigm neural responses to CS and US were studied in 20 medicated patients, and similar findings were demonstrated (93): attenuated activation to CS but intact responses to US were reported in the amygdala. Within patients, CS-related activation in the midbrain was correlated with delusion severity in a way that stronger CS-related responses in neutral trials predicted a higher degree of delusional symptoms (93). The authors additionally implemented a temporal-difference model to quantify neural correlates of prediction errors. Notably, the model's free parameter, the learning rate, was fixed for the entire sample and not fitted individually to behavioral or physiological responses [which were shown to vary, according reaction times and skin conductance e.g., Ref. (94, 95)]. Romaniuk and colleagues found no aversive prediction error correlate in the midbrain of schizophrenia patients as was observed in healthy controls. When modeling prediction errors for neutral events, they found a neural correlate of these prediction errors in patients' midbrain but not in controls (93).

With regard to appetitive classical conditioning with monetary reward, one study investigated neural activation to reward-associated CS in 25 medicated patients. They reported that relatively lower ventral-striatal and ventro-medial-prefrontal activation depended on the degree of anhedonia (96), which is in line with previous findings using the MID task (17). Another study examined appetitive classical conditioning in thirsty participants (15 medicated patients) using water as reward. The analysis focused on reward delivery and found blunted ventral striatal activation in patients to be correlated with negative symptoms (97). Further, functional connectivity of the dopaminergic midbrain with the insula was reduced in patients. Another appetitive classical conditioning paradigm with monetary reward was used in a study by Diaconescu et al. (98) in 18 medicated patients. While patients and controls were similarly able to recall reward contingencies in explicit ratings, implicit measures (skin conductance) did not differ between reward CS and neutral CS in patients. The analysis of fMRI data also focused on CS and revealed that increased activation in striatal and prefrontal areas of healthy controls to reward CS was accompanied by stronger effective connectivity between VS and orbitofrontal cortex as assessed using structural equation modeling (98). Crucially, this pattern was reversed in patients for the neutral CS. This is an important finding, as it has long been described that neural correlates of learning spread over nodes of a network and thereby drive changes in plasticity. A disturbance of such a mechanism was also proposed to be at the heart of the pathophysiology of schizophrenia (99–101). We will return to this issue in the final section.

INSTRUMENTAL LEARNING

We now proceed with further studies that investigated neural correlates during instrumental learning. In line with evidence for aberrant learning from classical conditioning, a recent multimodal imaging study using the instrumental "salience attribution task" [(55); for behavioral results see previous section] found that ventral striatal activation to irrelevant stimulus features were positively correlated to delusion-like symptom severity in 18 unmedicated people with an at-risk mental state for psychosis (55). Furthermore, hippocampal responses to irrelevant features were differently correlated with dopamine synthesis capacity in VS revealing a positive relationship in controls and a negative relationship in people with an at-risk mental state.

One exemplary study that assessed the association between impaired reinforcement learning and brain activation in dopaminergic target brain areas of first-episode schizophrenia patients ($n = 13$, 8 medicated) used an instrumental learning task with two choice options: one signaled a potential monetary feedback and the other a potential neutral feedback (43). In contrast to several other studies (see previous section), the groups did not differ in terms of acquisition of reward contingencies, which may be due to the rather small sample size of this pioneer study. In line with another study (59), patients responded faster on neutral trials in the study by Murray et al. (43). A Q-learner was fitted to the observed data based on maximum-likelihood estimates of parameters. Both groups did not differ in terms of model parameters. To generate regressors for fMRI data analysis, one set of parameters was fitted for the entire sample (fixed-effects). Model-derived prediction errors were used as a parametric modulator of feedback events. Prediction error correlates in bilateral midbrain, right VS, hippocampus, insula, and cingulate cortex were significantly stronger in controls than in patients. In patients, midbrain correlates of prediction errors appeared slightly augmented in neutral trials (43). A more complicated "allergy prediction" task design enabled Corlett et al. (102) to investigate different stages of learning in 14 patients, most of whom were medicated. For event-related fMRI analysis, an event was defined to start at the beginning of each stimulus presentation and to end after outcome delivery lasting a total time of 4 s. Compared to controls, patients did not activate the left caudate during the training stage, which was followed by revaluation of stimuli pairs that were either ambiguous or well learned pairs of cues during training. The comparison of these pairs revealed a failure to activate substantia nigra and right PFC. In the last phase, expectations about the outcome based on the trained stimulus pairs were violated. Here, predictable events elicited an augmented response in right PFC in patients versus controls, while an attenuated response was found for unexpected events (102). This lack of differentiation between expected- and unexpectedness events correlated with the level of unusual thought content. Notably, the analysis strategy chosen in this design makes it hard to interpret the findings in terms of prediction error or expected value signals because the whole trial period was modeled in the single-subject of the fMRI data. Similar results were reported in another study that investigated 20 medicated patients while performing a guessing–gambling paradigm at different levels of uncertainty but analyzed expectation-related and reward-related activation separately (103). Expectation-related brain activation at time of motor responses revealed increased activation with lower predictability in a fronto-parietal network, and this effect was diminished in dorsolateral PFC and anterior cingulate cortex of schizophrenia patients. Reward-associated activation was analyzed in relation to levels of predictability (assumed to mirror prediction error related brain activation), and patients showed reduced activation in putamen, dorsal cingulate, and superior frontal cortex (104). One study assessed probabilistic category learning ("weather prediction task") in medicated schizophrenia patients ($n = 40$) during fMRI. Albeit impaired performance in all patients, a small number of patients were able to apply a similar strategy to the task as controls did (105). When comparing fMRI data of these matched groups ($n = 8$ patients) during the presentation of stimulus combinations, patients displayed reduced activation in striatum and dorsolateral PFC. Patients exhibited stronger activation in a more rostral region of dlPFC and parietal cortex. Results from this task are hard to compare with instrumental reinforcement learning tasks due to the experimental design that primarily tests classification learning at different levels of difficulty.

In another study on instrumental learning, Gradin et al. (106) examined 15 medicated patients. Temporal-difference modeling was applied to the task that delivered water as reward. Random-effects parameters were initially estimated with maximum-likelihood, and the obtained parameters were subsequently used as empirical priors to regularize the possible range parameters to avoid extreme values of parameter estimates [also compare: Ref. (53, 106)]. Although patients differed in the amount of delivered water, no difference on model parameters was observed. To generate regressors for fMRI analysis, a single set of parameters was fitted for the entire sample (fixed-effects). Model-derived prediction errors were analyzed as parametric modulators of reward delivery, and model-derived values were included as modulators of expectation-related activation at the trial onset. Compared to controls, no correlation with prediction errors was observed in striatum, thalamus, amygdala-hippocampal complex, and insula of medicated schizophrenia patients. A trend-wise reduction in midbrain correlated with positive symptoms in patients. Patients also displayed reduced coding of value-related activation in the amygdala-hippocampal complex and this, again, was correlated with positive symptoms. Importantly, this study also included another psychiatric patient group, medicated depressed patients, and this group also exhibited blunted neural correlates of expected-reward values and prediction errors in slightly different regions. The strength of this reduction was correlated with anhedonia severity in dopaminergic core areas. In combination with detailed computational modeling, Schlagenhauf et al. (77) studied reversal learning (compare previous section) in 24 unmedicated patients. Analysis of fMRI focused on the time of reward delivery and included different model-derived modulations of this onset. The authors found reduced ventral striatal coding of model-derived reward prediction errors in patients. This finding remained trend-wise significant when restricting the group comparison to patients who had insight into the underlying task structure as defined by their beliefs about the states of the task based on a Hidden–Markov-Model ($n = 12$). A second fMRI analysis based on the latter model was applied to define subjective informative punishment trials, i.e., when participants believed that a change in reward contingencies had appeared. Both patients with good and poor task insight showed reduced ventral striatal activation during these trials (77). Reduced ventral striatal activation was also reported in another recent fMRI study on reversal learning in 28 medicated, chronic schizophrenia patients (76). In the study by Schlagenhauf et al. (77), patients with good task insight displayed relatively stronger activation of ventro-lateral and dorso-medial PFC than patients with poor insight. Well performing patients were not distinguishable from controls with respect to activation in these prefrontal regions. This result may reflect compensatory PFC processes in schizophrenia patients similar to that which has been described for the neural correlates of working memory deficits (107, 108).

In summary, several studies revealed reduced activation of brain areas typically encoding errors of reward prediction, most prominently the VS. This was reported consistently across classical and instrumental conditioning tasks, despite the fact that most of these studies differ enormously with regard to experimental designs and analysis strategies. Prediction errors arise when a reward is delivered and are typically thought to train expected values of stimuli or associated actions (42). Therefore, functional neuroimaging studies that studied learning during scanning have so far helped to elucidate the underlying dynamics of previous findings derived from studies using the MID or similar tasks. That is, neuronal teaching signals are not coded in ventral striatal activation of medicated and unmedicated patients to a similar extent as in controls. Only five imaging studies have applied reinforcement learning models to describe this process on a trial-by-trial level and these vary considerably in terms of the implemented models, inference of model parameters and the application of model-derived measures to the imaging data. We will further comment on these issues in the subsequent section. These studies comprised 78 medicated patients and 24 unmedicated patients. Studies in unmedicated patients are still rare. Nevertheless, the finding of reduced prediction error coding in dopaminergic core areas may indeed build a common ground for impaired learning of stimulus or decision values. In addition, such impaired coding might be closely related to the elevated levels of presynaptic dopamine synthesis capacity in schizophrenia reported in meta-analyses of PET studies (4, 5, 109). An important question remains how this stable marker of the dopamine system, probably reflecting tonic or rather stable aspects of dopaminergic neurotransmission (3), relates to event-related changes during learning. Studies approaching this question are discussed in Section "Functional Imaging Studies of Reinforcement Learning with Additional Neurochemical Measures or Pharmacological Challenges of the Dopamine System" of this article. Furthermore, it has been proposed that a hyperdopaminergic state in schizophrenia may result in imprecise and inefficient cortical information processing as a potential mechanism for cognitive impairments observed in patients as well as their first-degree relatives and in people at-risk mental states (9, 110, 111). This idea is compatible with the proposal of a deficit in prefrontal value representation shown to be related to negative symptoms. However, exact cognitive and affective correlates of such deficits remain to be explored. We will return to this in the final section.

The emerging picture is less clear with regard to evidence provided in favor of the aberrant salience hypothesis, in particular regarding the extent to which reduced neural correlates of prediction errors are linked to processes of aberrant salience attribution. Notably, the idea of aberrant salience may also account for reduced value-related anticipatory dopaminergic signals, in patients who exhibit high levels of positive and negative symptoms (for example). In this case, a lack of activation to cues associated with monetary as well as, probably, social reward may reflect reduced motivational or incentive salience in terms of apathy or other dimensions of negative symptoms, which may be a result of aberrant salience attribution. However, this requires more systematic studies along symptom dimensions. Evidence for neural correlates of aberrant learning was demonstrated in fMRI studies on classical conditioning that showed elevated striatal activation to cues indicating the delivery of a neutral event (92, 93, 98) and in one specific instrumental task design, the "salience attribution task" (55, 112). Studies using this specifically designed task point toward a relationship with positive symptoms, particularly delusions. Consequently, symptom and medication states of included patients may be crucially important. Indeed, a study on reversal learning in unmedicated patients with more pronounced positive symptoms showed that a subgroup of patients was not able to infer the task structure and this was best explained by individual levels of positive symptoms (77). Therefore, it is important to consider the amount of variance in symptom ratings and different medication states to better understand variability related to aberrant aspects of neural learning signals. Furthermore, when reviewing clinical data of several studies summarized in this article, it is compelling that even in medicated patients there is considerable variability in the extent of positive symptoms across studies varying from high levels to nearly no positive symptoms. Future studies are needed to address the question whether blunted learning signals indeed reflect aberrant salience attribution – and if this is a schizophrenia specific feature or a dimension of positive psychotic symptoms – which may then consequently also emerge in other psychiatric diseases and to some extent even in the at-risk healthy population or healthy people with some degree of psychotic experience.

METHODOLOGICAL REMARKS

The combination of model-derived learning signals with functional brain measures is very promising. This mechanistically informed quantification of signals reflecting learning processes provides a more fine-grained insight into neural trial-by-trial correlates of learning mechanisms and disease-specific alterations as compared to standard event-related fMRI analyses which rather rely on event definitions such as correct responses or experimenter-defined changes in reward contingencies. In fact, the latter may not always reflect the way study participants solve these tasks. On the other hand, a small number of healthy volunteers, in most studies, exhibit behavior that cannot be described better than chance by any reinforcement learning model. This may indicate the need to extend from standard reinforcement learning models to other types of models, for example Bayesian learners (94, 113, 114). Such non-fitters should be reported more clearly, in particular in clinical between-group studies, because this may crucially impair the between-group analysis of model parameters and comparisons of neural correlates based on model-derived measures between groups: in fact, underlying parameters of non-fitters are meaningless in terms of the mechanism that is described by the model [compare Ref. (77)]. Although studies which actually apply reinforcement learning modeling are the minority of those reported in this review article (seven studies, for an overview see **Table 1**), there is considerable variability on how these few studies inferred the models' parameters (some did and others did not fit parameters) and how (or if any) model selection was applied.

Further, the generation of trial-by-trial model-derived time-series for fMRI data analysis is sometimes performed based on random-effects parameters (individual parameters for each subject) or based on one set of parameters (fixed-effects). One group recommends the latter approach for studies in healthy volunteers by arguing for more robust correlations of BOLD signal with model-derived regressors (53). On the other hand, this appears questionable for group studies in which group differences in parameters may be causally linked to the disease status. We have the impression that model comparison techniques are of key importance (115). Even in the simple case that no alternative models are fitted, it may be informative to include a report of model fit based on the likelihood that the observed data is given by the parameters. To our mind, a situation where the individual model fit (expressed via the likelihood of the data given by the parameters) does not differ between groups exemplifies a desirable case: even if parameters differ between groups in this case, model-derived regressors are readily applicable to fMRI data because they do not differ in terms of the likelihood that the modeled strategy captures important aspects of the observed raw responses. Based on the sparsely available papers on these issues, the application of fixed-effects parameters to fMRI data rather appears as a workaround based on the observation that noisy parameters based on maximum-likelihood estimates potentially add further noise when fitting a hemodynamic model with model-derived time-series as parametric modulators to the imaging data [compare Ref. (53)]. In the case of clinical between-group studies, the use of fixed-effects parameters results in a situation where the observed behavior is relatively well explained by those parameters. Consequently, differences in terms of model parameters will then be expressed via the correlation between the regressor and the signal. This can be minimized by using parameters that closely match the observed individual's behavior to generate regressors. Unfortunately, no systematic studies of these questions are available involving either healthy volunteers only, or comparisons between psychiatric patients and healthy controls. Consequently, it appears to be desirable to develop methodological guidelines for these techniques, as it was published for other modeling approaches, for example for dynamic causal modeling for fMRI (116).

FUNCTIONAL IMAGING STUDIES OF REINFORCEMENT LEARNING WITH ADDITIONAL NEUROCHEMICAL MEASURES OR PHARMACOLOGICAL CHALLENGES OF THE DOPAMINE SYSTEM

In this last section, we describe research that pharmacologically manipulated the dopamine system during reinforcement learning or acquired an additional molecular measurement (PET) of dopamine. There are a substantial number of groups researching these questions in healthy volunteers, and this section does not aim to present a complete picture of all such studies. We will instead refer to studies that are particularly important for a better understanding of the above reviewed studies in patients.

A highly influential study was conducted by Pessiglione et al. (117). An instrumental learning task with a reward-approach (win or no win) and a punishment–avoidance (loss or no loss) condition was used (117). A similar design was recently applied in a behavioral study of medicated schizophrenia patients (64). Pessiglione et al. (117) demonstrated that dopamine medication, L-DOPA, and haloperidol, have opposing effects on behavior and neural correlates of model-derived prediction errors, and that these effects are selective for the reward-approach condition: L-DOPA administration enhanced reward-approaching behavior and associated ventral striatal reward prediction errors whereas haloperidol reduced such effects (117). The same direction of medication effects was reported in a study using aversive Pavlovian conditioning under amphetamine, haloperidol, or placebo (118). In addition, ventral striatal reward anticipation as in the MID task appears to be conveyed by reward-induced dopamine release (27) and can be blunted by massive dopamine release, based on dose-dependent effects of psychostimulants (26, 28). In line with this, a recent study applied the same reward-approach task as in Murray et al. (43) and found that methamphetamine blunts both reward prediction errors in VS and expected value representation in ventro-medial PFC (119). The strength of the disruption of value representation in ventro-medial PFC was correlated with amphetamine-induced psychotic symptoms. A third condition, amisulpride-pretreatment, did not affect amphetamine-induced blunting of learning signals. It is important to note that the reducing effects of haloperidol on striatal reward prediction error encoding can explain reduced prediction error related activation in medicated schizophrenia patients, whereas the blunting effects of amphetamine may potentially mirror a subcortical hyperdopaminergic state, as was demonstrated in unmedicated schizophrenia patients (2, 3). Therefore studies in unmedicated patients are crucially important to remove this confound. FGAs and SGAs strongly differ in their dopamine receptor affinity, and, based on two MID studies, it was shown that they also affect reward anticipation differently. These results point toward the idea that SGAs may help to remediate reward-related anticipatory brain activation (20–22) which nevertheless requires random assignment in a clinical-trial-type design. Such studies have not yet been conducted with learning tasks. In unmedicated patients, a reduction of ventral-striatal prediction error coding was recently demonstrated during reversal learning (77). Elevated presynaptic dopamine levels may account for this reduced activation, similar to that observed for Parkinson patients on L-DOPA medication, affecting the VS (early in the illness less degenerated) in an overdosing manner (120). Here, a long-lasting increase of presynaptic dopamine function may "drown" value-related and error-related phasic learning signals. Multimodal imaging studies combining fMRI with PET radiotracers that assess presynaptic dopamine function can link individual differences in neurochemical parameters with functional activation. For example, PET with FDOPA may be an important target for application in multimodal imaging studies, since this measure has been demonstrated in meta-analyses to best characterize the subcortical hyperdopaminergic state of patients [for meta-analyses see: Ref. (4, 5)]. Supporting this idea, another study demonstrated that ventral-striatal prediction errors are indeed negatively correlated with dopamine synthesis capacity in healthy controls (121). This negative correlation suggests that long-lasting increases in presynaptic dopamine function, as observed in schizophrenia patients, may reduce phasic learning signals, hypothetically via presynaptic D2-autoreceptors which regulate presynaptic activity of DOPA-decarboxylase activity to ensure homeostasis within the dopaminergic system (46, 121). Animal studies (122, 123) and other functional human imaging studies (36, 124, 125) also support the idea of this interplay of differential aspects of dopamine neurotransmission. In line with this, it has also been shown that behavioral effects of a dopamine-enhancing drug during reversal learning indeed depend on baseline levels of dopamine synthesis capacity (126): Participants with lower dopamine synthesis capacity benefit behaviorally from a dopamine agonist, while the same drug dose seemed to be disadvantageous for participants with rather high levels of dopamine synthesis capacity. Therefore, dopamine effects in learning and cognition appear to be a fine-tuned and optimized non-linear system where rather low and rather high levels result in inefficient neural processing (127, 128). This view is also supported by one of the few clinical multimodal imaging studies using FDOPA PET in combination with a working memory task during fMRI in controls and in people with an at-risk mental state for psychosis (129). At the same working memory load, they found a positive linear relationship of dopamine synthesis capacity and working memory related activation in dorsolateral PFC of healthy controls, while this relationship was negative in people with an at-risk mental state, indicating that potentially "too" high levels of dopamine synthesis may promote lower dorsolateral PFC activation during the same working memory load at which both groups coped with comparable performance. This observation can be reconciled with the observation of prefrontal efficiency during working memory when examining cognitive performance and dorsolateral PFC activation (130, 131): different dorsolateral PFC activation may primarily reflect different performance. Patients are assumed to reach maximum limits of dorsolateral PFC activation earlier reflecting a general impairment in this cognitive domain [see also: Ref. (108)]. A step further, there is also evidence that a reduction of working-memory-dependent effective connectivity from dorsolateral PFC to parietal cortex may be the potential mechanism underlying this inefficiency (108). Connectivity may indeed be an important target and it has also been demonstrated that functional connectivity during aversive conditioning is shifted differently by a dopamine agonist versus a dopamine antagonist (132).

CONCLUSION, REMARKS, OUTLOOK

In this review article we summarized studies that provide evidence for behavioral and neural correlates of impaired reinforcement learning in schizophrenia. Two main hypotheses guided this review: (1) Aberrant prediction errors drive learning of otherwise irrelevant stimuli and actions in schizophrenia, and that there is a potentially close link between this mechanism and the emergence of positive psychotic symptoms, in particular delusions. (2) A deficit of expected value representation may characterize patients suffering from schizophrenia, and this may fundamentally contribute to the formation of negative symptoms.

There is evidence for aberrant learning with most specific findings derived from the salience attribution task (54, 55). Although there is still limited evidence and future studies are needed for clarification, it seems conceivable that aberrant learning is involved in the formation of delusions and can therefore be observed in patients with prominent positive symptoms. Whether this sensitization to otherwise neutral stimuli is indeed dopamine mediated and actually blunts learning signals elicited by regularly salient cues remains to be further explored (9).

Our summary of fMRI studies during reinforcement learning clearly demonstrates that a reduction of these learning signals, namely blunted coding of ventral-striatal prediction errors, was consistently observed across studies. This deficit may actually be involved in aberrant learning as well as in a failure of value representation depending on fluctuating symptom states. During acute psychotic clinical states this may provide a conduit for aberrant learning, while the persistence of a noisy learning signals may provide the ground for a failure of building value expectations, ultimately contributing to the development and progress of detrimental negative symptoms. A large body of evidence from behavioral studies supports the hypothesis of a deficit in value representation and that this impairment is pronounced in patients with high levels of negative symptoms (11, 64). Nevertheless, antipsychotic medication was shown to contribute to the severity of negative symptoms based on the degree of striatal D2-receptor blockade (133) and may therefore also exacerbate impairments in value representation.

The psychosis spectrum has been characterized by imprecise and inefficient cortical information processing as a potential mechanism for cognitive impairments observed in patients and their first-degree relatives as well as in at-risk mental states. As a potential mechanism behind this, a disrupted cortico-cortical synaptic plasticity was suggested by a comprehensive biological hypothesis of schizophrenia, the "dysconnectivity" hypothesis (100, 101). This hypothesis focuses on aberrant experience-driven control of synaptic plasticity via *N*-methyl-D-aspartate receptors (NMDAR). Abnormal modulation of NMDAR-induced plasticity by neurotransmitter systems such as dopamine, acetylcholine, or serotonin are at the heart of this idea. In the present article, we have described a close link between reinforcement learning, symptom dimensions of schizophrenia and dopamine, which acts as a neuromodulator of NMDAR-function: Animal research demonstrated that D1-receptor agonists and D2-receptor antagonists facilitate NMDAR-dependent long-term plasticity while D2-receptor agonist suppress it (134, 135). Earlier in the manuscript, we have discussed the role of these receptors during reward and punishment as well as go-nogo learning (87, 88). Further, these receptors are targets of current antipsychotic treatment strategies. Stephan and colleagues conclude "... it is not plasticity *per se* that is abnormal but its modulation during reinforcement and perceptual learning." (100) These modulatory influences of NMDAR-function are thought to contribute to cortical representations of environmental states (136) and the consistently described reduction of ventral-striatal prediction errors could be crucially involved in a deficient shaping of such cortical representations (137, 138). Here, it is important to underline that aberrant neuromodulation can indeed be formulated via computational models of learning-induced plasticity.

So far, there is converging evidence that dysconnectivity may indeed account for the repeatedly described prefrontal inefficiency observed in schizophrenia during the performance of cognitive tasks: Using models of effective connectivity for fMRI, reduced working-memory-dependent prefrontal-parietal connectivity was reported, initially in medicated patients (108) and subsequently replicated in medication-naïve first-episode patients and in people with an at-risk mental state (139). Based on parameters of these models, a clustering analysis was able to identify three mechanistically informed subgroups of patients (91). These subgroups were found to be biologically distinct in terms of connectivity profiles and mapped on different levels of negative symptom severity (91). This observation also appears to be in accordance with the proposal of a deficit in value representation, which was demonstrated to be pronounced at high levels of negative symptoms (64). Therefore, it appears desirable to study the effect of neural learning signals at various levels in neural networks. It is important to note that studying the interaction of model-free learning signals and model-based neural representations of cognitive processes on the level of neural networks in a computational framework clearly has the potential to move beyond the evidence provided by standard cognitive tasks, such as working memory, even if some of the identified deficits overlap. The contribution of such an approach can be to gain more mechanistic information when studying these processes by applying detailed computational modeling to behavioral and neurobiological data. The focus of this idea is that different types of computational processes described in terms of different models may help us to improve our understanding of how patients actually solve certain tasks beyond the observation of being impaired or not. This may offer a unique source for mechanistically informed subtyping based on how patient subgroups deal differently with challenging tasks and in particular how these abilities are implemented in neural networks. Such subgroups require clinical validation in terms of longitudinal predictions (e.g., treatment responses). Promising future research in this field may strongly benefit from an integration of different modeling techniques for reinforcement as well as perceptual learning and brain connectivity [e.g., dynamic causal modeling; (140)]. It has been demonstrated in healthy volunteers that such an experimental approach is feasible (94, 141, 142) and therefore presents a highly promising venue for schizophrenia research. Finally, this may result in a dissection of the heterogeneous clinical entity of schizophrenia into biologically informed subgroups, thereby providing a framework for a better understanding of cognitive deficits, where a deficit of learning expectations about sensory inputs and future actions may constitute a potential key mechanism of the disorder.

ACKNOWLEDGMENTS

This study was supported by funding from the German Research Foundation (Deutsche Forschungsgemeinschaft, DFG) to Florian Schlagenhauf SCHL1969/1-1.

REFERENCES

1. Carlsson A. Does dopamine have a role in schizophrenia? *Biol Psychiatry* (1978) **13**:3–21.
2. Abi-Dargham A, Gil R, Krystal J, Baldwin RM, Seibyl JP, Bowers M, et al. Increased striatal dopamine transmission in schizophrenia: confirmation in a second cohort. *Am J Psychiatry* (1998) **155**:761–7.
3. Kumakura Y, Cumming P, Vernaleken I, Buchholz HG, Siessmeier T, Heinz A, et al. Elevated [18F]fluorodopamine turnover in brain of patients with schizophrenia: an [18F]fluorodopa/positron emission tomography study. *J Neurosci* (2007) **27**:8080–7. doi:10.1523/JNEUROSCI.0805-07.2007
4. Howes OD, Kambeitz J, Kim E, Stahl D, Slifstein M, Abi-Dargham A, et al. The nature of dopamine dysfunction in schizophrenia and what this means for treatment. *Arch Gen Psychiatry* (2012) **69**:776–86. doi:10.1001/archgenpsychiatry.2012.169
5. Fusar-Poli P, Meyer-Lindenberg A. Striatal presynaptic dopamine in schizophrenia, part II: meta-analysis of [(18)F/(11)C]-DOPA PET studies. *Schizophr Bull* (2013) **39**:33–42. doi:10.1093/schbul/sbr180
6. Schultz W, Dayan P, Montague PR. A neural substrate of prediction and reward. *Science* (1997) **275**:1593–9. doi:10.1126/science.275.5306.1593
7. Bayer HM, Glimcher PW. Midbrain dopamine neurons encode a quantitative reward prediction error signal. *Neuron* (2005) **47**:129–41. doi:10.1016/j.neuron.2005.05.020
8. Steinberg EE, Keiflin R, Boivin JR, Witten IB, Deisseroth K, Janak PH. A causal link between prediction errors, dopamine neurons and learning. *Nat Neurosci* (2013) **16**:966–73. doi:10.1038/nn.3413
9. Heinz A. Dopaminergic dysfunction in alcoholism and schizophrenia – psychopathological and behavioral correlates. *Eur Psychiatry* (2002) **17**:9–16. doi:10.1016/S0924-9338(02)00628-4
10. Kapur S. Psychosis as a state of aberrant salience: a framework linking biology, phenomenology, and pharmacology in schizophrenia. *Am J Psychiatry* (2003) **160**:13–23. doi:10.1176/appi.ajp.160.1.13
11. Gold JM, Waltz JA, Prentice KJ, Morris SE, Heerey EA. Reward processing in schizophrenia: a deficit in the representation of value. *Schizophr Bull* (2008) **34**:835–47. doi:10.1093/schbul/sbn068
12. Montague PR, Dayan P, Sejnowski TJ. A framework for mesencephalic dopamine systems based on predictive Hebbian learning. *J Neurosci* (1996) **16**:1936–47.
13. Friston KJ, Frith CD. Schizophrenia: a disconnection syndrome? *Clin Neurosci* (1995) **3**:89–97.
14. Friston KJ. The disconnection hypothesis. *Schizophr Res* (1998) **30**:115–25. doi:10.1016/S0920-9964(97)00140-0
15. Knutson B, Adams CM, Fong GW, Hommer D. Anticipation of increasing monetary reward selectively recruits nucleus accumbens. *J Neurosci* (2001) **21**:RC159.
16. Breiter HC, Aharon I, Kahneman D, Dale A, Shizgal P. Functional imaging of neural responses to expectancy and experience of monetary gains and losses. *Neuron* (2001) **30**:619–39. doi:10.1016/S0896-6273(01)00303-8
17. Juckel G, Schlagenhauf F, Koslowski M, Wustenberg T, Villringer A, Knutson B, et al. Dysfunction of ventral striatal reward prediction in schizophrenia. *Neuroimage* (2006) **29**:409–16. doi:10.1016/j.neuroimage.2005.07.051
18. Esslinger C, Englisch S, Inta D, Rausch F, Schirmbeck F, Mier D, et al. Ventral striatal activation during attribution of stimulus saliency and reward anticipation is correlated in unmedicated first episode schizophrenia patients. *Schizophr Res* (2012) **140**:114–21. doi:10.1016/j.schres.2012.06.025
19. Nielsen MO, Rostrup E, Wulff S, Bak N, Lublin H, Kapur S, et al. Alterations of the brain reward system in antipsychotic naive schizophrenia patients. *Biol Psychiatry* (2012) **71**:898–905. doi:10.1016/j.biopsych.2012.02.007
20. Juckel G, Schlagenhauf F, Koslowski M, Filonov D, Wustenberg T, Villringer A, et al. Dysfunction of ventral striatal reward prediction in schizophrenic patients treated with typical, not atypical, neuroleptics. *Psychopharmacology (Berl)* (2006) **187**:222–8. doi:10.1007/s00213-006-0405-4
21. Schlagenhauf F, Juckel G, Koslowski M, Kahnt T, Knutson B, Dembler T, et al. Reward system activation in schizophrenic patients switched from typical neuroleptics to olanzapine. *Psychopharmacology (Berl)* (2008) **196**:673–84. doi:10.1007/s00213-007-1016-4
22. Nielsen MO, Rostrup E, Wulff S, Bak N, Broberg BV, Lublin H, et al. Improvement of brain reward abnormalities by antipsychotic monotherapy in schizophrenia. *Arch Gen Psychiatry* (2012) **69**:1195–204. doi:10.1001/archgenpsychiatry.2012.847
23. Walter H, Kammerer H, Frasch K, Spitzer M, Abler B. Altered reward functions in patients on atypical antipsychotic medication in line with the revised dopamine hypothesis of schizophrenia. *Psychopharmacology (Berl)* (2009) **206**:121–32. doi:10.1007/s00213-009-1586-4
24. Simon JJ, Biller A, Walther S, Roesch-Ely D, Stippich C, Weisbrod M, et al. Neural correlates of reward processing in schizophrenia – relationship to apathy and depression. *Schizophr Res* (2010) **118**:154–61. doi:10.1016/j.schres.2009.11.007
25. Waltz JA, Schweitzer JB, Ross TJ, Kurup PK, Salmeron BJ, Rose EJ, et al. Abnormal responses to monetary outcomes in cortex, but not in the basal ganglia, in schizophrenia. *Neuropsychopharmacology* (2010) **35**:2427–39. doi:10.1038/npp.2010.126
26. Knutson B, Gibbs SE. Linking nucleus accumbens dopamine and blood oxygenation. *Psychopharmacology (Berl)* (2007) **191**:813–22. doi:10.1007/s00213-006-0686-7
27. Schott BH, Minuzzi L, Krebs RM, Elmenhorst D, Lang M, Winz OH, et al. Mesolimbic functional magnetic resonance imaging activations during reward anticipation correlate with reward-related ventral striatal dopamine release. *J Neurosci* (2008) **28**:14311–9. doi:10.1523/JNEUROSCI.2058-08.2008
28. Knutson B, Bjork JM, Fong GW, Hommer D, Mattay VS, Weinberger DR. Amphetamine modulates human incentive processing. *Neuron* (2004) **43**:261–9. doi:10.1016/j.neuron.2004.06.030
29. Heinz A, Schlagenhauf F. Dopaminergic dysfunction in schizophrenia: salience attribution revisited. *Schizophr Bull* (2010) **36**:472–85. doi:10.1093/schbul/sbq031
30. Pankow A, Friedel E, Sterzer P, Seiferth N, Walter H, Heinz A, et al. Altered amygdala activation in schizophrenia patients during emotion processing. *Schizophr Res* (2013) **150**:101–6. doi:10.1016/j.schres.2013.07.015
31. Schlagenhauf F, Sterzer P, Schmack K, Ballmaier M, Rapp M, Wrase J, et al. Reward feedback alterations in unmedicated schizophrenia patients: relevance for delusions. *Biol Psychiatry* (2009) **65**:1032–9. doi:10.1016/j.biopsych.2008.12.016
32. Waltz JA, Schweitzer JB, Gold JM, Kurup PK, Ross TJ, Salmeron BJ, et al. Patients with schizophrenia have a reduced neural response to both unpredictable and predictable primary reinforcers. *Neuropsychopharmacology* (2009) **34**:1567–77. doi:10.1038/npp.2008.214
33. Morris RW, Vercammen A, Lenroot R, Moore L, Langton JM, Short B, et al. Disambiguating ventral striatum fMRI-related bold signal during reward prediction in schizophrenia. *Mol Psychiatry* (2011) **17**:280–9. doi:10.1038/mp.2011.75
34. Kapur S, Remington G, Jones C, Wilson A, Dasilva J, Houle S, et al. High levels of dopamine D2 receptor occupancy with low-dose haloperidol treatment: a PET study. *Am J Psychiatry* (1996) **153**:948–50.
35. Kapur S, Zipursky R, Jones C, Shammi CS, Remington G, Seeman P. A positron emission tomography study of quetiapine in schizophrenia: a preliminary finding of an antipsychotic effect with only transiently high dopamine D2 receptor occupancy. *Arch Gen Psychiatry* (2000) **57**:553–9. doi:10.1001/archpsyc.57.6.553
36. Vernaleken I, Kumakura Y, Cumming P, Buchholz HG, Siessmeier T, Stoeter P, et al. Modulation of [18F]fluorodopa (FDOPA) kinetics in the brain of healthy volunteers after acute haloperidol challenge. *Neuroimage* (2006) **30**:1332–9. doi:10.1016/j.neuroimage.2005.11.014
37. Vernaleken I, Kumakura Y, Buchholz HG, Siessmeier T, Hilgers RD, Bartenstein P, et al. Baseline [18F]-FDOPA kinetics are predictive of haloperidol-induced changes in dopamine turnover and cognitive performance: a positron emission tomography study in healthy subjects. *Neuroimage* (2008) **40**:1222–31. doi:10.1016/j.neuroimage.2007.12.045
38. Insel TR, Scolnick EM. Cure therapeutics and strategic prevention: raising the bar for mental health research. *Mol Psychiatry* (2006) **11**:11–7. doi:10.1038/sj.mp.4001777
39. Insel TR, Wang PS. Rethinking mental illness. *JAMA* (2010) **303**:1970–1. doi:10.1001/jama.2010.555
40. Huys QJ, Moutoussis M, Williams J. Are computational models of any use to psychiatry? *Neural Netw* (2011) **24**:544–51. doi:10.1016/j.neunet.2011.03.001

41. Montague PR, Dolan RJ, Friston KJ, Dayan P. Computational psychiatry. *Trends Cogn Sci* (2012) **16**:72–80. doi:10.1016/j.tics.2011.11.018
42. Sutton RS, Barto AG. *Reinforcement Learning: An Introduction.* Cambridge, MA: MIT Press (1998).
43. Murray GK, Corlett PR, Clark L, Pessiglione M, Blackwell AD, Honey G, et al. Substantia nigra/ventral tegmental reward prediction error disruption in psychosis. *Mol Psychiatry* (2008) **13**(239):267–76. doi:10.1038/sj.mp.4002058
44. Robinson TE, Berridge KC. The neural basis of drug craving: an incentive-sensitization theory of addiction. *Brain Res Brain Res Rev* (1993) **18**:247–91. doi:10.1016/0165-0173(93)90013-P
45. King R, Barchas JD, Huberman BA. Chaotic behavior in dopamine neurodynamics. *Proc Natl Acad Sci U S A* (1984) **81**:1244–7. doi:10.1073/pnas.81.4.1244
46. Grace AA. Phasic versus tonic dopamine release and the modulation of dopamine system responsivity: a hypothesis for the etiology of schizophrenia. *Neuroscience* (1991) **41**:1–24. doi:10.1016/0306-4522(91)90196-U
47. Frank MJ. Schizophrenia: a computational reinforcement learning perspective. *Schizophr Bull* (2008) **34**:1008–11. doi:10.1093/schbul/sbn123
48. Smith A, Li M, Becker S, Kapur S. Dopamine, prediction error and associative learning: a model-based account. *Network* (2006) **17**:61–84. doi:10.1080/09548980500361624
49. Roesch MR, Esber GR, Li J, Daw ND, Schoenbaum G. Surprise! Neural correlates of Pearce-Hall and Rescorla-Wagner coexist within the brain. *Eur J Neurosci* (2012) **35**:1190–200. doi:10.1111/j.1460-9568.2011.07986.x
50. Metereau E, Dreher JC. Cerebral correlates of salient prediction error for different rewards and punishments. *Cereb Cortex* (2013) **23**:477–87. doi:10.1093/cercor/bhs037
51. Barch DM, Dowd EC. Goal representations and motivational drive in schizophrenia: the role of prefrontal-striatal interactions. *Schizophr Bull* (2010) **36**:919–34. doi:10.1093/schbul/sbq068
52. O'Doherty JP, Hampton A, Kim H. Model-based fMRI and its application to reward learning and decision making. *Ann N Y Acad Sci* (2007) **1104**:35–53. doi:10.1196/annals.1390.022
53. Daw ND. Trial-by-trial data analysis using computational models. In: Phelps EA, Robbins TW, Delgado M editors. *In Affect, Learning and Decision Making, Attention and Performance XXIII.* New York: Oxford University Press (2009) p. 3–38.
54. Roiser JP, Stephan KE, Den Ouden HE, Barnes TR, Friston KJ, Joyce EM. Do patients with schizophrenia exhibit aberrant salience? *Psychol Med* (2009) **39**:199–209. doi:10.1017/S0033291708003863
55. Roiser JP, Howes OD, Chaddock CA, Joyce EM, Mcguire P. Neural and behavioral correlates of aberrant salience in individuals at risk for psychosis. *Schizophr Bull* (2012) **39**:1328–36. doi:10.1093/schbul/sbs147
56. Heerey EA, Gold JM. Patients with schizophrenia demonstrate dissociation between affective experience and motivated behavior. *J Abnorm Psychol* (2007) **116**:268–78. doi:10.1037/0021-843X.116.2.268
57. Dowd EC, Barch DM. Anhedonia and emotional experience in schizophrenia: neural and behavioral indicators. *Biol Psychiatry* (2010) **67**:902–11. doi:10.1016/j.biopsych.2009.10.020
58. Ursu S, Kring AM, Gard MG, Minzenberg MJ, Yoon JH, Ragland JD, et al. Prefrontal cortical deficits and impaired cognition-emotion interactions in schizophrenia. *Am J Psychiatry* (2011) **168**:276–85. doi:10.1176/appi.ajp.2010.09081215
59. Heerey EA, Robinson BM, Mcmahon RP, Gold JM. Delay discounting in schizophrenia. *Cogn Neuropsychiatry* (2007) **12**:213–21. doi:10.1080/13546800601005900
60. Ahn WY, Rass O, Fridberg DJ, Bishara AJ, Forsyth JK, Breier A, et al. Temporal discounting of rewards in patients with bipolar disorder and schizophrenia. *J Abnorm Psychol* (2011) **120**:911–21. doi:10.1037/a0023333
61. Heerey EA, Matveeva TM, Gold JM. Imagining the future: degraded representations of future rewards and events in schizophrenia. *J Abnorm Psychol* (2011) **120**:483–9. doi:10.1037/a0021810
62. Wing VC, Moss TG, Rabin RA, George TP. Effects of cigarette smoking status on delay discounting in schizophrenia and healthy controls. *Addict Behav* (2012) **37**:67–72. doi:10.1016/j.addbeh.2011.08.012
63. Heerey EA, Bell-Warren KR, Gold JM. Decision-making impairments in the context of intact reward sensitivity in schizophrenia. *Biol Psychiatry* (2008) **64**:62–9. doi:10.1016/j.biopsych.2008.02.015
64. Gold JM, Waltz JA, Matveeva TM, Kasanova Z, Strauss GP, Herbener ES, et al. Negative symptoms and the failure to represent the expected reward value of actions: behavioral and computational modeling evidence. *Arch Gen Psychiatry* (2012) **69**:129–38. doi:10.1001/archgenpsychiatry.2011.1269
65. Somlai Z, Moustafa AA, Keri S, Myers CE, Gluck MA. General functioning predicts reward and punishment learning in schizophrenia. *Schizophr Res* (2011) **127**:131–6. doi:10.1016/j.schres.2010.07.028
66. Yilmaz A, Simsek F, Gonul AS. Reduced reward-related probability learning in schizophrenia patients. *Neuropsychiatr Dis Treat* (2012) **8**:27–34. doi:10.2147/NDT.S26243
67. Gold JM, Strauss GP, Waltz JA, Robinson BM, Brown JK, Frank MJ. Negative symptoms of schizophrenia are associated with abnormal effort-cost computations. *Biol Psychiatry* (2013) **74**:130–6. doi:10.1016/j.biopsych.2012.12.022
68. Kasanova Z, Waltz JA, Strauss GP, Frank MJ, Gold JM. Optimizing vs. matching: response strategy in a probabilistic learning task is associated with negative symptoms of schizophrenia. *Schizophr Res* (2011) **127**:215–22. doi:10.1016/j.schres.2010.12.003
69. Elliott R, Mckenna PJ, Robbins TW, Sahakian BJ. Neuropsychological evidence for frontostriatal dysfunction in schizophrenia. *Psychol Med* (1995) **25**:619–30. doi:10.1017/S0033291700033523
70. Pantelis C, Barber FZ, Barnes TR, Nelson HE, Owen AM, Robbins TW. Comparison of set-shifting ability in patients with chronic schizophrenia and frontal lobe damage. *Schizophr Res* (1999) **37**:251–70. doi:10.1016/S0920-9964(98)00156-X
71. Waltz JA, Gold JM. Probabilistic reversal learning impairments in schizophrenia: further evidence of orbitofrontal dysfunction. *Schizophr Res* (2007) **93**:296–303. doi:10.1016/j.schres.2007.03.010
72. Prentice KJ, Gold JM, Buchanan RW. The Wisconsin card sorting impairment in schizophrenia is evident in the first four trials. *Schizophr Res* (2008) **106**:81–7. doi:10.1016/j.schres.2007.07.015
73. McKirdy J, Sussmann JE, Hall J, Lawrie SM, Johnstone EC, Mcintosh AM. Set shifting and reversal learning in patients with bipolar disorder or schizophrenia. *Psychol Med* (2009) **39**:1289–93. doi:10.1017/S0033291708004935
74. Murray GK, Cheng F, Clark L, Barnett JH, Blackwell AD, Fletcher PC, et al. Reinforcement and reversal learning in first-episode psychosis. *Schizophr Bull* (2008) **34**:848–55. doi:10.1093/schbul/sbn078
75. Leeson VC, Robbins TW, Matheson E, Hutton SB, Ron MA, Barnes TR, et al. Discrimination learning, reversal, and set-shifting in first-episode schizophrenia: stability over six years and specific associations with medication type and disorganization syndrome. *Biol Psychiatry* (2009) **66**:586–93. doi:10.1016/j.biopsych.2009.05.016
76. Waltz JA, Kasanova Z, Ross TJ, Salmeron BJ, Mcmahon RP, Gold JM, et al. The roles of reward, default, and executive control networks in set-shifting impairments in schizophrenia. *PLoS One* (2013) **8**:e57257. doi:10.1371/journal.pone.0057257
77. Schlagenhauf F, Huys QJM, Deserno L, Rapp MA, Beck A, Heinze HJ, et al. Striatal dysfunction during reversal learning in unmedicated schizophrenia patients. *Neuroimage* (2013). doi:10.1016/j.neuroimage.2013.11.034
78. Hampton AN, Bossaerts P, O'Doherty JP. The role of the ventromedial prefrontal cortex in abstract state-based inference during decision making in humans. *J Neurosci* (2006) **26**:8360–7. doi:10.1523/JNEUROSCI.1010-06.2006
79. Glascher J, Daw N, Dayan P, O'Doherty JP. States versus rewards: dissociable neural prediction error signals underlying model-based and model-free reinforcement learning. *Neuron* (2010) **66**:585–95. doi:10.1016/j.neuron.2010.04.016
80. Daw ND, Gershman SJ, Seymour B, Dayan P, Dolan RJ. Model-based influences on humans' choices and striatal prediction errors. *Neuron* (2011) **69**:1204–15. doi:10.1016/j.neuron.2011.02.027
81. Collins AG, Frank MJ. How much of reinforcement learning is working memory, not reinforcement learning? A behavioral, computational, and neurogenetic analysis. *Eur J Neurosci* (2012) **35**:1024–35. doi:10.1111/j.1460-9568.2011.07980.x
82. Otto AR, Gershman SJ, Markman AB, Daw ND. The curse of planning: dissecting multiple reinforcement-learning systems by taxing the central executive. *Psychol Sci* (2013) **24**:751–61. doi:10.1177/0956797612463080
83. Waltz JA, Frank MJ, Robinson BM, Gold JM. Selective reinforcement learning deficits in schizophrenia support predictions from computational models of

striatal-cortical dysfunction. *Biol Psychiatry* (2007) **62**:756–64. doi:10.1016/j.biopsych.2006.09.042

84. Morris SE, Heerey EA, Gold JM, Holroyd CB. Learning-related changes in brain activity following errors and performance feedback in schizophrenia. *Schizophr Res* (2008) **99**:274–85. doi:10.1016/j.schres.2007.08.027
85. Waltz JA, Frank MJ, Wiecki TV, Gold JM. Altered probabilistic learning and response biases in schizophrenia: behavioral evidence and neurocomputational modeling. *Neuropsychology* (2011) **25**:86–97. doi:10.1037/a0020882
86. Frank MJ, O'Reilly RC. A mechanistic account of striatal dopamine function in human cognition: psychopharmacological studies with cabergoline and haloperidol. *Behav Neurosci* (2006) **120**:497–517. doi:10.1037/0735-7044.120.3.497
87. Frank MJ, Seeberger LC, O'Reilly RC. By carrot or by stick: cognitive reinforcement learning in parkinsonism. *Science* (2004) **306**:1940–3. doi:10.1126/science.1102941
88. Kravitz AV, Tye LD, Kreitzer AC. Distinct roles for direct and indirect pathway striatal neurons in reinforcement. *Nat Neurosci* (2012) **15**:816–8. doi:10.1038/nn.3100
89. Strauss GP, Frank MJ, Waltz JA, Kasanova Z, Herbener ES, Gold JM. Deficits in positive reinforcement learning and uncertainty-driven exploration are associated with distinct aspects of negative symptoms in schizophrenia. *Biol Psychiatry* (2011) **69**:424–31. doi:10.1016/j.biopsych.2010.10.015
90. Brodersen KH, Schofield TM, Leff AP, Ong CS, Lomakina EI, Buhmann JM, et al. Generative embedding for model-based classification of fMRI data. *PLoS Comput Biol* (2011) **7**:e1002079. doi:10.1371/journal.pcbi.1002079
91. Brodersen KH, Deserno L, Schlagenhauf F, Lin Z, Penny WD, Buhmann JM, et al. Dissecting psychiatric spectrum disorders by generative embedding. *Neuroimage Clin* (2014) **4**:98–111. doi:10.1016/j.nicl.2013.11.002
92. Jensen J, Willeit M, Zipursky RB, Savina I, Smith AJ, Menon M, et al. The formation of abnormal associations in schizophrenia: neural and behavioral evidence. *Neuropsychopharmacology* (2008) **33**:473–9. doi:10.1038/sj.npp.1301437
93. Romaniuk L, Honey GD, King JR, Whalley HC, Mcintosh AM, Levita L, et al. Midbrain activation during Pavlovian conditioning and delusional symptoms in schizophrenia. *Arch Gen Psychiatry* (2010) **67**:1246–54. doi:10.1001/archgenpsychiatry.2010.169
94. den Ouden HE, Daunizeau J, Roiser J, Friston KJ, Stephan KE. Striatal prediction error modulates cortical coupling. *J Neurosci* (2010) **30**:3210–9. doi:10.1523/JNEUROSCI.4458-09.2010
95. Li J, Schiller D, Schoenbaum G, Phelps EA, Daw ND. Differential roles of human striatum and amygdala in associative learning. *Nat Neurosci* (2011) **14**:1250–2. doi:10.1038/nn.2904
96. Dowd EC, Barch DM. Pavlovian reward prediction and receipt in schizophrenia: relationship to anhedonia. *PLoS One* (2012) **7**:e35622. doi:10.1371/journal.pone.0035622
97. Gradin VB, Waiter G, O'Connor A, Romaniuk L, Stickle C, Matthews K, et al. Salience network-midbrain dysconnectivity and blunted reward signals in schizophrenia. *Psychiatry Res* (2013) **211**:104–11. doi:10.1016/j.pscychresns.2012.06.003
98. Diaconescu AO, Jensen J, Wang H, Willeit M, Menon M, Kapur S, et al. Aberrant effective connectivity in schizophrenia patients during appetitive conditioning. *Front Hum Neurosci* (2011) **4**:239. doi:10.3389/fnhum.2010.00239
99. Wernicke C. *Grundrisse der Psychiatrie*. Leipzig: Thieme (1906).
100. Stephan KE, Baldeweg T, Friston KJ. Synaptic plasticity and dysconnection in schizophrenia. *Biol Psychiatry* (2006) **59**:929–39. doi:10.1016/j.biopsych.2005.10.005
101. Stephan KE, Friston KJ, Frith CD. Dysconnection in schizophrenia: from abnormal synaptic plasticity to failures of self-monitoring. *Schizophr Bull* (2009) **35**:509–27. doi:10.1093/schbul/sbn176
102. Corlett PR, Murray GK, Honey GD, Aitken MR, Shanks DR, Robbins TW, et al. Disrupted prediction error signal in psychosis: evidence for an associative account of delusions. *Brain* (2007) **130**:2387–400. doi:10.1093/brain/awm173
103. Koch K, Schachtzabel C, Wagner G, Schikora J, Schultz C, Reichenbach JR, et al. Altered activation in association with reward-related trial-and-error learning in patients with schizophrenia. *Neuroimage* (2010) **50**:223–32. doi:10.1016/j.neuroimage.2009.12.031
104. Koch K, Schachtzabel C, Wagner G, Reichenbach JR, Sauer H, Schlosser R. The neural correlates of reward-related trial-and-error learning: an fMRI study with a probabilistic learning task. *Learn Mem* (2008) **15**:728–32. doi:10.1101/lm.1106408
105. Weickert TW, Goldberg TE, Callicott JH, Chen Q, Apud JA, Das S, et al. Neural correlates of probabilistic category learning in patients with schizophrenia. *J Neurosci* (2009) **29**:1244–54. doi:10.1523/JNEUROSCI.4341-08.2009
106. Gradin VB, Kumar P, Waiter G, Ahearn T, Stickle C, Milders M, et al. Expected value and prediction error abnormalities in depression and schizophrenia. *Brain* (2011) **134**:1751–64. doi:10.1093/brain/awr059
107. Tan HY, Callicott JH, Weinberger DR. Dysfunctional and compensatory prefrontal cortical systems, genes and the pathogenesis of schizophrenia. *Cereb Cortex* (2007) **17**(Suppl 1):i171–81. doi:10.1093/cercor/bhm069
108. Deserno L, Sterzer P, Wustenberg T, Heinz A, Schlagenhauf F. Reduced prefrontal-parietal effective connectivity and working memory deficits in schizophrenia. *J Neurosci* (2012) **32**:12–20. doi:10.1523/JNEUROSCI.3405-11.2012
109. Fusar-Poli P, Meyer-Lindenberg A. Striatal presynaptic dopamine in schizophrenia, part I: meta-analysis of dopamine active transporter (DAT) density. *Schizophr Bull* (2013) **39**:22–32. doi:10.1093/schbul/sbr111
110. Weinberger DR. Implications of normal brain development for the pathogenesis of schizophrenia. *Arch Gen Psychiatry* (1987) **44**:660–9. doi:10.1001/archpsyc.1987.01800190080012
111. Fusar-Poli P, Borgwardt S, Bechdolf A, Addington J, Riecher-Rossler A, Schultze-Lutter F, et al. The psychosis high-risk state: a comprehensive state-of-the-art review. *JAMA Psychiatry* (2013) **70**:107–20. doi:10.1001/jamapsychiatry.2013.269
112. Roiser JP, Stephan KE, Den Ouden HE, Friston KJ, Joyce EM. Adaptive and aberrant reward prediction signals in the human brain. *Neuroimage* (2010) **50**:657–64. doi:10.1016/j.neuroimage.2009.11.075
113. Behrens TE, Woolrich MW, Walton ME, Rushworth MF. Learning the value of information in an uncertain world. *Nat Neurosci* (2007) **10**:1214–21. doi:10.1038/nn1954
114. Mathys C, Daunizeau J, Friston KJ, Stephan KE. A bayesian foundation for individual learning under uncertainty. *Front Hum Neurosci* (2011) **5**:39. doi:10.3389/fnhum.2011.00039
115. Stephan KE, Penny WD, Daunizeau J, Moran RJ, Friston KJ. Bayesian model selection for group studies. *Neuroimage* (2009) **46**:1004–17. doi:10.1016/j.neuroimage.2009.03.025
116. Stephan KE, Penny WD, Moran RJ, Den Ouden HE, Daunizeau J, Friston KJ. Ten simple rules for dynamic causal modeling. *Neuroimage* (2010) **49**:3099–109. doi:10.1016/j.neuroimage.2009.11.015
117. Pessiglione M, Seymour B, Flandin G, Dolan RJ, Frith CD. Dopamine-dependent prediction errors underpin reward-seeking behaviour in humans. *Nature* (2006) **442**:1042–5. doi:10.1038/nature05051
118. Menon M, Jensen J, Vitcu I, Graff-Guerrero A, Crawley A, Smith MA, et al. Temporal difference modeling of the blood-oxygen level dependent response during aversive conditioning in humans: effects of dopaminergic modulation. *Biol Psychiatry* (2007) **62**:765–72. doi:10.1016/j.biopsych.2006.10.020
119. Bernacer J, Corlett PR, Ramachandra P, Mcfarlane B, Turner DC, Clark L, et al. Methamphetamine-induced disruption of frontostriatal reward learning signals: relation to psychotic symptoms. *Am J Psychiatry* (2013) **170**:1326–34. doi:10.1176/appi.ajp.2013.12070978
120. Cools R, Lewis SJ, Clark L, Barker RA, Robbins TW. L-DOPA disrupts activity in the nucleus accumbens during reversal learning in Parkinson's disease. *Neuropsychopharmacology* (2007) **32**:180–9. doi:10.1038/sj.npp.1301153
121. Schlagenhauf F, Rapp MA, Huys QJ, Beck A, Wustenberg T, Deserno L, et al. Ventral striatal prediction error signaling is associated with dopamine synthesis capacity and fluid intelligence. *Hum Brain Mapp* (2013) **34**:1490–9. doi:10.1002/hbm.22000
122. Cumming P, Ase A, Laliberte C, Kuwabara H, Gjedde A. In vivo regulation of DOPA decarboxylase by dopamine receptors in rat brain. *J Cereb Blood Flow Metab* (1997) **17**:1254–60. doi:10.1097/00004647-199711000-00014
123. Bello EP, Mateo Y, Gelman DM, Noain D, Shin JH, Low MJ, et al. Cocaine supersensitivity and enhanced motivation for reward in mice lacking dopamine D2 autoreceptors. *Nat Neurosci* (2011) **14**:1033–8. doi:10.1038/nn.2862
124. Buckholtz JW, Treadway MT, Cowan RL, Woodward ND, Benning SD, Li R, et al. Mesolimbic dopamine reward system hypersensitivity in individuals with psychopathic traits. *Nat Neurosci* (2010) **13**:419–21. doi:10.1038/nn.2510
125. Ito H, Kodaka F, Takahashi H, Takano H, Arakawa R, Shimada H, et al. Relation between presynaptic and postsynaptic dopaminergic functions measured by

positron emission tomography: implication of dopaminergic tone. *J Neurosci* (2011) **31**:7886–90. doi:10.1523/JNEUROSCI.6024-10.2011

126. Cools R, Frank MJ, Gibbs SE, Miyakawa A, Jagust W, D'Esposito M. Striatal dopamine predicts outcome-specific reversal learning and its sensitivity to dopaminergic drug administration. *J Neurosci* (2009) **29**:1538–43. doi:10.1523/JNEUROSCI.4467-08.2009
127. Goldman-Rakic PS. The physiological approach: functional architecture of working memory and disordered cognition in schizophrenia. *Biol Psychiatry* (1999) **46**:650–61. doi:10.1016/S0006-3223(99)00130-4
128. Cools R, D'Esposito M. Inverted-U-shaped dopamine actions on human working memory and cognitive control. *Biol Psychiatry* (2011) **69**:e113–25. doi:10.1016/j.biopsych.2011.03.028
129. Fusar-Poli P, Howes OD, Allen P, Broome M, Valli I, Asselin MC, et al. Abnormal frontostriatal interactions in people with prodromal signs of psychosis: a multimodal imaging study. *Arch Gen Psychiatry* (2010) **67**:683–91. doi:10.1001/archgenpsychiatry.2010.77
130. Tan HY, Sust S, Buckholtz JW, Mattay VS, Meyer-Lindenberg A, Egan MF, et al. Dysfunctional prefrontal regional specialization and compensation in schizophrenia. *Am J Psychiatry* (2006) **163**:1969–77. doi:10.1176/appi.ajp.163.11.1969
131. Potkin SG, Turner JA, Brown GG, Mccarthy G, Greve DN, Glover GH, et al. Working memory and DLPFC inefficiency in schizophrenia: the FBIRN study. *Schizophr Bull* (2009) **35**:19–31. doi:10.1093/schbul/sbn162
132. Diaconescu AO, Menon M, Jensen J, Kapur S, Mcintosh AR. Dopamine-induced changes in neural network patterns supporting aversive conditioning. *Brain Res* (2010) **1313**:143–61. doi:10.1016/j.brainres.2009.11.064
133. Heinz A, Knable MB, Coppola R, Gorey JG, Jones DW, Lee KS, et al. Psychomotor slowing, negative symptoms and dopamine receptor availability – an IBZM SPECT study in neuroleptic-treated and drug-free schizophrenic patients. *Schizophr Res* (1998) **31**:19–26. doi:10.1016/S0920-9964(98)00003-6
134. Centonze D, Usiello A, Costa C, Picconi B, Erbs E, Bernardi G, et al. Chronic haloperidol promotes corticostriatal long-term potentiation by targeting dopamine D2L receptors. *J Neurosci* (2004) **24**:8214–22. doi:10.1523/JNEUROSCI.1274-04.2004
135. Tseng KY, O'Donnell P. Dopamine-glutamate interactions controlling prefrontal cortical pyramidal cell excitability involve multiple signaling mechanisms. *J Neurosci* (2004) **24**:5131–9. doi:10.1523/JNEUROSCI.1021-04.2004
136. Friston K. A theory of cortical responses. *Philos Trans R Soc Lond B Biol Sci* (2005) **360**:815–36. doi:10.1098/rstb.2005.1622
137. Braver TS, Cohen JD. Dopamine, cognitive control, and schizophrenia: the gating model. *Prog Brain Res* (1999) **121**:327–49. doi:10.1016/S0079-6123(08)63082-4
138. Rolls ET, Loh M, Deco G, Winterer G. Computational models of schizophrenia and dopamine modulation in the prefrontal cortex. *Nat Rev Neurosci* (2008) **9**:696–709. doi:10.1038/nrn2462
139. Schmidt A, Smieskova R, Aston J, Simon A, Allen P, Fusar-Poli P, et al. Brain connectivity abnormalities predating the onset of psychosis: correlation with the effect of medication. *JAMA Psychiatry* (2013) **70**:903–12. doi:10.1001/jamapsychiatry.2013.117
140. Friston KJ, Harrison L, Penny W. Dynamic causal modelling. *Neuroimage* (2003) **19**:1273–302. doi:10.1016/S1053-8119(03)00202-7
141. den Ouden HE, Friston KJ, Daw ND, Mcintosh AR, Stephan KE. A dual role for prediction error in associative learning. *Cereb Cortex* (2009) **19**:1175–85. doi:10.1093/cercor/bhn161
142. Iglesias S, Mathys C, Brodersen KH, Kasper L, Piccirelli M, Den Ouden HE, et al. Hierarchical prediction errors in midbrain and basal forebrain during sensory learning. *Neuron* (2013) **80**:519–30. doi:10.1016/j.neuron.2013.09.009
143. Li J, Daw ND. Signals in human striatum are appropriate for policy update rather than value prediction. *J Neurosci* (2011) **31**:5504–11. doi:10.1523/JNEUROSCI.6316-10.2011

7

A Critical Review of Pro-Cognitive Drug Targets in Psychosis: Convergence on Myelination and Inflammation

Rune A. Kroken[1]*, Else-Marie Løberg[1,2], Tore Drønen[1], Renate Grüner[3,4], Kenneth Hugdahl[1,2,3,5], Kristiina Kompus[2], Silje Skrede[5,6,7] and Erik Johnsen[1,8]

[1] Division of Psychiatry, Haukeland University Hospital, Bergen, Norway
[2] Department of Biological and Medical Psychology, University of Bergen, Bergen, Norway
[3] Department of Radiology, Haukeland University Hospital, Bergen, Norway
[4] Department of Physics and Technology, University of Bergen, Bergen, Norway
[5] NORMENT Center of Excellence, University of Bergen, Bergen, Norway
[6] Dr. Einar Martens' Research Group for Biological Psychiatry, Centre for Medical Genetics and Molecular Medicine, Haukeland University Hospital, Bergen, Norway
[7] Department of Clinical Science, K.G. Jebsen Centre for Psychosis Research, University of Bergen, Bergen, Norway
[8] Department of Clinical Medicine, University of Bergen, Bergen, Norway

Correspondence:
Rune A. Kroken, Division of Psychiatry, Haukeland University Hospital, PB 1400, N-5021 Bergen, Norway
e-mail: rune.kroken@helse-bergen.no

Antipsychotic drugs have thus far focused on dopaminergic antagonism at the D2 receptors, as counteracting the hyperdopaminergia in nigrostriatal and mesolimbic projections has been considered mandatory for the antipsychotic action of the drugs. Current drugs effectively target the positive symptoms of psychosis such as hallucinations and delusions in the majority of patients, whereas effect sizes are smaller for negative symptoms and cognitive dysfunctions. With the understanding that neurocognitive dysfunction associated with schizophrenia have a greater impact on functional outcome than the positive symptoms, the focus in pharmacotherapy for schizophrenia has shifted to the potential effect of future drugs on cognitive enhancement. A major obstacle is, however, that the biological underpinnings of cognitive dysfunction remain largely unknown. With the availability of increasingly sophisticated techniques in molecular biology and brain imaging, this situation is about to change with major advances being made in identifying the neuronal substrates underlying schizophrenia, and putative pro-cognitive drug targets may be revealed. In relation to cognitive effects, this review focuses on evidence from basic neuroscience and clinical studies, taking two separate perspectives. One perspective is the identification of previously under-recognized treatment targets for existing antipsychotic drugs, including myelination and mediators of inflammation. A second perspective is the development of new drugs or novel treatment targets for well-known drugs, which act on recently discovered treatment targets for cognitive enhancement, and which may complement the existing drugs. This might pave the way for personalized treatment regimens for patients with schizophrenia aimed at improved functional outcome. The review also aims at identifying major current constraints for pro-cognitive drug development for patients with schizophrenia.

Keywords: schizophrenia, cognition, glutamate, myelin, inflammation, immunology, connectivity, neuroimaging

INTRODUCTION

Schizophrenia is a severe mental disorder with typical onset in the late teens or early adulthood and a chronically relapsing remitting course in the majority of cases (1). Schizophrenia remains a leading cause of years lived with disability (2), and active psychosis has been ranked among the most disabling disorders by severity in the general population (3).

The clinical picture of schizophrenia is heterogeneous, but in the vast majority of patients, cognitive dysfunctions are present with adverse impact on daily functioning (1). Antipsychotic drugs have for six decades been a cornerstone in the treatment of the disorder but a fundamental limitation is their small effect sizes in the cognitive symptom domain (4) as the drugs are primarily effective against the positive symptoms of psychosis including hallucinations and delusions (4). Since the serendipitous discovery of chlorpromazine's antipsychotic properties, dopaminergic antagonism has served as a template for all subsequent antipsychotics through counteracting subcortical hyperdopaminergia (5). The drugs following chlorpromazine are usually classified as typical or first generation antipsychotics (FGAs), whereas clozapine much later became the prototype for the atypical or second-generation antipsychotic (SGA) drugs that were developed in the 1990s onward (4, 6). Only modest differences in antipsychotic efficacy have been found among FGAs and SGAs (7), but the SGAs seem to display a broader therapeutic repertoire including also pro-cognitive properties, although of a small magnitude (8). Pharmacologically, the FGAs have strong affinities for the dopamine type 2 (D2) receptor, whereas the SGAs are characterized by a more pronounced 5-HT2A antagonism than FGAs, and a lower potency for the D2 receptor (9, 10). The narrow focus on the dopaminergic system and striatal hyperdopaminergia in particular has most likely contributed to the limited evolvement of more effective drug treatment options as it has become increasingly clear that dopaminergic disturbances account for only parts of the clinical picture (particularly for positive symptoms) (11–13), and hyperdopaminergia is not present in all schizophrenia patients (14).

Recognizing the large impact that the schizophrenia associated cognitive dysfunctions have on functional outcome (15, 16), the efforts to improve the pharmacological treatment have moved toward cognitive enhancement, and pro-cognitive effects have been proposed as primary targets in future drug studies (17, 18). A major obstacle restricting hypothesis-driven pro-cognitive drug development has been the lacking knowledge of the structural and functional brain alterations underlying cognitive dysfunction in patients with schizophrenia (19, 20). Major scientific advances in unveiling the neurobiology of schizophrenia have emerged in recent years, however. The knowledge of transmitter dysfunctions especially is widened (21), accompanied by evidence of disturbances of myelination and inflammation/immunology in the pathophysiology of schizophrenia (22, 23). Thus, going beyond the neurotransmitter disturbances associated with schizophrenia, the present work reviews the latest evidence on myelin alterations, and the involvement of neuroinflammation/immunology in schizophrenia, with putative relevance for pro-cognitive drug effects in schizophrenia and related psychotic disorders. Moreover, these areas seem at least partly inter-related and the review aims at integrating the evidence from key publications in a joint model. Increased insight into the relevant functional and structural alterations might pave the way for more efficacious, targeted, and personalized pro-cognitive drug treatment opportunities aimed at improving real-world functioning. The review focuses on both previously unknown treatment targets for existing antipsychotic drugs, and potentially novel pro-cognitive drugs addressing extra-dopaminergic treatment targets, and gives an update also commenting on current constraints of pro-cognitive drug development for patients with schizophrenia.

COGNITIVE DYSFUNCTION IN PATIENTS WITH SCHIZOPHRENIA

Cognitive function may be understood in terms of inter-related complex neural networks, influenced by different neurotransmitters, cytokines, and other substances including brain-derived neurotropic factor (BDNF) acting as neuromodulators (24).

Cognitive deficits are viewed as core characteristics of schizophrenia, with clinically significant cognitive impairments observed in a large majority of patients, and most patients experience lower cognitive functioning than would be expected from parental levels of education (16, 25). Cognitive deficits are seen before the development of psychosis (25–28), and cognitive decline and intellectual stagnation have been suggested to constitute a risk phenotype for developing schizophrenia (25). Furthermore, cognitive deficits are relatively stable after psychotic breakthrough and still present when the symptoms of psychosis have been treated (29, 30). A general cognitive dysfunction across cognitive domains is present, with additional selective deficits in working memory, executive function, attention, verbal fluency, episodic memory, and processing speed (15, 31). The effect size of the cognitive dysfunction compared to healthy subjects is close to 1.0 (32, 33), and in several neurocognitive dimensions the impairment is between 1 and 2 SDs, indicating a clinically significant loss of function (25, 34–37). Cognitive functioning has greater impact than positive psychotic symptoms in determining the patient's real-world functional outcome (15, 38–41), and relationships between more specific cognitive domains and functional domains have also been reported (38, 40, 42). Thus, cognitive impairment has been put forward as the main target for novel treatment interventions in schizophrenia (25).

A significant challenge has been to develop clinical meaningful measures of cognitive dysfunction for pro-cognitive drug advancement. A major contribution to establish a standardized and manageable test battery for measuring cognition in schizophrenia has been the development of the Measurement and Treatment Research to Improve Cognition in Schizophrenia (MATRICS) Consensus Cognitive Battery (MCCB) (43). The MCCB composite score has been suggested as the best outcome measure based on findings of low practice effects, high test–retest reliability, and good external validity (44), while a recent factor analysis identified a three factor model of processing speed, attention/working memory, and learning as the best representations of data in this particular study (45).

DOES ABNORMAL MYELINATION CAUSE COGNITIVE DYSFUNCTIONS IN PATIENTS WITH SCHIZOPHRENIA?

Myelin, the main constituent of white matter, is essential for controlling and regulating conduction velocities along axons and thus the synchronicity of brain signals across different brain regions, and for controlling synapse plasticity (46). Decreased myelin integrity might accordingly alter normal signal transduction. In the following, we will focus on one major line of recent achievements in schizophrenia research, namely the rapidly expanding knowledge of abnormal central nervous myelination in patients with schizophrenia and the possibilities to prevent or repair myelin pathology. White matter brain alterations and functional connectivity problems that have been linked to cognitive dysfunctions in schizophrenia will be briefly described, followed by in-depth descriptions of new findings of myelin alterations linked to cognition. Again, a major problem is to identify manageable tests/measures of myelinization and myelin integrity that can be used in drug discovery programs in a reliable way. Finally, we will discuss candidate drug treatments counteracting deficits of myelinization in patients with schizophrenia

WHITE MATTER CHANGES AND COGNITION

Several distinct alterations in gray and white matter are well established for schizophrenia patients as a group (47). Reviews of white matter tract pathology in patients with schizophrenia [mostly studies based on voxel-based morphometry (VBM) and diffusion tensor imaging (DTI)] have identified widespread and, in many studies, progressive changes (47). A meta-analysis of 15 DTI studies by Ellison-Wright and Bullmore (48) identified reductions (in all studies) of left frontal deep white matter and left temporal white matter. Thus, the authors suggested that two different networks may be affected; one connecting the frontal lobe with thalamus and cingulate gyrus, the other connecting the temporal lobe with, e.g., insula, amygdala, hippocampus, and the frontal lobe. A review by Walterfang et al. (49) of white matter pathology in patients with schizophrenia identified changes in the left uncinate fasciculi as the most replicated finding, furthermore that deficits of information processing was associated with volume reductions in the uncinate and inferior longitudinal fasciculi, anterior internal capsule, and corpus callosum (49). White matter pathology related to cognition has also been found in first-episode patients with psychosis. For example, Rigucci and colleagues (50) reported a relationship between speed of processing and visual memory and white matter fractional anisotropy (FA) in fronto-temporal tracts. Focusing on intra-cortical white matter, several clusters of superficial white matter (SWM) composed of U-shaped fibers connecting neighboring gyri together with intra-cortical axons and fibers from deep matter pathways displayed reduced FA in a study comparing patients with schizophrenia to healthy controls. The correlations between SWM-FA and cognition displayed in healthy controls were missing in patients (51).

FUNCTIONAL CONNECTIVITY STUDIES

Recently, also related to myelination, the search for brain alterations underlying the psychopathology of schizophrenia has refocused to examine neuronal dysconnectivity, i.e., abnormal communication between local and distributed neuronal circuits or disrupted integration of brain activation (52–54). Fornito et al. (53) reviewed data on brain connectivity, and concluded that schizophrenia is associated with: (1) a widespread and possibly context-independent connectivity deficits, (2) additional transient states of hyper- and/or hypo-connectivity related to specific tasks.

Disturbed connectivity within the frontal lobes has been found to be related to working memory and to executive functioning (52, 54). This includes abnormal connectivity in fronto-parietal, fronto-cerebellar, and fronto-hippocampal networks (52). Verbal processing deficits have been shown to be related to circuits in the language areas of the brain, particularly to fronto-temporal dysfunction (52, 54). Indeed, theories have been developed concentrating on the effect of reduced executive cognitive control over the language processing in the temporal lobes as central to the development of the symptoms of psychosis, for instance auditory verbal hallucination (55).

Of future interest may be the influence of antipsychotic drugs on the dynamic interaction between large-scale cortical networks related to resting and effort-mode states (56). Using fMRI, Hugdahl et al. (57) found overlapping activation in a large-scale network to occur with a range of different cognitive tasks implicating the prefrontal cortex [see also Ref. (58)] suggesting that effective cognitive processing would require down-regulation of the resting-state network in situations with increasing demands for the up-regulation of the effort-mode network, and that cognitive impairment in schizophrenia may result from failure of network up- and down-regulation dynamics. Thus, based on brain imaging results, therapeutic agents inducing stabilization and, ideally, normalization of large-scale cortical network dynamics could possibly have pro-cognitive effects. However, thus far no drug has been reported to enhance connectivity (52).

The major question related to the structural basis of functional dysconnectivity was addressed in the review by Fornito et al. (53). The authors concluded with major overlaps between functional and structural findings, but also differences, which could at least partly be caused by intrinsic problems of the methods of structural measurements (see Measuring Myelination).

MEASURING MYELINATION

Several methodological issues need consideration regarding the use of imaging techniques for myelin assessments. The DTI signal may reveal changes in white matter integrity but has limitations in identifying the exact nature of these changes, as the FA reflects different processes like demyelination, axonal swelling, or atrophy, and is sensitive to confounding effects of fiber crossings (59). In a recent review by Du and Öngür (60), two novel MR-based approaches – diffusion tensor spectroscopy (DTS) and magnetization transfer ratio (MTR) – were reviewed as measures of axonal diameter (DTS) and myelin volume (MTR). Combining MTR with DTI, Palaniyappan et al. (61) recently showed that the degree of FA reduction in areas with decreased myelin volume predicted impaired processing speed, leading the authors to suggest that combined DTI/MTR could be used as a treatment measure in the development of pro-cognitive drugs.

A study applying graph theory to analyze data from DTI combined with MTR showed that patients with schizophrenia have a weaker globally integrated structural brain network when compared to healthy controls (62). The same study concluded that the frontal hubs had a less central role than in healthy controls, which is in accordance with a reduced structural capacity to integrate information across brain regions. Moreover, a new study combining DTI and resting-state fMRI comparing patients with schizophrenia to healthy controls identified a selective disruption of brain connectivity among central hub regions with a potential communication capacity reduction and brain dynamics alterations (63).

MYELIN DEFICIENCIES IN SCHIZOPHRENIA

Compelling evidence from several different lines of research has, in recent years, implicated dysfunctional myelin and oligodendrocytes, the cells responsible for wrapping myelin around neuronal axons in the brain, in the pathology of schizophrenia and related psychoses (22, 64–66). Sources of evidence include genetics and pharmacogenetic studies, post-mortem studies, and as briefly reviewed in the previous subsections of brain imaging studies, particularly DTI studies.

Normal myelination starts in the late part of fetal life and occurs most rapidly during the first 2 years after birth, but continues to adulthood in a region- and brain matter-specific manner (22, 65, 67). Initial myelination occurs subcortically, thus increasing the conduction velocities across different brain regions while leaving the intra-cortical portion of the axon unmyelinated during childhood (65). Interestingly, maturation of white matter in the prefrontal cortex and in fronto-temporal tracts occurs later, in late adolescence and early adult life, coinciding in time with the peak age of schizophrenia onset (1). Possibly, disturbances in the maturation of myelin around the end of the myelination stage could be one of the events contributing to the peak debut incidence of schizophrenia in this age group (66). The prefrontal cortex is one of the regions most robustly implicated in schizophrenia pathology, and working memory performance, which engages this region, has been found to be positively associated with the level of white matter maturation (67). Later intra-cortical myelination occurs for the most part in adulthood and is associated with the refinement of cognitive functions and brain plasticity (65). Importantly, myelination is a dynamic process, and oligodendrocyte progenitor cells continue to differentiate throughout life (68). In schizophrenia, intra-cortical myelin deficits seems to be more pronounced than subcortical deficits, which have been found to be more strongly associated with the duration of illness. Indeed, evidence suggests that myelin integrity is closely related to both cognitive functioning and to the symptoms of a variety of psychiatric and neurological disorders (22, 46).

Alterations particularly in dopaminergic transmission (69, 70), and also in the glutamatergic system, (11, 71) have been robustly implicated in the pathology of schizophrenia for several decades. Glutamatergic *N*-methyl-D-aspartate (NMDA) receptor antagonists, such as phencyclidine (PCP) and ketamine, have the potential to induce not only positive symptoms of psychosis but also negative symptoms and cognitive dysfunction resembling those seen in schizophrenia (11, 71). This has given rise to the NMDA receptor hypofunction hypothesis of schizophrenia (21, 72). The hypothesis has been extensively investigated in animal models but several limitations related to how well evidence from preclinical studies translate into schizophrenia patients have been pointed to (72). Seemingly, paradoxically another model of schizophrenia-related cognitive dysfunction is that of glutamatergic hyperactivity (73). The model is based on other observations of increased prefrontal glutamate release following NMDA receptor antagonism. The apparent paradoxical glutamate findings might be explained by different NMDA receptor properties related to the different locations and/or sub-compositions of the different NMDA receptors as elaborated by Zhou et al. (74). Interestingly, there are several points of convergence between myelin deficits and neurotransmitter alterations. Firstly, glutamate is excitotoxic when in excess, and oligodendrocyte progenitor cells display great vulnerability for glutamatergic excitotoxicity (68). Increased glutamate levels have been found in some phases of schizophrenia (75–77). Secondly, there is emerging evidence that dysfunctional myelin and oligodendrocytes could increase striatal dopamine levels, see Ref. (22) for details. One example could be that if glutamatergic projections from the prefrontal cortex to brainstem areas suffer from myelin damage, this might lead to lower excitatory input at inhibitory brainstem GABAergic interneurons, resulting in less inhibition of dopaminergic mesolimbic projections and consequently striatal hyperdopaminergia as outlined by Schwartz et al. (78).

MYELIN AS DRUG TARGET FOR PRESENT ANTIPSYCHOTICS

Animal studies suggest that myelin-protecting and oligodendrocyte-stimulating properties may be a therapeutically relevant mechanism of action for at least some SGAs (61, 79, 80). In a DTI study of schizophrenia patients in exacerbation, Garver et al. (81) found increased diffusibility consistent with decreased myelin integrity during acute psychosis. After initial examination, patients were treated with the SGAs risperidone or ziprasidone, or the FGA haloperidol, with partial restoration of myelin integrity after 4 weeks in the subgroup that responded to treatment. Bartzokis et al. found higher volumes of intra-cortical myelin in schizophrenia patients treated with oral risperidone compared to those treated with the FGA fluphenazine decanoate (82). In a recent study by the same group, the long acting injection formulation of risperidone was associated with increased intra-cortical myelin volume compared to the oral formulation of the same compound (64). Myelin primarily consists of lipids, particularly cholesterol, which are mainly synthesized *de novo* in the brain. Interestingly, several antipsychotic agents have been demonstrated to directly induce lipogenesis through the sterol regulatory element binding protein (SREBP) system, and these lipogenic effects have been suggested to contribute to myelin-stimulating effects of antipsychotic agents (83–85). In this regard, it is highly interesting that clozapine, with its superior clinical efficacy, is also among the antipsychotics associated with the most pronounced metabolic adverse effects; in fact, a correlation between clinical improvement and increase in serum lipid levels has repeatedly been demonstrated (86–88). Summing up, a small but consistent body of evidence indicates that some current SGAs have positive effects on myelin volume, with possible distinctions among drugs and drug formulations.

OTHER POTENTIAL "MYELIN-ENHANCING" TREATMENT OPTIONS

In a clinical randomized controlled trial (RCT) by Amminger et al. (89), a markedly decreased progression rate to psychosis was found in at risk subjects receiving high-dose polyunsaturated fatty acids (PUFAs). PUFAs are involved in the myelination process, and peripheral PUFA levels have been found to be decreased in schizophrenia (90, 91). A recent DTI study in early-phase psychosis patients found an association between level of PUFAs in peripheral erythrocytes and white matter integrity (90). Possibly, PUFA distribution is altered in patients at risk for psychosis, with a link between PUFA levels and white matter integrity. Free radicals can damage membrane PUFAs, and disturbances in fatty acids and membrane phospholipid identified in patients with schizophrenia may be caused by increased oxidative stress according to a review by Yao and Keshavan (92). The same authors point to disruption of antioxidative systems related to schizophrenia, with reduced amounts of non-enzymatic plasma antioxidant components [e.g., albumin, bilirubin, uric acid, ascorbic acid (vitamin C), α-tocopherol (vitamin E)], see also the recent clinical study by Zhang et al. demonstrating a reduced plasma total antioxidant status in a sample of schizophrenia patients (93). Interestingly, PUFAs also have mild anti-inflammatory effects, see Section "Additional Drugs with Anti-Inflammatory Action as Add-on Treatments for Patients with Schizophrenia."

INFLAMMATION AND IMMUNOLOGY IN SCHIZOPHRENIA

IMPLICATING INFLAMMATORY SYSTEMS IN SCHIZOPHRENIA

Several findings point to a link between inflammatory processes and the pathophysiology of schizophrenia: (1) activated peripheral inflammatory system and neuroinflammation in patients with schizophrenia (94, 95), (2) evidence from genetic studies of correlation between schizophrenia and genes encoding for different components of the immune system (96–98), (3) post-mortem studies demonstrating up-regulated immune genes in the prefrontal cortex of patients with schizophrenia (99), (4) findings that the raised risk of schizophrenia seen after maternal infections acts via immunological mechanism (23), and (5) psychotic symptoms and cognitive dysfunction caused by immunological neurological syndromes (100), e.g., the interesting line of pathophysiological evidence based on findings in autoimmune synaptic encephalitis (limbic encephalitis), where antibody formation against NMDA receptors is associated with a wide range of psychiatric symptoms, in some patients also with syndromes resembling schizophrenia (100). Binding of NMDA antibodies has been found predominantly in the hippocampus (101). Also, in systemic autoimmune disorders such as systemic lupus erythematosus (SLE), patients can suffer from various psychiatric syndromes, but the pathophysiology has yet to be characterized in detail (102). A recent remarkable finding is that the levels of soluble receptors for the pro-inflammatory cytokine tumor necrosis factor (TNF)-α correlates with function in patients with schizophrenia compared to healthy individuals (103), the same study also found increased levels of TNF-α in the treatment resistant group compared to treatment responders.

In the following sections, we highlight some of the main findings related to inflammation/immunology and schizophrenia, with the specific purpose of evaluating the status of immune-modulating treatment with cognitive-enhancing effects.

CYTOKINES

In the context of inflammatory changes in schizophrenia, the majority of findings stem from the innate system, but components of the adaptive immunology system have also been implicated. The macrophages of the innate system induce the release of acute-phase proteins [e.g., C-reactive protein (CRP) from hepatocytes] as well as producing and releasing cytokines (97), all markers of inflammation (104). Cytokines are also produced by peripherally activated endothelial cells and monocyte-derived dendritic cells (97).

PERIPHERAL INFLAMMATORY FINDINGS IN SCHIZOPHRENIA

Multiple studies have shown low-grade disturbances in the peripheral inflammatory system in patients with schizophrenia, see recent reviews (105–107). Pro-inflammatory changes include elevated serum measures of pro-inflammatory cytokines [interleukin (IL)-1β, IL-6, IL-8, TNF-α] and other pro-inflammatory factors [prostaglandin E_2 (PGE_2), CRP] and elevated monocyte counts and activated immune cells have been associated with schizophrenia (108). Interestingly, some cytokines [IL-12, IFN-γ, TNF-α, soluble IL-2 receptor (sIL-2R)] may be trait markers for schizophrenia, while others are raised during phases of intensified symptoms (IL-1β, IL-6, and TGF-β) (106, 108). Furthermore, some anti-inflammatory substances are elevated in subgroups of patients with schizophrenia [soluble IL-1 receptor antagonist (sIL-1RA), soluble IL-2 receptor antagonist (sIL-2RA), soluble TNF receptors (sTNFRs)1, sTNFR2 (109), IL-10 (a cytokine with anti-inflammatory properties), and transforming growth factor (TGF)-β] (105). A review (110) identified decreased levels of IL-2 in patients with schizophrenia. IL-2 serves important functions in T-cell-mediated immunologic reactions. Although the findings of disturbances in the peripheral inflammatory system are not without inconsistencies, and the measurements of cytokines are sensible to a wide range of confounders (e.g., the influence of antipsychotic medication and metabolic status), there is firm evidence for a mixed picture of peripheral pro- and anti-inflammatory changes in a large proportion of patients with schizophrenia.

CENTRAL INFLAMMATORY FINDINGS IN PATIENTS WITH SCHIZOPHRENIA

Brain neuroinflammation, in contrast to inflammation in other parts of the body, does not lead to leukocyte recruitment, but is characterized by activated microglia, the mononuclear phagocytes of the brain (111). Microglia develop from primitive myeloid progenitors, and have various roles in the developing human brain including synaptic pruning, remodeling of axons, neuronal differentiation, and programed cell death (112). PET studies using (R)[11C]PK11195 (95, 113) have found microglial activation in schizophrenia, in addition to post-mortem studies demonstrating increased density and activation of microglia, though some of these studies have yielded conflicting evidence (112). Activated microglia have increased levels of the translocator protein (TPSO) located at the mitochondrial membrane, and the binding of TPSO to the (R)[11C]PK11195 is utilized in PET studies as a measure of neuroinflammation, while other PET ligands for activated microglia are under development (113). Free-water imaging (114) is another mode of neuroinflammation imaging, and studies using this novel method have indicated widespread brain inflammation and early signs of neurodegeneration in first-episode patients with schizophrenia (115).

Microglia, astrocytes, and the kynurenine pathway

Activated microglia have many important functions besides phagocytosis, including cytokine production (IL-1β, IL-12, and TNF-α) (94, 111), most importantly crosstalk with the serotonin and glutamate neurotransmitter systems, involving the kynurenine pathway (116). Activated microglia also induce functional changes in brain astrocytes, which release IL-6, IL-10, and TGF-β (94). In the presence of pro-inflammatory cytokines, e.g., IFN-γ and TNF-α, tryptophan catabolism to kynurenins in microglia and astrocytes is induced, resulting in the production of quinolinic acid (QUIN) in microglia and KYNA in astrocytes. QUIN is an NMDA agonist and potentially excitotoxic, while KYNA is an NMDA antagonist and also blocks the α7 nicotinic acetylcholine receptor (α7nAChR) (94, 116). **Figure 1** summarizes major points of the activated inflammatory responses in schizophrenia. The demonstration of elevated levels of KYNA in the cerebrospinal fluid (CSF) of patients with schizophrenia by two independent groups (117, 118) in 2001 boosted research in brain inflammatory-related processes implicated in schizophrenia. Elevation of KYNA in the CSF and prefrontal cortex in patients with schizophrenia is now an established finding, and is probably a consequence of peripheral inflammation according to a recent review by Schwarcz et al. (119). Elevated levels of KYNA are associated with decreased cognitive performance in animal models, including altered pre-pulse inhibition of the auditory startle

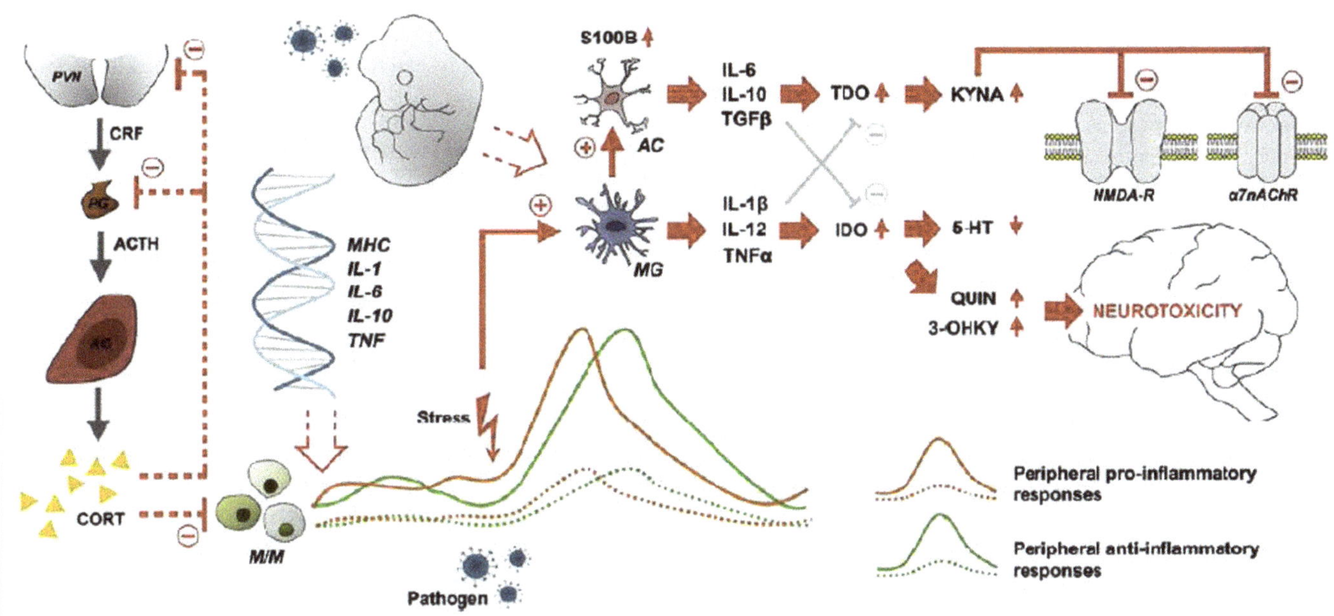

FIGURE 1 | Characteristics, sources, and neuronal consequences of activated inflammatory responses in schizophrenia. Abnormal expression of inflammatory genes in monocytes/macrophages (M/M) results in peripheral low-grade inflammation (patients: solid orange and green lines-healthy subjects: dashed lines). Stress and/or pathogen exposure may lead to an over-activation of microglia (MG), which activates astrocytes (AC) and the consequent release of cytokines (IL-6, IL-10, TGF-β) that stimulate the production of kynurenic acid (KYNA). KYNA blocks signaling at the NMDA receptor and the α7 nicotinic acetylcholine receptor (α7nAChR). MGs releases cytokines (IL-1β, IL-12, TNF-α) that weaken the biosynthesis of serotonin and promotes the production of quinolinic acid (QUIN) and 3-hydroxykynurenine (3-OHKY), both neurotoxic substances. Abnormal HPA axis function may further contribute to the development of low-grade inflammation as the normal feed-back exerted by cortisol is not working properly. Furthermore, prenatal immune priming by *in utero* exposure to infection may provide a developmental source of long-term immune abnormalities to schizophrenia. With permission from Meyer et al. (84).

response, deficits of working memory, and attentional set-shifting paradigms (120, 121), while reducing KYNA resulted in improved cognitive performance in a wide range of tasks (121). Adding to this, the kynurenic pathway also offers a possible explanation of how stress induces psychotic symptoms and cognitive dysfunction in schizophrenia by linking increased levels of glucocorticoids to the production of kynurenine in liver, subsequently converted to KYNA in the brain (121). The kynurenic pathway offers several potential drug targets for the reduction of brain KYNA levels, which could improve cognitive function in schizophrenia. Candidate pharmacological agents related to schizophrenia treatment block, e.g., the enzyme kynurenine aminotransferase (KAT), which transforms kynurenine into KYNA. Most KYNA-lowering drugs still lack behavioral data (122), while cerebrolysin, a peptidergic drug manufactured from purified porcine brain preparations, which lower brain tissue KYNA levels *in vitro* (123) also have been found to improve cognition (124). Interestingly, in a double blind RCT of patients with schizophrenia cerebrolysin (intravenous infusion) as add-on treatment to risperidone was found to improve scores at the Wechsler Adult Intelligence Scale and the Wechsler Memory Scale (124). Cerebrolysin is generally well-tolerated (125) and has also demonstrated pro-cognitive effects in patients with dementia (126, 127) and traumatic brain injury (128). In another recent study, D-cycloserine (DSC), a partial agonist at the glycine site of the NMDA receptor, was also found to reduce the levels of KYNA in human post-mortem frontal cortex homogenates by dose-dependently blocking KAT (129). DSC has also been found to improve memory consolidation and to reduce delusions in combination with cognitive behavioral therapy (130).

IL-1β, S100B, BDNF

In addition to elevated KYNA/QUIN, other aspects of an activated brain immune system can also have clinically important effects in schizophrenia. The proinflammatory cytokine IL-1β has been linked to glutamatergic excitotoxicity (131), and close dynamic interactions between IL-1β and the NMDA receptor was the recently demonstrated (132). Pro-inflammatory cytokines (e.g., IL-1) are also candidate causal agents implicated in the cerebral myelin damages discussed above, see (133, 134). The protein S100B, produced by astrocytes, is a marker of astrocyte activation. Serving as an example of the pleiotropic effects associated with many inflammatory factors at low concentration, S100B has beneficial effects, limiting microglia activation, stress-related neuronal damage, and increase glutamate uptake by astrocytes, while at higher concentration it has detrimental effects, including induction of microglial TNF-α secretion and induced production of, e.g., COX2/PGE-2, IL-1β, etc. (135). A meta-analysis concluded that serum levels of S100B may be elevated in schizophrenia, and disruptions of the blood–brain barrier (BBB) and/or active secretion by astrocytes were suggested as possible causes (136).

The neurotrophin BDNF is among the substances secreted by immune cells during inflammation and immune responses (137), and an inverse relationship between levels of BDNF and certain cytokines has been found (138). BDNF has been implicated in widespread processes relevant to the pathophysiology of schizophrenia including neurodevelopment, synapse regulation, and neuroplasticity, as well as effects on cognition, see for example (138–140). BDNF has been found to be reduced in schizophrenia in both drug-naïve and chronic patients, although findings are not entirely consistent across studies. Furthermore, an association has been found between reduced neurocognitive function and reduced serum BDNF levels (139). BDNF interacts with dopaminergic, glutamatergic, and serotonergic systems in the brain, see Nurjono et al. (138) for a recent update. Regarding BDNF as a drug target, FGAs have been reported to lower peripheral BDNF, whereas SGAs either have no effect or increase BDNF, while antidepressants have been shown to increase BDNF (140).

STRUCTURAL AND FUNCTIONAL CORRELATES OF INFLAMMATORY DISTURBANCES IN PATIENTS WITH SCHIZOPHRENIA

Structural brain alterations associated with immune-related genetic polymorphisms were recently reviewed by Fineberg and Ellman (107). The review identified associations between variability in the IL-1 gene complex and white and gray matter volume reductions in temporal and frontal brain regions, together with enlarged ventricles in patients with schizophrenia. Furthermore, this review discussed associations of IL-1 gene variations with decreased dorsolateral prefrontal function during different neurocognitive tasks (107). In another review, Meyer (105) found evidence for a positive correlation between the severity of cognitive deficits and the peripheral levels of IL-1β, IL-6, TNF-α, CRP, and S100B. While the correlation of the inflammatory disturbances with specific cognitive effects is not clarified in patients with schizophrenia, findings from animal studies and studies in non-schizophrenic individuals reveal associations of inflammatory disturbances with executive function, sustained attention, and working memory according to the review by Meyer et al. (105).

ANTI-INFLAMMATORY EFFECTS OF ANTIPSYCHOTIC DRUGS

Monji et al. (141) recently reviewed studies (mostly *in vitro* and animal studies) concerning the capability of antipsychotic drugs to influence activated microglia. The review identified several studies showing that antipsychotic drugs significantly reduce the secretion of TNF-α, nitric oxide, IL-1β, and IL-2 from activated microglia. Furthermore, some drugs were found to have stronger inhibitory effects, e.g., risperidone, which inhibited the secretion of several cytokines from activated microglia more than haloperidol, and indications of clozapine-specific effects have also been reported. Moreover, in the context of the kynurenine pathway, one animal study demonstrated that chronic treatment with antipsychotic drugs reduces brain KYNA (142). Meyer et al. (94) reviewed the influence of antipsychotic treatment on peripheral cytokines in clinical populations and found that antipsychotics reduced the level of proinflammatory cytokines (IL-1β, IL-6, sIL-6R, TNF-α) while increasing peripheral production of anti-inflammatory substances such as (sIL-1RA, sIL-2R and IL-10). Here, SGAs seemed to have the most pronounced effects and a possible relation between the ability to normalize immune function and clinical effects were identified. Brain imaging studies investigating antipsychotic drug treatment in brain imaging paradigms capable of showing effects on neuroinflammation (e.g., PET/"free water" MRI) would truly improve this field of research, but we have not been able to identify any such studies.

THE EFFECTS OF ANTI-INFLAMMATORY/IMMUNE-MODULATING DRUGS IN THE TREATMENT OF SCHIZOPHRENIA

Non-steroid anti-inflammatory drugs

Based on the notion of activated immune responses in the brain and/or peripheral tissues, a few clinical studies have evaluated the effects of non-steroid anti-inflammatory drugs (NSAIDs) in schizophrenia. The pooled effects size in reducing total Positive and Negative Syndrome Scale (PANSS) score according to a recent meta-analysis of the effect of add-on treatment with NSAIDs [eight studies, two with aspirin ($n = 270$), six with celecoxib ($n = 504$)] to different antipsychotics showed non-significant benefit over placebo (143). Treatment with aspirin alone was superior to placebo, while treatment with celecoxib was not; these conclusions were also drawn in a meta-analysis of Sommer et al. (144). When the studies were categorized according to disease phase, the pooled analyses of all eight studies revealed positive effects of NSAIDs vs. placebo for first-episode patients. The authors concluded that the present data do not lend significant support to NSAIDs as add-on therapy to antipsychotic treatment for patients with schizophrenia. Another review agreed that indiscriminately suppressing inflammation seems not to be the optimal way of treating immunological disturbances associated with schizophrenia, and that treatment should aim at reversing glial loss, upregulating beneficial microglial activation and proliferation (MAP) together with other neuroprotective measures, while ideally downregulating harmful aspects of MAP (135). At present, studies more precisely aiming to elucidate the putative pro-cognitive effects of treatment with NSAIDs in patients with schizophrenia are lacking, although non-significant effects were demonstrated in a small study (145).

Erythropoietin

Erythropoietin (EPO) is a cytokine with several identified functions in the brain (146). In a 12-week, placebo-controlled study ($n = 39$) with stable schizophrenia patients, treatment with recombinant human EPO (40000 IU/week) improved neurocognitive function compared to placebo in the domains of delayed memory, language-semantic fluency, attention and perseverative errors (147). An evaluation of gray matter development in the same study showed that gray matter loss was significantly less pronounced in the group treated with EPO (148). Animal studies have supported a pro-cognitive effect of EPO treatment (146). A systematic review identified multiple putative beneficial brain targets of EPO treatment, e.g., modulation of inflammation, neuroprotection, neurotransmission regulation, effects on BBB permeability, but the use of EPO can be limited by adverse effects such as thrombosis and cancer (149). EPO has also been found to improve cognitive function in studies of patients with Parkinson's disease (150) and multiple sclerosis (151).

Minocycline

The tetracycline antibiotic drug minocycline has also been tested as an add-on treatment for patients with schizophrenia, based on evidence from animal studies that showed minocycline to have multiple actions including inhibition of microglial activation and the attenuation of adaptive immunity through the reduction of activity and expression of matrix metalloproteinases (MMPs). MMPs enable T-cells to migrate through the BBB by altering its permeability, a process associated with myelin degradation (152). In a placebo-controlled, 6-month trial in patients with schizophrenia (54 patients receiving 200 mg minocycline and 26 patients receiving placebo), cognitive function (and negative symptoms) improved significantly in the minocycline-treated group, particularly in the domains of working memory, cognitive flexibility, and planning (153). Chaudry et al. (154) reported the results of a 1-year RCT of 155 early schizophrenia patients performed in Brazil and Pakistan, where minocycline reduced negative symptoms (adjusted difference 95% confidence interval 1.55–5.51 at the PANSS negative subscale), but no significant effects of treatment were found in tests for cognitive function. The meta-analysis of Sommer et al. (144) identified four RCT studies with $n = 182$ patients given minocycline, and $n = 166$ on placebo, the effects on cognition were not reported, but no significant effects on overall symptom severity were identified.

Additional drugs with anti-inflammatory action as add-on treatments for patients with schizophrenia

The meta-analysis by Sommer et al. (144) also investigated the effect of additional anti-inflammatory treatments. The outcome measure was the mean change in PANSS (155) or the Brief Psychiatric Rating Scale (156), and significant improvements of treatment with *n*-acetylcysteine ($n = 140$), aspirin ($n = 270$), and estrogens ($n = 262$) were identified, while studies with davunetide and PUFAs (eicosapentanoic acid and docosahexanoic acids) did not show significant effects.

SUMMING UP PRO-COGNITIVE EFFECTS OF IMMUNOMODULATING/ANTI-INFLAMMATORY DRUG TREATMENT FOR PATIENTS WITH SCHIZOPHRENIA: CRITICAL METHODOLOGICAL PROBLEMS REMAIN

The involvement of inflammatory/immunological factors in the pathophysiology of a large portion of patients with schizophrenia is well established through different lines of research, and data point to several links between these factors and cognitive dysfunction. Presently, many drugs with anti-inflammatory or immunomodulatory action have been tested (as add-on to antipsychotic treatment) for patients with schizophrenia, and while some have shown positive effects for global schizophrenia symptoms, the effects on cognition were not possible to assess in the recent meta-analysis by Sommer et al. (144), as only 5 of 26 included studies reported data on cognitive tests and the heterogeneity of the cognitive tasks made it impossible to quantitatively review the effects. Furthermore, as highlighted by Sommer et al. the drugs tested that were shown to improve the symptoms of schizophrenia (*N*-acetylcysteine, estrogens, aspirin) have broad mechanisms of action, and it is not at all demonstrated that the improved symptoms are caused by anti-inflammatory actions. A further critical question to address in future drug research will be to establish reliable brain imaging methods to quantitatively assess neuroinflammation, as the levels of peripheral cytokines are only an indirect measure of brain neuroinflammation. PET studies with new ligands that specifically target activated microglia and the "free-water" MRI scanning seem promising, but extensive development remains before these methods are ready as outcome measures in drug discovery studies.

SUMMARY AND CONVERGENCE

At present, pharmacological treatment of schizophrenia relies on antipsychotic drugs, which predominantly relieve positive psychotic symptoms and have little effect on the cognitive dysfunctions restricting the functional level of patients. However, recent developments in brain imaging, including novel specific PET ligands and MRI paradigms specifically investigating myelin integrity, neurotransmitter levels, and neuroinflammation, facilitate the unraveling of mechanisms underlying cognitive dysfunction in schizophrenia. Accumulating evidence supports a combined model including all these areas of pathology underlying the cognitive deficits in schizophrenia, schematically exemplified by **Figure 2** for the interplay between prefrontal cortex, striatum, and brain stem. This joint model represents several potential pro-cognitive drug targets at the level of neurotransmitters, lipids, and inflammatory markers, however, no current drugs aimed at these targets are so far definitely proven to be clinically useful as pro-cognitive drugs for patients with schizophrenia. Studies concerning immunomodulatory drugs, including EPO, minocycline, celecoxib, aspirin, estrogens, *n*-acetylcysteine have shown promising results in single studies, but have not yielded straightforward support for the use in clinical practice to enhance cognition.

FUTURE PERSPECTIVES

Drugs that would reduce brain levels of KYNA (e.g., KAT inhibitors) are expected to improve cognitive dysfunctions in schizophrenia based on animal studies, but remain to be developed for clinical use. The possibility of pro-cognitive effects of drugs that have been used to treat other medical conditions for years, e.g., EPO, minocycline, and aspirin is attractive, also because the safety profile of many of these drugs are well known in neurological patients populations, reducing the costs of introducing the drugs as cognitive enhancers for schizophrenia patients. Several critical questions currently constraining progress remain to be solved, however. Firstly, uniformly accepted and standardized cognitive assessments for repeated measures must be agreed on for pro-cognitive drug studies in schizophrenia patients. Secondly, the refinement of brain imaging methods unto sufficient reliability and specificity (e.g., measuring neuroinflammation and myelin integrity) for use as outcome measures in pro-cognitive drug is essential for studies of putative cognition enhancers in humans. Thirdly, and at least of prominent importance in the field of further developments of pro-cognitive glutamatergic substances are the problems of translating findings in animal studies to human drug treatment.

However, even though the process of developing novel pharmacological agents is highly sophisticated, identifying novel treatment targets through thorough clinical and preclinical studies remains pivotal in the continued search for improved treatment of schizophrenia. The convergence of a disordered inflammatory system, disturbances in myelination/oligodendrocyte function,

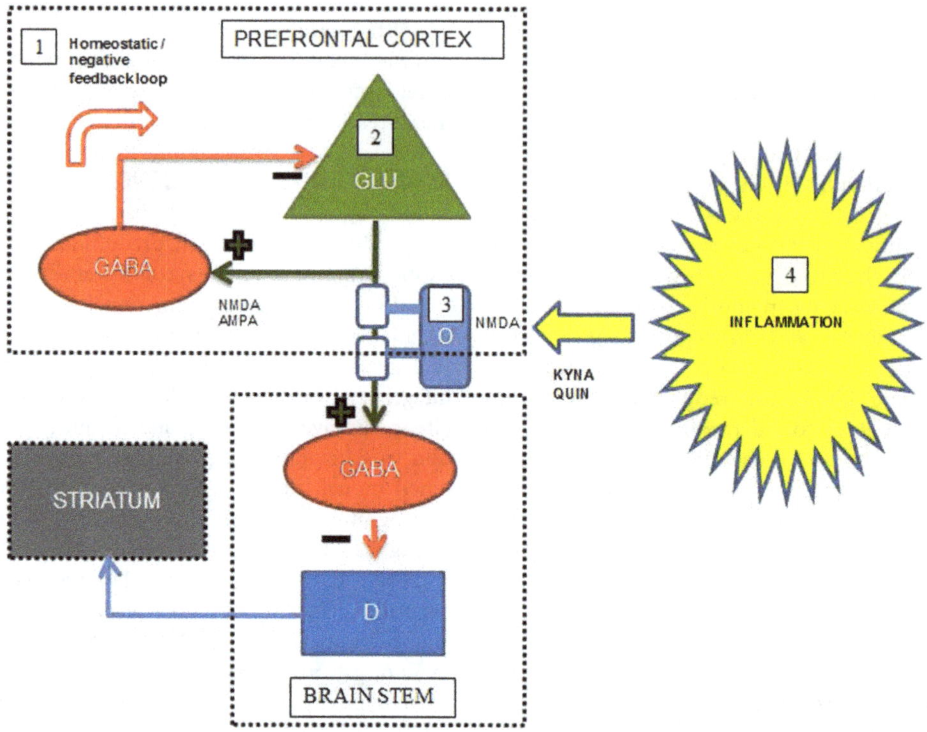

FIGURE 2 | Simplified putative interplay between selected neurotransmitters, oligodendrocytes, and inflammation in the pathology of cognitive dysfunctions in schizophrenia. Green cell = excitatory pyramidal glutamatergic (GLU) neuron; red cell = inhibitory GABAergic (GABA) interneuron; blue cell = modulatory dopaminergic (D) neuron; light blue cell = oligodendrocyte (O) with white myelin sheets enclosing the pyramidal cell axon; KYNA = kynurenic acid, QUIN = quinolinic acid. The figure displays some putative points of convergence between neurotransmitters, myelin, and neuroinflammation relevant to the cognitive dysfunctions of schizophrenia. Details are elaborated in the text. (1) In the prefrontal cortex, abnormal NMDA functioning on, and/or deficient GABA release and reuptake in a subset of GABAergic interneurons result in deficient negative feedback on pyramidal glutamatergic neurons, which may lead to glutamatergic hyperactivity, excitotoxicity, and disruption of coordinated firing of pyramidal cells. (2) Deficient glutamatergic neuronal activity leads to decreased excitatory input on GABAergic interneurons terminating on dopaminergic projections to striatum, leading to striatal hyperdopaminergia. The hyperdopaminergia may inversely influence cognitive functions located in the prefrontal cortex. (3) Reduced myelin integrity may inversely influence glutamatergic signaling leading to the same consequences as in the point above. Oligodendrocytes express NMDA receptors and are thus vulnerable for excitotoxicity from excess glutamate and QUIN. (4) During inflammation QUIN is produced in microglia and KYNA in astrocytes. QUIN is an NMDA agonist and potentially excitotoxic, while KYNA is an NMDA antagonist that could induce cognitive dysfunctions consistent with the NMDA receptor hypofunction hypothesis of schizophrenia. Adapted with permission from Lisman et al. (72) and Takahashi et al. (102).

and transmitter dysfunctions in schizophrenia open new paths for pro-cognitive drug discovery with putative large functional improvements to be achieved for patients with schizophrenia.

ACKNOWLEDGMENTS

Parts of the research were funded by grants to Erik Johnsen from the Research Council of Norway, project no. 213727, and several grants from Helse Vest. Parts of the research were funded by an ERC Advanced Grant and by the NORMENT SFF from the Research Council of Norway to Kenneth Hugdahl and Silje Skrede.

REFERENCES

1. Tandon R, Nasrallah HA, Keshavan MS. Schizophrenia, "just the facts" 4. Clinical features and conceptualization. *Schizophr Res* (2009) **110**:1–23. doi:10.1016/j.schres.2009.03.005
2. World Health Organization. *The World Health Report 2001 – Mental Health: New Understanding, New Hope*. Geneva: WHO (2001).
3. Ustun TB, Rehm J, Chatterji S, Saxena S, Trotter R, Room R, et al. Multiple-informant ranking of the disabling effects of different health conditions in 14 countries. WHO/NIH Joint Project CAR Study Group. *Lancet* (1999) **354**:111–5. doi:10.1016/S0140-6736(98)07507-2
4. Tandon R. Antipsychotics in the treatment of schizophrenia: an overview. *J Clin Psychiatry* (2011) **72**(Suppl 1):4–8. doi:10.4088/JCP.10075su1.01
5. Miyamoto S, Miyake N, Jarskog LF, Fleischhacker WW, Lieberman JA. Pharmacological treatment of schizophrenia: a critical review of the pharmacology and clinical effects of current and future therapeutic agents. *Mol Psychiatry* (2012) **17**(12):1206–27. doi:10.1038/mp.2012.47
6. Shen WW. A history of antipsychotic drug development. *Compr Psychiatry* (1999) **40**:407–14. doi:10.1016/S0010-440X(99)90082-2
7. Leucht S, Cipriani A, Spineli L, Mavridis D, Orey D, Richter F, et al. Comparative efficacy and tolerability of 15 antipsychotic drugs in schizophrenia: a multiple-treatments meta-analysis. *Lancet* (2013) **382**(9896):951. doi:10.1016/S0140-6736(13)60733-3
8. Meltzer HY. Update on typical and atypical antipsychotic drugs. *Annu Rev Med* (2012) **64**:393–406. doi:10.1146/annurev-med-050911-161504
9. Meltzer HY, Massey BW. The role of serotonin receptors in the action of atypical antipsychotic drugs. *Curr Opin Pharmacol* (2011) **11**:59–67. doi:10.1016/j.coph.2011.02.007

10. Meltzer HY, Matsubara S, Lee JC. Classification of typical and atypical antipsychotic drugs on the basis of dopamine D-1, D-2 and serotonin2 pKi values. *J Pharmacol Exp Ther* (1989) **251**:238–46.
11. Kantrowitz JT, Javitt DC. N-methyl-d-aspartate (NMDA) receptor dysfunction or dysregulation: the final common pathway on the road to schizophrenia? *Brain Res Bull* (2010) **83**:108–21. doi:10.1016/j.brainresbull.2010.04.006
12. Gray JA, Roth BL. The pipeline and future of drug development in schizophrenia. *Mol Psychiatry* (2007) **12**:904–22. doi:10.1038/sj.mp.4002062
13. Gray JA, Roth BL. Molecular targets for treating cognitive dysfunction in schizophrenia. *Schizophr Bull* (2007) **33**:1100–19. doi:10.1093/schbul/sbm074
14. Demjaha A, Egerton A, Murray RM, Kapur S, Howes OD, Stone JM, et al. Antipsychotic treatment resistance in schizophrenia associated with elevated glutamate levels but normal dopamine function. *Biol Psychiatry* (2013). doi:10.1016/j.biopsych.2013.06.011
15. Green MF. What are the functional consequences of neurocognitive deficits in schizophrenia? *Am J Psychiatry* (1996) **153**:321–30.
16. Palmer BW, Dawes SE, Heaton RK. What do we know about neuropsychological aspects of schizophrenia? *Neuropsychol Rev* (2009) **19**:365–84. doi:10.1007/s11065-009-9109-y
17. Chou H-H, Twamley E, Swerdlow N. Towards medication-enhancement of cognitive interventions in schizophrenia. In: Geyer MA, Gross G, editors. *Novel Antischizophrenia Treatments.* Berlin: Springer (2012). p. 81–111.
18. Lameh J, McFarland K, Ohlsson J, Ek F, Piu F, Burstein E, et al. Discovery of potential antipsychotic agents possessing pro-cognitive properties. *Naunyn Schmiedebergs Arch Pharmacol* (2012) **385**:313–23. doi:10.1007/s00210-011-0702-2
19. Insel TR, Voon V, Nye JS, Brown VJ, Altevogt BM, Bullmore ET, et al. Innovative solutions to novel drug development in mental health. *Neurosci Biobehav Rev* (2013) **37**(10 Pt 1):2438–44. doi:10.1016/j.neubiorev.2013.03.022
20. Williams M. Productivity shortfalls in drug discovery: contributions from the preclinical sciences? *J Pharmacol Exp Ther* (2011) **336**:3–8. doi:10.1124/jpet.110.171751
21. Marek GJ, Behl B, Bespalov AY, Gross G, Lee Y, Schoemaker H. Glutamatergic (N-methyl-d-aspartate receptor) hypofrontality in schizophrenia: too little juice or a miswired brain? *Mol Pharmacol* (2010) **77**:317–26. doi:10.1124/mol.109.059865
22. Takahashi N, Sakurai T, Davis KL, Buxbaum JD. Linking oligodendrocyte and myelin dysfunction to neurocircuitry abnormalities in schizophrenia. *Prog Neurobiol* (2011) **93**:13–24. doi:10.1016/j.pneurobio.2010.09.004
23. Anderson G, Berk M, Dodd S, Bechter K, Altamura AC, Dell'Osso B, et al. Immuno-inflammatory, oxidative and nitrosative stress, and neuroprogressive pathways in the etiology, course and treatment of schizophrenia. *Prog Neuropsychopharmacol Biol Psychiatry* (2013) **42**:1–4. doi:10.1016/j.pnpbp.2012.07.016
24. Millan MJ, Agid Y, Brüne M, Bullmore ET, Carter CS, Clayton NS, et al. Cognitive dysfunction in psychiatric disorders: characteristics, causes and the quest for improved therapy. *Nat Rev Drug Discov* (2012) **11**:141–68. doi:10.1038/nrd3628
25. Kahn RS, Keefe RE. Schizophrenia is a cognitive illness: time for a change in focus. *JAMA Psychiatry* (2013) **70**(10):1107–12. doi:10.1001/jamapsychiatry.2013.155
26. Weinberger DR. From neuropathology to neurodevelopment. *Lancet* (1995) **346**:552–7. doi:10.1016/S0140-6736(95)91386-6
27. Caspi A, Reichenberg A, Weiser M, Rabinowitz J, Kaplan Z, Knobler H, et al. Cognitive performance in schizophrenia patients assessed before and following the first psychotic episode. *Schizophr Res* (2003) **65**:87–94. doi:10.1016/S0920-9964(03)00056-2
28. Gschwandtner U, Aston J, Borgwardt S, Drewe M, Feinendegen C, Lacher D, et al. Neuropsychological and neurophysiological findings in individuals suspected to be at risk for schizophrenia: preliminary results from the Basel early detection of psychosis study – Fruherkennung von Psychosen (FEPSY). *Acta Psychiatr Scand* (2003) **108**:152–5. doi:10.1034/j.1600-0447.2003.00157.x
29. Heaton RK, Gladsjo J, Palmer BW, Kuck J, Marcotte TD, Jeste DV. Stability and course of neuropsychological deficits in schizophrenia. *Arch Gen Psychiatry* (2001) **58**:24–32. doi:10.1001/archpsyc.58.1.24
30. Rund BR. A review of longitudinal studies of cognitive functions in schizophrenia patients. *Schizophr Bull* (1998) **24**:425–35. doi:10.1093/oxfordjournals.schbul.a033337
31. Nuechterlein KH, Barch DM, Gold JM, Goldberg TE, Green MF, Heaton RK. Identification of separable cognitive factors in schizophrenia. *Schizophr Res* (2004) **72**:29–39. doi:10.1016/j.schres.2004.09.007
32. Dickinson D, Ramsey ME, Gold JM. Overlooking the obvious: a meta-analytic comparison of digit symbol coding tasks and other cognitive measures in schizophrenia. *Arch Gen Psychiatry* (2007) **64**:532–42. doi:10.1001/archpsyc.64.5.532
33. Heinrichs R, Zakzanis K. Neurocognitive deficit in schizophrenia: a quantitative review of the evidence. *Neuropsychology* (1998) **12**:426–45. doi:10.1037/0894-4105.12.3.426
34. Wilk CM, Gold JM, Bartko JJ, Dickerson F, Fenton WS, Knable M, et al. Test-retest stability of the repeatable battery for the assessment of neuropsychological status in schizophrenia. *Am J Psychiatry* (2002) **159**:838–44. doi:10.1176/appi.ajp.159.5.838
35. Wilk CM, Gold JM, Humber K, Dickerson F, Fenton WS, Buchanan RW. Brief cognitive assessment in schizophrenia: normative data for the repeatable battery for the assessment of neuropsychological status. *Schizophr Res* (2004) **70**:175–86. doi:10.1016/j.schres.2003.10.009
36. Gold MJ, Queern C, Iannone VN, Buchanan RW. Repeatable battery for the assessment of neuropsychological status as a screening test in schizophrenia I: sensitivity, reliability, and validity. *Am J Psychiatry* (1999) **156**:1944–50.
37. Keefe RS. Should cognitive impairment be included in the diagnostic criteria for schizophrenia? *World Psychiatry* (2008) **7**:22–8. doi:10.1002/j.2051-5545.2008.tb00142.x
38. Green MF, Kern RS, Braff DL, Mintz J. Neurocognitive deficits and functional outcome in schizophrenia: are we measuring the "right stuff"? *Schizophr Bull* (2000) **26**:119–36. doi:10.1093/oxfordjournals.schbul.a033430
39. Kaneda Y, Jayathilak K, Meltzer HY. Determinants of work outcome in schizophrenia and schizoaffective disorder: role of cognitive function. *Psychiatry Res* (2009) **169**:178–9. doi:10.1016/j.psychres.2008.08.003
40. Laes JR, Sponheim SR. Does cognition predict community function only in schizophrenia? A study of schizophrenia patients, bipolar affective disorder patients, and community control subjects. *Schizophr Res* (2006) **84**:121–31. doi:10.1016/j.schres.2005.11.023
41. Tsang HW, Leung AY, Chung RC, Bell M, Cheung WM. Review on vocational predictors: a systematic review of predictors of vocational outcomes among individuals with schizophrenia: an update since 1998. *Aust N Z J Psychiatry* (2010) **44**:495–504. doi:10.3109/00048671003785716
42. McClure MM, Bowie CR, Patterson TL, Heaton RK, Weaver C, Anderson H, et al. Correlations of functional capacity and neuropsychological performance in older patients with schizophrenia: evidence for specificity of relationships? *Schizophr Res* (2007) **89**:330–8. doi:10.1016/j.schres.2006.07.024
43. Nuechterlein K, Green M, Kern R, Baade L, Barch D, Cohen J, et al. The MATRICS consensus cognitive battery, part 1: test selection, reliability, and validity. *Am J Psychiatry* (2008) **165**:203–13. doi:10.1176/appi.ajp.2007.07010042
44. Keefe RS, Fox KH, Harvey PD, Cucchiaro J, Siu C, Loebel A. Characteristics of the MATRICS consensus cognitive battery in a 29-site antipsychotic schizophrenia clinical trial. *Schizophr Res* (2011) **125**:161–8. doi:10.1016/j.schres.2010.09.015
45. Burton CZ, Vella L, Harvey PD, Patterson TL, Heaton RK, Twamley EW. Factor structure of the MATRICS consensus cognitive battery (MCCB) in schizophrenia. *Schizophr Res* (2013) **146**:244–8. doi:10.1016/j.schres.2013.02.026
46. Fields RD. White matter in learning, cognition and psychiatric disorders. *Trends Neurosci* (2008) **31**:361–70. doi:10.1016/j.tins.2008.04.001
47. Puri BK. Progressive structural brain changes in schizophrenia. *Expert Rev Neurother* (2010) **10**:33–42. doi:10.1586/ern.09.142
48. Ellison-Wright I, Bullmore E. Meta-analysis of diffusion tensor imaging studies in schizophrenia. *Schizophr Res* (2009) **108**:3–10. doi:10.1016/j.schres.2008.11.021
49. Walterfang M, Wood SJ, Velakoulis D, Pantelis C. Neuropathological, neurogenetic and neuroimaging evidence for white matter pathology in schizophrenia. *Neurosci Biobehav Rev* (2006) **30**:918–48. doi:10.1016/j.neubiorev.2006.02.001
50. Rigucci S, Rossi-Espagnet C, Ferracuti S, De Carolis A, Corigliano V, Carducci F, et al. Comparelli, anatomical substrates of cognitive and clinical dimensions in first episode schizophrenia. *Acta Psychiatr Scand* (2012) **128**:261–70. doi:10.1111/acps.12051

51. Nazeri A, Mallar Chakravarty M, Felsky D, Lobaugh NJ, Rajji TK, Mulsant BH, et al. Alterations of superficial white matter in schizophrenia and relationship to cognitive performance. *Neuropsychopharmacology* (2013) **38**:1954–62. doi:10.1038/npp.2013.93
52. Ruiz S, Birbaumer N, Sitaram R. Abnormal neural connectivity in schizophrenia and fMRI-brain-computer interface as a potential therapeutic approach. *Front Psychiatry* (2013) **4**:17. doi:10.3389/fpsyt.2013.00017
53. Fornito A, Zalesky A, Pantelis C, Bullmore ET. Schizophrenia, neuroimaging and connectomics. *Neuroimage* (2012) **62**:2296–314. doi:10.1016/j.neuroimage.2011.12.090
54. Pettersson-Yeo W, Allen P, Benetti S, McGuire P, Mechelli A. Dysconnectivity in schizophrenia: where are we now? *Neurosci Biobehav Rev* (2011) **35**:1110–24. doi:10.1016/j.neubiorev.2010.11.004
55. Hugdahl K, Loberg EM, Nygard M. Left temporal lobe structural and functional abnormality underlying auditory hallucinations in schizophrenia. *Front Neurosci* (2009) **3**:34–45. doi:10.3389/neuro.01.001.2009
56. Raichle M. Two views of brain function. *Trends Cogn Sci* (2010) **14**:180–90. doi:10.1016/j.tics.2010.01.008
57. Hugdahl K, Løberg E-M, Nygård M. Left temporal lobe structural and functional abnormality underlying auditory hallucinations. *Front Neurosci* (2009) **3**(1):34–45. doi:10.3389/neuro.01.001.2009
58. Hugdahl K, Rund B, Lund A, Asbjørnsen A, Egeland J, Landrø N, et al. Brain activation measured with fMRI during a mental arithmetic task in schizophrenia and major depression. *Am J Psychiatry* (2004) **161**(2):286–93. doi:10.1176/appi.ajp.161.2.286
59. Alexander A, Lee J, Lazar M, Field A. Diffusion tensor imaging of the brain. *Neurotherapeutics* (2007) **4**:316–29. doi:10.1016/j.nurt.2007.05.011
60. Ongur D, Du F. Probing myelin and axon abnormalities separately in psychiatric disorders using MRI techniques. *Front Integr Neurosci* (2013) **7**:24. doi:10.3389/fnint.2013.00024
61. Kimoto S, Okuda A, Toritsuka M, Yamauchi T, Makinodan M, Okuda H, et al. Olanzapine stimulates proliferation but inhibits differentiation in rat oligodendrocyte precursor cell cultures. *Prog Neuropsychopharmacol Biol Psychiatry* (2011) **35**:1950–6. doi:10.1016/j.pnpbp.2011.07.011
62. van den Heuvel MP, Mandl RC, Stam CJ, Kahn RS, Hulshoff Pol HE. Aberrant frontal and temporal complex network structure in schizophrenia: a graph theoretical analysis. *J Neurosci* (2010) **30**:15915–26. doi:10.1523/JNEUROSCI.2874-10.2010
63. van den Heuvel MP, Sporns O, Collin G, Scheewe T, Mandl RC, Cahn W, et al. Abnormal rich club organization and functional brain dynamics in schizophrenia. *JAMA Psychiatry* (2013) **70**:783–92. doi:10.1001/jamapsychiatry.2013.1328
64. Bartzokis G, Lu PH, Raven EP, Amar CP, Detore NR, Couvrette AJ, et al. Impact on intracortical myelination trajectory of long acting injection versus oral risperidone in first-episode schizophrenia. *Schizophr Res* (2012) **140**:122–8. doi:10.1016/j.schres.2012.06.036
65. Bartzokis G. Neuroglialpharmacology: myelination as a shared mechanism of action of psychotropic treatments. *Neuropharmacology* (2012) **62**:2137–53. doi:10.1016/j.neuropharm.2012.01.015
66. Catts VS, Fung SJ, Long LE, Joshi D, Vercammen A, Allen KM, et al. Rethinking schizophrenia in the context of normal neurodevelopment. *Front Cell Neurosci* (2013) **7**:60. doi:10.3389/fncel.2013.00060
67. Fields RC, Aft RL, Gillanders WE, Eberlein TJ, Margenthaler JA. Treatment and outcomes of patients with primary breast sarcoma. *Am J Surg* (2008) **196**:559–61. doi:10.1016/j.amjsurg.2008.06.010
68. Walterfang M, Velakoulis D, Whitford TJ, Pantelis C. Understanding aberrant white matter development in schizophrenia: an avenue for therapy? *Expert Rev Neurother* (2011) **11**:971–87. doi:10.1586/ern.11.76
69. Howes OD, Kapur S. The dopamine hypothesis of schizophrenia: version III – the final common pathway. *Schizophr Bull* (2009) **35**:549–62. doi:10.1093/schbul/sbp006
70. Howes OD, Kambeitz J, Kim E, Stahl D, Slifstein M, Abi-Dargham A, et al. The nature of dopamine dysfunction in schizophrenia and what this means for treatment. *Arch Gen Psychiatry* (2012) **69**:776–86. doi:10.1001/archgenpsychiatry.2012.169
71. Snyder MA, Gao WJ. NMDA hypofunction as a convergence point for progression and symptoms of schizophrenia. *Front Cell Neurosci* (2013) **7**:31. doi:10.3389/fncel.2013.00031
72. Gilmour G, Dix S, Fellini L, Gastambide F, Plath N, Steckler T, et al. NMDA receptors, cognition and schizophrenia – testing the validity of the NMDA receptor hypofunction hypothesis. *Neuropharmacology* (2012) **62**:1401–12. doi:10.1016/j.neuropharm.2011.03.015
73. Javitt DC. Glutamate as a therapeutic target in psychiatric disorders. *Mol Psychiatry* (2004) **9**:984–97, 979. doi:10.1038/sj.mp.4001602
74. Zhou Q, Sheng M. NMDA receptors in nervous system diseases. *Neuropharmacology* (2013) **74**:69–75. doi:10.1016/j.neuropharm.2013.03.030
75. Theberge J, Bartha R, Drost DJ, Menon RS, Malla A, Takhar J, et al. Glutamate and glutamine measured with 4.0 T proton MRS in never-treated patients with schizophrenia and healthy volunteers. *Am J Psychiatry* (2002) **159**:1944–6. doi:10.1176/appi.ajp.159.11.1944
76. Olbrich HM, Valerius G, Rusch N, Buchert M, Thiel T, Hennig J, et al. Frontolimbic glutamate alterations in first episode schizophrenia: evidence from a magnetic resonance spectroscopy study. *World J Biol Psychiatry* (2008) **9**:59–63. doi:10.1080/15622970701227811
77. Ota M, Ishikawa M, Sato N, Hori H, Sasayama D, Hattori K, et al. Glutamatergic changes in the cerebral white matter associated with schizophrenic exacerbation. *Acta Psychiatr Scand* (2012) **126**:72–8. doi:10.1111/j.1600-0447.2012.01853.x
78. Schwartz TL, Sachdeva S, Stahl SM. Glutamate neurocircuitry: theoretical underpinnings in schizophrenia. *Front Pharmacol* (2012) **3**:195. doi:10.3389/fphar.2012.00195
79. Xiao L, Xu H, Zhang Y, Wei Z, He J, Jiang W, et al. Quetiapine facilitates oligodendrocyte development and prevents mice from myelin breakdown and behavioral changes. *Mol Psychiatry* (2008) **13**:697–708. doi:10.1038/sj.mp.4002064
80. Zhang Y, Xu H, Jiang W, Xiao L, Yan B, He J, et al. Quetiapine alleviates the cuprizone-induced white matter pathology in the brain of C57BL/6 mouse. *Schizophr Res* (2008) **106**:182–91. doi:10.1016/j.schres.2008.09.013
81. Garver DL, Holcomb JA, Christensen JD. Compromised myelin integrity during psychosis with repair during remission in drug-responding schizophrenia. *Int J Neuropsychopharmacol* (2008) **11**:49–61. doi:10.1017/S1461145707007730
82. Bartzokis G, Lu PH, Stewart SB, Oluwadara B, Lucas AJ, Pantages J, et al. In vivo evidence of differential impact of typical and atypical antipsychotics on intracortical myelin in adults with schizophrenia. *Schizophr Res* (2009) **113**:322–31. doi:10.1016/j.schres.2009.06.014
83. Ferno J, Raeder MB, Vik-Mo AO, Skrede S, Glambek M, Tronstad KJ, et al. Antipsychotic drugs activate SREBP-regulated expression of lipid biosynthetic genes in cultured human glioma cells: a novel mechanism of action? *Pharmacogenomics J* (2005) **5**:298–304. doi:10.1038/sj.tpj.6500323
84. Ferno J, Skrede S, Vik-Mo A, Havik B, Steen V. Drug-induced activation of SREBP-controlled lipogenic gene expression in CNS-related cell lines: marked differences between various antipsychotic drugs. *BMC Neurosci* (2006) **7**:69. doi:10.1186/1471-2202-7-69
85. Skrede S, Fernø J, Vázquez MJ, Fjær S, Pavlin T, Lunder N, et al. Olanzapine, but not aripiprazole, weight-independently elevates serum triglycerides and activates lipogenic gene expression in female rats. *Int J Neuropsychopharmacol* (2012) **15**:163–79. doi:10.1017/S1461145711001271
86. Leucht S, Cipriani A, Spineli L, Mavridis D, Örey D, Richter F, et al. Comparative efficacy and tolerability of 15 antipsychotic drugs in schizophrenia: a multiple-treatments meta-analysis. *Lancet* (2013) **382**:951–62. doi:10.1016/S0140-6736(13)60733-3
87. Procyshyn RM, Wasan KM, Thornton AE, Barr AM, Chen EY, Pomarol-Clotet E, et al. Changes in serum lipids, independent of weight, are associated with changes in symptoms during long-term clozapine treatment. *J Psychiatry Neurosci* (2007) **32**:331–8.
88. Lally J, Gallagher A, Bainbridge E, Avalos G, Ahmed M, McDonald C. Increases in triglyceride levels are associated with clinical response to clozapine treatment. *J Psychopharmacol* (2013) **27**:401–3. doi:10.1177/0269881112472568
89. Amminger GP, Schafer MR, Papageorgiou K, Klier CM, Cotton SM, Harrigan SM, et al. Long-chain omega-3 fatty acids for indicated prevention of psychotic disorders: a randomized, placebo-controlled trial. *Arch Gen Psychiatry* (2010) **67**:146–54. doi:10.1001/archgenpsychiatry.2009.192
90. Peters BD, Machielsen MW, Hoen WP, Caan MW, Malhotra AK, Szeszko PR, et al. Polyunsaturated fatty acid concentration predicts myelin integrity in

early-phase psychosis. *Schizophr Bull* (2013) **39**:830–8. doi:10.1093/schbul/sbs089
91. Kaddurah-Daouk R, McEvoy J, Baillie RA, Lee D, Yao JK, Doraiswamy PM, et al. Metabolomic mapping of atypical antipsychotic effects in schizophrenia. *Mol Psychiatry* (2007) **12**:934–45. doi:10.1038/sj.mp.4002000
92. Yao J, Keshavan M. Antioxidants, redox signaling, and pathophysiology in schizophrenia: an integrative view. *Antioxid Redox Signal* (2011) **15**:2011–35. doi:10.1089/ars.2010.3603
93. Zhang XY, Chen DC, Xiu MH, Tang W, Zhang F, Liu L, et al. Plasma total antioxidant status and cognitive impairments in schizophrenia. *Schizophr Res* (2012) **139**:66–72. doi:10.1016/j.schres.2012.04.009
94. Meyer U, Schwarz MJ, Muller N. Inflammatory processes in schizophrenia: a promising neuroimmunological target for the treatment of negative/cognitive symptoms and beyond. *Pharmacol Ther* (2011) **132**:96–110. doi:10.1016/j.pharmthera.2011.06.003
95. Doorduin J, de Vries EF, Willemsen AT, de Groot JC, Dierckx RA, Klein HC. Neuroinflammation in schizophrenia-related psychosis: a PET study. *J Nucl Med* (2009) **50**:1801–7. doi:10.2967/jnumed.109.066647
96. Ripke S, Sanders A, Kendler K, Levinson D, Sklar P, Holmans P, et al. Genome-wide association study identifies five new schizophrenia loci. *Nat Genet* (2011) **43**:969–76. doi:10.1038/ng.940
97. Debnath M, Cannon DM, Venkatasubramanian G. Variation in the major histocompatibility complex [MHC] gene family in schizophrenia: associations and functional implications. *Prog Neuropsychopharmacol Biol Psychiatry* (2013) **42**:49–62. doi:10.1016/j.pnpbp.2012.07.009
98. Pickard B. Progress in defining the biological causes of schizophrenia. *Expert Rev Mol Med* (2011) **13**:e25. doi:10.1017/S1462399411001955
99. Sequeira PA, Martin MV, Vawter MP. The first decade and beyond of transcriptional profiling in schizophrenia. *Neurobiol Dis* (2012) **45**:23–36. doi:10.1016/j.nbd.2011.03.001
100. Kayser M, Dalmau J. The emerging link between autoimmune disorders and neuropsychiatric disease. *J Neuropsychiatry Clin Neurosci* (2011) **23**:90–97. doi:10.1176/appi.neuropsych.23.1.90
101. Dalmau J, Gleichman AJ, Hughes EG, Rossi JE, Peng X, Lai M, et al. Anti-NMDA-receptor encephalitis: case series and analysis of the effects of antibodies. *Lancet Neurol* (2008) **7**:1091–8. doi:10.1016/S1474-4422(08)70224-2
102. American College of Rheumatology. The American College of Rheumatology nomenclature and case definitions for neuropsychiatric lupus syndromes. *Arthritis Rheum* (1999) **42**:599–608. doi:10.1002/1529-0131(199904)42:4<599::AID-ANR2>3.0.CO;2-F
103. Noto C, Gadelha A, Belangero SI, Spindola LM, Rocha NP, de Miranda AS, et al. Circulating levels of sTNFR1 as a marker of severe clinical course in schizophrenia. *J Psychiatr Res* (2013) **47**:467–71. doi:10.1016/j.jpsychires.2012.12.010
104. Dean B. Understanding the role of inflammatory-related pathways in the pathophysiology and treatment of psychiatric disorders: evidence from human peripheral studies and CNS studies. *Int J Neuropsychopharmacol* (2011) **14**:997–1012. doi:10.1017/S1461145710001410
105. Meyer U. Anti-inflammatory signaling in schizophrenia. *Brain Behav Immun* (2011) **25**:1507–18. doi:10.1016/j.bbi.2011.05.014
106. Miller B, Buckley P, Seabolt W, Mellor A, Kirkpatrick B. Meta-analysis of cytokine alterations in schizophrenia: clinical status and antipsychotic effects. *Biol Psychiatry* (2011) **70**:663–671. doi:10.1016/j.biopsych.2011.04.013
107. Fineberg AM, Ellman LM. Inflammatory cytokines and neurological and neurocognitive alterations in the course of schizophrenia. *Biol Psychiatry* (2013) **73**:951–66. doi:10.1016/j.biopsych.2013.01.001
108. Drexhage RC, Knijff EM, Padmos RC, Heul-Nieuwenhuijzen LV, Beumer W, Versnel MA, et al. The mononuclear phagocyte system and its cytokine inflammatory networks in schizophrenia and bipolar disorder. *Expert Rev Neurother* (2009) **10**:59–76. doi:10.1586/ern.09.144
109. Hope S, Melle I, Aukrust P, Steen NE, Birkenaes AB, Lorentzen S, et al. Similar immune profile in bipolar disorder and schizophrenia: selective increase in soluble tumor necrosis factor receptor I and von Willebrand factor. *Bipolar Disord* (2009) **11**:726–34. doi:10.1111/j.1399-5618.2009.00757.x
110. Potvin S, Stip E, Sepehry A, Gendron A, Bah R, Kouassi E. Inflammatory cytokine alterations in schizophrenia: a systematic quantitative review. *Biol Psychiatry* (2008) **63**:801–808. doi:10.1016/j.biopsych.2007.09.024
111. Anthony DC, Pitossi FJ. Special issue commentary: the changing face of inflammation in the brain. *Mol Cell Neurosci* (2013) **53**:1–5. doi:10.1016/j.mcn.2012.11.005
112. Beumer W, Gibney SM, Drexhage RC, Pont-Lezica L, Doorduin J, Klein HC, et al. The immune theory of psychiatric diseases: a key role for activated microglia and circulating monocytes. *J Leukoc Biol* (2012) **92**:959–75. doi:10.1189/jlb.0212100
113. van Berckel BN, Bossong MG, Boellaard R, Kloet R, Schuitemaker A, Caspers E, et al. Microglia activation in recent-onset schizophrenia: a quantitative (R)-[11C]PK11195 Positron Emission Tomography Study. *Biol Psychiatry* (2008) **64**:820–2. doi:10.1016/j.biopsych.2008.04.025
114. Pasternak O, Sochen N, Gur Y, Intrator N, Assaf Y. Free water elimination and mapping from diffusion MRI. *Magn Reson Med* (2009) **62**:717–30. doi:10.1002/mrm.22055
115. Pasternak O, Westin C, Bouix S, Seidman L, Goldstein J, Woo T, et al. Excessive extracellular volume reveals a neurodegenerative pattern in schizophrenia onset. *J Neurosci* (2012) **32**(48):17365–72. doi:10.1523/JNEUROSCI.2904-12.2012
116. Steiner J, Bogerts B, Sarnyai Z, Walter M, Gos T, Bernstein H-G, et al. Bridging the gap between the immune and glutamate hypotheses of schizophrenia and major depression: potential role of glial NMDA receptor modulators and impaired blood-brain barrier integrity. *World J Biol Psychiatry* (2012) **13**:482–92. doi:10.3109/15622975.2011.583941
117. Erhardt S, Blennow K, Nordin C, Skogh E, Lindström LH, Engberg G. Kynurenic acid levels are elevated in the cerebrospinal fluid of patients with schizophrenia. *Neurosci Lett* (2001) **313**:96–8. doi:10.1016/S0304-3940(01)02242-X
118. Schwarcz R, Rassoulpour A, Wu H-Q, Medoff D, Tamminga CA, Roberts RC. Increased cortical kynurenate content in schizophrenia. *Biol Psychiatry* (2001) **50**:521–30. doi:10.1016/S0006-3223(01)01078-2
119. Schwarcz R, Bruno JP, Muchowski PJ, Wu H-Q. Kynurenines in the mammalian brain: when physiology meets pathology. *Nat Rev Neurosci* (2012) **13**:465–77. doi:10.1038/nrn3257
120. Erhardt S, Schwieler L, Emanuelsson C, Geyer M. Endogenous kynurenic acid disrupts prepulse inhibition. *Biol Psychiatry* (2004) **56**:255–60. doi:10.1016/j.biopsych.2004.06.006
121. Stone TW, Darlington LG. The kynurenine pathway as a therapeutic target in cognitive and neurodegenerative disorders. *Br J Pharmacol* (2013) **169**:1211–27. doi:10.1111/bph.12230
122. Wonodi I, Schwarcz R. Cortical kynurenine pathway metabolism: a novel target for cognitive enhancement in schizophrenia. *Schizophr Bull* (2010) **36**:211–8. doi:10.1093/schbul/sbq002
123. Baran H, Kepplinger B. Cerebrolysin lowers kynurenic acid formation – an in vitro study. *Eur Neuropsychopharmacol* (2009) **19**:161–8. doi:10.1016/j.euroneuro.2008.09.003
124. Shifu X, Haibo X, Guanjun L, Chengmei Y, Xia L, Chao C, et al. Therapeutic effects of cerebrolysin added to risperidone in patients with schizophrenia dominated by negative symptoms. *Aust N Z J Psychiatry* (2012) **46**:153–60. doi:10.1177/0004867411433213
125. Thome J, Doppler E. Safety profile of cerebrolysin: clinical experience from dementia and stroke trials. *Drugs Today* (2012) **48**(Suppl A):63–9. doi:10.1358/dot.2012.48(Suppl.A).1739724
126. Alvarez XA, Cacabelos R, Sampedro C, Aleixandre M, Linares C, Granizo E, et al. Efficacy and safety of cerebrolysin in moderate to moderately severe Alzheimer's disease: results of a randomized, double-blind, controlled trial investigating three dosages of cerebrolysin. *Eur J Neurol* (2011) **18**:59–68. doi:10.1111/j.1468-1331.2010.03092.x
127. Plosker G, Gauthier S. Cerebrolysin. *Drugs Aging* (2009) **26**:893–915. doi:10.2165/11203320-000000000-00000
128. Chen C-C, Wei S-T, Tsaia S-C, Chen X-X, Cho D-Y. Cerebrolysin enhances cognitive recovery of mild traumatic brain injury patients: double-blind, placebo-controlled, randomized study. *Br J Neurosurg* (2013) **27**:803–7. doi:10.3109/02688697.2013.793287
129. Baran H, Kepplinger B. d-Cycloserine lowers kynurenic acid formation – new mechanism of action. *Eur Neuropsychopharmacol* (2013). doi:10.1016/j.euroneuro.2013.10.006
130. Goff DC. D-cycloserine: an evolving role in learning and neuroplasticity in schizophrenia. *Schizophr Bull* (2012) **38**:936–41. doi:10.1093/schbul/sbs012
131. Fogal B, Hewett SJ. Interleukin-1β: a bridge between inflammation and excitotoxicity? *J Neurochem* (2008) **106**:1–23. doi:10.1111/j.1471-4159.2008.05315.x
132. Gardoni F, Boraso M, Zianni E, Corsini E, Galli C, Cattabeni F, et al. Distribution of interleukin-1 receptor complex at the synaptic membrane driven by

interleukin-1beta and NMDA stimulation. *J Neuroinflammation* (2011) **8**:14. doi:10.1186/1742-2094-8-14
133. Chew LJ, Fusar-Poli P, Schmitz T. Oligodendroglial alterations and the role of microglia in white matter injury: relevance to schizophrenia. *Dev Neurosci* (2013) **35**:102–29. doi:10.1159/000346157
134. Schmitz T, Chew L-J. Cytokines and myelination in the central nervous system. *ScientificWorldJournal* (2008) **8**:1119–47. doi:10.1100/tsw.2008.140
135. Najjar S, Pearlman D, Alper K, Najjar A, Devinsky O. Neuroinflammation and psychiatric illness. *J Neuroinflammation* (2013) **1**(10):43. doi:10.1186/1742-2094-10-43
136. Schroeter ML, Abdul-Khaliq H, Krebs M, Diefenbacher A, Blasig IE. Neuron-specific enolase is unaltered whereas S100B is elevated in serum of patients with schizophrenia – original research and meta-analysis. *Psychiatry Res* (2009) **167**:66–72. doi:10.1016/j.psychres.2008.01.002
137. Kerschensteiner M, Stadelmann C, Dechant G, Wekerle H, Hohlfeld R. Neurotrophic cross-talk between the nervous and immune systems: implications for neurological diseases. *Ann Neurol* (2003) **53**:292–304. doi:10.1002/ana.10446
138. Nurjono M, Lee J, Chong SA. A review of brain-derived neurotrophic factor as a candidate biomarker in schizophrenia. *Clin Psychopharmacol Neurosci* (2012) **10**:61–70. doi:10.9758/cpn.2012.10.2.61
139. Nieto R, Kukuljan M, Silva H. BDNF and schizophrenia: from neurodevelopment to neuronal plasticity, learning, and memory. *Front Psychiatry* (2013) **4**:45. doi:10.3389/fpsyt.2013.00045
140. Goff DC. Future perspectives on the treatment of cognitive deficits and negative symptoms in schizophrenia. *World Psychiatry* (2013) **12**:99–107. doi:10.1002/wps.20026
141. Monji A, Kato TA, Mizoguchi Y, Horikawa H, Seki Y, Kasai M, et al. Neuroinflammation in schizophrenia especially focused on the role of microglia. *Prog Neuropsychopharmacol Biol Psychiatry* (2013) **42**:115–21. doi:10.1016/j.pnpbp.2011.12.002
142. Ceresoli-Borroni G, Rassoulpour A, Wu HQ, Guidetti P, Schwarcz R. Chronic neuroleptic treatment reduces endogenous kynurenic acid levels in rat brain. *J Neural Transm* (2006) **113**:1355–65. doi:10.1007/s00702-005-0432-z
143. Nitta M, Kishimoto T, Müller N, Weiser M, Davidson M, Kane JM, et al. Adjunctive use of nonsteroidal anti-inflammatory drugs for schizophrenia: a meta-analytic investigation of randomized controlled trials. *Schizophr Bull* (2013) **39**(6):1230–41. doi:10.1093/schbul/sbt070
144. Sommer IE, van Westrhenen R, Begemann MJ, de Witte LD, Leucht S, Kahn RS. Efficacy of anti-inflammatory agents to improve symptoms in patients with schizophrenia: an update. *Schizophr Bull* (2013) **40**(1):181–91. doi:10.1093/schbul/sbt139
145. Muller N, Riedel M, Schwarz MJ, Engel RR. Clinical effects of COX-2 inhibitors on cognition in schizophrenia. *Eur Arch Psychiatry Clin Neurosci* (2005) **255**:149–51. doi:10.1007/s00406-004-0548-4
146. Sirén A-L, Faßhauer T, Bartels C, Ehrenreich H. Therapeutic potential of erythropoietin and its structural or functional variants in the nervous system. *Neurotherapeutics* (2009) **6**:108–27. doi:10.1016/j.nurt.2008.10.041
147. Ehrenreich H, Hinze-Selch D, Stawicki S, Aust C, Knolle-Veentjer S, Wilms S, et al. Improvement of cognitive functions in chronic schizophrenic patients by recombinant human erythropoietin. *Mol Psychiatry* (2007) **12**:206–20. doi:10.1038/sj.mp.4001907
148. Wustenberg T, Begemann M, Bartels C, Gefeller O, Stawicki S, Hinze-Selch D, et al. Recombinant human erythropoietin delays loss of gray matter in chronic schizophrenia. *Mol Psychiatry* (2011) **16**:26–36. doi:10.1038/mp.2010.51
149. Fond G, Macgregor A, Attal J, Larue A, Brittner M, Ducasse D, et al. Treating patients with schizophrenia deficit with erythropoietin? *Psychiatry Clin Neurosci* (2012) **66**:375–82. doi:10.1111/j.1440-1819.2012.02359.x
150. Jang W, Park J, Shin KJ, Kim J-S, Kim JS, Youn J, et al. Safety and efficacy of recombinant human erythropoietin treatment of non-motor symptoms in Parkinson's disease. *J Neurol Sci* (2013). doi:10.1016/j.jns.2013.11.015
151. Sargin D, Friedrichs H, El-Kordi A, Ehrenreich H. Erythropoietin as neuroprotective and neuroregenerative treatment strategy: comprehensive overview of 12 years of preclinical and clinical research. *Best Pract Res Clin Anaesthesiol* (2010) **24**:573–94. doi:10.1016/j.bpa.2010.10.005
152. Domercq M, Matute C. Neuroprotection by tetracyclines. *Trends Pharmacol Sci* (2004) **25**:609–12. doi:10.1016/j.tips.2004.10.001
153. Levkovitz Y, Mendlovich S, Riwkes S, Braw Y, Levkovitch-Verbin H, Gal G, et al. A double-blind, randomized study of minocycline for the treatment of negative and cognitive symptoms in early-phase schizophrenia. *J Clin Psychiatry* (2010) **71**:138–149. doi:10.4088/JCP.08m04666yel
154. Chaudhry IB, Hallak J, Husain N, Minhas F, Stirling J, Richardson P, et al. Minocycline benefits negative symptoms in early schizophrenia: a randomised double-blind placebo-controlled clinical trial in patients on standard treatment. *J Psychopharmacol* (2012) **26**:1185–93. doi:10.1177/0269881112444941
155. Kay SR, Fiszbein A, Opler LA. The Positive and Negative Syndrome Scale (PANSS) for schizophrenia. *Schizophr Bull* (1987) **13**:261–76. doi:10.1093/schbul/13.2.261
156. Overall J, Gorham D. The Brief Psychiatric Rating Scale. *Psychol Rep* (1962) **10**:799–812. doi:10.2466/pr0.1962.10.3.799

8

Dysconnectivity in the Frontoparietal Attention Network in Schizophrenia

Jonathan P. Roiser[1]*†, Rebekah Wigton[2†], James M. Kilner[3,4], Maria A. Mendez[5], Nicholas Hon[6], Karl J. Friston[3] and Eileen M. Joyce[4]

[1] *Institute of Cognitive Neuroscience, University College London, London, UK*
[2] *Psychosis Studies, Cognition and Schizophrenia Imaging Lab, Institute of Psychiatry, King's College London, London, UK*
[3] *Wellcome Trust Centre for Neuroimaging, University College London, London, UK*
[4] *Institute of Neurology, University College London, London, UK*
[5] *Department of Forensic and Neurodevelopmental Sciences, Institute of Psychiatry, King's College London, London, UK*
[6] *Department of Psychology, National University of Singapore, Singapore*

Correspondence:
Jonathan P. Roiser, Institute of Cognitive Neuroscience, University College London, 17 Queen Square, London WC1N 3AR, UK
e-mail: j.roiser@ucl.ac.uk

†Jonathan P. Roiser and Rebekah Wigton have contributed equally to this work.

Cognitive impairment is common in patients with schizophrenia, and even those with relatively preserved function perform worse than healthy volunteers (HVs) on attentional tasks. This is consistent with the hypothesis that connectivity – in the frontoparietal network (FPN) activated during attention – is disrupted in schizophrenia. We examined attentional effects on connectivity in the FPN, in schizophrenia, using magnetoencephalography (MEG). Twenty-three HVs and 19 first-episode schizophrenia patients were scanned during a simple visual change test, known to activate the FPN, in which attention was monitored and directed with an orthogonal flicker-detection task. Dynamic causal modeling (DCM) of evoked responses was used to assess effective connectivity – and its modulation by changes in the attended stimulus dimension – in the following network: higher visual area; temporoparietal junction (TPJ); intraparietal sulcus (IPS); dorsal anterior cingulate cortex; and ventrolateral prefrontal cortex. The final MEG analysis included 18 HVs and 14 schizophrenia patients. While all participants were able to maintain attention, HVs responded slightly, but non-significantly, more accurately than schizophrenia patients. HVs, but not schizophrenia patients, exhibited greater cortical responses to attended visual changes. Bayesian model comparison revealed that a DCM with attention dependent changes in both top-down and bottom-up connections best explained responses by patients with schizophrenia, while in HVs the best model required only bottom-up changes. Quantitative comparison of connectivity estimates revealed a significant group difference in changes in the right IPS-TPJ connection: schizophrenia patients showed relative reductions in connectivity during attended stimulus changes. Crucially, this reduction predicted lower intelligence. These data are consistent with the hypothesis that functional dysconnections in the FPN contribute to cognitive impairment in schizophrenia.

Keywords: schizophrenia, frontoparietal, magnetoencephalography, dynamic causal modeling, dysconnectivity, DCM

INTRODUCTION

Patients with schizophrenia exhibit reliable impairments on almost all cognitive tests (1). They exhibit particular impairments on tests that depend on attention (2, 3) and working memory (4–6). This is a pattern observed even in patients whose cognitive performance is otherwise in the normal range. Generalized cognitive impairment, indexed by intelligence quotient (IQ), precedes the onset of psychosis and is detectable as far back as infancy (7). In addition, the severity of impairment is linearly related to the risk of developing psychosis and predicts functional outcome following illness onset (7, 8). Furthermore, supporting the notion that cognitive impairment represents a core feature of the syndrome in addition to positive and negative symptoms, it has also been reported in unaffected first degree relatives of patients with schizophrenia (9–15). This suggests that the neural abnormalities underlying impaired cognition reflect the neurodevelopmental susceptibility to schizophrenia. Cognitive impairment is thus a core feature of schizophrenia that significantly impacts on the course of illness; warranting a more detailed understanding of its generalized nature and neurobiological basis.

Functional neuroimaging has highlighted a core network of prefrontal and parietal regions that is activated during the performance of a variety of disparate cognitive tasks. For example, this frontoparietal network (FPN) is activated in tasks ranging from set-shifting (16) to feature selection (17) and object orientation (18) as well as recognition memory (19), working memory (20) and attention [for reviews see Ref. (21–23)]. One hypothesis is that the FPN serves as a "multiple demand system" which undertakes the information processing requirements common to different cognitive tasks, for example by updating and maintaining changes to attended stimuli (24). This system is supported by various attention networks such as the orientation network (25, 26) as well as global connectivity within this network (27). Furthermore, the development, and thus differences, of these specific attention systems – particularly in the FPN – are driven by interactions between cognition and our environment (28). This is further supported by the findings of an fMRI study by Hon et al. (29) using a task in which subjects were instructed to attend to a subset of visual stimuli and press a button when they detected a brief "flicker." This task robustly activated the FPN simply when attended visual stimuli changed, independent of any flickers or responses. Importantly, interposed unattended stimulus changes did not elicit FPN activation, thus implicating involvement of FPN specifically in task-relevant information processing.

The "multiple demand" hypothesis predicts that dysfunction of the FPN will adversely impact on the performance of a wide range of cognitive tasks. In schizophrenia, fMRI studies have shown that nodes in this network respond abnormally across different tasks such as attention, executive control, and working memory (19, 30, 31). However, no studies in schizophrenia have examined FPN integrity in the context of a task that recruits a fundamental attentional process – a process that is essential for the performance of many higher order tasks but which itself requires "minimal decision and control" (29, 32). We therefore investigated FPN function in schizophrenia using the task described by Hon et al. (29).

Regarding possible pathophysiological mechanisms underlying schizophrenia, the "dysconnection" hypothesis is one of the most influential (33–35). The central tenet of this model is that the symptoms observed in schizophrenia arise from abnormal regulation of *N*-methyl-D-aspartate (NMDA) receptor-dependent synaptic efficacy by modulatory transmitters, such as dopamine or acetylcholine (35). This is proposed to result in abnormal integration of neural processes, which can be measured in terms of effective connectivity, or the influence that one neural system has over another (36). Using dynamic causal modeling (DCM) – which estimates effective connectivity – prior studies have found that aberrant perceptual processes in schizophrenia are associated with such dysconnectivity (37, 38). These differences in effective connectivity are thought to reflect aberrant NMDA receptor-dependent regulation of synaptic efficacy; similar dysfunction may also occur in the FPN, resulting in dysfunctional processing in the multiple demand system and thus impairment on several different types of cognitive tests. Furthermore, disrupted connectivity assessed using DCM has also been reported during tasks that examined working memory and verbal fluency in individuals at risk for psychosis (39–41). However, most previous studies assessing differences in connectivity employed functional magnetic resonance imaging (fMRI), which precludes the use of detailed and neurophysiological plausible (neural mass) models, due to its low temporal resolution.

In this study we therefore measured neural responses in patients with schizophrenia and healthy volunteers (HVs) with magnetoencephalography (MEG) during a simple visual change task known to engage the FPN (29); we assessed effective connectivity in the FPN with DCM. MEG, in particular, provides more temporally precise data than fMRI. This detailed time course information enables the efficient estimation of much more realistic and detailed neural mass models – particularly models with different types of connection (i.e., forward; backward; and lateral) among distinct neuronal populations. Cortical areas previously reported to be activated by the task employed (using fMRI) were used as regions of interest (ROIs) when specifying the different neural network models for DCM [see Figure 2 and Table 2 of Ref. (29)]. DCM uses these co-ordinates as spatial priors when specifying the location of the electromagnetic sources that generate sensor-space responses. With these models, we were able to estimate how effective connectivity between nodes in the FPN – and its modulation by attended visual changes – differs between patients with schizophrenia and HVs. We predicted that patients with schizophrenia would show abnormal effective connectivity (and its modulation by attention), as reflected in the coupling estimates from DCM, and – crucially – that these would predict cognitive impairment (i.e., low IQ).

MATERIALS AND METHODS

PARTICIPANTS

Nineteen patients with schizophrenia were recruited from a longitudinal study of cognitive impairment in first-episode psychosis (6). The diagnosis was ascertained using a structured interview, the diagnostic module of the Diagnostic Interview for Psychosis (42), which includes items from the Operational Criteria Checklist for Psychosis (43) and the World Health Organisation Schedules for Clinical Assessment in Neuropsychiatry (44). Diagnoses were made at study entry and reviewed 1 year later. Twenty-three HVs were recruited via advertisement.

Exclusion criteria for all participants included: medical disorders likely to cause cognitive impairment; IQ less than 70; left-handedness; and recent illicit substance use. Additional exclusion criteria for HVs included: past or present psychiatric or neurological disorders; and any first degree relatives with a psychotic illness. All HVs were screened for Axis-I psychopathology using the Mini International Neuropsychiatric Interview (45). One healthy volunteer was excluded because he had a brother with psychosis; another was excluded for being left-handed. Three HVs and two patients with schizophrenia were excluded because we were unable to identify clear visual evoked responses. Two patients with schizophrenia were excluded due to failure to follow task instructions. One patient with schizophrenia was excluded because her diagnosis was subsequently changed to depression with psychosis. After exclusions, the final MEG analysis included 18 HVs (9 male, 9 female) and 14 patients with schizophrenia (10 male, 4 female), all right-handed.

Demographic and clinical data are presented in **Table 1**. The groups were similar in terms of age, premorbid IQ [estimated using the National Reading Test: (46)], and current IQ [estimated using the Wechsler scale of adult intelligence (WAIS)-III] (47). All patients but one were taking antipsychotic medication; four were also taking antidepressant medication; and one was only taking antidepressant medication. None of the HVs were taking any psychotropic medication. Symptom severity scores for the patients were measured using the Scale for Assessment of Negative Symptoms (SANS) (48) and the Scale for Assessment of Positive Symptoms (SAPS) (49). All participants provided written informed consent before the start of the experiment and were

Table 1 | Demographic and clinical sample characteristics.

	Patients with schizophrenia ($N=14$) [mean (SD)]	Healthy volunteers ($N=18$) [mean (SD)]	Statistics
Age (years)	25.21 (4.23)	24.11 (6.00)	$t(30)=0.584$, $P>0.1$
WAIS-III Byler IQ	101.43 (19.23)	106.83 (15.22)	$t(30)=0.888$, $P>0.1$
NART verbal IQ	101.57 (7.94)	99.33 (9.63)	$t(30)=0.703$, $P>0.1$
Gender	10M, 4F	9M, 9F	$\chi^2(1)=1.50$, $P>0.1$
Age at onset (years)	21.43 (4.85)	–	
Duration of illness (years)	3.79 (1.37)	–	
CPZ equivalents	247.62 (143.80)	–	
SANS global ratings		–	
Affective flattening or blunting	6.86 (8.47)	–	
Alogia	5.80 (6.76)	–	
Anhedonia-asociality	3.14 (4.31)	–	
Attention	0.21 (0.80)	–	
Overall	19.1 (21.9)	–	
SAPS global ratings		–	
Hallucinations	3.79 (6.13)	–	
Delusions	4.64 (5.73)	–	
Bizarre behavior	0.29 (1.07)	–	
Positive formal thought disorder	0.86 (2.48)	–	
Overall	9.6 (14.0)	–	

IQ, intelligence quotient; M, male; F, female.
WAIS, Wechsler adult intelligence scale; NART, national adult reading test; CPZ, chlorpromazine equivalent (72, 73); SANS, scale for assessment of negative symptoms; SAPS, scale for assessment of positive symptoms.

compensated for participation. The study was approved by Ealing and West London Local Research Ethics Committee.

COGNITIVE ACTIVATION PARADIGM

The paradigm was presented as described in Hon et al. (29), with the exception that all stimuli were black and white. Participants were presented with a series of complex, nonsense shapes, similar to those shown in **Figure 1**. The images were displayed to the left, right, top and bottom of a central box. Each stimulus on either the vertical or horizontal axis was a mirror reflection of the opposite image. The shapes were hand drawn to ensure that they did not resemble any familiar patterns or objects. Each stimulus was presented for a period of 1000 ms before an off period of 500 ms, during which only the central box appeared. All the images and lines appeared and disappeared at the same time. This task comprised two blocks, each consisting of 180 trials, and lasted four and a half minutes per block. For each trial, either: (1) the shapes on the horizontal axis changed, in relation to the previous trial but the shapes on the vertical axis remained the same (60 occurrences); or (2) the shapes on the vertical axis changed and the shapes on the horizontal axis remained the same (60 occurrences); or (3) no shape change occurred on either axis (60 occurrences). On one-third of trials (20 in each condition) either the horizontal or the vertical axis flickered briefly. Trial types were presented in a random order. In order to maintain stimulus novelty, no shape was reused in each block.

This task was chosen to be sufficiently straightforward so that patients with schizophrenia would be able to perform it to a high level of accuracy. Participants were instructed to maintain fixation on the box in the center of the screen, which was confirmed using concurrent eye-tracking. During each run, participants were instructed to watch either the horizontal axis or the vertical axis, and press a button on an MEG-compatible button-box with their right index finger only when a flicker occurred on the axis they were attending to. The order was counterbalanced across participants. Two runs were conducted for each participant, each lasting 4.5 min.

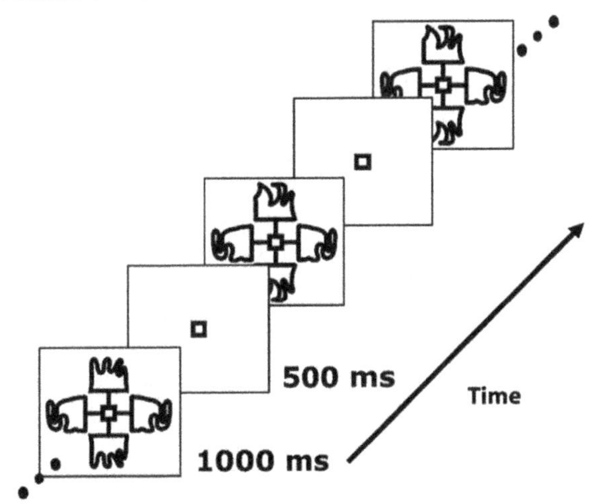

FIGURE 1 | Example of a stimulus sequence used in the task (29).

MAGNETOENCEPHALOGRAPHY

MEG data acquisition

Magnetoencephalography data were recorded using 275 first order axial gradiometers with the Omega275 CTF MEG system (VSMmedtech, Vancouver, Canada) at a 480 Hz sampling frequency. Data were recorded in a magnetically shielded room. Each participant's head was supported by a padded headrest to restrict head movement during recording. To monitor head motion, sensors were placed near the ears and nose. None of the participants included in the final analysis exceeded a threshold of 5 mm for head movement within a single run. Eye-tracking was also used to ensure that all participants attended continually to the visual stimuli.

MEG data analysis

Data analysis was performed using Statistical Parametric Mapping 12 (SPM12) (Wellcome Trust Centre for Neuroimaging, London, UK; www.fil.ion.ucl.ac.uk/spm) in MATLAB 12.1 (MathWorks Inc., Sherbon, MA, USA). Blocks with attended flicker-detection (hit) rates lower than 60% or incorrect response (false alarm) rates greater than 15%, were excluded from the analysis. The remaining data were epoched with a peristimulus window from −100 to 1300 ms. Data were processed using artifact detection routines to identify and exclude eye blinks or movement before bandpass filtering between 0.5 and 16 Hz. The data were then down sampled to 200 Hz and baseline corrected using the −100–0 ms period. One bad MEG channel was excluded from the analysis across all participants.

All flicker and false alarm trials (i.e., if the participant made a response when the attended axis had not flickered) were removed from further analysis. Robust averages were calculated for each event type (attended change, unattended change and no change) across all valid trials for each session – note that no trial included in the analysis featured a flicker stimulus or any response by the participant. Grand average responses were created for each participant for all sessions that met the performance criteria specified above. These average responses were interpolated into images and visually inspected for artifacts and the presence of visual evoked fields (VEFs). Data were excluded if a clear VEF could not be identified over occipital sensors. From these grand average images, contrast images were created for the following comparisons: (attended change minus unattended change); (attended change minus no change); and (unattended change minus no change). A smoothing kernel of (2 mm × 2 mm × 2 mm) was applied to each contrast image.

These sensor-space contrast images were combined at the group-level for random-effects analysis, which was performed across all sensors and all time points. For group comparisons, significant clusters were defined as those surviving an uncorrected voxel-level threshold of $P < 0.001$ with a cluster-level threshold corrected across the whole of sensor-space and peristimulus time, controlling the family-wise error (FWE) rate at $P < 0.05$. For within-group contrasts, which produced extensive activation in HVs, we used an uncorrected voxel-level threshold of $P < 0.0005$, again controlling the FWE rate at $P < 0.05$ at the cluster-level.

Dynamic causal modeling

Dynamic causal modeling was applied to assess effective connectivity. DCM uses the concept of effective connectivity, or the influence that one neural system has over another, to create a model of coupled neuronal populations that is used to explain evoked responses (50). The parameters (effective connectivity and other synaptic constants) are optimized by fitting responses generated by the model – in response to stimuli – to observed responses using standard Bayesian model inversion techniques (51). In addition, the evidence for a particular model (irrespective of the particular parameters) is evaluated in terms of model evidence through Bayesian model comparison (BMC) (52, 53). Crucially, DCM estimates not just the effective connectivity or coupling between sources of electromagnetic responses but also sets of experimental changes in coupling. This allows one to use BMC to assess the evidence for context dependent changes in connectivity – such as changes induced by the nature of the stimulus (attended versus unattended). This method incorporates an exceedance probability to determine the best fitting model or the likelihood that one model fit the data better than any of the other models.

The network architecture used for the DCM comprised sources that were previously identified as being activated in an fMRI study employing the same task (29). These sources were consistent with the most robust responses in the (attended change minus unattended change) analysis of sensor-space responses [see Figure 2 and Table 2 of Ref. (29)]. They included: higher visual area (HVA) ([48, −66, −4] and [−48, −66 −16]); temporoparietal junction (TPJ) ([64, −38, 6] and [−64, −38, 6]); intraparietal sulcus (IPS) ([26, −62, 42] and [−24, −66, 50]); ventrolateral prefrontal cortex (vlPFC) ([36, 35, −4] and [−44, 34, 6]); and dorsal anterior cingulate (dACC) ([14, 26, 44] and [−6, 14, 48]). All models had a fixed model architecture within each hemisphere (both forward and backward connections) as follows: between HVA and TPJ; between TPJ and IPS; between IPS and dACC; and between IPS and vlPFC. Furthermore, all models had fixed lateral connections between vlPFC and dACC, and inter-hemispherically between all corresponding regions (i.e., between left and right HVA, TPJ, IPS, vlPFC, and dACC) (see **Figure 2**). Using the above co-ordinates as spatial location priors, three DCMs were constructed, varying in relation to modulatory effects – the modulation attributable to a stimulus change on the attended dimension or axis – on forward connections (reflecting bottom-up effects), on backward connections (reflecting top-down effects), or on both forward and backward connections (see **Figure 2**). This approach is consistent with prior studies using DCM for MEG (38, 54). All models had driving inputs into the HVA, modeling subcortical visual input.

Each DCM was estimated at the subject level, but BMC was conducted at the group-level, in each group separately, to determine the most parsimonious explanation for the data in terms of attentional modulation of connectivity (models with the most evidence represent an accurate explanation of observed data with minimal complexity). To make quantitative inferences about differences in connection strengths, effective connectivity, and its modulation were compared using classical statistics at the group-level. Fixed and modulatory coupling estimate parameters (indicating the

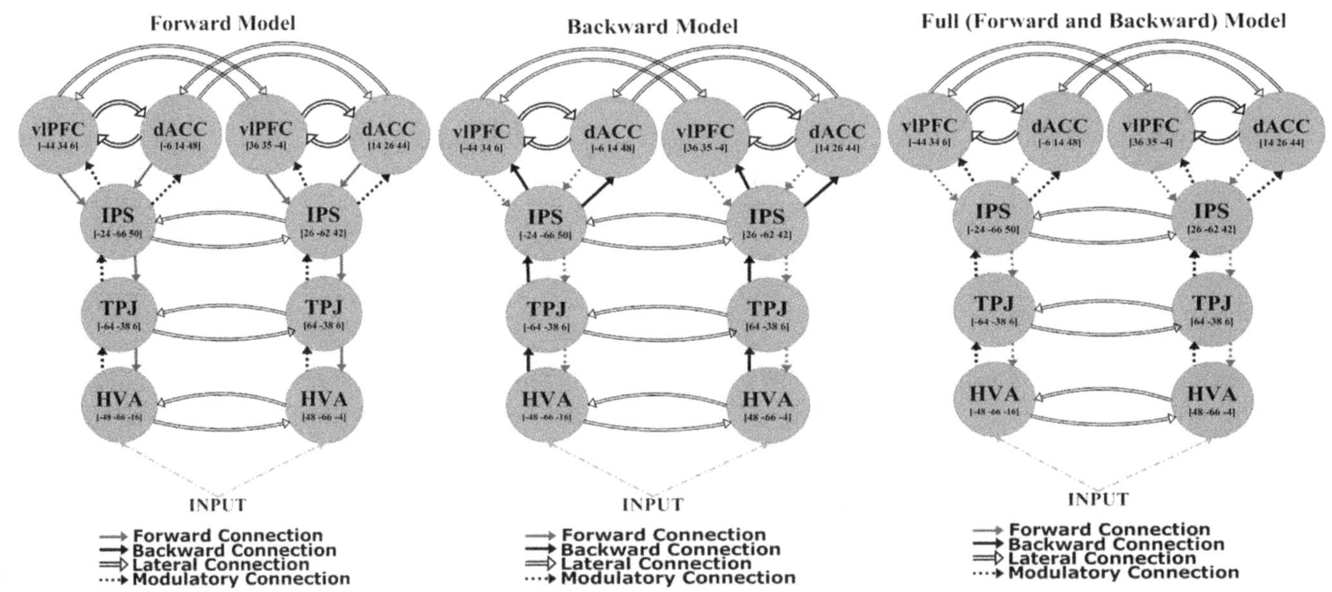

FIGURE 2 | Models used for the dynamic causal modeling analysis.

strength of each fixed connection and its modulation by attended visual change, respectively) were computed using random-effects Bayesian model averaging (BMA) (55), and submitted to analysis in SPSS 17 (SPSS Inc., Chicago, IL, USA). After BMA, we obtained connectivity parameters for all fixed and modulatory connections (only forward and backward) for each hemisphere as well as the intrahemispheric connections: total 46 parameters. However, we did not examine any of the intrahemispheric connections so this left a total of 36 connections that were examined for group differences.

Group differences were assessed with t-tests and relationships with demographic, clinical, and cognitive variables with Pearson's r correlation coefficients. These tests were not corrected for multiple comparisons. Since this was an exploratory analysis, and because our primary inference related to the BMC, an alpha level of 0.05 was adopted for all group comparisons. We refer to trend significance at a threshold of $0.05 < P < 0.1$. However, to reduce the number of correlations performed, only those coupling parameters that differed between the groups at least at a trend level were entered into correlation analyses.

RESULTS

BEHAVIORAL PERFORMANCE

Patients with schizophrenia responded slightly, but non-significantly, less accurately than HVs, with a lower hit rate (**Table 2**). There were no significant differences between the groups in terms of reaction times, false alarms or d'. Concurrent eye-tracking confirmed that all participants attended to the visual stimuli throughout the task.

MEG SENSOR-SPACE RESPONSES

The MEG grand average image in the healthy controls (**Figures 3A–C**) showed a consistent and sustained deviation in cortical responses between attended and unattended stimulus changes from approximately 200 ms after stimulus onset, primarily in right lateral frontal sensors. This increase was evident for almost 1 s. This deviation becomes statistically significant (cluster-level correction) at approximately 375 ms over right frontal sensors [peak at 395 ms: $t(17) = 4.87$, $P_{\mathrm{FWE}} = 0.039$]. The response at this peristimulus time is consistent with the P300 response often observed in oddball paradigms (56, 57), of which our task is a variant (with an attentional manipulation). Similar effects were observed later in peristimulus time over the same sensors, and over more anterior frontal sensors (see **Table 3**).

By contrast, the MEG responses from the patients with schizophrenia showed no difference between the attended change and unattended change conditions (**Figures 3D–F**). This finding was paralleled in the statistical analyses, where no differences in sensor-space responses were observed between any of the conditions, even when the threshold was lowered to $P < 0.001$ (uncorrected), extent threshold 10 voxels. However, patients with schizophrenia did, nonetheless, show a clear VEF across all conditions (**Figure 3F**), suggesting that they did engage with the task and have detectable electromagnetic responses.

Although patients with schizophrenia exhibited diminished cortical responses to attended visual change at frontal sensors in comparison to the controls (**Figures 3B,E**), no group differences survived stringent correction for multiple comparisons across the whole of sensor-space and peristimulus time at any time point (**Table 3**). However, at a more liberal threshold of $P < 0.001$ (uncorrected), extent threshold 10 voxels, diminished responses in the schizophrenia patients were detected over right frontal sensors at 260 ms [$t(30) = 3.78$, $P < 0.001$, uncorrected], 320 ms [$t(30) = 3.50$, $P < 0.001$, uncorrected], 360 ms [$t(30) = 3.55$, $P < 0.001$, uncorrected], and 375 ms [$t(30) = 3.60$, $P < 0.001$, uncorrected], and over left parietal sensors 755 ms

Table 2 | Behavioral data from the visual change task.

	Patients with schizophrenia, mean (SD)	Healthy volunteers, mean (SD)	Statistics
Correct hits (flickers detected) (%)	78.69 (9.90)	85.16 (8.96)	$t(30) = 1.943$, $P = 0.061$
False alarms (inappropriate responses) (%)	2.38 (2.24)	2.87 (2.90)	$t(30) = 0.521$, $P = 0.606$
Correct hit reaction time (ms)	499.02 (91.85)	466.51 (53.24)	$t(30) = 1.248$, $P = 0.218$
d'	2.88 (0.46)	3.21 (0.75)	$t(30) = 1.459$, $P = 0.155$

SD, standard deviation; ms, milliseconds.

[$t(30) = 3.85$, $P < 0.001$, uncorrected] (see **Table 3**). We report these results descriptively, noting that they require replication.

Neither group showed any activation in the (unattended change minus no change) contrast at a threshold of $P < 0.0005$ uncorrected, extent threshold 40 voxels. The (attended change minus no change) contrast produced similar results to the (attended change minus unattended change) contrast.

DYNAMIC CAUSAL MODELING

Bayesian model comparison

Using BMC, we were able to determine which model provided the most parsimonious explanation for the effects of attended stimulus changes in both groups. Different DCMs provided the best explanation in patients with schizophrenia and HVs, providing *prima facie* evidence for dysconnectivity during attentional processing in schizophrenia. In HVs, there was greatest evidence for the model with only forward modulations, with an exceedance probability of 99% over other models. In patients with schizophrenia there was greatest evidence for the model with both forward and backward modulations, with an exceedance probability of 75% over the other models (**Figure 4**).

Quantitative connectivity estimates

To understand better why the groups differed in terms of the most parsimonious architecture, we quantified the connectivity and its attentional modulation, using BMA (**Table 4**). This effectively weights the coupling estimates, under each model, according to the probability of that model and accommodates uncertainty about the underlying architectures.

Fixed connections. For the fixed connections, the left IPS-dACC fixed forward connection was marginally stronger in the HVs [$t(30) = 2.019$, $P = 0.052$]. This means that HVs show a trend toward being relatively more sensitive to parietal afferents to the dACC than schizophrenia patients, irrespective of whether the stimulus change was on the attended dimension or not.

Modulatory connections. For the modulatory connections (i.e., altered coupling elicited by attended visual change), only the right IPS-TPJ modulation differed significantly between the groups [$t(30) = 2.428$, $P = 0.021$]. This modulator was negative in schizophrenia and slightly positive in healthy subjects. In other words, the top-down afferents from the parietal source to the TPJ were reduced in their strength in schizophrenia, relative to HVs, only when the stimulus changed in the attended dimension. Note that a negative modulation corresponds to a reduction in connectivity (because connection strengths in DCM for electromagnetic responses are always positive – targeting excitatory and inhibitory neuronal populations).

There was also a trend toward a group difference in the right IPS-dACC modulation [$t(30) = 1.701$, $P = 0.099$], with a negative modulator in HVs but a positive modulator in schizophrenia patients.

Correlations with demographic, clinical, and cognitive measures

No correlations approaching significance were identified between the left IPS-dACC fixed connection, and behavior, current IQ, premorbid IQ, age, SAPS, SANS, or chlorpromazine equivalent dose. However, changes in the IPS-TPJ connectivity correlated positively with premorbid IQ score in the patient group ($r = 0.547$, $P = 0.043$) but not in the HVs ($r = -0.297$, $P = 0.231$; difference in correlation coefficients: Fisher's $Z = 2.32$, $P = 0.02$) (**Figure 5**). In other words, patients with the most (abnormal) decrease in this connection during attended stimulus change had the lowest premorbid IQ. Importantly, this modulation did not correlate significantly with the percentage of correct flicker-detections ($r = 0.127$, $P = 0.665$, in patients with schizophrenia and $r = -0.250$, $P = 0.318$ in HVs), suggesting that this difference does not simply reflect poor engagement in the task.

DISCUSSION

Using DCM, we found that patients with schizophrenia and HVs differ in their recruitment of the FPN during the processing of salient (attended) visual changes. Both inference about the architectures – and the connectivity of those architectures – pointed to an abnormality in top-down modulation of stimulus evoked responses, when stimulus changes were in the attended dimension or axis. In patients with schizophrenia the winning model featured modulation of both backwards (top-down) and forwards (bottom-up) connections. Specifically, patients with schizophrenia showed a relative failure (decreased connection strength) of the backward IPS-TPJ connection when processing attended visual changes.

Interestingly, this quantitative reduction was associated with lower premorbid IQ in schizophrenia patients only. In previous studies we showed that lower premorbid and current IQ (markers of general cognitive ability) at illness onset predicted poorer social function after 4 years (8). Another study also found that lower IQ and higher psychotic symptoms correlated with a loss in gray matter tissue (58). Previous studies also found that

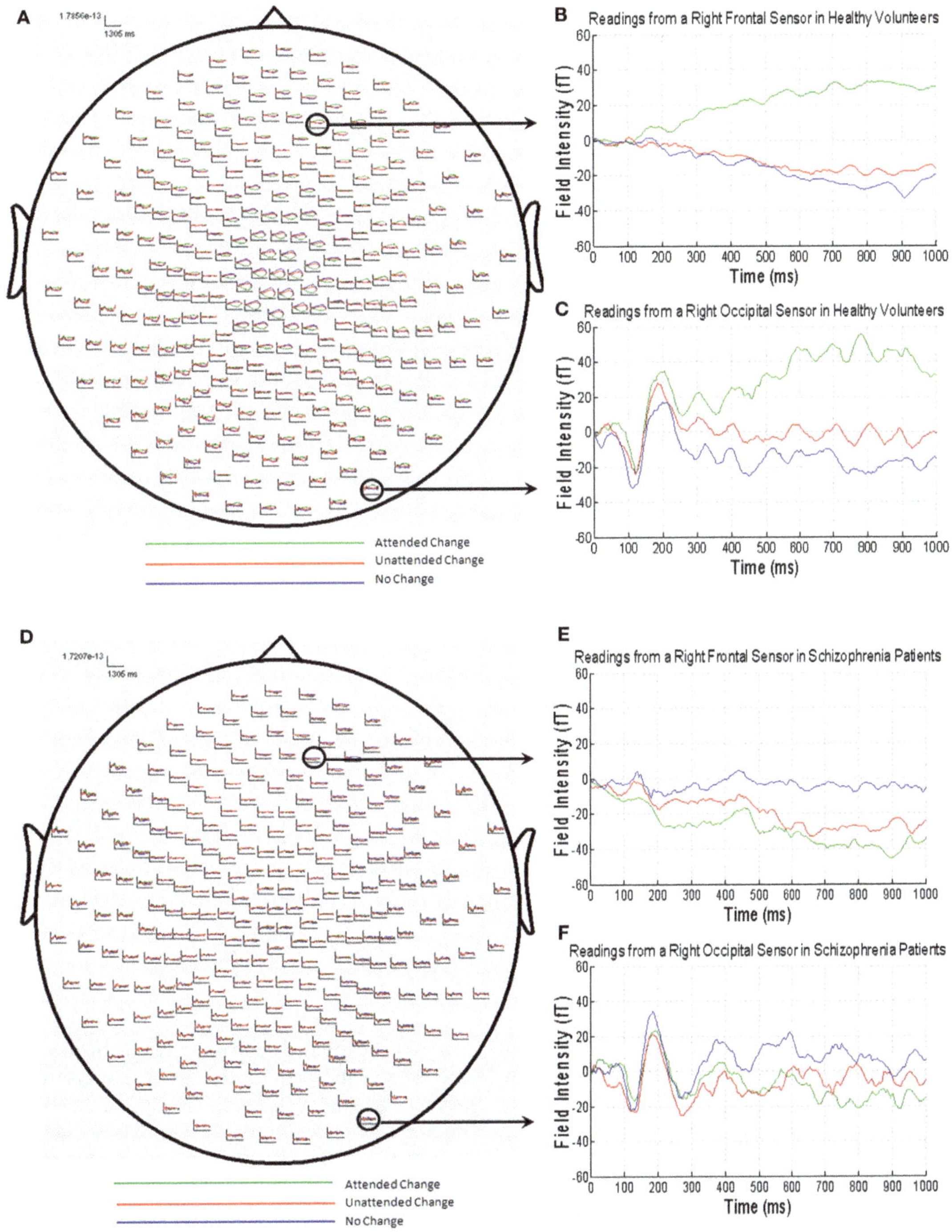

FIGURE 3 | (A) MEG responses averaged over all of the healthy volunteers with attended change trials in green, unattended change trials in red and no change trials in blue; **(B)** MEG data from a right frontal sensor; **(C)** MEG data from a right occipital sensor, showing the visual evoked field in response to stimulus presentation; **(D)** MEG responses averaged over all of the patients with schizophrenia (colors as above); **(E)** MEG data from a right frontal sensor; **(F)** MEG data from a right occipital sensor, showing the visual evoked field in response to stimulus presentation.

global connectivity within the FPN correlated negatively with IQ (27). We have also reported that in patients with schizophrenia, but not healthy controls, lower premorbid and current IQ was related to reduced frontotemporal cortical area and predicted progressive parietal cortical thinning over the following 3 years (59, Gutiérrez-Galve, unpublished observations). Although in the present study we did not find relationships with current IQ, taken together our findings support the hypothesis that FPN dysfunction is the basis of generalized cognitive impairment in schizophrenia (60).

Table 3 | Results for contrast images for MEG sensor-space responses.

Approximate location	Time (ms)	*k*	*Z*-score	*P* (cluster corrected)
Attended > unattended change for healthy volunteers[a]				
Right occipital/temporal	75	188	4.44	0.280
Mid frontal	685	284	4.07	0.091
Left parietal	755	173	4.02	0.333
Mid frontal	895	2066	3.98	<0.001*
Right frontal	715	380	3.90	0.031*
Mid frontal	905	155	3.88	0.409
Right frontal	395	359	3.80	0.039*
Right frontal	800	545	3.74	0.006*
Right frontal	540	264	3.73	0.115
Left frontal	315	137	3.69	0.498
Mid frontal	555	50	3.67	0.960
Mid frontal	710	61	3.59	0.923
Unattended > attended change for healthy volunteers[a]				
No clusters survived threshold				
Attended > unattended change for schizophrenia patients[a]				
No clusters survived threshold				
Unattended > attended change for schizophrenia patients[a]				
No clusters survived threshold				
Attended > unattended change for healthy volunteers > schizophrenia patients[b]				
Left parietal	755	14	3.45	0.999
Right frontal	260	22	3.39	0.999
Right frontal	375	14	3.25	0.999
Right frontal	320	12	3.18	0.999
Unattended > attended change for healthy volunteers > schizophrenia patients[b]				
No clusters survived threshold				
Attended > unattended change for schizophrenia patients > healthy volunteers[b]				
No clusters survived threshold				
Unattended > attended change for schizophrenia patients > healthy volunteers[b]				
No clusters survived threshold				

[a]*Analyses within groups thresholded at $P < 0.0005$, cluster size 40 voxels.*

[b]*Analyses between groups thresholded at $P < 0.001$, cluster size 10 voxels.*

**$P < 0.05$ FWE whole-brain cluster-level corrected.*

k = number of contiguous voxels.

Differences in connectivity were observed between the groups in several parts of the FPN, all involving parietal cortex connections. The left forward (bottom-up) IPS-dACC fixed connection showed a trend toward being stronger in HVs. This would be consistent with a relatively inefficient transmission of information from parietal to frontal regions in schizophrenia, and could explain the lack of frontal cortical activity elicited by attended visual changes in patients. We also identified a trend difference in the modulation of the right IPS-dACC forward (bottom-up) connection, which was negative only in HVs. However, we note that neither of these differences achieved statistical significance. The only effect to differ significantly between the groups was in the right IPS-TPJ backward (top-down) connection: this connection was lower in patients with schizophrenia.

These results were consistent with the sensor-space results which indicated reduced cortical responses to attended visual changes in patients with schizophrenia, consistent with prior reports of attenuated P300 responses in this group (61). Our DCM suggests that these attenuated responses are caused by selective differences in coupling between the TPJ, parietal cortex, and anterior cingulate. Importantly, the MEG results we observed are unlikely to reflect solely a lack of engagement with the task, as all patients included in the analysis could perform at a high level and, as a group, did not differ from the HVs in terms of reaction times or false alarms; although, we did observe a slight impairment in percentage correct flicker-detection. However, this measure did not correlate with any of the DCM parameters. Together, these results are consistent with the dysconnection hypothesis of schizophrenia – which proposes that aberrant cortical coupling arises due to aberrant regulation of NMDA-dependent synaptic plasticity. Within the FPN we speculate that this may lead to differences in the efficiency in which regions of the FPN are able to interact, resulting in altered effective connectivity, as assessed with MEG. Furthermore, these fit findings comfortably with recent computational accounts of dysconnectivity as a failure to adjust or contextualize

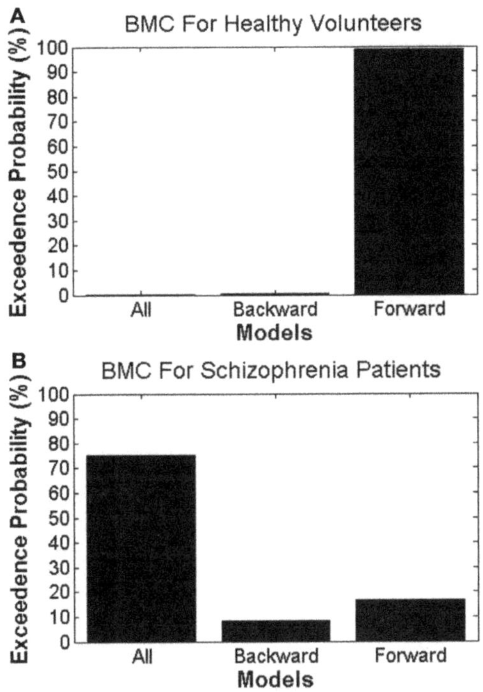

FIGURE 4 | Bayesian model comparison results for (A) healthy volunteers and (B) patients with schizophrenia, showing the exceedance probabilities for each DCM model.

the synaptic efficacy that underlies the routing of salient or precise sensory information (62).

It is interesting to interpret our results in relation to computational formulations of the dysconnection hypothesis – in particular, predictive coding models of hierarchical Bayesian inference. In these formulations, psychotic symptoms are understood in terms of the false inference that arises when the salience or precision afforded sensory information is aberrant (62–64). Formally, top-down or descending predictions in cortical hierarchies try to explain representations at lower levels by forming prediction errors at each level of the hierarchy. Ascending prediction errors are then passed forward to improve the representations at higher levels – and thereby minimize prediction error at every hierarchical level. Crucially, the influence prediction errors have on high level representations depends upon their precision (inverse variance or reliability), which itself has to be optimized (62, 65). Physiologically, precision is thought to be encoded by the postsynaptic neuromodulatory gain of superficial pyramidal cells reporting prediction error (66). Psychologically, the optimization of precision provides a simple explanation for attentional gain; in other words, the selection of ascending prediction errors that are considered salient of precise in any given context (65).

This formulation is particularly relevant here, for two reasons: first, it provides a computational account of dysconnection – that can be reduced to an abnormality of message passing during perceptual inference that rests explicitly on the aberrant modulation of synaptic efficacy (62). Second, it speaks to the important role of attentional deficits in disclosing this aberrant modulation. Although speculative, it is tempting to interpret our results from this computational perspective. The results of the DCM in HVs are entirely consistent with predictive coding; in that attention endows ascending prediction errors from lower (temporal) regions with greater precision and preferential access to higher (parietal) regions – resulting in an increase in forward effective connectivity (67). However, in schizophrenia it appears that the descending predictions – that are informed by ascending prediction errors – "fall on deaf ears," when descending to the temporal region. This is evidenced by a reduction in the backwards connection. Although this account is somewhat heuristic, it is consistent with the fact that backward connections target superficial cortical layers that are rich in NMDA receptors – receptors that are crucial for neuromodulatory effects and play a central role in the dysconnection hypothesis (35).

Prior studies have highlighted the importance of the interaction between the IPS and the TPJ in the detection of behaviorally salient events (23). The interaction between these two areas can be split between two proposed FPN systems: the dorsal FPN, which is responsible for the orientation and maintenance of selective attention (26, 68); and the ventral FPN, which acts to direct attention to salient events (23) – and aids in the application of attentional set (69). The dorsal FPN also plays an important role in the synchronization of activity between the visual cortex and other areas of the dorsal FPN as a means of mediating top-down visual attention (69) to exert control over tasks from bottom-up sensory signals (26). It is thought that these networks are co-activated during stimulus-driven reorientation when a salient and behaviorally relevant event occurs, and is highly right-lateralized (69). Differences in integration between these systems of the FPN are evident in the connection between the IPS and TPJ; where the IPS plays a greater role in the dorsal FPN and the TPJ is more involved in the ventral FPN (23, 69). The reduction in the strength in this connection in patients with schizophrenia during attended stimulus change could be interpreted as a relative failure of functional integration between these two regions. Furthermore, a failure of this backward (top-down modulation) in attentional processing of salient events may thus explain why patients with schizophrenia recruit a more complicated connectivity architecture during the processing of visual change. Due to this connection's role in both the dorsal and ventral FPN, we speculate this relative failure in top-down connectivity might contribute to the difficulty that patients with schizophrenia face in modifying behavior in response to salient stimuli, though this requires testing in future studies.

The groups included in this study were well matched in terms of their task performance and demographic variables. Although patients with schizophrenia made slightly fewer correct responses when detecting flickers, the false alarm rate and reaction times were similar to those of the healthy volunteer group, and the average performance in schizophrenia patients exceeded 75%. Despite performing well above chance and close to controls in being able to detect attended stimulus flickers, the activation of the FPN in schizophrenia patients to attended visual change was diminished. The implication of this finding is that the updating of attended information necessary to perform more complex tasks would be compromised due to dysconnectivity within this network, which could account for poor cognitive function more generally.

Table 4 | Connectivity estimates from Bayesian model averaging.

	Group difference statistic	Schizophrenia patients, mean (SD)	Healthy volunteers, mean (SD)
Fixed connections			
Forward			
Right HVA to TPJ	$t(30) = 0.687, P = 0.498$	−0.001 (0.130)	0.037 (0.178)
Left HVA to TPJ	$t(30) = 0.152, P = 0.880$	0.010 (0.179)	0.029 (0.172)
Right TPJ to IPS	$t(30) = 0.854, P = 0.400$	0.030 (0.232)	0.094 (0.192)
Left TPJ to IPS	$t(30) = 0.876, P = 0.388$	0.036 (0.131)	0.090 (0.204)
Right IPS to dACC	$t(30) = 1.678, P = 0.104$	0.065 (0.162)	−0.019 (0.119)
Left IPS to dACC	$t(30) = 2.019, P = 0.052$*	0.062 (0.188)	0.219 (0.240)
Right IPS to vlPFC	$t(30) = 0.932, P = 0.359$	0.118 (0.180)	0.061 (0.163)
Left IPS to vlPFC	$t(30) = 0.758, P = 0.455$	0.085 (0.170)	0.034 (0.206)
Backward			
Right TPJ to HVA	$t(30) = 1.352, P = 0.187$	0.010 (0.208)	−0.097 (0.233)
Left TPJ to HVA	$t(30) = 1.049\ P = 0.302$	0.038 (0.192)	−0.029 (0.172)
Right IPS to TPJ	$t(30) = 0.912, P = 0.514$	0.000 (0.109)	−0.027 (0.125)
Left IPS to TPJ	$t(30) = 0.300, P = 0.766$	0.018 (0.172)	0.003 (0.115)
Right dACC to IPS	$t(30) = 0.946, P = 0.351$	−0.035 (0.124)	0.030 (0.232)
Left dACC to IPS	$t(30) = 0.254, P = 0.801$	0.102 (0.307)	0.078 (0.216)
Right vlPFC to IPS	$t(30) = 1.666, P = 0.106$	0.104 (0.182)	0.004 (0.160)
Left vlPFC to IPS	$t(30) = 0.271, P = 0.788$	0.000 (0.167)	0.016 (0.168)
Lateral			
Right dACC to vlPFC	$t(30) = 0.476, P = 0.638$	−0.031 (0.126)	−0.008 (0.136)
Left dACC to vlPFC	$t(30) = 0.356, P = 0.724$	−0.056 (0.156)	−0.037 (0.150)
Right vlPFC to dACC	$t(30) = 0.425, P = 0.674$	0.034 (0.148)	0.015 (0.106)
Left vlPFC to dACC	$t(30) = 1.070, P = 0.293$	0.013 (0.142)	−0.038 (0.128)
Modulatory connections			
Forward			
Right HVA to TPJ	$t(30) = 0.352, P = 0.728$	−0.043 (0.209)	−0.013 (0.264)
Left HVA to TPJ	$t(30) = 0.725, P = 0.474$	−0.018 (0.255)	0.041 (0.207)
Right TPJ to IPS	$t(30) = 0.857, P = 0.398$	0.009 (0.189)	−0.057 (0.233)
Left TPJ to IPS	$t(30) = 1.165, P = 0.253$	0.014 (0.254)	−0.082 (0.219)
Right IPS to dACC	$t(30) = 1.701, P = 0.099$*	0.019 (0.172)	−0.092 (0.192)
Left IPS to dACC	$t(30) = 0.614, P = 0.544$	0.025 (0.149)	0.059 (0.163)
Right IPS to vlPFC	$t(30) = 1.236, P = 0.226$	0.060 (0.172)	−0.015 (0.166)
Left IPS to vlPFC	$t(30) = 0.087, P = 0.931$	−0.044 (0.200)	−0.050 (0.204)
Backward			
Right TPJ to HVA	$t(30) = 1.445, P = 0.159$	0.073 (0.236)	−0.030 (0.168)
Left TPJ to HVA	$t(30) = 1.002, P = 0.324$	−0.026 (0.254)	0.048 (0.161)
Right IPS to TPJ	$t(30) = 2.428, P = 0.021$**	−0.063 (0.116)	0.036 (0.115)
Left IPS to TPJ	$t(30) = 1.269, P = 0.214$	0.065 (0.188)	−0.010 (0.146)
Right dACC to IPS	$t(30) = 0.567, P = 0.575$	0.006 (0.178)	−0.023 (0.115)
Left dACC to IPS	$t(30) = 1.527, P = 0.137$	−0.017 (0.144)	0.069 (0.169)
Right vlPFC to IPS	$t(30) = 0.174, P = 0.863$	0.042 (0.164)	0.031 (0.178)
Left vlPFC to IPS	$t(30) = 1.133, P = 0.266$	0.053 (0.167)	−0.018 (0.178)
Input			
Right HVA	$t(30) = 1.073, P = 0.292$	−0.107 (0.207)	−0.026 (0.214)
Left HVA	$t(30) = 0.081. P = 0.936$	−0.063 (0.193)	−0.068 (0.168)

HVA, higher visual area; TPJ, temporoparietal junction; IPS, intraparietal sulcus; dACC, dorsal anterior cingulate cortex; vlPFC, ventrolateral prefrontal cortex.

**Trend toward significance ($P < 0.1$).*

***$P < 0.05$.*

Several limitations of our study merit comment. The first is the low number of participants that we were able to include in the final analysis. This affects the statistical sensitivity (Type-II error) of our analyses. It is possible that there are other differences between the groups that we did not have sufficient sensitivity to detect. Second, the relatively preserved task performance we observed is not

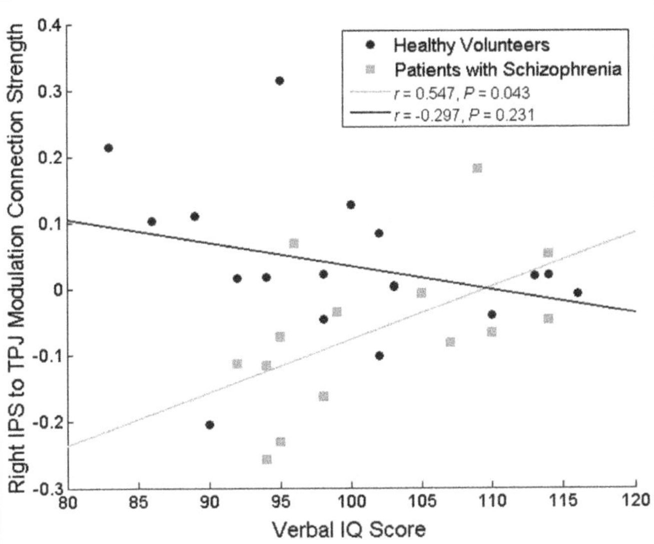

FIGURE 5 | Correlation between the attentional modulation of the IPS to TPJ backward connection and premorbid IQ. This relationship was significant only in patients with schizophrenia.

common to most studies of attention and working memory in schizophrenia (70), and indicates that the patients included in the present study were high-functioning. This subgroup of patients may not exhibit as extreme FPN network dysconnectivity as other groups, which would also raise the chance of Type-II error, and means that our results may not generalize to other schizophrenia patients. Third, patients with schizophrenia did exhibit a slight, non-significant impairment in their ability to detect flickers. It is therefore possible that the results that we report reflect a lack of attentional engagement during the task. However, the presence of a clear VEF in each MEG – as well as concurrent monitoring of eye-gaze – suggests that patients with schizophrenia did indeed engage with the task. Moreover, there was no relationship between DCM parameters and sensitivity to detect flickers. Fourth, all but one of the schizophrenia patients were taking antipsychotic medication, raising the possibility that group differences were either caused by or even masked by medication. A recent paper using DCM supports the latter possibility (71). In that study, both individuals at risk for psychosis and in a first-episode exhibited FPN dysconnectivity (assessed using fMRI); but this was normalized by antipsychotic medication. However, in the present study we did not detect any correlation between chlorpromazine equivalent dosage and behavioral performance or DCM coupling estimates. Finally, it is important to note that these results require replication, especially as the results for the between-group comparison in sensor-space did survive correction for multiple comparisons.

In summary, these data support the notion of FPN dysconnectivity in schizophrenia. This exists despite patients with schizophrenia being able to engage in the task and perform at a high standard on average. This dysconnectivity was mainly reflected in a reduction in top-down connectivity between the right IPS and TPJ in patients when processing attended stimuli. This reduction was associated with low premorbid IQ in the schizophrenia group, and may indicate aberrant integration between the dorsal and ventral components of the FPN. Future work should investigate the association between FPN dysconnection and impairment on specific neurocognitive measures, and assess the impact of antipsychotic medication.

ACKNOWLEDGMENTS

The authors thank John Duncan for helpful discussions. This study was funded by the Wellcome Trust (programme grant 064607/Z/01/Z to EMJ and Principal Research Fellowship 088130/Z/09/Z to KJF), and EMJ was funded by the UCLH Biomedical Research Centre. We are grateful to Isobel Harrison and Libby Matheson from the West London team for help with patient recruitment.

REFERENCES

1. Carroll R. Cognitive impairment in schizophrenia. *Adv Psychiatr Treat* (2000) **6**:161–8. doi:10.1192/apt.6.3.161
2. Morey RA, Inan S, Mitchell TV, Perkins DO, Lieberman JA, Belger A. Imaging frontostriatal function in ultra-high-risk, early, and chronic schizophrenia during executive processing. *Arch Gen Psychiatry* (2005) **62**:254–62. doi:10.1001/archpsyc.62.3.254
3. Dichter GS, Bellion C, Casp M, Belger A. Impaired modulation of attention and emotion in schizophrenia. *Schizophr Bull* (2010) **36**:595–606. doi:10.1093/schbul/sbn118
4. Barch DM, Sheline YI, Csernansky JG, Snyder AZ. Working memory and prefrontal cortex dysfunction: specificity to schizophrenia compared with major depression. *Biol Psychiatry* (2003) **53**:376–84. doi:10.1016/S0006-3223(02)01674-8
5. Manoach DS. Prefrontal cortex dysfunction during working memory performance in schizophrenia: reconciling discrepant findings. *Schizophr Res* (2003) **60**:285–98. doi:10.1016/S0920-9964(02)00294-3
6. Joyce EM, Hutton SB, Mutsatsa SH, Barnes TR. Cognitive heterogeneity in first-episode schizophrenia. *Br J Psychiatry* (2005) **187**:516–22. doi:10.1192/bjp.187.6.516
7. Khandaker GM, Zimbron J, Dalman C, Lewis G, Jones PB. Childhood infection and adult schizophrenia: a meta-analysis of population-based studies. *Schizophr Res* (2012) **139**:161–8. doi:10.1016/j.schres.2012.05.023
8. Leeson VC, Barnes TR, Hutton SB, Ron MA, Joyce EM. IQ as a predictor of functional outcome in schizophrenia: a longitudinal, four-year study of first-episode psychosis. *Schizophr Res* (2009) **107**:55–60. doi:10.1016/j.schres.2008.08.014
9. Chen WJ, Liu SK, Chang CJ, Lien YJ, Chang YH, Hwu HG. Sustained attention deficit and schizotypal personality features in nonpsychotic relatives of schizophrenic patients. *Am J Psychiatry* (1998) **155**:1214–20.
10. Sitskoorn MM, Aleman A, Ebisch SJ, Appels MC, Kahn RS. Cognitive deficits in relatives of patients with schizophrenia: a meta-analysis. *Schizophr Res* (2004) **71**:285–95. doi:10.1016/j.schres.2004.03.007
11. Snitz BE, Macdonald AW III, Carter CS. Cognitive deficits in unaffected first-degree relatives of schizophrenia patients: a meta-analytic review of putative endophenotypes. *Schizophr Bull* (2006) **32**:179–94. doi:10.1093/schbul/sbi048
12. Jabben N, Arts B, Van Os J, Krabbendam L. Neurocognitive functioning as intermediary phenotype and predictor of psychosocial functioning across the psychosis continuum: studies in schizophrenia and bipolar disorder. *J Clin Psychiatry* (2010) **71**:764–74. doi:10.4088/JCP.08m04837yel
13. Montag C, Neuhaus K, Lehmann A, Kruger K, Dziobek I, Heekeren HR, et al. Subtle deficits of cognitive theory of mind in unaffected first-degree relatives of schizophrenia patients. *Eur Arch Psychiatry Clin Neurosci* (2012) **262**:217–26. doi:10.1007/s00406-011-0250-2
14. Scala S, Lasalvia A, Cristofalo D, Bonetto C, Ruggeri M. Neurocognitive profile and its association with psychopathology in first-degree relatives of patients with schizophrenia. A case-control study. *Psychiatry Res* (2012) **200**:137–43. doi:10.1016/j.psychres.2012.05.006
15. Hill SK, Reilly JL, Keefe RS, Gold JM, Bishop JR, Gershon ES, et al. Neuropsychological impairments in schizophrenia and psychotic bipolar disorder: findings

from the bipolar-schizophrenia network on intermediate phenotypes (B-SNIP) study. *Am J Psychiatry* (2013) **170**:1275–84. doi:10.1176/appi.ajp.2013.12101298
16. Perianez JA, Maestu F, Barcelo F, Fernandez A, Amo C, Ortiz Alonso T. Spatiotemporal brain dynamics during preparatory set shifting: MEG evidence. *Neuroimage* (2004) **21**:687–95. doi:10.1016/j.neuroimage.2003.10.008
17. Greenberg AS, Esterman M, Wilson D, Serences JT, Yantis S. Control of spatial and feature-based attention in frontoparietal cortex. *J Neurosci* (2010) **30**:14330–9. doi:10.1523/JNEUROSCI.4248-09.2010
18. Corbetta M, Kincade JM, Ollinger JM, Mcavoy MP, Shulman GL. Voluntary orienting is dissociated from target detection in human posterior parietal cortex. *Nat Neurosci* (2000) **3**:292–7. doi:10.1038/73009
19. Weiss AP, Ellis CB, Roffman JL, Stufflebeam S, Hamalainen MS, Duff M, et al. Aberrant frontoparietal function during recognition memory in schizophrenia: a multimodal neuroimaging investigation. *J Neurosci* (2009) **29**:11347–59. doi:10.1523/JNEUROSCI.0617-09.2009
20. Coull JT, Frith CD, Frackowiak RS, Grasby PM. A fronto-parietal network for rapid visual information processing: a PET study of sustained attention and working memory. *Neuropsychologia* (1996) **34**:1085–95. doi:10.1016/0028-3932(96)00029-2
21. Kanwisher N, Wojciulik E. Visual attention: insights from brain imaging. *Nat Rev Neurosci* (2000) **1**:91–100. doi:10.1038/35040042
22. Kastner S, Ungerleider LG. Mechanisms of visual attention in the human cortex. *Annu Rev Neurosci* (2000) **23**:315–41. doi:10.1146/annurev.neuro.23.1.315
23. Corbetta M, Shulman GL. Control of goal-directed and stimulus-driven attention in the brain. *Nat Rev Neurosci* (2002) **3**:201–15. doi:10.1038/nrn755
24. Duncan J. The multiple-demand (MD) system of the primate brain: mental programs for intelligent behaviour. *Trends Cogn Sci* (2010) **14**:172–9. doi:10.1016/j.tics.2010.01.004
25. Posner MI, Petersen SE. The attention system of the human brain. *Annu Rev Neurosci* (1990) **13**:25–42. doi:10.1146/annurev.ne.13.030190.000325
26. Petersen SE, Posner MI. The attention system of the human brain: 20 years after. *Annu Rev Neurosci* (2012) **35**:73–89. doi:10.1146/annurev-neuro-062111-150525
27. Cole MW, Yarkoni T, Repovs G, Anticevic A, Braver TS. Global connectivity of prefrontal cortex predicts cognitive control and intelligence. *J Neurosci* (2012) **32**:8988–99. doi:10.1523/JNEUROSCI.0536-12.2012
28. Scerif G. Attention trajectories, mechanisms and outcomes: at the interface between developing cognition and environment. *Dev Sci* (2010) **13**:805–12. doi:10.1111/j.1467-7687.2010.01013.x
29. Hon N, Epstein RA, Owen AM, Duncan J. Frontoparietal activity with minimal decision and control. *J Neurosci* (2006) **26**:9805–9. doi:10.1523/JNEUROSCI.3165-06.2006
30. Wang K, Fan J, Dong Y, Wang CQ, Lee TM, Posner MI. Selective impairment of attentional networks of orienting and executive control in schizophrenia. *Schizophr Res* (2005) **78**:235–41. doi:10.1016/j.schres.2005.01.019
31. Backes V, Kellermann T, Voss B, Kramer J, Depner C, Schneider F, et al. Neural correlates of the attention network test in schizophrenia. *Eur Arch Psychiatry Clin Neurosci* (2011) **261**(Suppl 2):S155–60. doi:10.1007/s00406-011-0264-9
32. Minzenberg MJ, Laird AR, Thelen S, Carter CS, Glahn DC. Meta-analysis of 41 functional neuroimaging studies of executive function in schizophrenia. *Arch Gen Psychiatry* (2009) **66**:811–22. doi:10.1001/archgenpsychiatry.2009.91
33. Friston KJ. The disconnection hypothesis. *Schizophr Res* (1998) **30**:115–25. doi:10.1016/S0920-9964(97)00140-0
34. Stephan KE, Baldeweg T, Friston KJ. Synaptic plasticity and dysconnection in schizophrenia. *Biol Psychiatry* (2006) **59**:929–39. doi:10.1016/j.biopsych.2005.10.005
35. Stephan KE, Friston KJ, Frith CD. Dysconnection in schizophrenia: from abnormal synaptic plasticity to failures of self-monitoring. *Schizophr Bull* (2009) **35**:509–27. doi:10.1093/schbul/sbn176
36. Kiebel SJ, Garrido MI, Moran RJ, Friston KJ. Dynamic causal modelling for EEG and MEG. *Cogn Neurodyn* (2008) **2**:121–36. doi:10.1007/s11571-008-9038-0
37. Dima D, Dietrich DE, Dillo W, Emrich HM. Impaired top-down processes in schizophrenia: a DCM study of ERPs. *Neuroimage* (2010) **52**:824–32. doi:10.1016/j.neuroimage.2009.12.086
38. Dima D, Frangou S, Burge L, Braeutigam S, James AC. Abnormal intrinsic and extrinsic connectivity within the magnetic mismatch negativity brain network in schizophrenia: a preliminary study. *Schizophr Res* (2012) **135**:23–7. doi:10.1016/j.schres.2011.12.024
39. Allen P, Stephan KE, Mechelli A, Day F, Ward N, Dalton J, et al. Cingulate activity and fronto-temporal connectivity in people with prodromal signs of psychosis. *Neuroimage* (2010) **49**:947–55. doi:10.1016/j.neuroimage.2009.08.038
40. Dauvermann MR, Whalley HC, Romaniuk L, Valton V, Owens DG, Johnstone EC, et al. The application of nonlinear dynamic causal modelling for fMRI in subjects at high genetic risk of schizophrenia. *Neuroimage* (2013) **73**:16–29. doi:10.1016/j.neuroimage.2013.01.063
41. Schmidt A, Borgwardt S. Abnormal effective connectivity in the psychosis high-risk state. *Neuroimage* (2013) **81**:119–20. doi:10.1016/j.neuroimage.2013.05.035
42. Jablensky A, Mcgrath J, Herrman H, Castle D, Gureje O, Evans M, et al. Psychotic disorders in urban areas: an overview of the study on low prevalence disorders. *Aust N Z J Psychiatry* (2000) **34**:221–36. doi:10.1080/j.1440-1614.2000.00728.x
43. McGuffin P, Farmer A, Harvey I. A polydiagnostic application of operational criteria in studies of psychotic illness. Development and reliability of the OPCRIT system. *Arch Gen Psychiatry* (1991) **48**:764–70. doi:10.1001/archpsyc.1991.01810320088015
44. Wing JK, Babor T, Brugha T, Burke J, Cooper JE, Giel R, et al. SCAN. Schedules for clinical assessment in neuropsychiatry. *Arch Gen Psychiatry* (1990) **47**:589–93. doi:10.1001/archpsyc.1990.01810180089012
45. Sheehan DV, Lecrubier Y, Sheehan KH, Amorim P, Janavs J, Weiller E, et al. The Mini-International Neuropsychiatric Interview (M.I.N.I.): the development and validation of a structured diagnostic psychiatric interview for DSM-IV and ICD-10. *J Clin Psychiatry* (1998) **59**(Suppl 20):22–33.
46. Nelson HE. *The National Adult Reading Test (NART): Test Manual.* Windsor, UK: NFER-Nelson (1982).
47. Wechsler D. *Wechsler Adult Intelligence Scale-Third Edition.* San Antonio, TX: The Psychological Corporation (1997).
48. Andreasen NC. *Scale for the Assessment of Negative Symptoms.* Iowa City: University of Iowa (1983).
49. Andreasen NC. *Scale for the Assessment of Positive Symptoms.* Iowa City: University of Iowa (1984).
50. Kiebel SJ, Garrido MI, Moran R, Chen CC, Friston KJ. Dynamic causal modeling for EEG and MEG. *Hum Brain Mapp* (2009) **30**:1866–76. doi:10.1002/hbm.20775
51. Friston KJ, Harrison L, Penny W. Dynamic causal modelling. *Neuroimage* (2003) **19**:1273–302. doi:10.1016/S1053-8119(03)00202-7
52. Penny WD, Stephan KE, Mechelli A, Friston KJ. Comparing dynamic causal models. *Neuroimage* (2004) **22**:1157–72. doi:10.1016/j.neuroimage.2004.03.026
53. Penny WD, Stephan KE, Daunizeau J, Rosa MJ, Friston KJ, Schofield TM, et al. Comparing families of dynamic causal models. *PLoS Comput Biol* (2010) **6**:e1000709. doi:10.1371/journal.pcbi.1000709
54. Garrido MI, Kilner JM, Kiebel SJ, Stephan KE, Friston KJ. Dynamic causal modelling of evoked potentials: a reproducibility study. *Neuroimage* (2007) **36**:571–80. doi:10.1016/j.neuroimage.2007.03.014
55. Stephan KE, Penny WD, Daunizeau J, Moran RJ, Friston KJ. Bayesian model selection for group studies. *Neuroimage* (2009) **46**:1004–17. doi:10.1016/j.neuroimage.2009.03.025
56. Kasckow JW, Twamley E, Mulchahey JJ, Carroll B, Sabai M, Strakowski SM, et al. Health-related quality of well-being in chronically hospitalized patients with schizophrenia: comparison with matched outpatients. *Psychiatry Res* (2001) **103**:69–78. doi:10.1016/S0165-1781(01)00260-8
57. van der Stelt O, Frye J, Lieberman JA, Belger A. Impaired P3 generation reflects high-level and progressive neurocognitive dysfunction in schizophrenia. *Arch Gen Psychiatry* (2004) **61**:237–48. doi:10.1001/archpsyc.61.3.237
58. Moorhead TW, Stanfield AC, Mckechanie AG, Dauvermann MR, Johnstone EC, Lawrie SM, et al. Longitudinal gray matter change in young people who are at enhanced risk of schizophrenia due to intellectual impairment. *Biol Psychiatry* (2013) **73**:985–92. doi:10.1016/j.biopsych.2012.12.011
59. Gutierrez-Galve L, Wheeler-Kingshott CA, Altmann DR, Price G, Chu EM, Leeson VC, et al. Changes in the frontotemporal cortex and cognitive correlates in first-episode psychosis. *Biol Psychiatry* (2010) **68**:51–60. doi:10.1016/j.biopsych.2010.03.019
60. Joyce EM. Cognitive function in schizophrenia: insights from intelligence research. *Br J Psychiatry* (2013) **203**:161–2. doi:10.1192/bjp.bp.112.109553

61. Bramon E, Rabe-Hesketh S, Sham P, Murray RM, Frangou S. Meta-analysis of the P300 and P50 waveforms in schizophrenia. *Schizophr Res* (2004) **70**:315–29. doi:10.1016/j.schres.2004.01.004
62. Adams RA, Stephan KE, Brown HR, Frith CD, Friston KJ. The computational anatomy of psychosis. *Front Psychiatry* (2013) **4**:47. doi:10.3389/fpsyt.2013.00047
63. Kapur S. Psychosis as a state of aberrant salience: a framework linking biology, phenomenology, and pharmacology in schizophrenia. *Am J Psychiatry* (2003) **160**:13–23. doi:10.1176/appi.ajp.160.1.13
64. Fletcher PC, Frith CD. Perceiving is believing: a Bayesian approach to explaining the positive symptoms of schizophrenia. *Nat Rev Neurosci* (2009) **10**:48–58. doi:10.1038/nrn2536
65. Feldman H, Friston KJ. Attention, uncertainty, and free-energy. *Front Hum Neurosci* (2010) **4**:215. doi:10.3389/fnhum.2010.00215
66. Bastos AM, Usrey WM, Adams RA, Mangun GR, Fries P, Friston KJ. Canonical microcircuits for predictive coding. *Neuron* (2012) **76**:695–711. doi:10.1016/j.neuron.2012.10.038
67. Fries P, Womelsdorf T, Oostenveld R, Desimone R. The effects of visual stimulation and selective visual attention on rhythmic neuronal synchronization in macaque area V4. *J Neurosci* (2008) **28**:4823–35. doi:10.1523/JNEUROSCI.4499-07.2008
68. Shulman GL, Pope DL, Astafiev SV, Mcavoy MP, Snyder AZ, Corbetta M. Right hemisphere dominance during spatial selective attention and target detection occurs outside the dorsal frontoparietal network. *J Neurosci* (2010) **30**:3640–51. doi:10.1523/JNEUROSCI.4085-09.2010
69. Mangun G. *The Neuroscience of Attention.* New York, NY: Oxford University Press, Inc (2012).
70. Joyce EM, Roiser JP. Cognitive heterogeneity in schizophrenia. *Curr Opin Psychiatry* (2007) **20**:268–72. doi:10.1097/YCO.0b013e3280ba4975
71. Schmidt A, Smieskova R, Aston J, Simon A, Allen P, Fusar-Poli P, et al. Brain connectivity abnormalities predating the onset of psychosis: correlation with the effect of medication. *JAMA Psychiatry* (2013) **70**(9):903–12. doi:10.1001/jamapsychiatry.2013.117
72. Woods SW. Chlorpromazine equivalent doses for the newer atypical antipsychotics. *J Clin Psychiatry* (2003) **64**:663–7. doi:10.4088/JCP.v64n0607
73. Bazire S. *Psychotropic Drug Directory 2005: The Professionals' Pocket Handbook and Aide Memoire.* Salisbury, UK: Fivepin Publishing Limited (2005).

Connectivity, Pharmacology and Computation: Toward a Mechanistic Understanding of Neural System Dysfunction in Schizophrenia

Alan Anticevic[1,2,3,4,5,6]*, *Michael W. Cole*[7], *Grega Repovs*[8], *Aleksandar Savic*[9], *Naomi R. Driesen*[1], *Genevieve Yang*[1,4], *Youngsun T. Cho*[1], *John D. Murray*[10], *David C. Glahn*[1,5], *Xiao-Jing Wang*[10] and *John H. Krystal*[1,2,3,11]

[1] Department of Psychiatry, Yale University School of Medicine, New Haven, CT, USA
[2] NIAAA Center for the Translational Neuroscience of Alcoholism, New Haven, CT, USA
[3] Abraham Ribicoff Research Facilities, Connecticut Mental Health Center, New Haven, CT, USA
[4] Interdepartmental Neuroscience Program, Yale University, New Haven, CT, USA
[5] Olin Neuropsychiatry Research Center, Institute of Living, Hartford Hospital, Hartford, CT, USA
[6] Department of Psychology, Yale University, New Haven, CT, USA
[7] Department of Psychology, Washington University in St. Louis, St. Louis, MO, USA
[8] Department of Psychology, University of Ljubljana, Ljubljana, Slovenia
[9] Department of Psychiatry, University of Zagreb School of Medicine, Zagreb, Croatia
[10] Center for Neural Science, New York University, New York, NY, USA
[11] Department of Neurobiology, Yale University School of Medicine, New Haven, CT, USA

Correspondence:
Alan Anticevic, Department of Psychiatry, Yale University, 34 Park Street, New Haven, CT 06519, USA
e-mail: alan.anticevic@yale.edu

Neuropsychiatric diseases such as schizophrenia and bipolar illness alter the structure and function of distributed neural networks. Functional neuroimaging tools have evolved sufficiently to reliably detect system-level disturbances in neural networks. This review focuses on recent findings in schizophrenia and bipolar illness using resting-state neuroimaging, an advantageous approach for biomarker development given its ease of data collection and lack of task-based confounds. These benefits notwithstanding, neuroimaging does not yet allow the evaluation of individual neurons within local circuits, where pharmacological treatments ultimately exert their effects. This limitation constitutes an important obstacle in translating findings from animal research to humans and from healthy humans to patient populations. Integrating new neuroscientific tools may help to bridge some of these gaps. We specifically discuss two complementary approaches. The first is pharmacological manipulations in healthy volunteers, which transiently mimic some cardinal features of psychiatric conditions. We specifically focus on recent neuroimaging studies using the NMDA receptor antagonist, ketamine, to probe glutamate synaptic dysfunction associated with schizophrenia. Second, we discuss the combination of human pharmacological imaging with biophysically informed computational models developed to guide the interpretation of functional imaging studies and to inform the development of pathophysiologic hypotheses. To illustrate this approach, we review clinical investigations in addition to recent findings of how computational modeling has guided inferences drawn from our studies involving ketamine administration to healthy subjects. Thus, this review asserts that linking experimental studies in humans with computational models will advance to effort to bridge cellular, systems, and clinical neuroscience approaches to psychiatric disorders.

Keywords: schizophrenia, pharmacology, functional connectivity, computational modeling, thalamus, NMDA receptors, glutamate

INTRODUCTION

The human brain is a complex, dynamic system with computations occurring at several levels of organization, from individual synapses to networks that span multiple brain regions. These large-scale neural systems ultimately produce complex behaviors that are profoundly altered in the context of psychotropic drug administration or neuropsychiatric disease.

One example is schizophrenia – a common, multi-faceted, and heterogeneous neuropsychiatric syndrome (1) associated with disturbances in perception (2), belief (3), emotion (4), and cognition (5). A number of theoretical models of schizophrenia suggest that the clinical features of this disorder emerge from disturbances in neural connectivity and deficits in synaptic plasticity (6). Progress in explicating the pathophysiology of schizophrenia has been slowed by our limited understanding of the neurobiology of schizophrenia, shortcomings of animal models for this disorder, and the challenge of translating basic and clinical research approaches to this disorder. This knowledge gap has constrained our ability to develop new and more effective pharmacotherapies for schizophrenia (7), accounting for little change in the public health impact of this disease over the past two decades (8).

Disturbances in the structural and functional connectivity of the cerebral cortex are thought to be central to the neurobiology of schizophrenia (6) and are thought to impair the function of large-scale neural systems (9–13). Efforts have been made to reconcile these system-level observations with the cellular neuropathology of schizophrenia. One leading mechanistic model proposes that glutamate synaptic abnormalities associated with schizophrenia, mimicked in part by the effects of drugs that block the *N*-methyl-D-aspartate glutamate receptor (NMDAR) (7), disturb the local balance of excitation and inhibition and thereby contribute to alterations in large-scale neural system functional connectivity (14). This influential hypothesis is based on a key observation: sub-anesthetic doses of non-competitive NMDAR antagonists such as ketamine produce symptoms resembling those of schizophrenia in healthy humans (15). There is also growing evidence from pre-clinical (16), post-mortem (17), neuroimaging (18), and pharmacological experiments (15) illustrating that abnormal NMDA receptor function may be one pathophysiological mechanism occurring in people with schizophrenia. Alterations in synaptic function of gamma-aminobutyric acid (GABA) (19, 20) and dopamine (21) have also been implicated in schizophrenia, which likely affect local circuit computations (22). Collectively, this work provides insight into how disturbances in synaptic glutamate signaling (among other neurotransmitters) could contribute to producing schizophrenia symptoms (7). Nevertheless, there remains an important explanatory gap between mechanistic cellular-level hypotheses of schizophrenia and non-invasive neuroimaging studies that characterize the function of neural systems.

Functional neuroimaging has consistently revealed both region-specific and network alterations in schizophrenia across a number of cognitive measures (23). For instance, there is now substantial evidence suggesting profound alterations in networks supporting complex cognition in schizophrenia [e.g., working memory (WM) (24–26)]. This work has been complemented by a parallel focus on characterizing functional connectivity alterations in schizophrenia (27). Resting-state functional connectivity is based on the analysis of low-frequency fluctuations present in the blood-oxygenation-level-dependent (BOLD) signal (28, 29). These low-frequency fluctuations have been shown to be temporally correlated within spatially distinct but functionally related networks (30), establishing an intrinsic functional architecture (31) across species (32). The functional networks identified at rest also are correlated with other measures of structural and functional connectivity in healthy populations (33) and allow for characterization of distributed circuit abnormalities in neuropsychiatric illness (34, 35). Such approaches have been successfully applied to the study of schizophrenia and have increasingly revealed neuroimaging markers of this complex illness (12, 27, 36–38), which may be consistent with established theoretical models of this disease (39).

This review first focuses on resting-state functional connectivity MRI (rs-fcMRI) studies of schizophrenia that are providing distinct insights into cortical dysfunction associated with this disorder (37, 38). We highlight emerging connectivity strategies that deal with the complexity and heterogeneity of schizophrenia anatomy, physiology, and behavior (40). For instance, we articulate how data-driven tools that capture distributed connectivity abnormalities – such as global brain connectivity (GBC) – have the potential to avoid biases and identify network disturbances that traditional seed-based approaches may fail to detect. We next detail recent specific efforts to assay thalamo-cortical dysfunction in schizophrenia (38), long thought to be important to the clinical features of this disorder (41–43). We also discuss the potential utility of such data-driven approaches to discover variations in large-scale systems that may be altered across diagnostic categories (e.g., bipolar illness with psychosis and schizophrenia) and that may inform symptom-based or circuit-based diagnostic systems, such as the NIMH Research Domain Criteria (RDoC) (44–46).

The encouraging progress in understanding functional connectivity alterations in schizophrenia creates new opportunity to reconcile system-level findings with hypotheses emerging from molecular and cellular studies of this disorder. Failure to integrate these multiple levels of research undermines our understanding of the pathophysiology of this disorder and it will impede medications development. To this end, we next turn to studies using pharmacological models (47), such as the NMDAR antagonist ketamine, to test hypotheses related to the causes of circuit dysfunction in schizophrenia (18). Here we review a focused set of pharmacological neuroimaging (ph-fMRI) studies that utilized NMDAR antagonists to alter behavior and connectivity in healthy volunteers as a way to better understand schizophrenia (18, 48–54). These ph-fMRI investigations provide insight into how specific manipulations of synaptic function have effects that scale to produce both behavioral and system-level alterations that may be observed in patients. We articulate a set of directions for future studies that can capitalize on ph-fMRI as a tool to provide insight into specific illness-related mechanisms, especially when combined with advanced functional connectivity approaches.

Finally, we briefly articulate the utility of neuroscience theory and computational models for iteratively guiding our pharmacological and clinical experiments (55, 56). We focus on one type of computational modeling that may hold promise in this regard – namely, biophysically realistic computational models that contain cellular-level detail necessary to characterize specific synaptic disturbances that may occur in disease states (56, 57). This level of biophysical detail can provide a vital opportunity to test both hypothesized synaptic alterations in schizophrenia (55) and also possible pharmacotherapies that may attenuate such disturbances (58). Despite possible advantages, we note some key limitations of these modeling approaches, pertaining to the constrained behavioral repertoire and neural architectures that are currently effectively modeled in this way, largely owing to gaps in our basic understanding of neurobiology that can constrain such models. Therefore, we articulate a key objective for the future of schizophrenia research: biophysically realistic computational models need to be systematically developed and scaled to the level of neural systems (59), to inform fMRI-level observations in schizophrenia as well as those observed following pharmacological manipulations in healthy humans (**Figure 1**). We argue that this approach could be especially productive for the study of functional connectivity in psychiatric conditions, with the

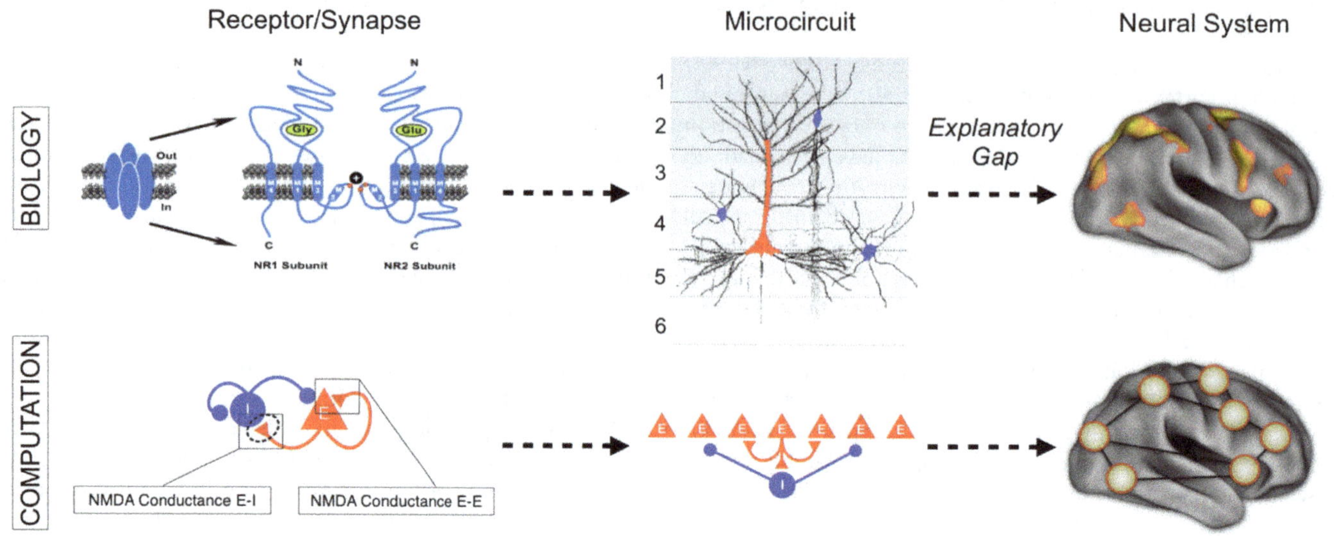

FIGURE 1 | Understanding complex mental illness from synapses to circuits to neural systems. A major challenge facing the field of clinical neuroscience is building the links across levels of inquiry, from the level of receptors and cells, to microcircuits, and ultimately scale to the level of neural systems and behavior. At present, there is a vast explanatory gap across these levels in our understanding of psychiatric symptoms (top panel). Bridging this gap represents a major effort in explaining how alterations of specific mechanisms across neural systems may produce complex behavioral alterations seen in serious mental illness. This challenge is also exemplified by the National Institute of Mental Health Research Domain Criteria (RDoC) initiative (45) in order to map the biology across levels of inquiry onto behavior in a more systematic and data-driven way. We argue that computational modeling approaches (55) combined with additional experimental tools such as functional neuroimaging and pharmacology (47) offer one possible path toward this objective (bottom panel). We detail emerging efforts in functional connectivity work that may present a unique opportunity in this regard (59). Note: top left receptor figure was adapted with permission from Kotermanski and Johnson (60).

ultimate aim of developing mechanistically derived biomarker predictions.

Building on these insights, we emphasize the need for efforts to translate our basic discoveries in neuroscience and cellular-level hypotheses in schizophrenia with system-level observations that may directly relate to the complex behavioral abnormalities observed in this illness. We highlight multiple complementary neuroscientific approaches, including recent clinical studies (37), pharmacological neuroimaging experiments (54), and theoretical/computational neuroscience approaches (18, 58) that can be synergistically harnessed to inform our understanding of underlying mechanisms and guide development of better pharmacotherapies for schizophrenia.

DEVELOPMENTS IN FUNCTIONAL CONNECTIVITY APPLICATIONS TO NEUROPSYCHIATRIC DISEASE

Nearly two decades ago Biswal and colleagues (61) demonstrated that coherent fluctuations in the BOLD signal exist across time and space, demarcating a functional network architecture in the human brain. Such early studies highlighted this phenomenon by focusing on the fluctuations between the left and right motor cortex. This key property of the BOLD signal has in turn generated a paradigm shift in non-invasive human neuroimaging and allowed for characterization of distributed neural networks across species in the absence of task-mediated effects (28–30, 32, 62). Importantly, a close correspondence between resting-state networks and task-based networks has been established within individual subjects and using meta-analytic techniques (31). The value of this approach has been enhanced by the subsequent emergence of analytic techniques that have provided insights into the component structure and regulation of distributed cortical networks (62). For instance, recent advances in graph-theoretical approaches have shown that cortical and subcortical networks can be segregated into unique community structures, providing a comprehensive data-driven mapping of human functional networks (63). Another set of studies has demonstrated the temporal non-stationary properties of the large-scale functional networks, delineating temporal functional modes of the human brain (64). In other words, there seem to be distinct and independent patterns of connectivity over both space and time. Although a comprehensive review of connectivity method developments is beyond the scope of this manuscript, we refer the reader to recent detailed reports on this topic (62). Here we specifically focus on select clinical applications in schizophrenia and bipolar illness.

Resting-state functional connectivity MRI approaches have been increasingly applied to neuropsychiatric illness (65). Use of this technique is built upon the hypothesis that specific neuropsychiatric conditions are brain disorders that affect computations across large-scale networks of regions or specific circuits in such a way that these alterations can be identified with functional connectivity measures. This hypothesis suggests that such disturbances in neural network function may reflect alterations in more basic cellular-level mechanisms. Thus, disturbances in molecular signaling or synaptic function would be hypothesized to scale and produce disturbances in large-scale neural systems (66). Such network-level disturbances in a given functional system may then reflect specific psychiatric symptoms (12, 27). This framework has guided the application of functional connectivity with the objective of identifying putative biomarkers via BOLD fMRI that could reveal neural system-level disturbances in neuropsychiatric conditions even in the absence of specific tasks. Such an approach may hold promise if its sensitivity and specificity is ultimately refined to the point of diagnostic utility.

Specific advantages of rs-fcMRI include: (i) speed, as the functional network architecture can be reliably assayed within 10 min of data acquisition (67), and perhaps even faster with recent advances in multi-band imaging technology (68, 69); (ii) possible cost-effectiveness. Task-based studies may require longer time for data acquisition, depending on the precise paradigm being imaged. (iii) Lack of performance confounds, which likely affects nearly every cognitive activation task when applied to a psychiatric population (70). (iv) In addition, when coupled with techniques such as GBC or independent component analyses (ICA), rs-fcMRI studies allow the unbiased, simultaneous examination of all neural networks (see below for more discussion). All of these features suggest that rs-fcMRI may be a feasible method for eventually guiding and tracking symptoms, illness progression and possibly response to pharmacotherapies and/or behavioral treatments.

The approach itself, however, is not without limitations. For instance, the size of the correlation coefficient is often used to examine the strength of coupling between different network nodes (71). While this is an analysis-level consideration, the majority of published studies use this technique. This approach may not be ideal for examining shared versus non-shared variance between regions and may obscure more complex differences that could occur in psychiatric conditions (71). For instance, it may be important to uniquely identify functional connectivity alterations that truly reflect altered neuronal communication between two network nodes, as opposed to the influence of a third region on both (a correlation-based approach could not disambiguate these possibilities). It is also important to emphasize that functional connectivity, as measured at rest, is purely correlational and therefore can only be used to make tentative causal inferences. That is, if there is evidence for an alteration in a given circuit, this alteration could be predictive of disease onset or could be a consequence of some upstream physiological alteration. Moreover, there are additional complications involved in the study of neuropsychiatric illness concerning what is a primary deficit, as opposed to a compensation or treatment effects. These potential confounds underscore the complementary value of causal experimental designs involving pharmacologic, neuro-stimulation, or cognitive manipulations of circuit activity. Finally, there are still notable differences in the methods used to analyze rs-fcMRI data. For instance, one ongoing controversial issue relates to removal of the global signal (i.e., global signal regression, GSR) from functional connectivity data (72, 73). This step effectively regresses out variance associated with global brain fluctuations, which can be large in magnitude and can perhaps obscure certain real functional relationships (74). Nonetheless, this step effectively shifts the mean of the connectivity distribution, resulting in a portion of correlations being moved into the negative range – thus spuriously inducing at least some anti-correlations. There is convincing evidence from electrophysiology experiments using animals that anti-correlations indeed exist (75, 76). However, GSR could still complicate some aspects of between-group comparisons and the interpretations of clinical studies (73), especially when examining system-level relationships across groups. Therefore, future studies should carefully continue to consider the possible impact of this step on between-group differences in clinical rs-fcMRI studies.

Another methodological issue pertains to how networks are identified. Many early functional connectivity studies both in healthy adults and in clinical populations used a seed-based approach, whereby the correlation from a given region of interest is examined with all other voxels in the brain. This approach has also been complemented by more complex graph theoretical and network-based methods (77). Seed-based approaches inherently assume a consistent difference across a set of regions in a clinical condition. However, the pattern of dysconnectivity for a single region could indeed be more variable both across subjects and within regions. Such spatial variability in functional networks across subjects may present a limitation of seed-based approaches when applied in studies of clinical populations (11, 40). This may be the case in complex mental illnesses such as schizophrenia. Therefore, detecting more complex patterns of dysconnectivity requires new approaches taking into account these confounds (78–80).

New methods are needed to detect more complex patterns of disorder-related disturbances in connectivity (80), illustrated by the GBC approach (11, 35, 40, 81). The GBC technique is specifically designed to consider connectivity from a given voxel or (area) to all other voxels (or areas) simultaneously by computing either average connectivity strength (weighted GBC) or by counting the number of connections above a given connection strength (unweighted GBC). Thus, this approach is data-driven and unbiased as to the location of connectivity disruption. That is, unlike typical seed-based approaches, GBC requires only the seed region to be relatively consistently located across subjects, while the target regions can vary substantially across subjects (**Figure 2**). For example, if a given area is perturbed in its functional connectivity consistently, irrespective of the overall network spatial configuration where the perturbation is, GBC will remain sensitive to this alteration. Further, unlike typical seed-based approaches, GBC involves one statistical test per voxel (or ROI) rather than one test per voxel-to-voxel pairing – substantially reducing multiple comparisons (e.g., 30,000 rather than ~900 million tests). These two improvements over typical seed-based approaches can dramatically increase the chance of identifying group differences in connectivity, or individual differences in connectivity correlated with behavioral symptoms (11, 35, 40, 81). Indeed, consistent with these proposed advantages, GBC has now been applied to identifying regions with large-scale disruptions in functional connectivity across a variety of mental illnesses, such as schizophrenia (11), bipolar disorder (35), and obsessive-compulsive disorder (OCD) (82). GBC is explicitly designed to address questions about brain connectivity that are qualitatively distinct from traditional seed-based functional connectivity analyses. For instance, areas of high GBC are "hubs" of connectivity in the brain that are maximally functionally connected with other areas and may play a role in coordinating large-scale patterns of brain activity (40). In that sense, a group difference in GBC may reflect areas and networks

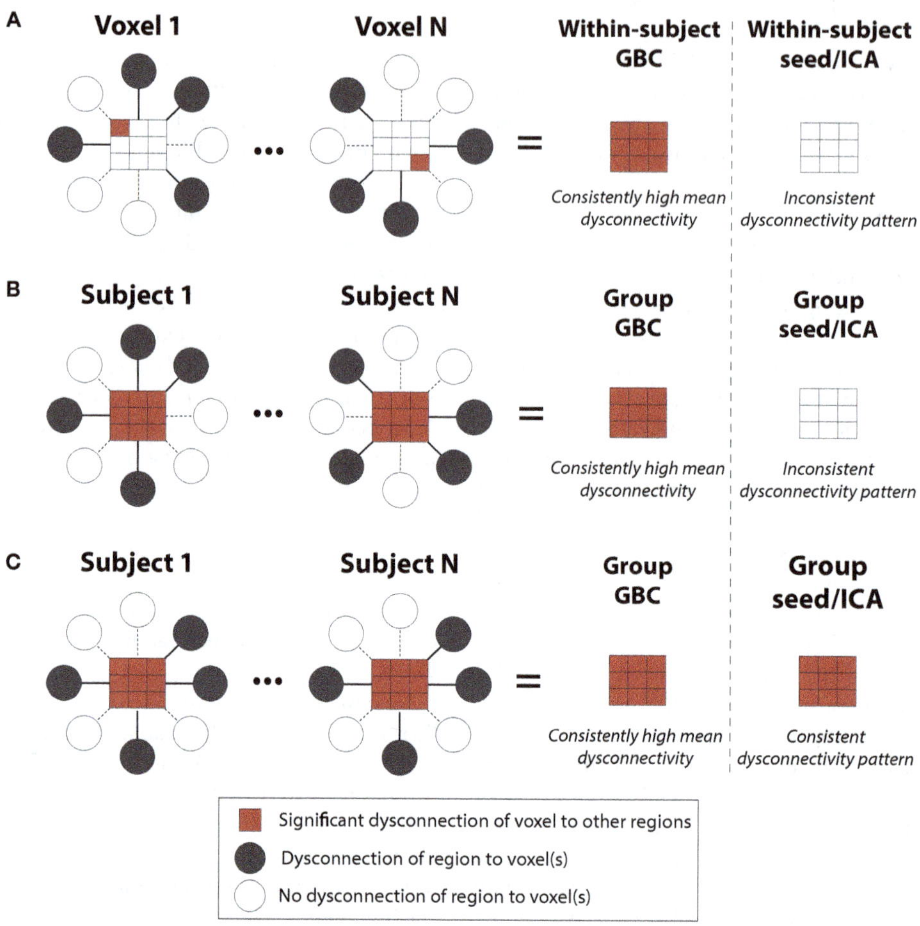

FIGURE 2 | Global brain connectivity identifies globally dysconnected regions despite substantial within or between subject variability. We hypothesized that some brain regions may have global variable disruptions in functional connectivity, which may contribute to individual differences in symptom severity in brain disorders. GBC can be used as a data-driven approach to search for such regions. GBC is computed as the average connectivity of each voxel to all others. Gray circles indicate regions with altered connectivity to the depicted red voxels. **(A)** GBC will identify a region with consistent global dysconnectivity even when there are substantial differences in connectivity patterns within the region. Seed or ICA approaches would be unable to identify dysconnectivity in such a region because of inconsistent dysconnectivity patterns across neighboring voxels. **(B)** GBC, unlike seed or ICA approaches, will identify a region with consistent global dysconnectivity even when there are substantial individual differences in connectivity across subjects. This allows the identification of regions with many individual differences in connectivity, which might correlate with individual differences in symptoms. **(C)** GBC is also sensitive to consistent group differences in connectivity that might be identified using seed or ICA approaches, though GBC might be more sensitive due to pooling of results for both consistent and inconsistent dysconnectivity. GBC, global brain connectivity; ICA, independent component analysis. Note: figure adapted with permission from Cole and colleagues (11).

in which the large-scale coordination of information processing is affected in the disease state. For instance, decreased GBC may reflect decreased participation of a brain region in broader networks. Conversely, increased GBC may suggest a pathological broadening or synchronization of functional networks. Related to this point, we have now published a manuscript examining distributed networks in OCD using GBC where specific striatal and orbitofrontal circuits have been implicated. Yet, GBC remains sensitive to alterations in neuropsychiatric conditions that may actually be associated with more focal deficits (which may be the case in OCD versus schizophrenia). In that sense, GBC is not necessarily more useful for "global" versus "restricted" deficits, but rather dysconnectivity to a given "hub" region that may be affected in its participation in wide-spread neural networks. These properties of GBC – detection of regions with large-scale functional connectivity disruptions along with tolerance for individual differences – makes this method particularly powerful for identifying regions with consistently large and distributed disruptions that have functional consequences reflected in individual differences in psychiatric symptoms. Continued refinement of graph-theoretical data-driven metrics such as GBC may allow a powerful path forward for delineating biomarkers within and across diagnostic categories.

Another data-driven method that has increasing applications in psychiatric neuroimaging involves ICA of BOLD signal fluctuations at rest. Here ICA provides a tool to identify spatially (78, 83) or temporally (64) independent modes of brain function. ICA has been successfully used to identify distributed network abnormalities in both schizophrenia and bipolar illness (84). In particular, temporal ICA (64) may provide a novel and powerful method to assay the non-stationary properties of distributed neural systems across different clinical conditions. It remains to be systematically tested if recently defined temporal functional modes exhibit alterations in neuropsychiatric illness. One possibility, given wide-spread neurotransmitter disruptions in schizophrenia, is that the temporal functional modes are substantially more non-stationary in this illness. Powerful new acquisition sequences [e.g., multi-band imaging (68)], that allow much finer temporal sampling, will provide critical technological innovations at the level of neuroimaging acquisition with direct clinical applications, in particular when using ICA-type measures.

Collectively, the continued success of these methods suggests that ongoing refinement of tools to examine functional connectivity remains vital for development of biomarkers for psychiatric illness. Next, we turn to specific findings in the field of schizophrenia and bipolar research. We detail recent methodological advances in connectivity work that have been directly applied to better understand network disruption in these psychiatric conditions.

EMERGING EVIDENCE SUGGESTS LARGE-SCALE DYSCONNECTIVITY IN SCHIZOPHRENIA

There are now a number of influential hypotheses suggesting that, at its core, schizophrenia may be a disorder of large-scale neural connectivity (6, 85), i.e., "dysconnectivity." Here we refer to dysconnectivity as an alteration in neural communication that specifically produces behavioral pathology, as opposed to a simple alteration in functional connectivity that deviates from the norm. The models proposing such dysconnectivity range from theoretical to formal computational hypotheses (42, 43, 66, 86–88). This work has inspired the search for connectivity biomarkers for schizophrenia and it broadly includes: (i) studies that use rs-fcMRI, that is investigations that study the intrinsic properties of BOLD signal fluctuations to delineate system-level alterations in psychiatric illness (27); (ii) studies that examine task-based dysconnectivity, that is alterations in connectivity during specific task contexts; (iii) pharmacological studies of individuals at rest or performing tasks, which we discuss in the upcoming section. While the literature on task-based connectivity has offered important clues regarding network alterations during specific cognitive processes (e.g., WM) (27, 89, 90), here we specifically detail emerging efforts to use rs-fcMRI to define biomarkers for schizophrenia. This is not to say that characterizing functional connectivity during cognitive processing is not important. In fact, such studies represent a vital effort to move our understanding beyond activation-based hypotheses regarding cognitive deficits in schizophrenia or regional hypotheses of specific symptoms. In the future, task-based functional connectivity studies will ultimately aid our understanding of network dysfunction with respect to specific symptoms or specific cognitive processes known to be profoundly affected in schizophrenia (e.g., WM) (26). Additionally, task-based studies of functional connectivity provide an important assurance that observed differences in resting-state functional connectivity do not merely reflect differences in the dynamics and content of mental processes subjects might engage in during rest, but rather stable disruptions in functional connectivity that persist across mental states (90). However, rs-fcMRI can be used to identify neural-system alterations even more broadly. With that in mind, we argue that rs-fcMRI offers a unique tool to identify distributed neural system alterations, extending beyond a given task context. Moreover, as noted above, this approach in particular bypasses task performance confounds which plague the task-based activation literature (70) and such concerns will likely extend to task-based connectivity work.

Despite its promise, a major obstacle in delineating successful neural markers for schizophrenia (or any other severe neuropsychiatric disease) using connectivity (or any other approach for that matter) has been the complexity of this illness and the vast range of behaviors it affects (91), as well as the complex temporal dynamics of its progression. That is, the apparent clinical complexity of schizophrenia is a major obstacle to biomarker development that may apply to all patients. In addition, the associated clinical heterogeneity (i.e., differences in symptoms across patients), the presence of numerous comorbidities and environmental modifiers, the ubiquitous confound of long-term antipsychotic treatment, and the wide range of affected behaviors collectively reduce the likelihood that a single biomarker would be applicable to the entire syndrome. Moreover, many researchers and clinicians would argue that schizophrenia is a theoretical construct used to label co-occurring symptoms whereby it may be challenging (or perhaps impossible) to map out a reliable and replicable marker of the entire syndrome in a parsimonious way [although theoretical models of the disease often consider it as one entity (66)]. We argue that functional connectivity tools offer a useful path forward in this regard by providing methods to test specific large-scale dysconnectivity patterns in relation to this heterogeneity that may be otherwise difficult to capture.

Certain studies using rs-fcMRI have, however, attempted to deal with clinical heterogeneity by focusing on the relationship between altered functional connectivity in specific pathways and linking those pathways to particular features of schizophrenia. For instance, studies by Hoffmann and colleagues have focused on better understanding alterations in connectivity specifically associated with auditory hallucinations (92), which many patients experience (1). They found compelling evidence for disruptions between regions associated with auditory processing. Specifically, they found that when they seeded Wernicke's area, there was significantly greater functional connectivity to Brodmann's areas 45/46 among hallucinating patients compared with non-hallucinating patients. In a subsequent analysis, they reported that the functional connectivity within a functional loop including the Wernicke's area, inferior frontal gyrus, and putamen was robustly greater for hallucinating patients compared with non-hallucinating patients. Vercammen and colleagues also found that patients with schizophrenia evidenced attenuated functional connectivity between the left TPJ (temporo-parietal junction) and the right Broca's area (93). These are examples where targeted seed-based approaches may identify alterations in circumscribed circuits associated with specific symptoms.

Another set of emerging studies have studied the "salience" and "control" systems, focused on striatal and insular dysconnectivity in schizophrenia (94, 95), particularly in relation to the "aberrant salience" hypothesis (96, 97). Briefly, the "aberrant salience" hypothesis has been linked to abnormal striatal dopamine function, suggesting that during psychotic states patients have a higher likelihood of forming inappropriate associations and respond excessively to random neutral events. Related to this issue a study by Tu and colleagues examined whether schizophrenia is associated with functional connectivity alterations within the cingulo-opercular (CO) network specifically (98). They identified significantly reduced functional connectivity in the bilateral putamen for patients with schizophrenia, which was related to cognitive performance in patients. The authors concluded that schizophrenia is associated with disconnection within cortico-striatal circuits. A complementary study by Moran and colleagues (99) focused on the anterior insula as a key node involved in modulation of distributed neural systems (as part of the CO system). The authors tested for disruptions in the functional relationships between the insula and control/default networks in patients with schizophrenia. Similarly, they examined a relationship between these network disturbances and cognitive deficits. Consistent with *a priori* predictions, Moran and colleagues found strong support for the disrupted relationship between the anterior insula and the control-executive and default-mode networks in schizophrenia, which again was predictive of cognitive performance. Most recently, a study by Palaniyappan and colleagues (100) also focused on the relationship between the salience (insular) system and the executive [lateral prefrontal cortex (PFC)] networks in schizophrenia. They explicitly tested for evidence of disrupted directional influence across the networks. In other words, similar to Moran and colleagues, they used an auto-regressive technique (i.e., Granger causality) to examine both feed-forward and reciprocal connectivity between the aforementioned networks. The authors reported significant differences in patients with regard to time-lagged functional relationships between executive and insular systems. The authors conclude that this "breakdown" in directional functional relationships may reflect aberrant processing of novel salient information. These studies provide compelling emerging evidence that there may indeed exist causal breakdowns across functional networks in schizophrenia. Nevertheless, it is important to note that lag-based causality measures in the context of BOLD signal analyses have not been without controversy (101–103), primarily because of systematic difference in the hemodynamic response function lags across areas. Given these concerns, the use of Granger causality in rs-fcMRI studies needs to be interpreted with caution [see Ref. (104) for a more detailed treatment of using auto-regression techniques with the BOLD signal]. Future studies using concurrent electrophysiology/fMRI protocols could provide convergent evidence to address issues regarding temporal dependencies across cortical networks when analyzing the BOLD signal.

We discussed studies that focused on either specific regions or networks that may be abnormal in schizophrenia. An alternative tactic, precisely because of the complexity of this illness, is to use data-driven methods to study large-scale connectivity alterations that may be difficult to pinpoint *a priori*. A number of prominent and well-established models of schizophrenia neuropathology implicate profound disruptions in PFC function (105), likely stemming from a confluence of glutamate, GABA, and dopamine alterations that could jointly affect PFC function (7, 19, 106–108) (see **Box 1**). One area that has been repeatedly implicated in schizophrenia neuropathology is the dorso-lateral PFC (23). However, this evidence has largely been marshaled through task-based studies such as those examining WM deficits in this illness (70). A deficit in task-evoked computations of a given region does not necessarily guarantee that the same node will show other forms of functional "dysconnectivity." Moreover, such evidence does not guarantee that this same area may be disrupted in its functional connectivity in the absence of a task (i.e., during resting-state). Nevertheless, PFC functional deficits have been considered a hallmark feature of the illness. Therefore, one promising approach is to examine global PFC dysconnectivity in a data-driven way.

As articulated above, the GBC functional connectivity approach is specifically designed to test the hypothesis that a given functional brain region has altered coupling with the rest of the brain (or a large anatomical portion of the brain, such as the PFC). To test the efficacy of this approach, Cole and colleagues (11) used a restricted GBC (rGBC) approach focused on PFC in particular in a sample of patients with chronic schizophrenia relative to demographically matched healthy comparison subjects. Cole and colleagues reported that bilateral regions centered on the lateral PFC showed reductions in their PFC rGBC, suggesting that these regions have profound alterations in their connectivity patterns with the rest of PFC. To further test the relationship between identified PFC rGBC alterations and cognitive deficits, Cole and colleagues quantified the relationship between IQ and the PFC global connectivity alterations. The authors found that greater connectivity between the identified lateral PFC and the rest of PFC predicted better cognitive performance, suggesting that a lower index of global PFC coupling may in part relate to cognitive deficits in schizophrenia. Moreover, the authors additionally examined the pattern of whole-brain coupling of the discovered right lateral PFC region using seed-based techniques. The authors found that patients diagnosed with schizophrenia showed increased coupling with sensory cortices (**Figure 3B**, posterior regions, shown in yellow-red). Patients also showed reduced connectivity with prefrontal and other higher-order temporal regions (**Figure 3B**, shown in blue). Collectively, this initial report demonstrates that data-driven functional connectivity approaches could identify regions previously implicated in schizophrenia using task-based methods. Moreover, these identified areas showed robust and complex alterations of connectivity with the rest of the brain and importantly, related to observed symptoms and other cognitive measures.

Similar data-driven efforts have been applied to study global connectivity alterations in other psychiatric conditions. Specifically, Anticevic and colleagues extended the approach to study bipolar patients with and without a history of psychotic symptoms (35). While examining neural system-level disturbances in schizophrenia is a vital objective, psychosis occurs across a number of diagnostic categories. For instance, many bipolar patients experience frank psychosis (121). Given this clinical observation, some studies divide bipolar patients based on the presence or absence of psychotic symptoms (122, 123). In that sense, there may be somewhat limited utility in predefined diagnostic boundaries for understanding variation in neural circuits that could possibly be affected across neuropsychiatric conditions (45). Recognizing this

Box 1 | Glutamate versus dopamine: upstream versus down-stream mechanisms in schizophrenia.

It is increasingly acknowledged that schizophrenia is associated with disturbances in multiple neurotransmitter systems, including alterations at the cortical microcircuit level in glutamate and γ-aminobutyric acid (GABA), as well as disturbances in dopaminergic neurotransmission along striatal-thalamic-cortical pathways (7, 106, 109). Additional studies have also implicated the glial system as possibly compromised in schizophrenia (110, 111) and other neuropsychiatric conditions (112). However, it remains unknown whether dopamine or glutamate alterations are the upstream causes or down-stream consequences of the disease process (109). Addressing this question has important implications for appropriately constraining computational models, both at the microcircuit level (58) and expanding those mechanisms to the system-level (18). There are two broad possibilities to consider: (i) there may be dissociable groups of patients each associated with a primary abnormality in one of the broad neurotransmitter systems, but as a consequence there may be secondary abnormalities in the other system due to shared pathways and functional loops (43, 88). (ii) One alternative possibility is that there are always primary alterations in only one of the two systems, followed by alterations in the other. Disambiguating between these causal possibilities can have important implications for developing optimized targeted pharmacotherapies for specific patient groups, which is a likely possibility given the heterogeneity of the illness. By extension, resolving these issues may have implications for optimized pharmacotherapies for a given phase of illness [if initial stages of schizophrenia are primary associated with hyper-glutamatergic neurotransmission (113)]. Also, these two possibilities have important implications for the utility of pharmacological models of psychosis (e.g., amphetamine versus the NMDAR antagonist challenge studies in healthy volunteers).

Here it is important to consider some key differences between the dopamine and glutamate hypotheses in schizophrenia in relation to pharmacological findings and their therapeutic effects: (i) dopaminergic medication has not proved successful at ameliorating the full range of impairing symptoms in schizophrenia, particularly cognitive deficits (26); (ii) pharmacological models of schizophrenia targeting the dopamine system (e.g., amphetamine challenge) have typically produced a clinical profile marked by acute psychosis, as opposed to a broader range of symptoms produced by pharmacological agents targeting the glutamate system (15, 114, 115). Therefore, while it is certainly important to acknowledge dopamine as a key component of disrupted neurotransmission in schizophrenia (21, 116, 117), it remains to be determined if dopamine is indeed a down-stream cause or a consequence of primary disruptions in glutamate (118). Relatedly, irrespective of cause or consequence arguments it will vital to consider the diversity of DA receptors (D1 versus D2) and their respective sites of influence in cortex (22, 119, 120) versus striatum (108), which in turn generates important constraints for computational modeling studies that incorporate dopaminergic and glutamatergic signaling mechanisms.

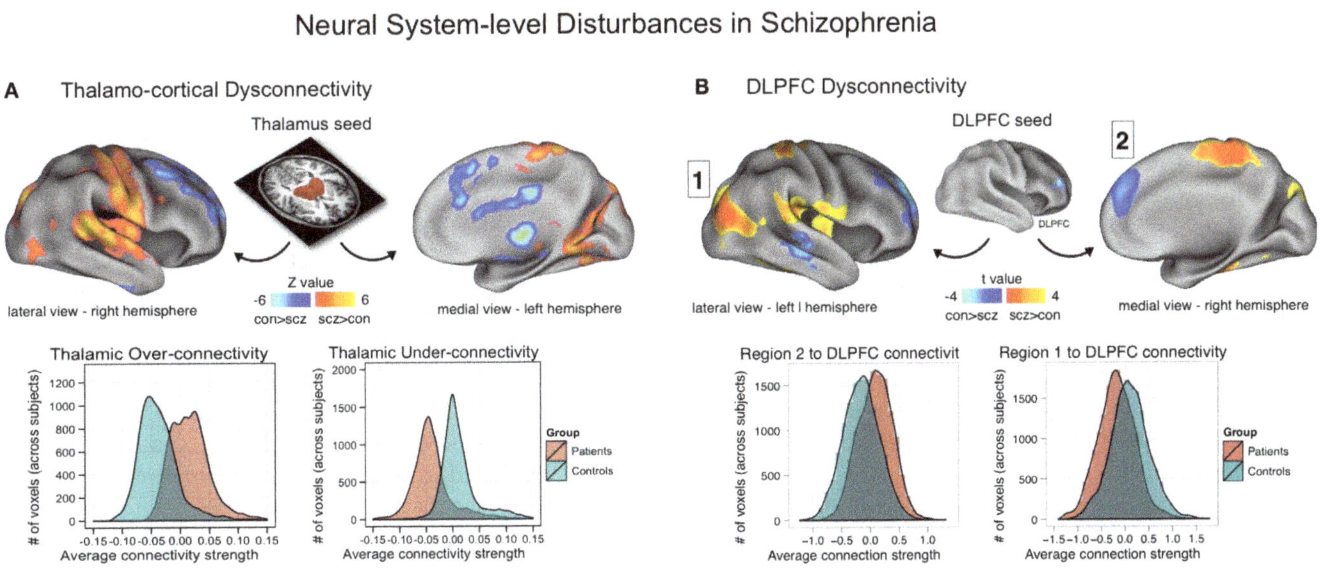

FIGURE 3 | Neural system-level dysconnectivity in schizophrenia – emerging biomarkers. (A) Results from a recent large connectivity investigation examining thalamo-cortical connectivity alterations in 90 patients diagnosed with schizophrenia relative to 90 matched healthy controls (38). Anticevic and colleagues found robust alterations in thalamo-cortical information flow in schizophrenia, whereby sensory-motor cortical regions showed over-connectivity in schizophrenia (regions shown in yellow-red), but prefrontal-striatal-cerebellar regions showed under connectivity in schizophrenia relative to controls (regions shown in blue). Anticevic and colleagues fully replicated this pattern in an independent sample. Woodward and colleagues, using complementary approaches, found highly comparable effects (37). **(B)** A similar pattern of over/under connectivity was identified in patients with schizophrenia when using a DLPFC seed region identified via GBC; as with the thalamic seed, there was increased coupling with sensory (posterior regions, shown in yellow-red) but reduced connectivity with prefrontal and other higher-order temporal regions (shown in blue). This over/under pattern recapitulated qualitatively the observations found for the thalamic analysis in **(A)**, as shown in the distribution plots on the bottom of each panel. Note: figures adapted with permission from Anticevic and colleagues (38) and Cole and colleagues (11).

limitation, there are emerging efforts to map common aspects of neural dysfunction across diagnostic categories.

Focusing on bipolar illness, Anticevic and colleagues examined the possibility that there are similar abnormalities in bipolar illness with a history of psychosis to those found in schizophrenia. Consistent with this hypothesis, Anticevic and colleagues found that bipolar illness is indeed associated with altered PFC rGBC specifically in a medial prefrontal/ventral cingulate region implicated in regulation of emotion (35). Importantly, this effect was primarily driven by a presence of psychosis history, and the magnitude of the observed PFC rGBC disruption was correlated with the severity of prior psychosis. This effect, however, was obtained in euthymic bipolar individuals (as opposed to symptomatic schizophrenia patients above), which suggests that at least some alterations in global connectivity may be a stable (trait) feature of the illness and may not necessarily only manifest in overtly symptomatic individuals. In that sense, data-driven functional connectivity may provide a tool to examine individual variability in both current and/or lifetime symptoms. Such data-driven approaches can also be used to establish alterations in functional neural architecture over time – namely, whether the observed disruptions in schizophrenia and bipolar illness change longitudinally as the illness progresses. This possibility is consistent with prominent neurodevelopmental models of severe psychiatric illness (14, 124–126), which suggest that there may be profound functional changes along the illness progression, to which these tools may be sensitive.

While promising, a key challenge facing data-driven approaches will be to establish whether identified effects consistently replicate across sites and samples. It may be possible that illness sample heterogeneity, illness stage, symptom severity, anatomical heterogeneity, or other factors will critically impact the patterns of data-driven effects across studies and samples. That is, it may be possible that different foci are detected as showing disruptions in different samples. Therefore, it will be critical to determine which of the identified data-driven global connectivity alterations are stable and replicable (perhaps capturing some core disturbances) and which alter as a function of other variables (perhaps capturing state effects). Such ongoing data-driven efforts should also continue to capitalize on recent advances in graph theory (80) as well as neuroimaging acquisition-level improvements (64, 69, 127) which could jointly improve the sensitivity of resting-state connectivity-derived metrics.

As described above, the PFC has been repeatedly implicated in schizophrenia neuropathology. However, despite data-driven efforts to map PFC dysfunction, the PFC remains a challenge in the study of schizophrenia, owing largely to the complex individual differences in function and anatomy of the PFC. Therefore, to ultimately establish a viable large-scale, brain-wide marker of neural alterations in schizophrenia, an alternative approach can be taken. One possible path is to start from the thalamus as a key region of interest (42). That is, while the PFC has classically been implicated in schizophrenia neuropathology, recent studies highlight disturbances in additional neural foci. In particular, the thalamus has emerged as an important disrupted locus in schizophrenia. While we presented some arguments against using seed-based approaches, the thalamus may present a unique opportunity in this case. Here we argue for the utility of specifying a seed when there is a specific theoretically guided hypothesis implicating a given area in the disease process. In this case, examining thalamic connectivity using rs-fcMRI in schizophrenia capitalizes on several key aspects of this subcortical region: (i) the thalamus is topographically connected to the entire cortex (128, 129), and may therefore represent a node particularly sensitive to network-level disturbances (42); and (ii) the thalamus contains anatomically and functionally segregated nuclei readily identifiable via neuroimaging (130) thus providing a lens for examining parallel yet distributed large-scale connectivity disturbances in neuropsychiatric disease.

Consistent with this view, a large body of evidence implicates significant thalamo-cortical communication disturbances in schizophrenia neuropathology (41, 42, 131–134). In fact, a fundamental aspect of large-scale brain organization preserved across mammalian species is thalamo-cortico-striatal sub-circuits that are thought to integrate various functions such as emotion processing and motor output (135–138). Such circuits may become profoundly dysregulated in schizophrenia, and the thalamus, as an organized hub of cortical and subcortical connections, may be especially sensitive to such dysregulation. Essentially, the thalamus serves as a nexus for parallel circuits through which diverse cortical and subcortical functions are integrated and distributed throughout the cortical mantle (128, 139, 140). These thalamic circuits have been implicated in schizophrenia pathophysiology on the basis of neuropathology studies (88, 141–143), pre-clinical lesion models (144, 145), structural imaging studies (146, 147), and computational models (43). Moreover, thalamic abnormalities are repeatedly implicated in sensory gating (148, 149) and filtering disruptions (150, 151) associated with this disorder (42). Indeed, one prominent model of schizophrenia neuropathology is centered on the thalamus as a key hub of disrupted computations in this illness. This "cognitive dysmetria" hypothesis articulates a distributed disruption in information processing across widespread cortical and subcortical nodes (39). In their seminal theoretical piece, Andreasen and colleagues argue that in order to explain the full range of schizophrenia symptoms, the field has to move away from region-specific models, but rather consider a distributed processing deficit, which could also parsimoniously explain a computational abnormality in a given node of a distributed complex system. In that sense, the thalamus is a uniquely positioned set of nuclei that communicates with virtually every cortical territory and is likely to be profoundly affected in schizophrenia.

Building on theoretical, pre-clinical, and anatomical work, recent studies of functional connectivity have begun to map thalamo-cortical alterations in schizophrenia. The first study to do so, by Welsh and colleagues (152), focused on the medio-dorsal nucleus of the thalamus as a seed region. This focused approach is justified given that specific thalamic nuclei in schizophrenia may show particularly profound functional connectivity disruptions. The medio-dorsal nucleus projects heavily to PFC regions (153, 154), and is thought to be compromised in schizophrenia (142, 144, 155). Welsh and colleagues found lower connectivity between the medio-dorsal nucleus and the PFC in patients with schizophrenia relative to healthy comparison subjects. However, this early investigation was based on a very small sample and could therefore be limited in its ability to provide conclusions regarding more subtle disruptions elsewhere. Moreover, Welsh and colleagues could not provide information regarding additional thalamic nuclei given the explicit focus on the medio-dorsal nucleus. In a subsequent study, Woodward and colleagues employed a substantially more powered sample ($N = 62$) and extended the approach to other thalamic nuclei (37). The authors used a parcellation scheme of thalamo-cortical connections at rest provided by Zhang and colleagues (129). In the study by Zhang and colleagues, cortical areas were clustered into subdivisions that exhibited unique functional connectivity with distinct thalamic nuclei based on the similarities in resting-state BOLD signal. Woodward and colleagues harnessed this segmentation scheme to test the hypothesis that unique thalamo-cortical circuits may show different patterns of disturbances in schizophrenia. Strikingly, Woodward and colleagues found that compared to healthy controls, the thalamic segmentations associated with the PFC showed reduced connectivity in schizophrenia. In contrast, cortical territories centered on sensory-motor regions showed increases in thalamic coupling in schizophrenia. This evidence suggests that there exists a profound alteration in thalamo-cortical information flow in schizophrenia but one that seems to follow an anatomical dissociation between sensory and higher order association regions. Building on this robust evidence for thalamo-cortical alterations in schizophrenia it is important to provide information about the specific connections being affected. Specifically, the cortical parcellation scheme, while a powerful initial demonstration, did not allow for examination of the cerebellum for instance. Cerebellum is a structure that, like the striatum, has projections to the cortex by way of the thalamus (156), and has been implicated in schizophrenia pathophysiology (39). Lastly, perhaps due to restricted power, the authors could not examine subtle relationships between symptoms and identified dysconnectivity.

A subsequent report by Anticevic and colleagues examined thalamo-cortical dysconnectivity in 90 patients diagnosed with schizophrenia relative to 90 matched healthy comparison subjects (38). The key objective of this investigation was to determine if thalamo-cortical disturbances span across diagnostic boundaries that share similar symptoms. This cross-diagnostic extension directly informs the objectives articulated by the NIMH RDoC initiative, which aims to develop biomarker-driven diagnostic systems (45). First, the authors replicated the core findings by Woodward and colleagues, demonstrating that schizophrenia is associated with increased coupling between the thalamus and all sensory-motor cortices. In contrast, frontal-striatal-cerebellar nodes showed reduced coupling with the thalamus in schizophrenia relative to healthy comparison subjects (**Figure 3A**). Both patterns were fully replicated in an independent and smaller sample of patients. Critically, further analyses demonstrated that these two sources of disturbance were functionally related. That is, those patients with the highest sensory-motor-thalamic coupling also showed the lowest prefrontal-striatal-cerebellar-thalamic coupling. This effect was most prominent for thalamic clusters centered on the medio-dorsal nucleus with known dense projections to the PFC, ruling out the possibility of pan-thalamic dysconnectivity that is uniform. Furthermore, the magnitude of the sensory-motor-thalamic over-connectivity was correlated with PANSS symptom severity across patients, confirming its functional relevance. The magnitude of this correlation, however, was small ($r = 0.23$) – indicating that the observed pattern explains only a small portion of the variance in symptom variation across subjects. An alternative possibility, given that the majority of patients were quite symptomatic, is that the small magnitude reflects a restricted range in symptoms whereby there was little variability in symptom severity across the patient sample.

The identified thalamic dysconnectivity was successfully used for diagnostic classification via multivariate pattern analysis (MVPA) (157) with high levels of sensitivity and specificity across both the discovery and replication samples. This implies that the identified dysconnectivity patterns, while not yet qualifying for a robust biomarker, may be refined and used to predict risk and assess treatment response. In particular, there are major ongoing improvements in neuroimaging acquisition (127) and processing (69) technology as a direct consequence of the Human Connectome Project (158) that can enable future studies to iteratively refine neuroimaging approaches. Such studies can focus on the identified patterns to ultimately improve methods and fine-tune the identified patterns for biomarker use.

Lastly, the authors found that the bipolar illness sample exhibited an "intermediate" pattern of disturbance such that the patterns of thalamo-cortical connectivity were "shifted" relative to healthy comparison subjects but not as severely altered as those identified in schizophrenia. This finding in particular offers promise for using neuroimaging markers to inform our understanding of shared disturbances in the underlying biology that cut across diagnostic categories (123). The next step will be to understand how such shared neural system-level "endophenotypes" (159, 160) map onto co-occurring behavioral disturbances (e.g., psychosis) as well as onto possibly shared alterations at the level of cortical microcircuits (which we discuss in the last section).

Most recently, Klingner and colleagues provided convergent results from a sample of 22 patients diagnosed with schizophrenia and 22 matched comparison subjects (161). In their study they separately examined the left and right thalamic seeds. They found robust evidence for increased thalamic connectivity with bilateral sensory-motor and auditory cortices. The authors conclude that their results suggest a possible "lack of thalamic control on motor/sensory information processing resulting in increased (and less filtered) forwarding of information to the prefrontal cortex." This hypothesis is consistent with findings from the two earlier and larger studies (37, 38). Interestingly, Klingner and colleagues did not observe notable reductions in thalamic coupling with frontal-striatal-cerebellar nodes in schizophrenia, reported by both aforementioned groups. There are at least two possible interpretations for this difference: (i) the sample size in the Klingner study was much smaller and possibly underpowered to find both sets of patterns (although the effect size analysis and replication analyses by Anticevic and colleagues argues against this possibility); and (ii) Klingner and colleagues may have employed techniques, such as using GSR as a preprocessing step, that could have led to different results (73). It remains to be systematically determined what the true contribution of the global signal is in these analyses, especially in the patient groups. One possibility is that the global signal carries biologically meaningful information regarding cortical-thalamic disruptions in schizophrenia that needs to be carefully characterized. Methodological issues notwithstanding, this emerging body of work strongly and consistently implicates disruptions in thalamo-cortical information flow as a neural system marker in schizophrenia.

While this initial progress in mapping thalamo-cortical disturbances in schizophrenia represents a promising advance in psychiatric neuroimaging research, there are still fundamental gaps in our understanding of how such findings relate to neuropathological mechanisms of this illness. There are a number of future directions that the field should pursue to better understand these observations. For instance, it remains unknown why there are dissociable disturbances across thalamic nuclei in schizophrenia. Future studies focused more exclusively on the medio-dorsal nucleus versus, say, the pulvinar (known to be more involved in visual processing) could begin to explain mechanism behind these differences. Although the original study by Welsh and colleagues provides clues here, follow-up studies with more power that focus on the medio-dorsal nucleus could provide finer-grained information regarding its patterns of dysconnectivity with the PFC.

Another complex issue that is not adequately resolved by any of the noted investigations relates to medication effects. For instance, there are considerations of medication dose, type of medications (given that patients are often treated with multiple drugs from different medication classes), and possible systematic differences in the medications received by patients carrying the diagnoses of schizophrenia, schizoaffective, and bipolar (e.g., mood stabilizers and anti-depressants). While all studies address this issue statistically to a certain extent (by computing chlorpromazine equivalents and then co-varying for the medication dose), future studies in un-medicated patients are needed. It is possible, however, that medication may not necessarily be a confound in this case – instead, antipsychotic medication could actually stabilize thalamo-cortical dysconnectivity. Studies explicitly aimed at testing medication effects on connectivity could provide more detailed insight into this issue. It also remains unknown if the identified patterns of large-scale thalamo-cortical dysconnectivity are characteristic only of chronic stages of schizophrenia or whether they already appear in the prodromal or early stages of the illness. Establishing the link between identified thalamo-cortical dysconnectivity and illness progression remains a vital effort to inform the viability of this marker for predicting and/or tracking risk and progression of the disease. While one of the studies noted above provides a functional link between sensory-motor-thalamic over-connectivity and PANSS symptoms, it remains unknown if these patterns relate to cognitive and executive functional deficits characteristic of the schizophrenia syndrome (26). It may be possible that alterations in thalamo-cortical function (especially the PFC component) in part relate to cognitive deficits observed in this illness.

Additional questions still exist pertaining to the cross-diagnostic relevance of these observations. As noted above, it was shown by Anticevic and colleagues that qualitatively similar patterns of thalamic dysconnectivity are apparent in bipolar illness (although smaller in magnitude than those found in schizophrenia). It remains to be determined if those bipolar patients with a history of co-occurring psychosis are quantitatively more similar to alterations identified in schizophrenia (123). Such finer-grained cross-diagnostic investigations have further potential to inform and refine the clinical relevance of the identified marker. These studies should be complemented with targeted efforts to improve the classification provided by Anticevic and colleagues and allow for even more precision in harnessing this putative biomarker. Recently Fox and Greicius discussed progress in neuropsychiatric studies using resting-state connectivity. They appropriately concluded at the time that in schizophrenia there has been remarkably little progress in producing replicable results (34), perhaps owing to the complexity and heterogeneity of this neuropsychiatric illness noted above. These recent studies reviewed here, which collectively focused on identifying patterns of thalamo-cortical disruption in schizophrenia, may be converging on a parsimonious final common pathway of this complex disease, at least at the neural systems level (43). In that sense, these effects may be one of the better-replicated findings in the schizophrenia connectivity literature to date, offering promise for biomarker development and refinement.

A longer-term goal will entail bridging this neural system-level marker of schizophrenia with evolving cellular-level hypotheses of schizophrenia neuropathology. It remains unknown how the identified neural system-level markers relate to hypotheses that propose disruptions at the cellular level in schizophrenia. For instance, Anticevic and colleagues articulate a possible role of the disruption in cortical excitation (E) and inhibition (I) balance within the cortical microcircuit in producing system-wide disruptions, which may occur in schizophrenia (see next section) and in turn affect cognition (162). It remains unknown, however, how such alterations can scale to produce the presently observed pattern of aberrant thalamo-cortical connectivity. A corollary of this hypothesis relates to observations in bipolar illness, which was associated with an intermediate pattern of thalamo-cortical alterations. In bipolar illness different cellular-level hypotheses have been proposed from those hypothesized to occur in schizophrenia (112, 163, 164) [although some authors have articulated shared disturbances in GABA interneuron function (165)]. Therefore, either distinct mechanisms operate in these different neuropsychiatric conditions that converge on the same alterations or there may be, at least in part, a shared alteration in some of the same mechanisms across the two conditions. That is, it is possible that some patients with bipolar illness share some of the features of cellular neuropathology that affect patients with schizophrenia (165), especially those bipolar patients who present with co-occurring psychosis (166). Moreover, alterations along a number of distinct neurotransmitter pathways, involving a confluence of glutamate (7, 167), GABA (19), and dopamine disturbance (106), could jointly converge on a profound disturbance in thalamo-cortical function. In the upcoming sections, we discuss additional neuroscientific tools, namely pharmacological neuroimaging and computational modeling, which can be combined to help elucidate the role of specific cellular and synaptic mechanisms in observed system-level disruptions that occur in schizophrenia.

PHARMACOLOGICAL NEUROIMAGING – TOWARD A MECHANISTIC UNDERSTANDING OF SYSTEM-LEVEL DISRUPTIONS IN PSYCHIATRIC ILLNESS

We presented evidence, supported by several emerging studies, for profound alterations in thalamo-cortical information flow in schizophrenia, as well as evidence for alterations in PFC connectivity. Yet, the mechanisms that could inform rationally guided pharmacotherapy for these disturbances in schizophrenia remain unknown. One leading mechanistic hypothesis proposes possible disruptions in the E/I balance in the cortical micro-circuitry resulting from hypo-function of the NMDAR (7), which might affect cortical computations, leading to large-scale dysconnectivity (14). A way to link such pharmacological mechanisms to neural system-level observations is to directly compare clinical patient studies and results following pharmacological manipulations, or to separately test the effects of pharmacological manipulations in healthy volunteers.

A powerful candidate approach is to use ketamine, a non-competitive NMDAR antagonist and a leading schizophrenia pharmacological model, which transiently, reversibly, and safely induces characteristic schizophrenia symptoms in healthy volunteers (7). Here pharmacological manipulations provide a method with which researchers can test the effects of a given neurotransmitter perturbation in a constrained, causal, and hypothesis-driven way. Moreover, such synaptic hypotheses can be implemented directly into computational models to generate experimental predictions (discussed in the last section). A prevailing hypothesis regarding ketamine's effects on cortical micro-circuitry proposes preferential antagonism of interneurons with subsequent disinhibition of pyramidal cells (168), a mechanism we implemented in a recent computational modeling investigation (58) (see below for a discussion). As an extension of this hypothesis, a cortex-wide disruption in E/I balance might de-stabilize thalamo-cortical information flow in ways observed in schizophrenia (or other neuropsychiatric conditions). It should be noted that it still remains unclear what the relative contribution is of NMDARs on pyramidal cells (169) versus interneurons (58) may be in relation to the hypothesized alterations in E/I balance. Understanding the relative contribution of such cell-specific receptor alterations remains an important future direction, which could inform targeted pharmacotherapies. Such detailed studies of how cellular-level alterations could give rise to thalamo-cortical alterations following pharmacological manipulations remain to be done. Nevertheless, there is emerging evidence from a few focused investigations detailing the effects of ketamine on large-scale cortical connectivity. These investigations provide preliminary clues for how ketamine's effects on large-scale systems may resemble effects seen in schizophrenia.

For instance, a recent resting-state connectivity study by Driesen and colleagues investigated the effects of acute ketamine administration to healthy volunteers on large-scale global cortical connectivity (**Figure 4A**). The authors use a resting-state connectivity approach similar to that applied by Cole and colleagues in chronic schizophrenia (40), extended to include the entire brain (i.e., all voxels without imposing a PFC restriction). A number of studies have demonstrated that NMDAR antagonist administration is associated with excessive pyramidal cell activity, increases extracellular glutamate levels (16), and increases in perfusion and cortical metabolism (48–51, 53). A logical extension of this hypothesis is that administration of ketamine may profoundly affect large-scale cortical connectivity. Consistent with pre-clinical studies, Driesen and colleagues found that NMDAR antagonist administration resulted in a global elevation of functional connectivity (i.e., everywhere in the brain). This observation is broadly consistent with cellular-level hypotheses of ketamine's effects on glutamate release, which may increase coupling of cortical circuits at rest by increasing the E/I ratio (i.e., decreasing cortical microcircuit inhibition). It is, however, critical to point out that chronic schizophrenia has typically been associated with reductions in cortical connectivity (170) and activation (70), especially in the PFC (11), as described above. Therefore, there are at least some evident discrepancies between the effects of pharmacological models such as ketamine and the actual illness (54). This important discrepancy between ketamine's effects on PFC circuits and observations in schizophrenia should be reconciled in prospective studies that directly compare pharmacological and clinical effects using resting-state connectivity measures. One possible factor that could explain differences between NMDAR antagonist effects and chronic schizophrenia is that such pharmacological models may be relevant only to specific patient subgroups or illness stages. One possibility is that the increased connectivity under ketamine is similar to the early stages of psychotic illness. This hypothesis is consistent with elevated glutamate levels reported early in the illness course (113, 171). It is also consistent with the observation that ketamine tends to produce symptoms associated with incipient illness stages, rather than auditory hallucinations that occur in frank psychosis and chronic schizophrenia (15, 49, 172–174). Moreover, significant functional dynamical changes may occur during schizophrenia progression (46) that could profoundly affect PFC function, structure, and integrity. This hypothesis is supported by recent meta-analytic findings reporting decreases in glutamate across the illness progression (113). Whether such alterations across the schizophrenia illness course are reflected in PFC connectivity changes remains unknown, as does ketamine's impact on PFC functional network architecture. Future pharmacological studies as well as cross-sectional and longitudinal clinical investigation are needed to test this hypothesis. In addition, careful pre-clinical experiments could possibly inform such hypotheses (118).

A complementary area of research has investigated the effects of ketamine on functional connectivity (177) in relation to its potential anti-depressant effects (178). While a comprehensive treatment of anti-depressant effects of ketamine is beyond the scope of this review, it is important to note that studies examining its effects on glutamateric pathways in the context of mood symptoms (178) may be highly informative for developing our understanding of its relevance to schizophrenia (111). Briefly, emerging models in this area postulate that ketamine may act as anti-depressant by promoting synaptic plasticity via intra-cellular signaling pathways, ultimately promoting brain-derived neurotrophic factor expression via synaptic potentiation (179) and in turns synaptic growth (178). In that sense, acute NMDAR antagonism may promote synaptic plasticity along specific pathways impacted in mood disorders, such as ventral medial PFC (180, 181, p. 916).

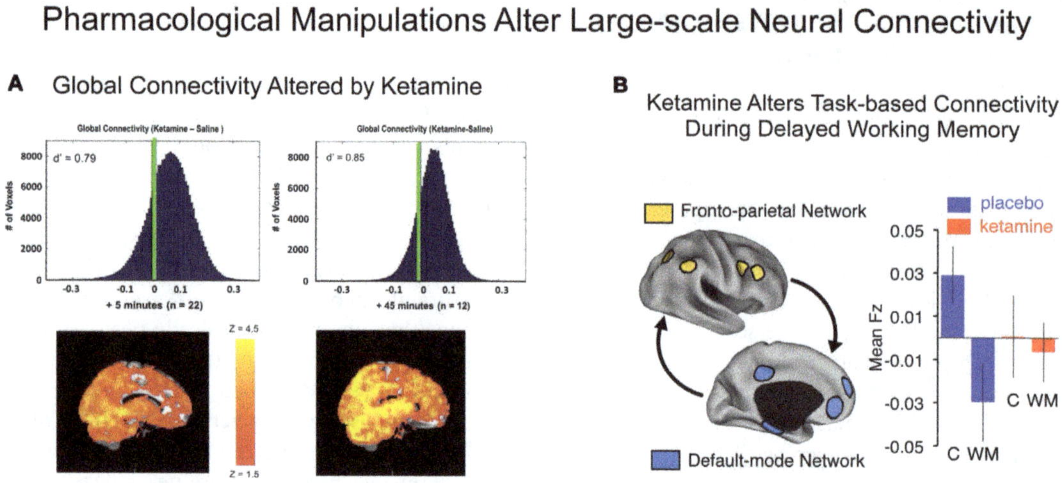

FIGURE 4 | Characterizing connectivity alterations using pharmacological neuroimaging. While functional connectivity neuroimaging alone has been a powerful tool for characterizing neural system-level alterations in schizophrenia, it is ultimately a correlational tool. That is, we are examining alterations in the associations as a function of illness presence or absence. To move toward understanding the possible role of specific neurotransmitter mechanisms in schizophrenia, however, neuroimaging studies can be combined with pharmacological manipulations (47, 175). Such causal experimental manipulations can shed light on the role of specific neurotransmitter systems in schizophrenia (15). **(A)** Driesen and colleagues have shown that administration of ketamine profoundly altered the global connectivity of the brain. Specifically they demonstrated that the GBC measure increased following ketamine administration, possibly reflecting a hyper-glutamatergic state or a state of cortical disinhibition (54) consistent with animal models (111, 176). Formal computational models are needed in order to provide a deeper intuition for such pharmacological effects on large-scale neural systems. **(B)** Anticevic and colleagues have shown that administration of an NMDAR antagonist, ketamine, alters the connectivity of large-scale anti-correlated neural systems during performance of a working memory task (18). Although this connectivity study was performed during task performance rather than rest, it illustrates a proof of concept for how a pharmacological challenge can alter connectivity in a causal way. Note: figures adapted with permission from Driesen and colleagues (54) and Anticevic and colleagues (18).

Conversely, when administered to patients diagnosed with schizophrenia, NMDAR antagonists seem to worsen their symptom profile (182), perhaps by "pushing" an already aberrantly elevated glutamatergic signaling profile upward. Collectively such dissociable effects of ketamine may imply that along distinct circuits there may be an inverted-U relationship between ketamine's effects and symptoms: depressed patients may be positioned on the low end of the inverted-U (178) and schizophrenia patents may be positioned on the higher end (183). Both task-based and resting-state functional connectivity techniques are well positioned to interrogate such system-level effects of NMDAR antagonists in humans.

As an example of such an approach, another study examining the effects of ketamine by Anticevic and colleagues focused on understanding the functional impact of NMDAR antagonism on the organization of the large-scale, anti-correlated neural systems (**Figure 4B**). This pharmacological neuroimaging investigation was explicitly focused on understanding ketamine effects on WM. However, in the context of this cognitive question, Anticevic and colleagues also assessed whether the task-based functional connectivity of large-scale neural systems is affected by ketamine administration. As we noted above, such task-based connectivity approaches can be useful to pinpoint how large-scale systems are affected during specific cognitive operations. The authors found that an acute administration of a low ketamine dose profoundly altered the typically observed anti-correlated structure of the large-scale neural systems – namely the task-positive fronto-parietal regions (184) and the task-negative regions (typically termed the default-mode network, DMN) (28). In line with this observed decrease in functional connectivity, Driesen and colleagues (185) also found a reduction in WM task-based functional connectivity along fronto-parietal areas (when using a DLPFC seed) following ketamine administration. The investigators reported *increased* functional connectivity of the DLPFC during rest using the exact same seed. This set of observations in particular sheds light on how a pharmacological manipulation such as NMDAR antagonism may have profoundly different effects in the context of a cognitive task (e.g., WM) and during rest. The mechanisms behind this observed difference are beyond the scope of this review and will be discussed in forthcoming studies.

Briefly, it may be possible that large-scale, network-level synchrony during WM is critically dependent on appropriate content-specific signals between neural subpopulations (186). In contrast, the BOLD fluctuations during rest likely relate to coupling between regions at the infra-slow-frequency ranges (187). It may be possible that a reduction in appropriate task-evoked synchrony by NMDAR antagonism reduces the ability of a network to form a coherent and optimal level of functional connectivity during WM. This may be exacerbated by an amplification of shared "noise" in the system, which is reflected in the apparent hyper-synchrony at rest (54). Collectively, therefore, an NMDAR antagonist may "disinhibit" the system, which gives rise to infra-slow, spatially distributed fluctuations across large areas of cortex that manifest in aberrant hyper-connectivity at rest. Precisely due to this elevated background noise, in combination with disrupted capacity for appropriate task-evoked synchrony, the net effect during WM may be a reduction in functional connectivity (which contrasts with observations at rest). Moreover, task-evoked activity can suppress the slow fluctuations associated with rest (188); if this suppression were weakened in schizophrenia, the "signal-to-noise" ratio would be degraded and task-based functional connectivity could be reduced. Because task-based and resting-state synchrony may be separated by timescale, EEG studies, combined with fMRI, could potentially address such hypotheses (189–191). Moreover, precisely because of such important differences between task and rest in certain contexts (e.g., ketamine manipulation) it remains important for task-based and resting-state investigations to inform one another. In the upcoming section, we explicitly discuss the recent developments in computational modeling that can provide a platform for formal integration of neuroscience theory both in the context of resting-state studies as well as formal task-based experiments.

BRIDGING LEVELS OF ANALYSIS VIA COMPUTATIONAL MODELING

Above we discussed recent clinical and pharmacological neuroimaging findings that shed light on the nature of large-scale neural system alterations in schizophrenia. In particular, the pharmacological experiments provide a causal method to explicitly manipulate specific neurotransmitter mechanisms that may be involved in schizophrenia. In that sense, these studies can begin to address given neurotransmitter contributions to neural system-level and behavioral alterations observed in schizophrenia. Still, these studies cannot measure synaptic and cellular-level phenomena alone. Therefore, one possible methodological integration involves a formal link between such pharmacological/clinical experiments and computational models that contain this level of functional detail. One branch of computational model that provides a particularly productive platform involves biophysically based models that contain the relevant synaptic mechanisms (57, 192) thought to be disrupted in neuropsychiatric illness (55). Such microcircuit models have been already harnessed to make predictions in the context of ketamine experimental manipulations of WM (58) (discussed more below). There is, however, an ongoing need to scale such models to the level of neural systems to provide relevant predictions for both resting-state and task-based clinical and pharmacological studies.

Recent computational models have been developed to explicitly capture how the global pattern of resting-state functional connectivity arises through cortico-cortical interactions (193). In particular, modeling studies in this area have focused on the extent to which functional connectivity can be predicted by long-range anatomical connectivity (**Figure 5A**). The dynamic interactions between neural populations will also shape functional connectivity. The starting point for these models is an anatomical coupling matrix reflecting long-range connections between cortical regions, derived either from tracer studies in macaque monkeys or from diffusion tractography in humans. The activity of a local region (a node in the large-scale network) follows some dynamics and is shaped by input from other areas, propagating via the long-range connections. Ongoing activity, either due to chaos or noise, produces fluctuations in the activity across the network. The functional connectivity of the model can then be calculated and compared to functional connectivity observed in experiments. Honey and colleagues (194) studied long-range chaotic synchronization when local nodes follow oscillatory dynamics, using connectivity from human diffusion tractography. They found that the global dynamics of the network could partially explain the presence of strong functional connections between regions that lack direct anatomical connection. Cabral and colleagues (195) used a similar oscillatory model with connectivity data from healthy subjects, and parametrically varied the overall strength of long-range connections. They found that decreasing long-range connection strength altered functional connectivity patterns in a manner similar to those observed in schizophrenia (9), with reduced overall functional connectivity strength and changes in certain graph-theoretic measures of the functional connectivity matrix.

Deco and colleagues (59, 193) extended this approach, deriving long-range connectivity from human diffusion tractography and implementing the local node dynamics with a biophysically based model of a cortical microcircuit. In particular, the local microcircuit incorporates recurrent excitation with realistic synaptic dynamics, and the strength of recurrent excitation enables multistable dynamics that can subserve cognitive computations such as WM (197, 198). Noisy background inputs to nodes induce fluctuations in activity that are shaped into correlated patterns by long-range coupling between nodes through the anatomically derived connectivity. Functional connectivity in the model is given by the pattern of these correlated fluctuations. The authors parametrically varied two global parameters with biophysical relevance: the strength of recurrent excitation within local nodes, and the strength of long-range connections between nodes. The strengths of local and long-range connections combine to provide recurrent excitation in the network. They found that the similarity between model and experimental functional connectivity patterns was maximized when the network's baseline state is near the boundary in parameter space between stability and instability induced by excess excitation. These studies reveal that the pattern of functional connectivity in the model is sensitive to both the pattern of anatomical connectivity and the physiological parameters that scale local and long-range connections. The biophysical basis of these models makes them directly applicable to address the dynamical consequences of anatomical and physiological changes induced by disease processes or pharmacological manipulation. Changes in the strengths of local and long-range connections may induce differential effects in the patterns of functional connectivity. Therefore, fitting models to functionally connectivity in patients could distinguish among distinct synaptic alterations. This approach could also potentially reveal the effects of complex drug actions on local circuit tuning and long-range interactions.

The models described above were explicitly constructed to simulate resting-state fluctuations, rather than to implement a particular function such as WM. Nevertheless, functional models can still make predictions that can be tested using functional connectivity, especially task-based functional connectivity (81). To this end, Anticevic and colleagues extended a microcircuit model of WM to study interactions between large-scale networks and

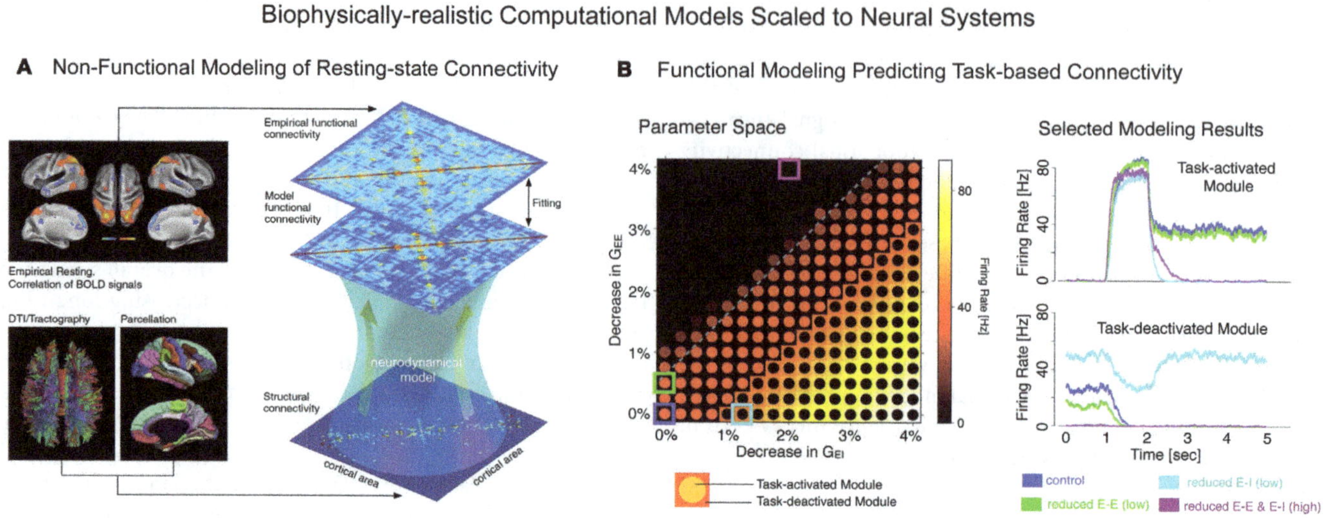

FIGURE 5 | Computational modeling of system-level effects via biophysically realistic computational approaches. While detailed microcircuit models have made an impact on our understanding of cortical dynamics (56), the challenge remains to scale such models to incorporate dynamic interactions across large-scale neural systems, which are likely profoundly affected in schizophrenia (and other severe neuropsychiatric conditions). **(A)** A recently published elegant study by Deco and colleagues (59) illustrates an approach where a biophysically realistic model of cortical computations has been applied to understand the generation of slow-frequency fluctuations in the BOLD signal. The authors used diffusion-spectrum imaging to anatomically constrain the model and in turn fitted the modeling results to empirically-derived resting-state functional connectivity data. The result illustrates that coherent fluctuations in the BOLD signal (i.e., resting functional connectivity) may emerge from a system that is at the edge of chaos, allowing linear but transient departures in neuronal firing rates. **(B)** Anticevic and colleagues have used a functional model of working memory, a cognitive process that is profoundly affected in schizophrenia (26), to better understand the role of NMDA receptor function in the interaction of large-scale anti-correlated neural systems. Specifically they studied the functional antagonism present during a cognitive task between the task-activated (fronto-parietal module) and task-deactivated (default-mode module) networks (196). Following a complete parameter sweep (left), the authors found that a small perturbation of the NMDARs on inhibitory interneurons within each cortical microcircuit captured the firing that was observed experimentally following ketamine administration in healthy volunteers (18). Collectively, these studies offer examples for how biologically constrained modeling approaches can be applied to understand large-scale neural system physiology in both resting-state (non-functional) and task-based (functional) settings. Note: **(A)** of the figure was adapted with permission from Deco and colleagues (59).

their disruption by synaptic perturbation (**Figure 5B**) (18). The biophysically based model consists of two modules of spiking microcircuits: one that is task-activated and capable of WM computations, and one that is task-deactivated from a high-activity baseline state (hypothesized to model the activity pattern of the default-mode network in the context of cognitive activation). The interactions between these modules are mutually suppressive, via long-range projections onto inhibitory interneurons, a feature founded on findings of anti-correlated fluctuations between task-positive and default-mode networks (30). Within the model authors specifically studied the functional impact of disinhibition via NMDA hypo-function on interneurons, to relate such microcircuit hypotheses to neural changes observed under ketamine administration. The authors found that disinhibition of the entire network results in a failure to shut off the default-mode module, impairing the pattern of activation and deactivation during WM tasks. This modeling study provides one example of how a microcircuit model of a specific cognitive process (i.e., WM) can be scaled to incorporate system-level interactions and make predictions relevant for task-based functional connectivity. In addition, one strength of computational models is the ability to systematically explore different operating regimes in the space of model parameters. For example, Anticevic and colleagues contrasted reductions in recurrent excitation onto interneurons versus pyramidal cells, generating testable predictions for elevated versus reduced excitation/inhibition balance. As a test of the model architecture and operation, the authors analyzed task-based functional connectivity between task-activated and task-deactivated networks, computed across trials during the delay period of a WM task. Under control conditions, the two networks exhibited robust negative correlation, in line with effective antagonistic interactions in the model. In contrast, under ketamine administration this negative correlation disappears (**Figure 4B**), in line with the model prediction that the task-positive module cannot effectively suppress the hyperactive default-mode module. Collectively, this study provides preliminary evidence that functional models can be directly related to functional connectivity predictions in the context of WM. Future computational/experimental studies should be designed to extend this framework to more complex processes and symptoms that may be disrupted in schizophrenia. We argue that such ongoing efforts for the integration of theory, pharmacological experiments and clinical work will be a vital path for the field of clinical neuroscience to provide testable and rationally guided advances for understanding disease mechanisms and putative treatments.

CONCLUDING REMARKS

Collectively, we articulated recent focused developments in three areas of clinical neuroscience of schizophrenia: (i) we reviewed methodological advances in resting-state functional connectivity that were directly translated to understand neural system-level disturbances in schizophrenia. We specifically focused on data-driven techniques that offer a promising way to detect disrupted connectivity while bypassing the likely complexity and regional heterogeneity of network alterations that are present in schizophrenia. We also discussed ongoing developments in studies of thalamo-cortical dysconnectivity in schizophrenia that are directly informed by influential theoretical models of the illness. (ii) We highlighted select pharmacological studies of the NMDARs that offer a causal way to understand neural system alterations in psychiatric illness. (iii) We articulated the developments in biophysically based computational modeling studies that provide a platform for testing specific synaptic alterations. In turn, we demonstrate that such models can potentially be scaled to the level of neural systems to make relevant predictions for both resting-state or task-based connectivity experiments. We argue that the ongoing blend of these three approaches can provide advances in the field of clinical neuroscience that create a final output that is much greater than the sum of its parts.

ACKNOWLEDGMENTS

Financial support for this study was provided by NIH grant DP5OD012109-01 (PI: Alan Anticevic), NIAAA grant 2P50AA012870-11 (PI: John H. Krystal), NIH grant MH096801 (PI: Michael W. Cole), NIH grant R01 MH062349 (PI: Xiao-Jing Wang) the National Alliance for Research on Schizophrenia and Depression (PIs: Alan Anticevic), the Fulbright Foundation (Aleksandar Savic), and the Yale Center for Clinical Investigation (YCCI, PI: Alan Anticevic). We thank Sharif Youssef for assistance with this manuscript.

REFERENCES

1. Walker E, Kestler L, Bollini A, Hochman KM. Schizophrenia: etiology and course. *Annu Rev Psychol* (2004) **55**:401–30. doi:10.1146/annurev.psych.55.090902.141950
2. Yoon JH, Tamir D, Minzenberg MJ, Ragland DJ, Ursu S, Carter CS. Multivariate pattern analysis of functional magnetic resonance imaging data reveals deficits in distributed representations in schizophrenia. *Biol Psychiatry* (2008) **64**:1035–41. doi:10.1016/j.biopsych.2008.07.025
3. Corlett PR, Honey GD, Fletcher PC. From prediction error to psychosis: ketamine as a pharmacological model of delusions. *J Psychopharmacol* (2007) **21**:238–52. doi:10.1177/0269881107077716
4. Holt DJ, Lakshmanan B, Freudenreich O, Goff DC, Rauch SL, Kuperberg GR. Dysfunction of a cortical midline network during emotional appraisals in schizophrenia. *Schizophr Bull* (2011) **37**:164–76. doi:10.1093/schbul/sbp067
5. Barch DM, Braver TS. Cognitive control in schizophrenia: psychological and neural mechanisms. In: Engle RW, Sedek G, von Hecker U, McIntosh AM, editors. *Cognitive Limitations in Aging and Psychopathology*. Cambridge: Cambridge University Press (2007). p. 122–59.
6. Stephan KE, Baldeweg T, Friston KJ. Synaptic plasticity and dysconnection in schizophrenia. *Biol Psychiatry* (2006) **59**:929–39. doi:10.1016/j.biopsych.2005.10.005
7. Krystal JH, D'Souza DC, Mathalon D, Perry E, Belger A, Hoffman R. NMDA receptor antagonist effects, cortical glutamatergic function, and schizophrenia: toward a paradigm shift in medication development. *Psychopharmacology (Berl)* (2003) **169**:215–33. doi:10.1007/s00213-003-1582-z
8. Murray CJ, Lopez AD, Harvard School of Public Health; World Health Organization; World Bank. *The Global Burden of Disease: A Comprehensive Assessment of Mortality and Disability from Diseases, Injuries, and Risk Factors in 1990 and Projected to 2020*. Cambridge, MA: Published by the Harvard School of Public Health on Behalf of the World Health Organization and the World Bank; Distributed by Harvard University Press (1996).
9. Lynall M-E, Bassett DS, Kerwin R, McKenna PJ, Kitzbichler M, Muller U, et al. Functional connectivity and brain networks in schizophrenia. *J Neurosci* (2010) **30**:9477–87. doi:10.1523/JNEUROSCI.0333-10.2010
10. van den Heuvel MP, Mandl RC, Stam CJ, Kahn RS, Pol HE. Aberrant frontal and temporal complex network structure in schizophrenia: a graph theoretical analysis. *J Neurosci* (2010) **30**:15915–26. doi:10.1523/JNEUROSCI.2874-10.2010
11. Cole MW, Anticevic A, Repovs G, Barch DM. Variable global dysconnectivity and individual differences in schizophrenia. *Biol Psychiatry* (2011) **70**:43–50. doi:10.1016/j.biopsych.2011.02.010
12. Fornito A, Yoon J, Zalesky A, Bullmore ET, Carter CS. General and specific functional connectivity disturbances in first-episode schizophrenia during cognitive control performance. *Biol Psychiatry* (2011) **70**:64–72. doi:10.1016/j.biopsych.2011.02.019
13. Salomon R, Bleich-Cohen M, Hahamy-Dubossarsky A, Dinstien I, Weizman R, Poyurovsky M, et al. Global functional connectivity deficits in schizophrenia depend on behavioral state. *J Neurosci* (2011) **31**:12972–81. doi:10.1523/JNEUROSCI.2987-11.2011
14. Uhlhaas PJ. Dysconnectivity, large-scale networks and neuronal dynamics in schizophrenia. *Curr Opin Neurobiol* (2013) **23**:283–90. doi:10.1016/j.conb.2012.11.004
15. Krystal JH, Karper LP, Seibyl JP, Freeman GK, Delaney R, Bremner JD, et al. Subanesthetic effects of the noncompetitive NMDA antagonist, ketamine, in humans. Psychotomimetic, perceptual, cognitive, and neuroendocrine responses. *Arch Gen Psychiatry* (1994) **51**:199–214. doi:10.1001/archpsyc.1994.03950030035004
16. Homayoun H, Moghaddam B. NMDA receptor hypofunction produces opposite effects on prefrontal cortex interneurons and pyramidal neurons. *J Neurosci* (2007) **27**:11496–500. doi:10.1523/JNEUROSCI.2213-07.2007
17. Gonzalez-Burgos G, Lewis DA. NMDA receptor hypofunction, parvalbumin-positive neurons and cortical gamma oscillations in schizophrenia. *Schizophr Bull* (2012) **38**(5):950–7. doi:10.1093/schbul/sbs010
18. Anticevic A, Gancsos M, Murray JD, Repovs G, Driesen NR, Ennis DJ, et al. NMDA receptor function in large-scale anti-correlated neural systems with implications for cognition and schizophrenia. *Proc Natl Acad Sci U S A* (2012) **109**:16720–5. doi:10.1073/pnas.1208494109
19. Lewis DA, Hashimoto T, Volk DW. Cortical inhibitory neurons and schizophrenia. *Nat Rev Neurosci* (2005) **6**:312–24. doi:10.1038/nrn1648
20. Lewis DA, Curley AA, Glausier JR, Volk DW. Cortical parvalbumin interneurons and cognitive dysfunction in schizophrenia. *Trends Neurosci* (2012) **35**:57–67. doi:10.1016/j.tins.2011.10.004
21. Toda M, Abi-Dargham A. Dopamine hypothesis of schizophrenia: making sense of it all. *Curr Psychiatry Rep* (2007) **9**:329–36. doi:10.1007/s11920-007-0041-7
22. Durstewitz D, Seamans JK. The computational role of dopamine D1 receptors in working memory. *Neural Netw* (2002) **15**:561–72. doi:10.1016/S0893-6080(02)00049-7
23. Glahn DC, Ragland JD, Abramoff A, Barrett J, Laird AR, Bearden CE, et al. Beyond hypofrontality: a quantitative meta-analysis of functional neuroimaging studies of working memory in schizophrenia. *Hum Brain Mapp* (2005) **25**:60–9. doi:10.1002/hbm.20138
24. Goldman-Rakic PS. Working memory dysfunction in schizophrenia. *J Neuropsychiatr* (1994) **6**:348–57.
25. Meyer-Lindenberg A, Poline JB, Kohn PD, Holt JL, Egan MF, Weinberger DR, et al. Evidence for abnormal cortical functional connectivity during working memory in schizophrenia. *Am J Psychiatry* (2001) **158**:1809–17. doi:10.1176/appi.ajp.158.11.1809
26. Barch DM, Ceaser A. Cognition in schizophrenia: core psychological and neural mechanisms. *Trends Cogn Sci* (2012) **16**:27–34. doi:10.1016/j.tics.2011.11.015
27. Fornito A, Zalesky A, Pantelis C, Bullmore ET. Schizophrenia, neuroimaging and connectomics. *Neuroimage* (2012) **62**:2296–314. doi:10.1016/j.neuroimage.2011.12.090

28. Raichle ME, Snyder AZ. A default mode of brain function: a brief history of an evolving idea. *Neuroimage* (2007) **37**:1083–90; discussion 1097–9. doi:10.1016/j.neuroimage.2007.02.041
29. Biswal BB, Mennes M, Zuo X-N, Gohel S, Kelly C, Smith SM, et al. Toward discovery science of human brain function. *Proc Natl Acad Sci U S A* (2010) **107**:4734–9. doi:10.1073/pnas.0911855107
30. Fox MD, Snyder AZ, Vincent JL, Corbetta M, Van Essen DC, Raichle ME. The human brain is intrinsically organized into dynamic, anticorrelated functional networks. *Proc Natl Acad Sci U S A* (2005) **102**:9673–8. doi:10.1073/pnas.0504136102
31. Smith SM, Fox PT, Miller KL, Glahn DC, Fox PM, Mackay CE, et al. Correspondence of the brain's functional architecture during activation and rest. *Proc Natl Acad Sci U S A* (2009) **106**:13040–5. doi:10.1073/pnas.0905267106
32. Vincent JL, Patel GH, Fox MD, Snyder AZ, Baker JT, Van Essen DC, et al. Intrinsic functional architecture in the anaesthetized monkey brain. *Nature* (2007) **447**:83–6. doi:10.1038/nature05758
33. Greicius MD, Supekar K, Menon V, Dougherty RF. Resting-state functional connectivity reflects structural connectivity in the default mode network. *Cereb Cortex* (2009) **19**:72–8. doi:10.1093/cercor/bhn059
34. Fox MD, Greicius M. Clinical applications of resting state functional connectivity. *Front Syst Neurosci* (2010) **4**:19. doi:10.3389/fnsys.2010.00019
35. Anticevic A, Brumbaugh MS, Winkler AM, Lombardo LE, Barrett J, Corlett PR, et al. Global prefrontal and fronto-amygdala dysconnectivity in bipolar I disorder with psychosis history. *Biol Psychiatry* (2012) **73**:565–73. doi:10.1016/j.biopsych.2012.07.031
36. Whitfield-Gabrieli S, Thermenos H, Milanovic S, Tsuang M, Faraone S, McCarley R, et al. Hyperactivity and hyperconnectivity of the default network in schizophrenia and in first-degree relatives of persons with schizophrenia. *Proc Natl Acad Sci U S A* (2009) **106**:1279–84. doi:10.1073/pnas.0809141106
37. Woodward ND, Karbasforoushan H, Heckers S. Thalamocortical dysconnectivity in schizophrenia. *Am J Psychiatry* (2012) **169**:1092–9. doi:10.1176/appi.ajp.2012.12010056
38. Anticevic A, Cole MW, Repovs G, Murray JD, Brumbaugh MS, Winkler AM, et al. Characterizing thalamo-cortical disturbances in schizophrenia and bipolar illness. *Cereb Cortex* (2013). doi:10.1093/cercor/bht165
39. Andreasen NC, Paradiso S, O'Leary DS. "Cognitive dysmetria" as an integrative theory of schizophrenia: a dysfunction in cortical-subcortical-cerebellar circuitry? *Schizophr Bull* (1998) **24**:203–18. doi:10.1093/oxfordjournals.schbul.a033321
40. Cole MW, Pathak S, Schneider W. Identifying the brain's most globally connected regions. *Neuroimage* (2010) **49**:3132–48. doi:10.1016/j.neuroimage.2009.11.001
41. Carlsson M, Carlsson A. Schizophrenia: a subcortical neurotransmitter imbalance syndrome? *Schizophr Bull* (1990) **16**:425–32. doi:10.1093/schbul/16.3.425
42. Andreasen NC. The role of the thalamus in schizophrenia. *Can J Psychiatry* (1997) **42**:27–33.
43. Lisman JE, Pi HJ, Zhang Y, Otmakhova NA. A thalamo-hippocampal-ventral tegmental area loop may produce the positive feedback that underlies the psychotic break in schizophrenia. *Biol Psychiatry* (2010) **68**:17–24. doi:10.1016/j.biopsych.2010.04.007
44. Insel TR, Cuthbert BN. Endophenotypes: bridging genomic complexity and disorder heterogeneity. *Biol Psychiatry* (2009) **66**:988–9. doi:10.1016/j.biopsych.2009.10.008
45. Cuthbert BN, Insel TR. Toward new approaches to psychotic disorders: the NIMH research domain criteria project. *Schizophr Bull* (2010) **36**:1061–2. doi:10.1093/schbul/sbq108
46. Insel TR. Rethinking schizophrenia. *Nature* (2010) **468**:187–93. doi:10.1038/nature09552
47. Honey G, Bullmore E. Human pharmacological MRI. *Trends Pharmacol Sci* (2004) **25**:366–74. doi:10.1016/j.tips.2004.05.009
48. Lahti AC, Holcomb HH, Medoff DR, Tamminga CA. Ketamine activates psychosis and alters limbic blood flow in schizophrenia. *Neuroreport* (1995) **6**:869–72. doi:10.1097/00001756-199504190-00011
49. Breier A, Malhotra AK, Pinals DA, Weisenfeld NI, Pickar D. Association of ketamine-induced psychosis with focal activation of the prefrontal cortex in healthy volunteers. *Am J Psychiatry* (1997) **154**:805–11.
50. Vollenweider FX, Leenders KL, Scharfetter C, Antonini A, Maguire P, Missimer J, et al. Metabolic hyperfrontality and psychopathology in the ketamine model of psychosis using positron emission tomography (PET) and [18F]fluorodeoxyglucose (FDG). *Eur Neuropsychopharmacol* (1997) **7**:9–24. doi:10.1016/S0924-977X(96)00039-9
51. Vollenweider FX, Vontobel P, Oye I, Hell D, Leenders KL. Effects of (S)-ketamine on striatal dopamine: a [11C]raclopride PET study of a model psychosis in humans. *J Psychiatr Res* (2000) **34**:35–43. doi:10.1016/S0022-3956(99)00031-X
52. Lahti AC, Weiler MA, Tamara Michaelidis BA, Parwani A, Tamminga CA. Effects of ketamine in normal and schizophrenic volunteers. *Neuropsychopharmacology* (2001) **25**:455–67. doi:10.1016/S0893-133X(01)00243-3
53. Lahti AC, Holcomb HH, Medoff DR, Weiler MA, Tamminga CA, Carpenter WT. Abnormal patterns of regional cerebral blood flow in schizophrenia with primary negative symptoms during an effortful auditory recognition task. *Am J Psychiatry* (2002) **158**:1797–808. doi:10.1176/appi.ajp.158.11.1797
54. Driesen NR, McCarthy G, Bhagwagar Z, Bloch MH, Calhoun VD, D'Souza DC, et al. Relationship of resting brain hyperconnectivity and schizophrenia-like symptoms produced by the NMDA receptor antagonist ketamine in humans. *Mol Psychiatry* (2013) **18**(11):1199–204. doi:10.1038/mp.2012.194
55. Wang X-J. Toward a prefrontal microcircuit model for cognitive deficits in schizophrenia. *Pharmacopsychiatry* (2006) **39**(Suppl 1):S80–7. doi:10.1055/s-2006-931501
56. Wang X-J. Neurophysiological and computational principles of cortical rhythms in cognition. *Physiol Rev* (2010) **90**:1195–268. doi:10.1152/physrev.00035.2008
57. Wang XJ. Synaptic reverberation underlying mnemonic persistent activity. *Trends Neurosci* (2001) **24**:455–63. doi:10.1016/S0166-2236(00)01868-3
58. Murray JD, Anticevic A, Gancsos M, Ichinose M, Corlett PR, Krystal JH. Linking microcircuit dysfunction to cognitive impairment: effects of disinhibition associated with schizophrenia in a cortical working memory model. *Cereb Cortex* (2012). doi:10.1093/cercor/bhs370
59. Deco G, Ponce-Alvarez A, Mantini D, Romani GL, Hagmann P, Corbetta M. Resting-state functional connectivity emerges from structurally and dynamically shaped slow linear fluctuations. *J Neurosci* (2013) **33**:11239–52. doi:10.1523/JNEUROSCI.1091-13.2013
60. Kotermanski SE, Johnson JW. Mg2+ imparts NMDA receptor subtype selectivity to the Alzheimer's drug memantine. *J Neurosci* (2009) **29**:2774–9. doi:10.1523/JNEUROSCI.3703-08.2009
61. Biswal B, Yetkin FZ, Haughton VM, Hyde JS. Functional connectivity in the motor cortex of resting human brain using echo-planar MRI. *Magn Reson Med* (1995) **34**:537–41. doi:10.1002/mrm.1910340409
62. Buckner RL, Krienen FM, Yeo BT. Opportunities and limitations of intrinsic functional connectivity MRI. *Nat Neurosci* (2013) **16**:832–7. doi:10.1038/nn.3423
63. Power JD, Cohen AL, Nelson SM, Wig GS, Barnes KA, Church JA, et al. Functional network organization of the human brain. *Neuron* (2011) **72**:665–78. doi:10.1016/j.neuron.2011.09.006
64. Smith SM, Miller KL, Moeller S, Xu J, Auerbach EJ, Woolrich MW, et al. Temporally-independent functional modes of spontaneous brain activity. *Proc Natl Acad Sci U S A* (2012) **109**:3131–6. doi:10.1073/pnas.1121329109
65. Greicius M. Resting-state functional connectivity in neuropsychiatric disorders. *Curr Opin Neurol* (2008) **21**:424–30. doi:10.1097/WCO.0b013e328306f2c5
66. Loh M, Rolls ET, Deco G. A dynamical systems hypothesis of schizophrenia. *PLoS Comput Biol* (2007) **3**:e228. doi:10.1371/journal.pcbi.0030228
67. Van Dijk KR, Hedden T, Venkataraman A, Evans KC, Lazar SW, Buckner RL. Intrinsic functional connectivity as a tool for human connectomics: theory, properties, and optimization. *J Neurophysiol* (2010) **103**:297–321. doi:10.1152/jn.00783.2009
68. Feinberg DA, Moeller S, Smith SM, Auerbach E, Ramanna S, Glasser MF, et al. Multiplexed echo planar imaging for sub-second whole brain fMRI and fast diffusion imaging. *PLoS One* (2010) **5**:e15710. doi:10.1371/journal.pone.0015710
69. Glasser MF, Sotiropoulos SN, Wilson JA, Coalson TS, Fischl B, Andersson JL, et al. The minimal preprocessing pipelines for the human connectome project. *Neuroimage* (2013) **80**:105–24. doi:10.1016/j.neuroimage.2013.04.127
70. Van Snellenberg JX, Torres IJ, Thornton AE. Functional neuroimaging of working memory in schizophrenia: task performance as a moderating variable. *Neuropsychology* (2006) **20**(5):497–510. doi:10.1037/0894-4105.20.5.497
71. Friston KJ. Functional and effective connectivity: a review. *Brain Connect* (2011) **1**:13–36. doi:10.1089/brain.2011.0008

72. Murphy K, Birn RM, Handwerker DA, Jones TB, Bandettini PA. The impact of global signal regression on resting state correlations: are anti-correlated networks introduced? *Neuroimage* (2009) **44**:893–905. doi:10.1016/j.neuroimage.2008.09.036
73. Saad ZS, Gotts SJ, Murphy K, Chen G, Jo HJ, Martin A, et al. Trouble at rest: how correlation patterns and group differences become distorted after global signal regression. *Brain Connect* (2012) **2**:25–32. doi:10.1089/brain.2012.0080
74. Fox M, Zhang D, Snyder A, Raichle M. The global signal and observed anticorrelated resting state brain networks. *J Neurophysiol* (2009) **101**:3270–83. doi:10.1152/jn.90777.2008
75. Mantini D, Gerits A, Nelissen K, Durand JB, Joly O, Simone L, et al. Default mode of brain function in monkeys. *J Neurosci* (2011) **31**:12954–62. doi:10.1523/JNEUROSCI.2318-11.2011
76. Keller CJ, Bickel S, Honey CJ, Groppe DM, Entz L, Craddock RC, et al. Neurophysiological investigation of spontaneous correlated and anticorrelated fluctuations of the BOLD signal. *J Neurosci* (2013) **33**:6333–42. doi:10.1523/JNEUROSCI.4837-12.2013
77. Bullmore E, Sporns O. Complex brain networks: graph theoretical analysis of structural and functional systems. *Nat Rev Neurosci* (2009) **10**:186–98. doi:10.1038/nrn2575
78. Calhoun VD, Sui J, Kiehl K, Turner J, Allen E, Pearlson G. Exploring the psychosis functional connectome: aberrant intrinsic networks in schizophrenia and bipolar disorder. *Front Psychiatry* (2011) **2**:75. doi:10.3389/fpsyt.2011.00075
79. Khadka S, Meda SA, Stevens MC, Glahn DC, Calhoun VD, Sweeney JA, et al. Is aberrant functional connectivity a psychosis endophenotype? A resting state functional magnetic resonance imaging study. *Biol Psychiatry* (2013) **74**(6):458–66. doi:10.1016/j.biopsych.2013.04.024
80. van den Heuvel MP, Sporns O, Collin G, Scheewe T, Mandl RC, Cahn W, et al. Abnormal rich club organization and functional brain dynamics in schizophrenia. *JAMA Psychiatry* (2013) **70**:783–92. doi:10.1001/jamapsychiatry.2013.1328
81. Cole MW, Yarkoni T, Repovs G, Anticevic A, Braver TS. Global connectivity of prefrontal cortex predicts cognitive control and intelligence. *J Neurosci* (2012) **32**:8988–99. doi:10.1523/JNEUROSCI.0536-12.2012
82. Anticevic A, Hu S, Zhang S, Savic A, Billingslea E, Wasylink S, et al. Global resting-state fMRI analysis identifies frontal cortex, striatal, and cerebellar dysconnectivity in obsessive-compulsive disorder. *Biol Psychiatry* (2013). doi:10.1016/j.biopsych.2013.10.021
83. Calhoun VD, Maciejewski PK, Pearlson GD, Kiehl KA. Temporal lobe and "default" hemodynamic brain modes discriminate between schizophrenia and bipolar disorder. *Hum Brain Mapp* (2008) **29**:1265–75. doi:10.1002/hbm.20463
84. Meda SA, Gill A, Stevens MC, Lorenzoni RP, Glahn DC, Calhoun VD, et al. Differences in resting-state functional magnetic resonance imaging functional network connectivity between schizophrenia and psychotic bipolar probands and their unaffected first-degree relatives. *Biol Psychiatry* (2012) **71**:881–9. doi:10.1016/j.biopsych.2012.01.025
85. Friston KJ, Frith CD. Schizophrenia: a disconnection syndrome? *Clin Neurosci* (1995) **2**:1–9.
86. Rolls ET, Loh M, Deco G, Winterer G. Computational models of schizophrenia and dopamine modulation in the prefrontal cortex. *Nat Rev Neurosci* (2008) **9**:696–709. doi:10.1038/nrn2462
87. Rolls ET, Deco G. A computational neuroscience approach to schizophrenia and its onset. *Neurosci Biobehav Rev* (2010) **35**(8):1644–53. doi:10.1016/j.neubiorev.2010.09.001
88. Lisman J. Excitation, inhibition, local oscillations, or large-scale loops: what causes the symptoms of schizophrenia? *Curr Opin Neurobiol* (2012) **22**:537–44. doi:10.1016/j.conb.2011.10.018
89. Repovs G, Csernansky JG, Barch DM. Brain network connectivity in individuals with schizophrenia and their siblings. *Biol Psychiatry* (2011) **15**:967–73. doi:10.1016/j.biopsych.2010.11.009
90. Repovs G, Barch DM. Working memory related brain network connectivity in individuals with schizophrenia and their siblings. *Front Hum Neurosci* (2012) **6**:137. doi:10.3389/fnhum.2012.00137
91. Anticevic A, Corlett PR. Cognition-emotion dysinteraction in schizophrenia. *Front Psychol* (2012) **3**:392. doi:10.3389/fpsyg.2012.00392
92. Hoffman RE, Fernandez T, Pittman B, Hampson M. Elevated functional connectivity along a corticostriatal loop and the mechanism of auditory/verbal hallucinations in patients with schizophrenia. *Biol Psychiatry* (2011) **69**:407–14. doi:10.1016/j.biopsych.2010.09.050
93. Vercammen A, Knegtering H, den Boer JA, Liemburg EJ, Aleman A. Auditory hallucinations in schizophrenia are associated with reduced functional connectivity of the temporo-parietal area. *Biol Psychiatry* (2010) **67**:912–8. doi:10.1016/j.biopsych.2009.11.017
94. Palaniyappan L. Does the salience network play a cardinal role in psychosis? An emerging hypothesis of insular dysfunction. *J Psychiatry Neurosci* (2012) **37**:17–27. doi:10.1503/jpn.100176
95. Palaniyappan L, White TP, Liddle PF. The concept of salience network dysfunction in schizophrenia: from neuroimaging observations to therapeutic opportunities. *Curr Top Med Chem* (2012) **12**:2324–38. doi:10.2174/156802612805289881
96. Kapur S. Psychosis as a state of aberrant salience: a framework linking biology, phenomenology, and pharmacology in schizophrenia. *Am J Psychiatry* (2003) **160**:13–23. doi:10.1176/appi.ajp.160.1.13
97. Kapur S, Mizrahi R, Li M. From dopamine to salience to psychosis-linking biology, pharmacology and phenomenology of psychosis. *Schizophr Res* (2005) **79**(1):59–68. doi:10.1016/j.schres.2005.01.003
98. Tu PC, Hsieh JC, Li CT, Bai YM, Su TP. Cortico-striatal disconnection within the cingulo-opercular network in schizophrenia revealed by intrinsic functional connectivity analysis: a resting fMRI study. *Neuroimage* (2012) **59**(1):238–47. doi:10.1016/j.neuroimage.2011.07.086.
99. Moran LV, Tagamets MA, Sampath H, O'Donnell A, Stein EA, Kochunov P, et al. Disruption of anterior insula modulation of large-scale brain networks in schizophrenia. *Biol Psychiatry* (2013) **74**:467–74. doi:10.1016/j.biopsych.2013.02.029
100. Palaniyappan L, Simmonite M, White TP, Liddle EB, Liddle PF. Neural primacy of the salience processing system in schizophrenia. *Neuron* (2013) **79**:814–28. doi:10.1016/j.neuron.2013.06.027
101. Schippers MB, Renken R, Keysers C. The effect of intra- and inter-subject variability of hemodynamic responses on group level Granger causality analyses. *Neuroimage* (2011) **57**:22–36. doi:10.1016/j.neuroimage.2011.02.008
102. Smith SM, Bandettini PA, Miller KL, Behrens T. The danger of systematic bias in group-level FMRI-lag-based causality estimation. *Neuroimage* (2012) **59**(2):1228–9. doi:10.1016/j.neuroimage.2011.08.015
103. Wen X, Rangarajan G, Ding M. Is Granger causality a viable technique for analyzing fMRI data? *PLoS One* (2013) **8**:e67428. doi:10.1371/journal.pone.0067428
104. Smith SM, Miller KL, Salimi-Khorshidi G, Webster M, Beckmann CF, Nichols TE, et al. Network modelling methods for FMRI. *Neuroimage* (2011) **54**:875–91. doi:10.1016/j.neuroimage.2010.08.063
105. Goldman-Rakic PS. Prefrontal cortical dysfunction in schizophrenia: the relevance of working memory. In: Carroll BJ, Barrett JE, editors. *Psychopathology and the Brain.* New York: Raven Press, Ltd. (1991). p. 1–23.
106. Laruelle M, Kegeles LS, Abi-Dargham A. Glutamate, dopamine, and schizophrenia: from pathophysiology to treatment. *Ann N Y Acad Sci* (2003) **1003**:138–58. doi:10.1196/annals.1300.063
107. Guillin O, Abi-Dargham A, Laruelle M. Neurobiology of dopamine in schizophrenia. *Int Rev Neurobiol* (2007) **78**:1–39. doi:10.1016/S0074-7742(06)78001-1
108. Howes OD, Kambeitz J, Kim E, Stahl D, Slifstein M, Abi-Dargham A, et al. The nature of dopamine dysfunction in schizophrenia and what this means for treatment: meta-analysis of imaging studies. *Arch Gen Psychiatry* (2012) **69**(8):776–86. doi:10.1001/archgenpsychiatry.2012.169
109. Coyle JT. Glutamate and schizophrenia: beyond the dopamine hypothesis. *Cell Mol Neurobiol* (2006) **26**(4–6):365–84. doi:10.1007/s10571-006-9062-8
110. Bernstein H-G, Steiner J, Bogerts B. Glial cells in schizophrenia: pathophysiological significance and possible consequences for therapy. *Expert Rev Neurother* (2009) **9**:1059–71. doi:10.1586/ern.09.59
111. Moghaddam B, Javitt D. From revolution to evolution: the glutamate hypothesis of schizophrenia and its implication for treatment. *Neuropsychopharmacology* (2011) **37**(1):4–15. doi:10.1038/npp.2011.181
112. Ongur D, Drevets WC, Price JL. Glial reduction in the subgenual prefrontal cortex in mood disorders. *Proc Natl Acad Sci U S A* (1998) **95**:13290–5. doi:10.1073/pnas.95.22.13290

113. Marsman A, van den Heuvel MP, Klomp DW, Kahn RS, Luijten PR, Hulshoff Pol HE. Glutamate in schizophrenia: a focused review and meta-analysis of 1H-MRS studies. *Schizophr Bull* (2013) **39**:120–9. doi:10.1093/schbul/sbr069
114. Krystal JH, Perry EB, Gueorguieva R, Belger A, Madonick SH, Abi-Dargham A, et al. Comparative and interactive human psychopharmacologic effects of ketamine and amphetamine: implications for glutamatergic and dopaminergic model psychoses and cognitive function. *Arch Gen Psychiatry* (2005) **62**:985–94. doi:10.1001/archpsyc.62.9.985
115. Stone JM, Dietrich C, Edden R, Mehta MA, De Simoni S, Reed LJ, et al. Ketamine effects on brain GABA and glutamate levels with 1H-MRS: relationship to ketamine-induced psychopathology. *Mol Psychiatry* (2012) **17**:664–5. doi:10.1038/mp.2011.171
116. Laruelle M, Abi-Dargham A, Gil R, Kegeles L, Innis R. Increased dopamine transmission in schizophrenia: relationship to illness phases. *Biol Psychiatry* (1999) **46**:56–72. doi:10.1016/S0006-3223(99)00067-0
117. Kegeles LS, Abi-Dargham A, Zea-Ponce Y, Rodenhiser-Hill J, Mann JJ, Van Heertum RL, et al. Modulation of amphetamine-induced striatal dopamine release by ketamine in humans: implications for schizophrenia. *Biol Psychiatry* (2000) **48**:627–40. doi:10.1016/S0006-3223(00)00976-8
118. Schobel SA, Chaudhury NH, Khan UA, Paniagua B, Styner MA, Asllani I, et al. Imaging patients with psychosis and a mouse model establishes a spreading pattern of hippocampal dysfunction and implicates glutamate as a driver. *Neuron* (2013) **10**:81–93. doi:10.1016/j.neuron.2013.02.011
119. Durstewitz D, Kelc M, Gunturkun O. A neurocomputational theory of the dopaminergic modulation of working memory functions. *J Neurosci* (1999) **19**:2807–22.
120. Durstewitz D, Seamans JK, Sejnowski TJ. Dopamine-mediated stabilization of delay-period activity in a network model of prefrontal cortex. *J Neurophysiol* (2000) **83**(3):1733–50.
121. Goodwin FK, Jamison KR. *Manic Depressive Illness*. New York: Oxford University Press (1990).
122. Pearlson GD, Wong DF, Tune LE, Ross CA, Chase GA, Links JM, et al. In vivo D2 dopamine receptor density in psychotic and non-psychotic patients with bipolar disorder. *Arch Gen Psychiatry* (1995) **52**:471–7. doi:10.1001/archpsyc.1995.03950180057008
123. Glahn DC, Bearden CE, Barguil M, Barrett J, Reichenberg A, Bowden CL, et al. The neurocognitive signature of psychotic bipolar disorder. *Biol Psychiatry* (2007) **62**:910–6. doi:10.1016/j.biopsych.2007.02.001
124. Weinberger DR. Implications of normal brain development for the pathogenesis of schizophrenia. *Arch Gen Psychiatry* (1987) **44**:660–9. doi:10.1001/archpsyc.1987.01800190080012
125. Lewis DA, Lieberman JA. Catching up on schizophrenia: natural history and neurobiology. *Neuron* (2000) **28**:325–34. doi:10.1016/S0896-6273(00)00111-2
126. Uhlhaas PJ, Singer W. Abnormal neural oscillations and synchrony in schizophrenia. *Nat Rev Neurosci* (2010) **11**:100–13. doi:10.1038/nrn2774
127. Van Essen DC, Ugurbil K, Auerbach E, Barch DM, Behrens TE, Bucholz R, et al. The human connectome project: a data acquisition perspective. *Neuroimage* (2012) **62**:2222–31. doi:10.1016/j.neuroimage.2012.02.018
128. Behrens TE, Johansen-Berg H, Woolrich MW, Smith SM, Wheeler-Kingshott CA, Boulby PA, et al. Non-invasive mapping of connections between human thalamus and cortex using diffusion imaging. *Nat Neurosci* (2003) **6**:750–7. doi:10.1038/nn1075
129. Zhang D, Snyder AZ, Shimony JS, Fox MD, Raichle ME. Noninvasive functional and structural connectivity mapping of the human thalamocortical system. *Cereb Cortex* (2010) **20**:1187–94. doi:10.1093/cercor/bhp182
130. Fischl B, Salat DH, van der Kouwe AJ, Makris N, Ségonne F, Quinn BT, et al. Sequence-independent segmentation of magnetic resonance images. *Neuroimage* (2004) **23**(Suppl 1):S69–84. doi:10.1016/j.neuroimage.2004.07.016
131. Carlsson M, Carlsson A. Interactions between glutamatergic and monoaminergic systems within the basal ganglia – implications for schizophrenia and Parkinson's disease. *Trends Neurosci* (1990) **13**:272–6. doi:10.1016/0166-2236(90)90108-M
132. Andreasen NC, Arndt S, Swayze V, Cizadlo T, Flaum M, O'Leary D, et al. Thalamic abnormalities in schizophrenia visualized through magnetic resonance image averaging. *Science* (1994) **266**:294–8. doi:10.1126/science.7939669
133. Carlsson A, Waters N, Holm-Waters S, Tedroff J, Nilsson M, Carlsson ML. Interactions between monoamines, glutamate, and GABA in schizophrenia: new evidence. *Annu Rev Pharmacol Toxicol* (2001) **41**:237–60. doi:10.1146/annurev.pharmtox.41.1.237
134. Lewis DA, Cruz DA, Melchitzky DS, Pierri JN. Lamina-specific deficits in parvalbumin-immunoreactive varicosities in the prefrontal cortex of subjects with schizophrenia: evidence for fewer projections from the thalamus. *Am J Psychiatry* (2001) **158**:1411–22. doi:10.1176/appi.ajp.158.9.1411
135. Alexander GE, Delong MR, Strick PL. Parallel organization of functionally segregated circuits linking basal ganglia and cortex. *Annu Rev Neurosci* (1986) **9**:357–81. doi:10.1146/annurev.ne.09.030186.002041
136. Guillery RW, Sherman SM. Thalamic relay functions and their role in corticocortical communication: generalizations from the visual system. *Neuron* (2002) **33**:163–75. doi:10.1016/S0896-6273(01)00582-7
137. Sherman SM. The thalamus is more than just a relay. *Curr Opin Neurobiol* (2007) **17**:417–22. doi:10.1016/j.conb.2007.07.003
138. Sherman SM. Thalamocortical interactions. *Curr Opin Neurobiol* (2012) **22**:575–9. doi:10.1016/j.conb.2012.03.005
139. Haber S, McFarland NR. The place of the thalamus in frontal cortical-basal ganglia circuits. *Neuroscientist* (2001) **7**:315–24. doi:10.1177/107385840100700408
140. Johansen-Berg H, Behrens TE, Sillery E, Ciccarelli O, Thompson AJ, Smith SM, et al. Functional-anatomical validation and individual variation of diffusion tractography-based segmentation of the human thalamus. *Cereb Cortex* (2005) **15**:31–9. doi:10.1093/cercor/bhh105
141. Pakkenberg B. Pronounced reduction of total neuron number in mediodorsal thalamic nucleus and nucleus accumbens in schizophrenics. *Arch Gen Psychiatry* (1990) **47**:1023–8. doi:10.1001/archpsyc.1990.01810230039007
142. Lewis DA. Is there a neuropathology of schizophrenia? Recent findings converge on altered thalamic-prefrontal cortical connectivity. *Neuroscientist* (2000) **6**:208–18. doi:10.1177/107385840000600311
143. Cronenwett WJ, Csernansky J. Thalamic pathology in schizophrenia. *Curr Top Behav Neurosci* (2010) **4**:509–28. doi:10.1007/7854_2010_55
144. Volk DW, Lewis DA. Effects of a mediodorsal thalamus lesion on prefrontal inhibitory circuitry: implications for schizophrenia. *Biol Psychiatry* (2003) **53**:385–9. doi:10.1016/S0006-3223(02)01547-0
145. Selemon LD, Begovic A, Rakic P. Selective reduction of neuron number and volume of the mediodorsal nucleus of the thalamus in macaques following irradiation at early gestational ages. *J Comp Neurol* (2009) **515**:454–64. doi:10.1002/cne.22078
146. Csernansky JG, Schindler MK, Splinter NR, Wang L, Gado M, Selemon LD, et al. Abnormalities of thalamic volume and shape in schizophrenia. *Am J Psychiatry* (2004) **161**:896–902. doi:10.1176/appi.ajp.161.5.896
147. Harms MP, Wang L, Mamah D, Barch DM, Thompson PA, Csernansky JG. Thalamic shape abnormalities in individuals with schizophrenia and their nonpsychotic siblings. *J Neurosci* (2007) **27**:13835–42. doi:10.1523/JNEUROSCI.2571-07.2007
148. Geyer MA, Krebs-Thomson K, Braff DL, Swerdlow NR. Pharmacological studies of prepulse inhibition models of sensorimotor gating deficits in schizophrenia: a decade in review. *Psychopharmacology* (2001) **156**:117–54. doi:10.1007/s002130100811
149. Turetsky BI, Calkins ME, Light GA, Olincy A, Radant AD, Swerdlow NR. Neurophysiological endophenotypes of schizophrenia: the viability of selected candidate measures. *Schizophr Bull* (2007) **33**:69–94. doi:10.1093/schbul/sbl060
150. Oltmanns TF, Neale JM. Schizophrenic performance when distractors are present: attentional deficit or differential task difficulty? *J Abnorm Psychol* (1975) **84**:205–9. doi:10.1037/h0076721
151. Anticevic A, Repovs G, Corlett PR, Barch DM. Negative and non-emotional interference with visual working memory in schizophrenia. *Biol Psychiatry* (2011) **70**:1159–68. doi:10.1016/j.biopsych.2011.07.010
152. Welsh RC, Chen AC, Taylor SF. Low-frequency BOLD fluctuations demonstrate altered thalamocortical connectivity in schizophrenia. *Schizophr Bull* (2010) **36**:713–22. doi:10.1093/schbul/sbn145
153. Giguere M, Goldman-Rakic PS. Mediodorsal nucleus: areal, laminar, and tangential distribution of afferents and efferents in the frontal lobe of rhesus monkeys. *J Comp Neurol* (1988) **277**:195–213. doi:10.1002/cne.902770204
154. Ray JP, Price JL. The organization of projections from the mediodorsal nucleus of the thalamus to orbital and medial prefrontal cortex in macaque monkeys. *J Comp Neurol* (1993) **337**:1–31. doi:10.1002/cne.903370102

155. Parnaudeau S, O'Neill PK, Bolkan SS, Ward RD, Abbas AI, Roth BL, et al. Inhibition of mediodorsal thalamus disrupts thalamofrontal connectivity and cognition. *Neuron* (2013) **77**:1151–62. doi:10.1016/j.neuron.2013.01.038
156. Rouiller EM, Liang F, Babalian A, Moret V, Wiesendanger M. Cerebellothalamocortical and pallidothalamocortical projections to the primary and supplementary motor cortical areas: a multiple tracing study in macaque monkeys. *J Comp Neurol* (1994) **345**(2):185–213.
157. Norman KA, Polyn SM, Detre GJ, Haxby JV. Beyond mind-reading: multi-voxel pattern analysis of fMRI data. *Trends Cogn Sci* (2006) **10**:424–30. doi:10.1016/j.tics.2006.07.005
158. Van Essen DC, Ugurbil K. The future of the human connectome. *Neuroimage* (2012) **62**:1299–310. doi:10.1016/j.neuroimage.2012.01.032
159. Gottesman II, Gould TD. The endophenotype concept in psychiatry: etymology and strategic intentions. *Am J Psychiatry* (2003) **160**:636–45. doi:10.1176/appi.ajp.160.4.636
160. Meyer-Lindenberg A. From maps to mechanisms through neuroimaging of schizophrenia. *Nature* (2010) **468**:194–202. doi:10.1038/nature09569
161. Klingner CM, Langbein K, Dietzek M, Smesny S, Witte OW, Sauer H, et al. Thalamocortical connectivity during resting state in schizophrenia. *Eur Arch Psychiatry Clin Neurosci* (2013). doi:10.1007/s00406-013-0417-0
162. Anticevic A, Cole MW, Murray JD, Corlett PR, Wang XJ, Krystal JH. The role of default network deactivation in cognition and disease. *Trends Cogn Sci* (2012) **16**:584–92. doi:10.1016/j.tics.2012.10.008
163. Drevets WC, Price JL, Simpson JR Jr, Todd RD, Reich T, Vannier M, et al. Subgenual prefrontal cortex abnormalities in mood disorders. *Nature* (1997) **386**:824–7. doi:10.1038/386824a0
164. Drevets WC, Savitz J, Trimble M. The subgenual anterior cingulate cortex in mood disorders. *CNS Spectr* (2008) **13**(8):663–81.
165. Benes FM, Berretta S. GABAergic interneurons: implications for understanding schizophrenia and bipolar disorder. *Neuropsychopharmacology* (2001) **25**:1–27. doi:10.1016/S0893-133X(01)00225-1
166. Keshavan MS, Clementz BA, Pearlson GD, Sweeney JA, Tamminga CA. Reimagining psychoses: an agnostic approach to diagnosis. *Schizophr Res* (2013) **146**:10–6. doi:10.1016/j.schres.2013.02.022
167. MacDonald AW III, Chafee MV. Translational and developmental perspective on N-methyl-D-aspartate synaptic deficits in schizophrenia. *Dev Psychopathol* (2006) **18**(3):853–76. doi:10.1017/S0954579406060421
168. Greene R. Circuit analysis of NMDAR hypofunction in the hippocampus, in vitro, and psychosis of schizophrenia. *Hippocampus* (2001) **11**:569–77. doi:10.1002/hipo.1072
169. Wang M, Yang Y, Wang CJ, Gamo NJ, Jin LE, Mazer JA, et al. NMDA receptors subserve persistent neuronal firing during working memory in dorsolateral prefrontal cortex. *Neuron* (2013) **77**:736–49. doi:10.1016/j.neuron.2012.12.032
170. Cho RY, Konecky RO, Carter CS. Impairments in frontal cortical gamma synchrony and cognitive control in schizophrenia. *Proc Natl Acad Sci U S A* (2006) **103**:19878–83. doi:10.1073/pnas.0609440103
171. de la Fuente-Sandoval C, León-Ortiz P, Favila R, Stephano S, Mamo D, Ramírez-Bermúdez J, et al. Higher levels of glutamate in the associative-striatum of subjects with prodromal symptoms of schizophrenia and patients with first-episode psychosis. *Neuropsychopharmacology* (2011) **36**:1781–91. doi:10.1038/npp.2011.65
172. Adler CM, Malhotra AK, Elman I, Goldberg T, Egan M, Pickar D, Comparison of ketamine-induced thought disorder in healthy volunteers and thought disorder in schizophrenia. *Am J Psychiatry* (1999) **156**(10):1646–9.
173. Thomas LE, Woods SW. The schizophrenia prodrome: a developmentally informed review and update for psychopharmacologic treatment. *Child Adolesc Psychiatr Clin N Am* (2006) **15**(1):109–33. doi:10.1016/j.chc.2005.08.011
174. Moore JW, Cambridge VC, Morgan H, Giorlando F, Adapa R, Fletcher PC. Time, action and psychosis: using subjective time to investigate the effects of ketamine on sense of agency. *Neuropsychologia* (2013) **51**:377–84. doi:10.1016/j.neuropsychologia.2012.07.005
175. Honey RA, Honey GD, O'Loughlin C, Sharar SR, Kumaran D, Bullmore ET, et al. Acute ketamine administration alters the brain responses to executive demands in a verbal working memory task: an FMRI study. *Neuropsychopharmacology* (2004) **29**:1203–4. doi:10.1038/sj.npp.1300438
176. Moghaddam B, Adams B, Verma A, Daly D. Activation of glutamatergic neurotransmission by ketamine: a novel step in the pathway from NMDA receptor blockade to dopaminergic and cognitive disruptions associated with the prefrontal cortex. *J Neurosci* (1997) **17**:2921–7.
177. Scheidegger M, Walter M, Lehmann M, Metzger C. Ketamine decreases resting state functional network connectivity in healthy subjects: implications for antidepressant drug action. *PLoS One* (2012) **7**(9):e44799. doi:10.1371/journal.pone.0044799
178. Krystal JH, Sanacora G, Duman RS. Rapid-acting glutamatergic antidepressants: the path to ketamine and beyond. *Biol Psychiatry* (2013) **73**(12):1133–41. doi:10.1016/j.biopsych.2013.03.026
179. Cornwell BR, Salvadore G, Furey M, Marquardt CA, Brutsche NE, Grillon C, et al. Synaptic potentiation is critical for rapid antidepressant response to ketamine in treatment-resistant major depression. *Biol Psychiatry* (2012) **72**:555–61. doi:10.1016/j.biopsych.2012.03.029
180. Nugent AC, Diazgranados N, Carlson PJ, Ibrahim L, Luckenbaugh DA, Brutsche N, et al. Neural correlates of rapid antidepressant response to ketamine in bipolar disorder. *Bipolar Disord* (2013). doi:10.1111/bdi.12118
181. Sheline YI, Barch DM, Price JL, Rundle MM, Vaishnavi SN, Snyder AZ, et al. The default mode network and self-referential processes in depression. *Proc Natl Acad Sci U S A* (2009) **106**:1942–7. doi:10.1073/pnas.0812686106
182. Moghaddam B, Krystal JH. Capturing the angel in "angel dust": twenty years of translational neuroscience studies of NMDA receptor antagonists in animals and humans. *Schizophr Bull* (2012) **38**:942–9. doi:10.1093/schbul/sbs075
183. Moghaddam B. Bringing order to the glutamate chaos in schizophrenia. *Neuron* (2003) **40**:881–4. doi:10.1016/S0896-6273(03)00757-8
184. Fornito A, Harrison BJ, Zalesky A, Simons JS. Competitive and cooperative dynamics of large-scale brain functional networks supporting recollection. *Proc Natl Acad Sci U S A* (2012) **109**(31):12788–93. doi:10.1073/pnas.1204185109
185. Driesen NR, McCarthy G, Bhagwagar Z, Bloch MH, Calhoun VD, D'Souza DC, et al. The impact of NMDA receptor blockade on human working memory-related prefrontal function and connectivity. *Neuropsychopharmacology* (2013) **38**(13):2613–22. doi:10.1038/npp.2013.170
186. Salazar RF, Dotson NM, Bressler SL, Gray CM. Content-specific fronto-parietal synchronization during visual working memory. *Science* (2012) **338**:1097–100. doi:10.1126/science.1224000
187. Pan WJ, Thompson GJ, Magnuson ME, Jaeger D, Keilholz S. Infraslow LFP correlates to resting-state fMRI BOLD signals. *Neuroimage* (2013) **74**:288–97. doi:10.1016/j.neuroimage.2013.02.035
188. He BJ. Spontaneous and task-evoked brain activity negatively interact. *J Neurosci* (2013) **33**:4672–82. doi:10.1523/JNEUROSCI.2922-12.2013
189. Musso F, Brinkmeyer J, Ecker D, London MK, Thieme G, Warbrick T, et al. Ketamine effects on brain function – simultaneous fMRI/EEG during a visual oddball task. *Neuroimage* (2011) **58**:508–25. doi:10.1016/j.neuroimage.2011.06.045
190. Schmidt A, Bachmann R, Kometer M, Csomor PA, Stephan KE, Seifritz E, et al. Mismatch negativity encoding of prediction errors predicts S-ketamine-induced cognitive impairments. *Neuropsychopharmacology* (2012) **37**:865–75. doi:10.1038/npp.2011.261
191. Gil-da-Costa R, Stoner GR, Fung R, Albright TD. Nonhuman primate model of schizophrenia using a noninvasive EEG method. *Proc Natl Acad Sci U S A* (2013) **110**:15425–30. doi:10.1073/pnas.1312264110
192. Wang X-J, Tegnér J, Constantinidis C, Goldman-Rakic PS. Division of labor among distinct subtypes of inhibitory neurons in a cortical microcircuit of working memory. *Proc Natl Acad Sci U S A* (2004) **101**:1368–73. doi:10.1073/pnas.0305337101
193. Deco G, Jirsa VK, McIntosh A. Emerging concepts for the dynamical organization of resting-state activity in the brain. *Nat Rev Neurosci* (2011) **12**:43–56. doi:10.1038/nrn2961
194. Honey CJ, Sporns O, Cammoun L, Gigandet X, Thiran JP, Meuli R, et al. Predicting human resting-state functional connectivity from structural connectivity. *Proc Natl Acad Sci U S A* (2009) **106**:2035–40. doi:10.1073/pnas.0811168106
195. Cabral J, Hugues E, Kringelbach ML, Deco G. Modeling the outcome of structural disconnection on resting-state functional connectivity. *Neuroimage* (2012) **62**:1342–53. doi:10.1016/j.neuroimage.2012.06.007
196. Buckner RL, Andrews-Hanna JR, Schacter DL. The brain's default network: anatomy, function, and relevance to disease. *Ann N Y Acad Sci* (2008) **1124**:1–38. doi:10.1196/annals.1440.011

197. Brunel N, Wang XJ. Effects of neuromodulation in a cortical network model of object working memory dominated by recurrent inhibition. *J Comput Neurosci* (2001) **11**:63–85. doi:10.1023/A:1011204814320
198. Wong KF, Wang XJ. A recurrent network mechanism of time integration in perceptual decisions. *J Neurosci* (2006) **26**:1314–28. doi:10.1523/JNEUROSCI.3733-05.2006

10

Near-Infrared Spectroscopy in Schizophrenia: A Possible Biomarker for Predicting Clinical Outcome and Treatment Response

***Shinsuke Koike*[1,2]*, *Yukika Nishimura*[2], *Ryu Takizawa*[2,3], *Noriaki Yahata*[4] and *Kiyoto Kasai*[2]**

[1] *Office for Mental Health Support, Division for Counseling and Support, The University of Tokyo, Tokyo, Japan*
[2] *Department of Neuropsychiatry, Graduate School of Medicine, The University of Tokyo, Tokyo, Japan*
[3] *Social, Genetic and Developmental Psychiatry Centre, Institute of Psychiatry, King's College London, London, UK*
[4] *Department of Youth Mental Health, Graduate School of Medicine, The University of Tokyo, Tokyo, Japan*

***Correspondence:**
Shinsuke Koike, Office for Mental Health Support, Division for Counseling and Support, The University of Tokyo, 7-3-1 Hongo, Bunkyo-ku, Tokyo 113-0033, Japan
e-mail: skoike-tky@umin.ac.jp

Functional near-infrared spectroscopy (fNIRS) is a relatively new technique that can measure hemoglobin changes in brain tissues, and its use in psychiatry has been progressing rapidly. Although it has several disadvantages (e.g., relatively low spatial resolution and the possibility of shallow coverage in the depth of brain regions) compared with other functional neuroimaging techniques (e.g., functional magnetic resonance imaging and positron emission tomography), fNIRS may be a candidate instrument for clinical use in psychiatry, as it can measure brain activity in naturalistic position easily and non-invasively. fNIRS instruments are also small and work silently, and can be moved almost everywhere including schools and care units. Previous fNIRS studies have shown that patients with schizophrenia have impaired activity and characteristic waveform patterns in the prefrontal cortex during the letter version of the verbal fluency task, and part of these results have been approved as one of the Advanced Medical Technologies as an aid for the differential diagnosis of depressive symptoms by the Ministry of Health, Labor and Welfare of Japan in 2009, which was the first such approval in the field of psychiatry. Moreover, previous studies suggest that the activity in the frontopolar prefrontal cortex is associated with their functions in chronic schizophrenia and is its next candidate biomarker. Future studies aimed at exploring fNIRS differences in various clinical stages, longitudinal changes, drug effects, and variations during different task paradigms will be needed to develop more accurate biomarkers that can be used to aid differential diagnosis, the comprehension of the present condition, the prediction of outcome, and the decision regarding treatment options in schizophrenia. Future fNIRS researches will require standardized measurement procedures, probe settings, analytical methods and tools, manuscript description, and database systems in an fNIRS community.

Keywords: near-infrared spectroscopy, verbal fluency task, biological markers, early intervention, clinical outcome

INTRODUCTION

Techniques that allow the easier and less invasive measurement of brain structure and activity, such as magnetic resonance imaging (MRI), functional MRI, and positron emission tomography (PET), have progressed rapidly over the past 20 years. There has been considerable expectation regarding the clinical application of neuroimaging techniques to psychological conditions and psychiatric illnesses (1, 2). Biological markers measured using neuroimaging instruments would clarify the pathophysiological features of psychiatric disorders, inform patients and family members regarding their actual conditions, and improve general impression of psychiatric disorders, by more easily giving the explanation of their conditions and discussing their assumed prognoses.

Functional near-infrared spectroscopy (fNIRS) is a functional brain imaging tool that can measure hemoglobin changes over the surface of the brain easily and non-invasively (**Figure 1**) (3–5). fNIRS technique was found in 1977 (6), and has been applied to measure brain hemodynamic activity through the scalp (7, 8). The release of commercial fNIRS machines that are small, movable, and work silently during the last decade (**Figure 1B**) has allowed the progress of fNIRS research in the field of psychiatry (9). In 2012, more than 100 studies were published on this subject; among these, about 20 articles pertained to the field of psychiatry (9). Part of the results of those fNIRS studies has been approved as one of the Advanced Medical Technologies as an aid for the differential diagnosis of depressive symptoms by the Ministry of Health, Labor and Welfare of Japan in 2009 (10–12), as the presence of different characteristic waveform patterns in the prefrontal cortex (PFC) during a verbal fluency task (VFT) has been reported among patients with major depressive illness (4, 12–17), bipolar disorder (12, 13), and schizophrenia (4, 5, 12). This was the first such approval in the field of psychiatry in Japan (see the "Application to supplementary diagnostic tool for psychiatric disorders" subsection). Here, we reviewed fNIRS research that focused on schizophrenia, which

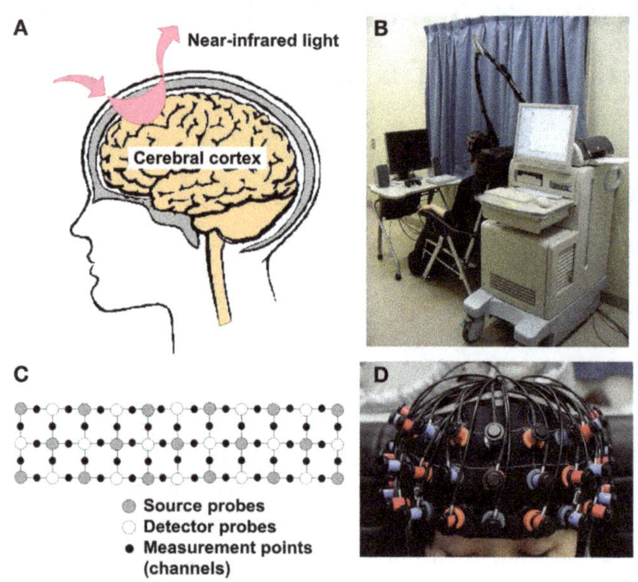

FIGURE 1 | Theoretical background and measurement settings of fNIRS. **(A)** Illustration of a simple source and detector probe set. When near-infrared light is emitted from a source probe onto the human scalp, it passes and scatters through brain tissues with relatively low absorption. Subsequently, part of this light is absorbed by blood hemoglobin in small vessels. A detector probe, normally placed 3 cm away from the source probe in adults, can detect scattered near-infrared light reflected by the surface of the cortex. **(B)** fNIRS measurement setting (ETG-4000, Hitachi Medical Corporation). Commercial fNIRS machines are small, movable, and work silently, so that they are easy to use in clinical settings. **(C,D)** 3 × 11 Probe attachment and fitting condition. Multi-channel fNIRS machines use multiple sources and detector probes and are able to measure brain activity between the probes. **(A–C)** Was approved by Hitachi Medical Corporation.

is currently the most published topic in the application of fNIRS in the field of psychiatry, and address future investigations that are needed for the clinical application of this technique as an aid for the differential diagnosis, comprehension of present conditions, prediction of outcome, and decision regarding treatment options in schizophrenia.

PRINCIPLES OF BRAIN ACTIVITY MEASUREMENT USING NEAR-INFRARED LIGHT

THEORETICAL BACKGROUND OF THE MEASUREMENT OF BRAIN ACTIVITY USING fNIRS INSTRUMENTS

Near-infrared light, especially that with a wavelength of 650–1000 nm, has characteristics that include a relatively high absorption through hemoglobin, as well as a relatively high penetration through bone and skin, compared with light with other wavelengths. The emission of near-infrared light from a source probe on the human scalp leads to its passing and scattering through brain tissues with relatively low absorption, followed by the absorption of part of this light by blood hemoglobin in small vessels (<1 mm) (18). A detector probe, which is normally placed 3 cm away from the source probe in adults, can detect scattered near-infrared light that is reflected by the surface of the cortex (**Figure 1A**). Therefore, the region located between the source and the detector probes is generally set as a measurement area that is often called a "channel" (**Figure 1C**). fNIRS instruments can measure oxygenated hemoglobin (O_2Hb) and deoxygenated hemoglobin (HHb), as well as total hemoglobin (tHb) by summing up O_2Hb and HHb, by using near-infrared light with two or more different wavelengths that are slightly different from the absorption rates of O_2Hb and HHb. In accordance with light manipulation, fNIRS instruments are roughly divided into three types: continuous wave (CW), frequency domain (FD), and time domain (TD) instruments. Although CW-type fNIRS machines are unable to measure absolute hemoglobin concentration in tissues, they are relatively small, have low installation and maintenance costs, and are able to perform measurements at a high sampling rate compared with FD- and TD-type fNIRS machines (18). Therefore, recent clinical studies have used CW-type fNIRS machines (19, 20). The theoretical details of all types of fNIRS instruments were reviewed elsewhere (18, 20, 21).

ADVANTAGES AND DISADVANTAGES OF fNIRS COMPARED WITH OTHER FUNCTIONAL IMAGING INSTRUMENTS

The advantages and disadvantages of CW-type fNIRS compared with other functional imaging instruments (fMRI, PET, and EEG) are shown in **Table 1**. fNIRS has the following advantages: (1) non-invasiveness, which allows repetitive measurements, even in infants (21, 22); (2) easy setting; (3) small size and portability; (4) high temporal resolution compared with fMRI and PET (18, 20); (5) possibility of performing measurements in a non-restrained position, such that participants can sit on a chair, talk, and move their hands; and (6) possibility of relatively easily combining measurements with other neuroimaging techniques, such as EEG (23, 24), MRI (25–30), PET (31–33), and magnetoencephalography (MEG) (34, 35). Conversely, fNIRS has the following disadvantages: (1) low spatial resolution (10–30 mm); (2) possibility of performing measurements only at the surface of the cortex; (3) inability to measure absolute hemoglobin value (CW-type); and (4) the data obtained can be influenced by scalp, muscle, skull, and cerebrospinal fluid factors in addition to hemodynamic changes in the cortex (20).

Other than task-related hemoglobin changes derived from neural activities under neurovascular coupling, fNIRS signals vary depending on task-related blood pressure changes and skin blood flow, as well as spontaneous brain activity related to heart rate, respiration, and physiological oscillations (20, 21). Simultaneous measurements by fNIRS and pulse Doppler sonography or by fNIRS with different probe distances [e.g., shallow (5 mm) and deep (30 mm)] allow the distinction of fNIRS signals from the cortex from those of other brain tissues. A study based on fNIRS with different probe distances and laser Doppler velocimetry showed that hemoglobin changes from the cortex during the VFT may contain only 6% of fNIRS data in the PFC, and that most signal changes may arise from changes in skin blood flow (36). The results OPF simultaneous fNIRS, fMRI, MR angiography, and peripheral physiological measurements suggested that task-evoked sympathetic arterial vasoconstriction affected fNIRS signal changes substantially (37). However, a subsequent study in which simultaneous measurements using multiple fNIRS probe

Table 1 | Comparison of CW-type fNIRS machines with other neuroimaging tools.

		fNIRS	fMRI	PET	EEG	MEG
Theoretical background	Signal property	Scattered near-infrared light	Magnetic property	Uptake of ligand marked positron	Collection of neural activity	Magnetic fields produced by brain's electrical activity
	Measurement area	Surface of the cortex	**Whole brain region**	**Whole brain region**	Surface of the cortex unless using depth EEG	Surface of the cortex
	Time resolution (s)	1	2–3	≥10	**0.01**	**0.01**
	Spatial resolution (mm)	20	**5**	10	20	10
	Effect of extra-cortical tissue	Some	**Little**	**Little**	Some	None
Measurement setting	Invasiveness	**No**	**No**	Intravenous injection of radioactive ligand	**No**	**No**
	Body movement	**Tolerable**	No	No	No	No
	Head restraint	**No**	Yes	Yes	**No**	Yes
Instrument	Size	**Small, movable**	Large, fix	Large, fix	Large in research use	Large, fix
	Transportability	**Yes**	No	No	Limited	No
	Initial cost	**300,000–400,000 USD**[a]	Several million USD	Several million USD	**100,000–300,000 USD**	Several million USD
	Measurement and maintenance cost	**Reasonable**	Moderate	Very expensive (positron ligand)	**Reasonable**	Moderate

Bold shows advantages compared to other neuroimaging tools.
[a] *ETG-4000 (Hitachi Medical Corporation).*

distances and laser Doppler flowmetry were performed suggested that about 50% of fNIRS signals contributed to the fNIRS signal component in the deep layer, mostly measured in the cortex, during several cognitive tasks, including the VFT (38). A study of simultaneous measurement using fMRI, fNIRS, and lase Doppler flowmeter showed that the prefrontal fNIRS signals were significantly correlated with the blood oxygenation level-dependent (BOLD) signals in the gray matter rather than those in the soft tissue or the laser Doppler signals (39). Previous studies have suggested that the ratio of fNIRS signal changes in the cortex varies from 6 to 60%, and the variation has been considered as being caused by differences in measuring instruments, estimation methods, and brain areas measured (20, 36–38, 40–44). Several studies have provided filtering methods that allow raising the ratio of task-related hemoglobin changes in the cortex to in the extra-cortical tissues; however, these systems require additional probes and complex analytical methodologies because of different near-infrared absorption and scattering coefficients in each tissue and anatomic characteristics throughout the light path in each brain area (25, 38, 40, 41). Therefore, fNIRS is a reliable tool for research based on the group-level and/or channel-cluster-level investigations, although its reliability at the individual and single-channel levels is not sufficient (18, 45–48). Few studies in clinical psychiatry have considered these filtering methods because of the limitations of measurement time and setting. Future studies will be needed to improve the signal-to-noise ratio for application over wide measurement areas without losing the advantage of fNIRS instruments.

COMPARISON OF fNIRS HEMOGLOBIN CHANGES WITH BOLD SIGNALS IN fMRI

The measurement of brain activity using the fMRI technique has progressed during the last two decades. The BOLD signal is thought to represent the differences in the magnetic properties of deoxygenated hemoglobin concentration under T2-weighted measurement conditions when cerebral blood flow (CBF) increases and HHb decreases in small vessels (49). The theoretical model of BOLD compared with fNIRS signals was reviewed in detail elsewhere (18). Briefly, localized O_2Hb decreases and HHb increases occur (i.e., initial dip) when neurons are activated in a specific region. Several seconds later, the blood flow system is triggered to request glucose to the region (i.e., hemodynamic response), which is followed by a CBF increase and peripheral vascular bed dilation, leading to tHb increase and HHb decrease in small vessels, and O_2Hb increase in blood capillaries and vascular bed. As this neurovascular coupling that occurs in the activated area is thought to vary according to brain area and vessel diameter, and to be sensitive to persistent neural activity, the relationship between hemoglobin changes and BOLD/fNIRS signals has a complex variation pattern.

Other than the difference in spatio-temporal measurement characteristics between BOLD and fNIRS signals, the BOLD signal is thought to detect mainly changes in the magnetic properties of small vessels, whereas the fNIRS signal is thought to detect changes in near-infrared light absorption in blood capillaries (50). Therefore, several discrepancies may occur between BOLD and fNIRS signals. Previous fNIRS studies have yielded inconsistent results compared with other imaging tools. Simultaneous fNIRS and fMRI studies have shown that the BOLD signal in a specific region was associated with the O_2Hb of fNIRS signal changes in the corresponding region (25, 29, 39, 51) or with HHb changes (26–28, 30, 51). One of the explanations for these inconsistent correlation results is that most fNIRS studies have been conducted using block-designed tasks, whereas fMRI studies have mainly used an event-related design. In addition, the analysis of fMRI data by software such as Statistical Parametric Mapping (SPM) uses a hypothesis that fits a probable activation model, whereas most fNIRS studies have analyzed average signal intensity during the whole task period without any probable activation model. Differences in acquired signal handling may result in discrepancies regarding regions with significant brain activity. As O_2Hb data generally exhibit larger changes compared with HHb during cognitive activity, most clinical fNIRS studies have mainly been analyzed using O_2Hb data.

ESTIMATION OF BRAIN AREA

As more studies have focused on the spatial characteristics of brain activity using multi-channel fNIRS instruments, the need to clarify the estimated location of each probe in the cortex and each channel on the scalp has arisen. As reviewed by Tsuzuki et al. recently (52), several methodologies can estimate brain areas at each probe and channel, such as structural MRI measurement using fNIRS probe marks for each participant (53, 54), a probabilistic registration method using a 3D digitizer (55), and a probabilistic virtual registration method without any additional instrument (56). As the virtual registration method enables the estimation of brain areas based on standard brain images at each probe and channel by defining only probe setting based on the 10–20 system electrode locations, and because this method has similar accuracy compared with other estimation methodologies (56), most fNIRS studies have applied this method to estimate the measurement brain areas of channels. fNIRS software can also use the virtual registration method as a toolbox (http://www.jichi.ac.jp/brainlab/tools.html) (57). There are several standard stereotaxic coordinate systems such as the Montreal Neurological Institute (MNI) and the Talairach Daemon. The LONI Probabilistic Brain Atlas (LPBA40) (58) system has been often used in fNIRS studies based on probabilistic registration methods (3, 52, 59, 60).

APPLICATION OF fNIRS IN SCHIZOPHRENIA RESEARCH

Schizophrenia is a syndrome that is characterized by positive and negative symptoms and cognitive dysfunction with enduring social deficits. Moreover, it affects approximately 0.7% of the general population (2). The World Health Organization reported that the estimated burden of schizophrenia accounts for 2.3% of all diseases worldwide, and its disability-adjusted life year ranks ninth among all non-communicable diseases (61). However, effective treatments and objective indices for all symptoms and functions of schizophrenia have not been fully met.

Since the first fNIRS report of altered activation patterns in schizophrenia compared with healthy controls was published in 1994 (62), fNIRS research focusing on schizophrenia has been the most published topic in the field of psychiatry (9). We reviewed systematically research articles published up to April 1, 2013, by searching PubMed and Web of Science. As in previous systematic reviews (9, 18), we used "[(near infrared) OR (optical topography)] AND (schizo* OR psycho*) AND (brain OR cortex)" as a search term. Two hundred and sixty articles were extracted, among which 29 explored brain activity in patients with schizophrenia. Half of these articles (15 articles, including 4 studies of genetic variants) adopted a VFT as an activation cognitive battery during measurement.

VERBAL FLUENCY TASK

The VFT is a popular cognitive task that is used in neuropsychological tests and neuroimaging measurements to explore various cognitive functions during verbal recall, retrieval, working memory, attention, and inhibition (avoiding inappropriate words) (63, 64). During the task, participants are instructed to say as many words from a given paradigm as possible in a given time (usually 60 s). This paradigm is roughly divided into semantic (category fluency task, CFT), such as fruits, or phonological (letter fluency task, LFT), such as words that begin with the letter "p." Neuropsychological studies have revealed that patients with schizophrenia have worse VFT performances compared with healthy controls (65). Although fMRI and fNIRS studies have shown that relatively global brain activity occurs during the VFT compared with a task that requires specific cognitive domains, such as the n-back working-memory task (28, 66) and the go/no-go task (67), most participants (including patients with chronic schizophrenia) can perform the task (10, 11, 19, 63, 64).

Eleven previous VFT studies are listed in **Table 2**. Watanabe and Kato firstly described that patients with schizophrenia had reduced O_2Hb and HHb changes in the left PFC during the LFT compared with healthy controls (68). This study also demonstrated that patients who were medicated with atypical antipsychotics had better task performances and similar O_2Hb changes compared with controls, suggesting that typical antipsychotics may impair task response and brain activity. However, that study did not explore whether impaired O_2Hb changes were derived from impaired task response or functional impairment in the PFC, which may be ameliorated by atypical antipsychotics. Suto et al. firstly described the spatio-temporal activity patterns in the PFC and temporal cortex among patients with depression and schizophrenia and healthy controls using two 24-channel fNIRS machines (4). In that study, a modified task procedure was adopted in which three initial syllables changed in turn every 20 s during a 60 s task period, to help participants avoid silence and reduce differences in task performances among groups. Patients with schizophrenia had lower activity in the bilateral PFC and temporal cortex at the start of the task period compared with controls, whereas patients with depression had lower activity in the bilateral PFC and temporal cortex across the task period. These results were irrespective of task performance, and the task paradigm used in that study was used widely in further studies. In addition, this result was based on the Advanced Medical Technologies in Japan (10–12). Using a larger cohort, Takizawa et al. replicated the observation that patients with schizophrenia had slower and inappropriate activity after the task period compared with healthy controls (5). Furthermore, activities in the frontopolar prefrontal cortex (FPC) region were positively

Table 2 | Previous fNIRS studies in schizophrenia using verbal fluency tasks.

Reference	Place	fNIRS instrument		Case demographics			
		Model[a]	Number of analyzed channels	Number of cases (M/F)	Mean age in cases (SD)	Medication	Recruitment places
Shimodera et al. (73)	Kochi	OMM-3000/16	42	32 (12/19)	42.4 (15.7)	All	University hospital
Koike et al. (3)	Tokyo	ETG-4000	52	38 (22/16)[b]	31.3 (6.1)[b]	All[b]	University hospital, psychiatric hospital, health service center, and clinics
Takeshi et al. (72)	Tokyo (Toho University)	OMM-3000/16	24	18 (7/11)	25.4 (5.8)	All	NA
Azechi et al. (70)	Osaka	OMM-3000/16	2	30 (16/14)[c]	39.6 (13.1)[c]	All	University hospital
Quaresima et al. (69)	L'Aquila	NIRO-300	2	9 (5/4)	32.1 (8.3)	All	NA
Ikezawa et al. (71)	Osaka	NIRO-200	2	30 (12/18)	38.7 (11.7)	Two patients drug naïve[d]	University hospital
Takizawa et al. (5)	Tokyo	ETG-4000	52	55 (26/29)	40.1 (11.1)	All	University hospital
Ehlis et al. (74)	Wuerzburg	ETG-100	22	12 (9/3)	34.2 (10.4)	One patient drug naïve	NA
Kubota et al. (75)	Cleveland	NIRO-300	2	16 (8/8)	37.5 (13.0)	All	NA
Suto et al. (4)	Gunma	ETG-100	48	13 (9/4)	37.9 (12.0)	All	University hospital
Watanabe and Kato (68)	Ehime	HEO-200	1	62 (30/32)	40.1 (12.3)	All	Psychiatric hospital

Reference	Task setting			Results[e]		
	Pre-task condition	Task condition	Post-task condition	Patients compared to controls	Estimated regions for group differences	Multiple analysis correlation
Shimodera et al. (73)	30-s Rest	30-s × 2 Letter sets	70-s Rest	↓	Bilateral FPC, DLPFC, and VLPFC regions	Bonferroni
Koike et al. (3)	60-s Vowel repeats	20-s × 3 Letter sets	70-s Vowel repeats	↓[f]	Bilateral FPC, DLPFC, and VLPFC regions[f]	FDR
Takeshi et al. (72)	60-s Vowel repeats	20-s × 3 Letter sets	70-s Vowel repeats	↓	Bilateral dorsal FPC and DLPFC	No
Azechi et al. (70)	30-s Vowel repeats	20-s × 3 Letter/category sets	60-s Vowel repeats	↓[g]	Bilateral FPC	No
Quaresima et al. (69)	120-s Rest	30-s × 4 Letter sets	No setting	↓	Bilateral FPC	No
Ikezawa et al. (71)	30-s Vowel repeats	20-s × 3 Letter/category sets	60-s Vowel repeats	↓[g]	Bilateral FPC	ANCOVA
Takizawa et al. (5)	60-s Vowel repeats	20-s × 3 Letter sets	70-s Vowel repeats	↓	Bilateral FPC, DLPFC, and VLPFC regions	FDR
Ehlis et al. (74)	10-s Rest	30-s Letter/category and 30-s rest × 2 sets	30-s Control task (repeatedly say weekdays) and 30-s rest between the sets of task conditions	↓[g]	Left DLPFC and VLPFC	ANOVA

(Continued)

Table 2 | Continued

Reference	Task setting			Results[e]		
	Pre-task condition	Task condition	Post-task condition	Patients compared to controls	Estimated regions for group differences	Multiple analysis correlation
Kubota et al. (75)	20-s A vowel repeats	15-s × 6 Letter/category sets	No setting	↓[g]	Bilateral FPC	ANOVA
Suto et al. (4)	30-s Vowel repeats	20-s × 3 Letter sets	60-s Vowel repeats	–	–	ANOVA
Watanabe and Kato (68)	15-s No detailed description	60-s One letter set	15-s No detailed description	↓	Left FPC	ANOVA

Reference	Correlational analysis between clinical variables and fNIRS signals		
	GAF	Other clinical variables	Medication
Shimodera et al. (73)	NA	n.s.	NA
Koike et al. (3)	Positive association in the FPC region in the chronic schizophrenia group	Positive association with PANSS positive or negative scores in the FEP group	n.s. (including no difference between UHR individuals with and without medication)
Takeshi et al. (72)	n.s., But positive association in the FPC during an idea fluency task	NA	NA
Azechi et al. (70)	NA	n.s.	n.s.
Quaresima et al. (69)	NA	NA	NA
Ikezawa et al. (71)	NA	n.s.	n.s.
Takizawa et al. (5)	Positive association in the FPC and right DLPFC regions	Negative correlation with age at measurement, positive correlation with PANSS positive score, and negative correlation with PANSS general psychopathology score in schizophrenia	n.s.
Ehlis et al. (74)	NA	NA	n.s.
Kubota et al. (75)	NA	NA	NA
Suto et al. (4)	NA	NA	NA
Watanabe and Kato (68)	NA	n.s.	n.s.

Excluded previous gene association studies.

NA, not applicable; n.s., no significant correlation; FPC, the frontopolar prefrontal cortex; DLPFC, dorsolateral prefrontal cortex; VLPFC, ventrolateral prefrontal cortex; FDR, false discovery rate; GAF, the global assessment of functioning; PANSS, the positive and negative symptom scale; FEP, first-episode psychosis, UHR, ultra-high risk.

[a] *OMM-3000/16, Shimadzu Corporation; ETG-4000 and ETG-100, Hitachi Medical Corporation; NIRO-300 and NIRO-200, Hamamatsu Photonics Corporation; HEO-200, Omron Healthcare Corporation.*

[b] *Exhibit case in the chronic schizophrenia group. Sixteen UHR and 2 FEP individuals were antipsychotics naïve and 8 UHR and 1 FEP individuals were drug naïve.*

[c] *As Azechi et al. (70) used the same sample from Ikezawa et al. (71) as the First group, we describe for the Second group.*

[d] *By Azechi et al. (70).*

[e] *Results from brain activity during the whole of the task period.*

[f] *Results in the chronic schizophrenia group.*

[g] *Results during the letter fluency tasks.*

associated with global assessment of functioning scores in schizophrenia. Quaresuma et al. replicated the finding of reduced brain activity in schizophrenia during the LFT, whereas no significant change was observed during a visual spatial working memory task (69). Ikezawa et al. and Azechi et al. showed the efficacy of the LFT task in fNIRS (70, 71). Ikezawa et al. measured hemoglobin changes in the PFC using a two-channel fNIRS instrument during the LFT, CFT, Tower of Hanoi (TOH), the Sternberg task, and the Stroop task, and showed that brain activities during the LFT and TOH were significantly different between patients with schizophrenia and healthy controls (71). Azechi et al. explored this further using discrimination analysis and showed that 88.3% of participants correctly discriminated between patients and controls based on task performance on the TOH, LFT, and CFT, and on fNIRS signals during the VFT (70). This result confirmed that 75% of independent participants were able to discriminate correctly using the same procedure. Koike et al. explored the signal differences among different clinical stages of schizophrenia (ultra-high risk, first-episode psychosis, and chronic schizophrenia) and showed that the activities in the FPC, ventrolateral PFC (VLPFC), and temporal cortex were lower in patients than they were in controls, whereas the activities in the dorsolateral PFC (DLPFC) decreased with advancing clinical stage (3). Those authors also replicated the finding that the activity in the FPC region was positively associated with global assessment of functioning scores in chronic schizophrenia, implying that it may be a candidate biomarker for the assessment of psychological condition in schizophrenia (3, 5). Takeshi et al. measured brain activity during the idea fluency task, which is thought to require more executive function, and showed that patients with schizophrenia had decreased activity in the ventral area of the PFC (72). Furthermore, these signal changes were positively associated with the global assessment of functioning scores, whereas O_2Hb changes during the LFT were not. Shimodera et al. replicated the characteristic waveforms in schizophrenia, such as smaller initial activity at the start of the task period, reduced activity during the task period, and inappropriate activity after the task period, and used a numerical calculation (73).

The CFT has also been used in fNIRS studies, which often compare this task to the LFT. Kubota et al. used a two-channel fNIRS instrument to show for the first time that healthy controls had larger activity in the PFC during the LFT than in the CFT under similar task performances, whereas patients with schizophrenia had smaller activity during the LFT than during the CFT (75). Patients with schizophrenia had smaller activity than did healthy controls under similar task performances between the groups. This result is consistent with those of other studies (70, 71). Ehlis et al. used a multi-channel fNIRS instrument that covered the left frontotemporal region and found that healthy controls had larger and spatially wider activities during the LFT compared with the CFT (74), which was then replicated by measuring wider areas of the bilateral prefrontal/temporal cortices (76). Ehlis et al. also replicated the finding that patients with schizophrenia had significantly reduced activities compared with healthy controls during LFT, but not during the CFT.

APPLICATION OF fNIRS AS A SUPPLEMENTARY DIAGNOSIS TOOL FOR PSYCHIATRIC DISORDERS

As described above, previous studies using a block-design LFT have indicated that patients with schizophrenia have not only reduced activity, but also inappropriate activity timing, especially at the start of the task period and post-task period, compared with healthy controls (4, 5). Subsequently, the Joint Project for Psychiatric Application of Near-Infrared Spectroscopy (JPSY-NIRS) Group has applied to these results and improved in the applicable way for clinical settings. The integral value (the size of the fNIRS signal area during the task period) and centroid value (the centroid time of the fNIRS signal area throughout the task) were determined by using averaged brain signals estimated in the frontopolar cortex. This group showed preliminarily that 69% of patients with MDD and 69% of patients with schizophrenia, and 69% MDD patients and 81% BP patients were correctly differentiated under an algorithm using these two values (10, 11). A part of these results was approved as one of the Advanced Medical Technologies as an aid for the differential diagnosis of depressive symptoms in 2009, which was the first such approval in the field of psychiatry in Japan (10, 11). Several criticisms have arisen regarding the limited replication in various clinical settings and the lack of consensus for application to mental health (77, 78). However, paper published recently on JPSY-NIRS replicated previous results (12). Using this algorithm, fNIRS can differentiate patients with depressive symptoms between major depressive disorder and psychotic disorders (bipolar disorder and schizophrenia), with a high classification rate (74.6 and 85.5%, respectively).

OTHER COGNITIVE TASKS AND MEASUREMENT SETTINGS

Three studies have explored the differences in brain activity during a random generation task (RNG) between patients with schizophrenia and healthy controls. Sinba et al. used a two-channel fNIRS instrument to describe for the first time that patients with schizophrenia had reduced brain activity in the PFC and worse task performances during the RNG compared with healthy controls, which represented different features during ruler-catching and sequential finger-to-thumb tasks (79). As healthy controls with better RNG task performances had greater brain activity, it remained unclear whether low brain activity was derived from worse task execution and/or functional impairment in schizophrenia. Hoshi et al. used time-resolved spectroscopy and two-channel fNIRS instruments to show that patients with schizophrenia, particularly those with a longer duration of illness, had reduced hemoglobin concentration during the resting state, and that this may cause altered activity during the RNG task (80). Koike et al. used a multi-channel fNIRS instrument to show that patients with schizophrenia had significantly reduced activity in the bilateral DLPFC and VLPFC regions, and that the activity in the right DLPFC region was associated with an earlier age at onset (81).

Okada et al. firstly showed the presence of altered brain activity in schizophrenia using a two-channel fNIRS instrument (62). Patients with schizophrenia had an aberrant task-related response pattern during a mirror drawing task, which was thought to be derived from a disrupted interhemispheric integration. Fallgatter et al. also showed the presence of altered frontal lateralization in schizophrenia during a continuous performance task using a two-channel fNIRS instrument (82). Folley et al. explored brain activity in patients with schizophrenia, individuals with schizotypal personality, and healthy controls during a divergent-thinking task using a two-channel fNIRS instrument, and showed that individuals with schizotypal personality had enhanced divergent-thinking ability and greater brain activity in the right PFC compared with patients with schizophrenia and healthy controls (83). Lee et al.

showed alternations in brain activity using fMRI and 24-channel fNIRS (not simultaneously) during the same event-related spatial working-memory task: patients with schizophrenia recruited the bilateral PFC, whereas healthy controls recruited only the right PFC (28). Zhu et al. used a 48-channel fNIRS instrument to show that patients with first-episode schizophrenia had reduced brain activity over the PFC during the Tower of London task (84). Nishimura et al. used a 52-channel fNIRS instrument during a go-no-go task to show that healthy controls had a significant decrease in activity in the DLPFC during the no-go condition, whereas patients with schizophrenia exhibited no changes (67). Furthermore, the high excitement score observed in patients with schizophrenia was associated with brain activity in the FPC and right DLPFC. Taniguchi et al. used a 24-channel fNIRS instrument to show that patients with schizophrenia had reduced brain activity in the PFC compared with healthy controls during a kana Stroop task, with similar task performances, whereas both patients and controls showed lack of activity during a kanji Stroop task, with significantly worse performance observed in the schizophrenia group (85).

Other than cognitive tasks, Fujita et al. explored hemoglobin changes through an electroconvulsive therapy using a two-channel fNIRS instrument, and showed that patients with schizophrenia had asymmetric hemoglobin changes in the PFC compared with patients with depression (86).

GENETIC VARIATION

Although schizophrenia is a syndrome, has been considered as a consolidation of several pathophysiological features, and has high genetic heritability, no crucial genetic risk factor has been found (87, 88). The results of genome-wide association studies that used a large sample size have suggested that schizophrenia risk genes are unable to be determined by specific gene variants but are thought to consist of common variants; furthermore, these risk genes had a substantial influence on environmental effects that occurred before the onset of schizophrenia. To clarify the impact of specific genes related to schizophrenia on the brain, imaging/genetics studies were performed to explore the relationship between brain structure and activity and genetic variants.

Five studies have explored the relationship between genetic variants and brain activity using fNIRS instruments. Takizawa et al. firstly reported that the val108/158met polymorphism of the catechol-*O*-methyltransferase (*COMT*) gene affected brain activity in the PFC only in schizophrenia patients (and not in healthy controls) (89). Schizophrenia patients with the Met variant (Val/Met and Met/Met) had significantly greater activation in the bilateral FPC and DLPFC during the LFT than did Val/Val carriers, implying that the inverted U curve shift of dopamine availability in schizophrenia might have an effect on the brain activity in the PFC (89). Regarding the Gln/Pro polymorphism of the sigma-1 receptor gene, Takizawa et al. reported that patients with the Gln/Gln genotype had significantly greater brain activity in the FPC and left DLPFC during the LFT than did Pro allele carriers; however, no significant differences were observed in healthy controls (90). However, Ohi et al. later used a two-channel fNIRS machine and a larger sample set to show that this genotype effect occurred in both the schizophrenia and control groups (91). Ohi et al. also reported that individuals with a longer cytosine/adenine/guanine (CAG) repeat in the spinocerebellar ataxia type 17 gene had reduced activity in the bilateral PFC during the TOH task in both the schizophrenia and control groups (92). Regarding the rs41279104 polymorphism of the nitric oxide synthase-I gene, Reif et al. showed that patients who were A allele carriers had significantly reduced activity in the right PFC during a VFT compared with those who had the GG genotype (93).

As recent methodological progress in gene analysis allows the exploration of whole genetic alterations between cases and controls using more than 10,000 samples, imaging/genetics studies should be performed using methods that enable the analysis of numerical data sets, such as bioinformatics and machine learning methods (94). Conversely, the investigation of the relationship between brain activity and relevant target genes (e.g., DLPFC function under dopamine regulation and *COMT* variants) may provide another imaging/genetics study strategy. The analysis of altered gene function in the brain among psychiatric illnesses may clarify the pathophysiology of specific psychiatric disorders and identify new treatment options.

EFFECT OF MEDICATION ON BRAIN ACTIVITY

As previous clinical fNIRS studies have mostly explored patients in the chronic stage and receiving medication, the effect of medication on brain function was a limitation of these studies. Although an inconsistent effect of medication on fNIRS signal has been reported (68, 70, 71, 79), most previous fNIRS studies have reported an absence of association between brain activity and medication dose (3, 5, 12, 74, 81, 84–86) or different brain activity between individuals with ultra-high risk for psychosis with and without medication (3) (**Table 1**). However, all of those studies were cross-sectional, and a previous randomized and controlled trial showed that the administration of mirtazapine increased brain activity compared with trazodone and placebo in healthy volunteers (95). Controlled trials and/or longitudinal investigation to elucidate specific drug effects will be needed.

LIMITATIONS OF PREVIOUS STUDIES AND FURTHER DIRECTIONS

The previous fNIRS studies of schizophrenia had several limitations; therefore, we propose further directions for future investigation (**Table 3**). First, as most previous studies have performed cross-sectional measurements in chronic and stable patients receiving medication, symptomatic, and functional changes were not fully explored. As fNIRS is able to perform measurements relatively easily in unstable patients, such as those with acute or recurrent conditions, longitudinal studies aimed at investigating changes in clinical symptoms and social function will be needed (3, 96). Although previous studies have revealed a negligible medication effect on fNIRS signals, investigations of drug-naïve patients or of those receiving controlling treatment (e.g., specific drugs, electroconvulsive therapy, and neurofeedback) will be needed to allow further clinical applications of fNIRS (60, 86, 97). The use of the easy portability of fNIRS machines may allow measurements in earlier clinical stages in cohort settings, such as adolescents with psychotic-like experiences, which may reveal the alterations in brain development in the PFC (98).

Table 3 | Limitation of previous fNIRS studies and further implication.

Limitation of previous studies	Further implications
Cross-sectional measurement for chronic and stable patients with medication	Measure in different clinical stages (e.g., UHR, FEP, recurrent phase) Measure longitudinally to explore the relationship between clinical changes and fNIRS signals Measure in drug-naïve patients to explore drug effect Measure in a specific treatment response (e.g., medication, electroconvulsive therapy, neurofeedback) Measure in cohort setting (e.g., psychotic-like experiences)
One-sided task procedure (block-designed VFTs)	Use of other cognitive tasks Adopt event-related design Adopt more naturalistic task (e.g., driving, conversation)
Small sample size in single institute	Make consortium with the same instrument and measurement procedure (e.g., task paradigm, probe setting) Adopt more sophisticated analytical methods (e.g., measurement tools, bioinformatics, machine learning) Standardize manuscript description Construct fNIRS community

UHR, ultra-high risk; FEP, first-episode psychosis.

Second, half of the previous studies of schizophrenia adopted block-design VFTs for cognitive activation. Although one of the major disadvantages of fNIRS is the inability to measure brain activity in deep brain tissues, and the block-design VFT is appropriate for elucidating brain activity over the PFC, other cognitive tasks, and event-related design will be helpful to explore brain pathology in schizophrenia and to compare signal differences between fNIRS and other neuroimaging tools, such as fMRI and PET. Conversely, the exploration of brain activity in a more naturalistic position and during natural activities, such as driving and conversation, is suitable for future investigations using the advantages of fNIRS (99, 100).

Third, as fNIRS allows easy and repetitive measurements, a study including a large number of samples has been conducted (12). To analyze such a large data set, the same measurement procedure regarding task paradigm and probe setting and more sophisticated analytical methods, such as measurement tools (e.g., NIRS-SPM) (101), bioinformatics methods, and machine learning (94), will be needed. Standardized manuscript description and a database system will be needed for further comparisons and meta-analyses (102). The construction of an fNIRS community is expected to provide this type of background in NIRS research (18).

CONCLUSION

Functional near-infrared spectroscopy has been progressing rapidly in the field of psychiatry, as it provides several advantages, such as small size, portability, silent functioning, and the achievement of easy and non-invasive measurements. A part of these results was approved in 2009 as one of the Advanced Medical Technologies as an aid for the differential diagnosis of depressive symptoms (10–12), which was the first such approval in the field of psychiatry in Japan. Future investigations aimed at exploring fNIRS differences in various clinical stages, longitudinal changes, drug effects, and variations during different task paradigms will be needed to develop more accurate biomarkers that can be used to aid differential diagnosis, the comprehension of the present condition, the prediction of outcome, and the decision regarding treatment options in schizophrenia. Future fNIRS research environments will require standardized measurement procedures, probe settings, analytical methods and tools, manuscript description, and database systems in a n fNIRS community.

ACKNOWLEDGMENTS

I would like to thank Mika Yamagishi and Hanako Sakurada for substantial support in article search. This study was supported by grants from the Ministry of Health, Labor, and Welfare (Health and Labor Science Research Grant for Comprehensive Research on Disability Health and Welfare H22-seishin-ippan-015 to Kiyoto Kasai) and from the JSPS/MEXT (No. 25870143 to Shinsuke Koike, and Grant-in-Aid for Scientific Research on Innovative Areas [Comprehensive Brain Science Network and Adolescent Mind and Self-Regulation (23118001 and 23118004) to Kiyoto Kasai], and National Bioscience Database Center (NBDC) of Japan Science and Technology Agency (JST) to Kiyoto Kasai. A portion of this study was also the result of a project entitled "Development of biomarker candidates for social behavior" carried out under the Strategic Research Program for Brain Sciences by the MEXT.

REFERENCES

1. Anonymous. A decade for psychiatric disorders. *Nature* (2010) **463**:9. doi:10.1038/463009a
2. Insel TR. Rethinking schizophrenia. *Nature* (2010) **468**:187–93. doi:10.1038/nature09552
3. Koike S, Takizawa R, Nishimura Y, Takano Y, Takayanagi Y, Kinou M, et al. Different hemodynamic response patterns in the prefrontal cortical sub-regions according to the clinical stages of psychosis. *Schizophr Res* (2011) **132**:54–61. doi:10.1016/j.schres.2011.07.014
4. Suto T, Fukuda M, Ito M, Uehara T, Mikuni M. Multichannel near-infrared spectroscopy in depression and schizophrenia: cognitive brain activation study. *Biol Psychiatry* (2004) **55**:501–11. doi:10.1016/j.biopsych.2003.09.008
5. Takizawa R, Kasai K, Kawakubo Y, Marumo K, Kawasaki S, Yamasue H, et al. Reduced frontopolar activation during verbal fluency task in schizophrenia: a multi-channel near-infrared spectroscopy study. *Schizophr Res* (2008) **99**:250–62. doi:10.1016/j.schres.2007.10.025
6. Jobsis FF. Noninvasive, infrared monitoring of cerebral and myocardial oxygen sufficiency and circulatory parameters. *Science* (1977) **198**:1264–7. doi:10.1126/science.929199
7. Hoshi Y, Tamura M. Dynamic multichannel near-infrared optical imaging of human brain activity. *J Appl Physiol* (1993) **75**:1842–6.

8. Kato T, Kamei A, Takashima S, Ozaki T. Human visual cortical function during photic stimulation monitoring by means of near-infrared spectroscopy. *J Cereb Blood Flow Metab* (1993) **13**:516–20. doi:10.1038/jcbfm.1993.66
9. Ehlis AC, Schneider S, Dresler T, Fallgatter AJ. Application of functional near-infrared spectroscopy in psychiatry. *Neuroimage* (2013). doi:10.1016/j.neuroimage.2013.03.067
10. Fukuda M. Near-infrared spectroscopy in psychiatry. *Brain Nerve* (2012) **64**:175–83.
11. Fukuda M, Mikuni M. Clinical application of near-infrared spectroscopy (NIRS) in psychiatry: the advanced medical technology for differential diagnosis of depressive state. *Seishin Shinkeigaku Zasshi* (2012) **114**:801–6.
12. Takizawa R, Fukuda M, Kawasaki S, Kasai K, Mimura M, Pu S, et al. Neuroimaging-aided differential diagnosis of the depressive state. *Neuroimage* (2013). doi:10.1016/j.neuroimage.2013.05.126
13. Kameyama M, Fukuda M, Yamagishi Y, Sato T, Uehara T, Ito M, et al. Frontal lobe function in bipolar disorder: a multichannel near-infrared spectroscopy study. *Neuroimage* (2006) **29**:172–84. doi:10.1016/j.neuroimage.2005.07.025
14. Noda T, Yoshida S, Matsuda T, Okamoto N, Sakamoto K, Koseki S, et al. Frontal and right temporal activations correlate negatively with depression severity during verbal fluency task: a multi-channel near-infrared spectroscopy study. *J Psychiatr Res* (2012) **46**:905–12. doi:10.1016/j.jpsychires.2012.04.001
15. Ohta H, Yamagata B, Tomioka H, Takahashi T, Yano M, Nakagome K, et al. Hypofrontality in panic disorder and major depressive disorder assessed by multi-channel near-infrared spectroscopy. *Depress Anxiety* (2008) **25**:1053–9. doi:10.1002/da.20463
16. Pu S, Matsumura H, Yamada T, Ikezawa S, Mitani H, Adachi A, et al. Reduced frontopolar activation during verbal fluency task associated with poor social functioning in late-onset major depression: multi-channel near-infrared spectroscopy study. *Psychiatry Clin Neurosci* (2008) **62**:728–37. doi:10.1111/j.1440-1819.2008.01882.x
17. Pu S, Nakagome K, Yamada T, Yokoyama K, Matsumura H, Mitani H, et al. The relationship between the prefrontal activation during a verbal fluency task and stress-coping style in major depressive disorder: a near-infrared spectroscopy study. *J Psychiatr Res* (2012) **46**:1427–34. doi:10.1016/j.jpsychires.2012.08.001
18. Ferrari M, Quaresima V. A brief review on the history of human functional near-infrared spectroscopy (fNIRS) development and fields of application. *Neuroimage* (2012) **63**:921–35. doi:10.1016/j.neuroimage.2012.03.049
19. Dieler AC, Tupak SV, Fallgatter AJ. Functional near-infrared spectroscopy for the assessment of speech related tasks. *Brain Lang* (2012) **121**:90–109. doi:10.1016/j.bandl.2011.03.005
20. Scholkmann F, Kleiser S, Metz AJ, Zimmermann R, Mata Pavia J, Wolf U, et al. A review on continuous wave functional near-infrared spectroscopy and imaging instrumentation and methodology. *Neuroimage* (2013). doi:10.1016/j.neuroimage.2013.05.004
21. Minagawa-Kawai Y, Mori K, Hebden JC, Dupoux E. Optical imaging of infants' neurocognitive development: recent advances and perspectives. *Dev Neurobiol* (2008) **68**:712–28. doi:10.1002/dneu.20618
22. Homae F, Watanabe H, Otobe T, Nakano T, Go T, Konishi Y, et al. Development of global cortical networks in early infancy. *J Neurosci* (2010) **30**:4877–82. doi:10.1523/JNEUROSCI.5618-09.2010
23. Ehlis AC, Ringel TM, Plichta MM, Richter MM, Herrmann MJ, Fallgatter AJ. Cortical correlates of auditory sensory gating: a simultaneous near-infrared spectroscopy event-related potential study. *Neuroscience* (2009) **159**:1032–43. doi:10.1016/j.neuroscience.2009.01.015
24. Herrmann MJ, Huter T, Plichta MM, Ehlis AC, Alpers GW, Muhlberger A, et al. Enhancement of activity of the primary visual cortex during processing of emotional stimuli as measured with event-related functional near-infrared spectroscopy and event-related potentials. *Hum Brain Mapp* (2008) **29**:28–35. doi:10.1002/hbm.20368
25. Heinzel S, Haeussinger FB, Hahn T, Ehlis AC, Plichta MM, Fallgatter AJ. Variability of (functional) hemodynamics as measured with simultaneous fNIRS and fMRI during intertemporal choice. *Neuroimage* (2013) **71**:125–34. doi:10.1016/j.neuroimage.2012.12.074
26. Huppert TJ, Hoge RD, Diamond SG, Franceschini MA, Boas DA. A temporal comparison of BOLD, ASL, and NIRS hemodynamic responses to motor stimuli in adult humans. *Neuroimage* (2006) **29**:368–82. doi:10.1016/j.neuroimage.2005.08.065
27. Kleinschmidt A, Obrig H, Requardt M, Merboldt KD, Dirnagl U, Villringer A, et al. Simultaneous recording of cerebral blood oxygenation changes during human brain activation by magnetic resonance imaging and near-infrared spectroscopy. *J Cereb Blood Flow Metab* (1996) **16**:817–26. doi:10.1097/00004647-199609000-00006
28. Lee J, Folley BS, Gore J, Park S. Origins of spatial working memory deficits in schizophrenia: an event-related FMRI and near-infrared spectroscopy study. *PLoS One* (2008) **3**:e1760. doi:10.1371/journal.pone.0001760
29. Strangman G, Culver JP, Thompson JH, Boas DA. A quantitative comparison of simultaneous BOLD fMRI and NIRS recordings during functional brain activation. *Neuroimage* (2002) **17**:719–31. doi:10.1006/nimg.2002.1227
30. Toronov V, Walker S, Gupta R, Choi JH, Gratton E, Hueber D, et al. The roles of changes in deoxyhemoglobin concentration and regional cerebral blood volume in the fMRI BOLD signal. *Neuroimage* (2003) **19**:1521–31. doi:10.1016/S1053-8119(03)00152-6
31. Hock C, Villringer K, Muller-Spahn F, Wenzel R, Heekeren H, Schuh-Hofer S, et al. Decrease in parietal cerebral hemoglobin oxygenation during performance of a verbal fluency task in patients with Alzheimer's disease monitored by means of near-infrared spectroscopy (NIRS) – correlation with simultaneous rCBF-PET measurements. *Brain Res* (1997) **755**:293–303. doi:10.1016/S0006-8993(97)00122-4
32. Hoshi Y, Onoe H, Watanabe Y, Andersson J, Bergstrom M, Lilja A, et al. Non-synchronous behavior of neuronal activity, oxidative metabolism and blood supply during mental tasks in man. *Neurosci Lett* (1994) **172**:129–33. doi:10.1016/0304-3940(94)90679-3
33. Ohmae E, Ouchi Y, Oda M, Suzuki T, Nobesawa S, Kanno T, et al. Cerebral hemodynamics evaluation by near-infrared time-resolved spectroscopy: correlation with simultaneous positron emission tomography measurements. *Neuroimage* (2006) **29**:697–705. doi:10.1016/j.neuroimage.2005.08.008
34. Sander TH, Liebert A, Burghoff M, Wabnitz H, Macdonald R, Trahms L. Cross-correlation analysis of the correspondence between magnetoencephalographic and near-infrared cortical signals. *Methods Inf Med* (2007) **46**(2):164–8.
35. Seki Y, Miyashita T, Kandori A, Maki A, Koizumi H. Simultaneous measurement of neuronal activity and cortical hemodynamics by unshielded magnetoencephalography and near-infrared spectroscopy. *J Biomed Opt* (2012) **17**(10):107001. doi:10.1117/1.JBO.17.10.107001
36. Takahashi T, Takikawa Y, Kawagoe R, Shibuya S, Iwano T, Kitazawa S. Influence of skin blood flow on near-infrared spectroscopy signals measured on the forehead during a verbal fluency task. *Neuroimage* (2011) **57**:991–1002. doi:10.1016/j.neuroimage.2011.05.012
37. Kirilina E, Jelzow A, Heine A, Niessing M, Wabnitz H, Bruhl R, et al. The physiological origin of task-evoked systemic artefacts in functional near infrared spectroscopy. *Neuroimage* (2012) **61**:70–81. doi:10.1016/j.neuroimage.2012.02.074
38. Funane T, Atsumori H, Katura T, Obata AN, Sato H, Tanikawa Y, et al. Quantitative evaluation of deep and shallow tissue layers' contribution to fNIRS signal using multi-distance optodes and independent component analysis. *Neuroimage* (2013). doi:10.1016/j.neuroimage.2013.02.026
39. Sato H, Yahata N, Funane T, Takizawa R, Katura T, Atsumori H, et al. A NIRS-fMRI investigation of prefrontal cortex activity during a working memory task. *Neuroimage* (2013) **83**:158–73. doi:10.1016/j.neuroimage.2013.06.043
40. Gagnon L, Yücel MA, Boas DA, Cooper RJ. Further improvement in reducing superficial contamination in NIRS using double short separation measurements. *Neuroimage* (2013). doi:10.1016/j.neuroimage.2013.01.073
41. Gagnon L, Cooper RJ, Yucel MA, Perdue KL, Greve DN, Boas DA. Short separation channel location impacts the performance of short channel regression in NIRS. *Neuroimage* (2011) **59**:2518–28. doi:10.1016/j.neuroimage.2011.08.095
42. Gagnon L, Yucel MA, Dehaes M, Cooper RJ, Perdue KL, Selb J, et al. Quantification of the cortical contribution to the NIRS signal over the motor cortex using concurrent NIRS-fMRI measurements. *Neuroimage* (2012) **59**(4):3933–40. doi:10.1016/j.neuroimage.2011.10.054
43. Haeussinger FB, Heinzel S, Hahn T, Schecklmann M, Ehlis AC, Fallgatter AJ. Simulation of near-infrared light absorption considering individual head and prefrontal cortex anatomy: implications for optical neuroimaging. *PLoS One* (2011) **6**:e26377. doi:10.1371/journal.pone.0026377
44. Kohri S, Hoshi Y, Tamura M, Kato C, Kuge Y, Tamaki N. Quantitative evaluation of the relative contribution ratio of cerebral tissue to near-infrared signals in the adult human head: a preliminary study. *Physiol Meas* (2002) **23**:301–12. doi:10.1088/0967-3334/23/2/306

45. Kakimoto Y, Nishimura Y, Hara N, Okada M, Tanii H, Okazaki Y. Intrasubject reproducibility of prefrontal cortex activities during a verbal fluency task over two repeated sessions using multi-channel near-infrared spectroscopy. *Psychiatry Clin Neurosci* (2009) **63**:491–9. doi:10.1111/j.1440-1819.2009.01988.x
46. Kono T, Matsuo K, Tsunashima K, Kasai K, Takizawa R, Rogers MA, et al. Multiple-time replicability of near-infrared spectroscopy recording during prefrontal activation task in healthy men. *Neurosci Res* (2007) **57**:504–12. doi:10.1016/j.neures.2006.12.007
47. Plichta MM, Herrmann MJ, Baehne CG, Ehlis AC, Richter MM, Pauli P, et al. Event-related functional near-infrared spectroscopy (fNIRS): are the measurements reliable? *Neuroimage* (2006) **31**:116–24. doi:10.1016/j.neuroimage.2005.12.008
48. Schecklmann M, Ehlis AC, Plichta MM, Fallgatter AJ. Functional near-infrared spectroscopy: a long-term reliable tool for measuring brain activity during verbal fluency. *Neuroimage* (2008) **43**:147–55. doi:10.1016/j.neuroimage.2008.06.032
49. Ogawa S, Lee TM, Kay AR, Tank DW. Brain magnetic resonance imaging with contrast dependent on blood oxygenation. *Proc Natl Acad Sci U S A* (1990) **87**:9868–72. doi:10.1073/pnas.87.24.9868
50. Yamamoto T, Kato T. Paradoxical correlation between signal in functional magnetic resonance imaging and deoxygenated haemoglobin content in capillaries: a new theoretical explanation. *Phys Med Biol* (2002) **47**:1121–41. doi:10.1088/0031-9155/47/7/309
51. Cui X, Bray S, Bryant DM, Glover GH, Reiss AL. A quantitative comparison of NIRS and fMRI across multiple cognitive tasks. *Neuroimage* (2011) **54**:2808–21. doi:10.1016/j.neuroimage.2010.10.069
52. Tsuzuki D, Dan I. Spatial registration for functional near-infrared spectroscopy: from channel position on the scalp to cortical location in individual and group analyses. *Neuroimage* (2013). doi:10.1016/j.neuroimage.2013.07.025
53. Okamoto M, Dan H, Sakamoto K, Takeo K, Shimizu K, Kohno S, et al. Three-dimensional probabilistic anatomical cranio-cerebral correlation via the international 10-20 system oriented for transcranial functional brain mapping. *Neuroimage* (2004) **21**:99–111. doi:10.1016/j.neuroimage.2003.08.026
54. Schroeter ML, Zysset S, Kupka T, Kruggel F, Yves von Cramon D. Near-infrared spectroscopy can detect brain activity during a color-word matching Stroop task in an event-related design. *Hum Brain Mapp* (2002) **17**:61–71. doi:10.1002/hbm.10052
55. Singh AK, Okamoto M, Dan H, Jurcak V, Dan I. Spatial registration of multichannel multi-subject fNIRS data to MNI space without MRI. *Neuroimage* (2005) **27**:842–51. doi:10.1016/j.neuroimage.2005.05.019
56. Tsuzuki D, Jurcak V, Singh AK, Okamoto M, Watanabe E, Dan I. Virtual spatial registration of stand-alone fNIRS data to MNI space. *Neuroimage* (2007) **34**:1506–18. doi:10.1016/j.neuroimage.2006.10.043
57. Katura T, Sato H, Fuchino Y, Yoshida T, Atsumori H, Kiguchi M, et al. Extracting task-related activation components from optical topography measurement using independent components analysis. *J Biomed Opt* (2008) **13**:054008. doi:10.1117/1.2981829
58. Shattuck DW, Mirza M, Adisetiyo V, Hojatkashani C, Salamon G, Narr KL, et al. Construction of a 3D probabilistic atlas of human cortical structures. *Neuroimage* (2008) **39**:1064–80. doi:10.1016/j.neuroimage.2007.09.031
59. Heinzel S, Metzger FG, Ehlis AC, Korell R, Alboji A, Haeussinger FB, et al. Aging-related cortical reorganization of verbal fluency processing: a functional near-infrared spectroscopy study. *Neurobiol Aging* (2013) **34**:439–50. doi:10.1016/j.neurobiolaging.2012.05.021
60. Monden Y, Dan H, Nagashima M, Dan I, Kyutoku Y, Okamoto M, et al. Clinically-oriented monitoring of acute effects of methylphenidate on cerebral hemodynamics in ADHD children using fNIRS. *Clin Neurophysiol* (2012) **123**:1147–57. doi:10.1016/j.clinph.2011.10.006
61. World Health Organization (WHO). *Global Burden of Disease*. New York: World Health Organization (2004).
62. Okada F, Tokumitsu Y, Hoshi Y, Tamura M. Impaired interhemispheric integration in brain oxygenation and hemodynamics in schizophrenia. *Eur Arch Psychiatry Clin Neurosci* (1994) **244**:17–25. doi:10.1007/BF02279807
63. Cabeza R, Nyberg L. Imaging cognition II: an empirical review of 275 PET and fMRI studies. *J Cogn Neurosci* (2000) **12**:1–47. doi:10.1162/08989290051137585
64. Curtis VA, Bullmore ET, Brammer MJ, Wright IC, Williams SC, Morris RG, et al. Attenuated frontal activation during a verbal fluency task in patients with schizophrenia. *Am J Psychiatry* (1998) **155**:1056–63.
65. Green MF, Nuechterlein KH, Gold JM, Barch DM, Cohen J, Essock S, et al. Approaching a consensus cognitive battery for clinical trials in schizophrenia: the NIMH-MATRICS conference to select cognitive domains and test criteria. *Biol Psychiatry* (2004) **56**:301–7. doi:10.1016/j.biopsych.2004.06.023
66. Koike S, Takizawa R, Nishimura Y, Kinou M, Kawasaki S, Kasai K. Reduced but broader prefrontal activity in patients with schizophrenia during n-back working memory tasks: a multi-channel near-infrared spectroscopy study. *J Psychiatr Res* (2013) **47**(9):1240–6. doi:10.1016/j.jpsychires.2013.05.009
67. Nishimura Y, Takizawa R, Muroi M, Marumo K, Kinou M, Kasai K. Prefrontal cortex activity during response inhibition associated with excitement symptoms in schizophrenia. *Brain Res* (2011) **1370**:194–203. doi:10.1016/j.brainres.2010.11.003
68. Watanabe A, Kato T. Cerebrovascular response to cognitive tasks in patients with schizophrenia measured by near-infrared spectroscopy. *Schizophr Bull* (2004) **30**:435–44. doi:10.1093/oxfordjournals.schbul.a007090
69. Quaresima V, Giosue P, Roncone R, Casacchia M, Ferrari M. Prefrontal cortex dysfunction during cognitive tests evidenced by functional near-infrared spectroscopy. *Psychiatry Res* (2009) **171**:252–7. doi:10.1016/j.pscychresns.2008.02.002
70. Azechi M, Iwase M, Ikezawa K, Takahashi H, Canuet L, Kurimoto R, et al. Discriminant analysis in schizophrenia and healthy subjects using prefrontal activation during frontal lobe tasks: a near-infrared spectroscopy. *Schizophr Res* (2010) **117**:52–60. doi:10.1016/j.schres.2009.10.003
71. Ikezawa K, Iwase M, Ishii R, Azechi M, Canuet L, Ohi K, et al. Impaired regional hemodynamic response in schizophrenia during multiple prefrontal activation tasks: a two-channel near-infrared spectroscopy study. *Schizophr Res* (2009) **108**:93–103. doi:10.1016/j.schres.2008.12.010
72. Takeshi K, Nemoto T, Fumoto M, Arita H, Mizuno M. Reduced prefrontal cortex activation during divergent thinking in schizophrenia: a multi-channel NIRS study. *Prog Neuropsychopharmacol Biol Psychiatry* (2010) **34**:1327–32. doi:10.1016/j.pnpbp.2010.07.021
73. Shimodera S, Imai Y, Kamimura N, Morokuma I, Fujita H, Inoue S, et al. Mapping hypofrontality during letter fluency task in schizophrenia: a multi-channel near-infrared spectroscopy study. *Schizophr Res* (2012) **136**:63–9. doi:10.1016/j.schres.2012.01.039
74. Ehlis AC, Herrmann MJ, Plichta MM, Fallgatter AJ. Cortical activation during two verbal fluency tasks in schizophrenic patients and healthy controls as assessed by multi-channel near-infrared spectroscopy. *Psychiatry Res* (2007) **156**:1–13. doi:10.1016/j.pscychresns.2006.11.007
75. Kubota Y, Toichi M, Shimizu M, Mason RA, Coconcea CM, Findling RL, et al. Prefrontal activation during verbal fluency tests in schizophrenia – a near-infrared spectroscopy (NIRS) study. *Schizophr Res* (2005) **77**:65–73. doi:10.1016/j.schres.2005.01.007
76. Tupak SV, Badewien M, Dresler T, Hahn T, Ernst LH, Herrmann MJ, et al. Differential prefrontal and frontotemporal oxygenation patterns during phonemic and semantic verbal fluency. *Neuropsychologia* (2012) **50**:1565–9. doi:10.1016/j.neuropsychologia.2012.03.009
77. Anonymous. First do no harm. *Nature* (2011) **469**:132. doi:10.1038/469132a
78. Cyranoski D. Neuroscience: thought experiment. *Nature* (2011) **469**:148–9. doi:10.1038/469148a
79. Shinba T, Nagano M, Kariya N, Ogawa K, Shinozaki T, Shimosato S, et al. Near-infrared spectroscopy analysis of frontal lobe dysfunction in schizophrenia. *Biol Psychiatry* (2004) **55**:154–64. doi:10.1016/S0006-3223(03)00547-X
80. Hoshi Y, Shinba T, Sato C, Doi N. Resting hypofrontality in schizophrenia: a study using near-infrared time-resolved spectroscopy. *Schizophr Res* (2006) **84**:411–20. doi:10.1016/j.schres.2006.03.010
81. Koike S, Takizawa R, Nishimura Y, Marumo K, Kinou M, Kawakubo Y, et al. Association between severe dorsolateral prefrontal dysfunction during random number generation and earlier onset in schizophrenia. *Clin Neurophysiol* (2011) **122**:1533–40. doi:10.1016/j.clinph.2010.12.056
82. Fallgatter AJ, Strik WK. Reduced frontal functional asymmetry in schizophrenia during a cued continuous performance test assessed with near-infrared spectroscopy. *Schizophr Bull* (2000) **26**:913–9. doi:10.1093/oxfordjournals.schbul.a033505
83. Folley BS, Park S. Verbal creativity and schizotypal personality in relation to prefrontal hemispheric laterality: a behavioral and near-infrared optical imaging study. *Schizophr Res* (2005) **80**:271–82. doi:10.1016/j.schres.2005.06.016
84. Zhu Y, Liu X, Wang H, Jiang T, Fang Y, Hu H, et al. Reduced prefrontal activation during tower of London in first-episode schizophrenia: a multi-channel

near-infrared spectroscopy study. *Neurosci Lett* (2010) **478**:136–40. doi:10.1016/j.neulet.2010.05.003

85. Taniguchi K, Sumitani S, Watanabe Y, Akiyama M, Ohmori T. Multi-channel near-infrared spectroscopy reveals reduced prefrontal activation in schizophrenia patients during performance of the kana Stroop task. *J Med Invest* (2012) **59**:45–52. doi:10.2152/jmi.59.45
86. Fujita Y, Takebayashi M, Hisaoka K, Tsuchioka M, Morinobu S, Yamawaki S. Asymmetric alternation of the hemodynamic response at the prefrontal cortex in patients with schizophrenia during electroconvulsive therapy: a near-infrared spectroscopy study. *Brain Res* (2011) **1410**:132–40. doi:10.1016/j.brainres.2011.06.052
87. Purcell SM, Wray NR, Stone JL, Visscher PM, O'Donovan MC, Sullivan PF, et al. Common polygenic variation contributes to risk of schizophrenia and bipolar disorder. *Nature* (2009) **460**:748–52. doi:10.1038/nature08185
88. Shi JX, Levinson DF, Duan JB, Sanders AR, Zheng YL, Pe'er I, et al. Common variants on chromosome 6p22.1 are associated with schizophrenia. *Nature* (2009) **460**:753–7. doi:10.1038/nature08192
89. Takizawa R, Tochigi M, Kawakubo Y, Marumo K, Sasaki T, Fukuda M, et al. Association between catechol-O-methyltrasferase Val108/158Met genotype and prefrontal hemodynamic response in schizophrenia. *PLoS One* (2009) **4**:e5495. doi:10.1371/journal.pone.0005495
90. Takizawa R, Hashimoto K, Tochigi M, Kawakubo Y, Marumo K, Sasaki T, et al. Association between sigma-1 receptor gene polymorphism and prefrontal hemodynamic response induced by cognitive activation in schizophrenia. *Prog Neuropsychopharmacol Biol Psychiatry* (2009) **33**:491–8. doi:10.1016/j.pnpbp.2009.01.014
91. Ohi K, Hashimoto R, Yasuda Y, Fukumoto M, Yamamori H, Umeda-Yano S, et al. The SIGMAR1 gene is associated with a risk of schizophrenia and activation of the prefrontal cortex. *Prog Neuropsychopharmacol Biol Psychiatry* (2011) **35**:1309–15. doi:10.1016/j.pnpbp.2011.04.008
92. Ohi K, Hashimoto R, Yasuda Y, Kiribayashi M, Iike N, Yoshida T, et al. TATA box-binding protein gene is associated with risk for schizophrenia, age at onset and prefrontal function. *Genes Brain Behav* (2009) **8**:473–80. doi:10.1111/j.1601-183X.2009.00497.x
93. Reif A, Schecklmann M, Eirich E, Jacob CP, Jarczok TA, Kittel-Schneider S, et al. A functional promoter polymorphism of neuronal nitric oxide synthase moderates prefrontal functioning in schizophrenia. *Int J Neuropsychopharmacol* (2011) **14**:887–97. doi:10.1017/S1461145710001677
94. Koutsouleris N, Meisenzahl EM, Davatzikos C, Bottlender R, Frodl T, Scheuerecker J, et al. Use of neuroanatomical pattern classification to identify subjects in at-risk mental states of psychosis and predict disease transition. *Arch Gen Psychiatry* (2009) **66**:700–12. doi:10.1001/archgenpsychiatry.2009.62
95. Kohmura K, Iwamoto K, Aleksic B, Sasada K, Kawano N, Katayama H, et al. Effects of sedative antidepressants on prefrontal cortex activity during verbal fluency task in healthy subjects: a near-infrared spectroscopy study. *Psychopharmacology (Berl)* (2013) **226**:75–81. doi:10.1007/s00213-012-2885-8
96. Koike S, Takano Y, Iwashiro N, Satomura Y, Suga M, Nagai T, et al. A multimodal approach to investigate biomarkers for psychosis in a clinical setting: the integrative neuroimaging studies in schizophrenia targeting for early intervention and prevention (IN-STEP) project. *Schizophr Res* (2013) **143**:116–24. doi:10.1016/j.schres.2012.11.012
97. Mihara M, Miyai I, Hattori N, Hatakenaka M, Yagura H, Kawano T, et al. Neurofeedback using real-time near-infrared spectroscopy enhances motor imagery related cortical activation. *PLoS One* (2012) **7**:e32234. doi:10.1371/journal.pone.0032234
98. Nishida A, Tanii H, Nishimura Y, Kajiki N, Inoue K, Okada M, et al. Associations between psychotic-like experiences and mental health status and other psychopathologies among Japanese early teens. *Schizophr Res* (2008) **99**:125–33. doi:10.1016/j.schres.2007.11.038
99. Suda M, Takei Y, Aoyama Y, Narita K, Sato T, Fukuda M, et al. Frontopolar activation during face-to-face conversation: an in situ study using near-infrared spectroscopy. *Neuropsychologia* (2010) **48**:441–7. doi:10.1016/j.neuropsychologia.2009.09.036
100. Tomioka H, Yamagata B, Takahashi T, Yano M, Isomura AJ, Kobayashi H, et al. Detection of hypofrontality in drivers with Alzheimer's disease by near-infrared spectroscopy. *Neurosci Lett* (2009) **451**(3):252–6. doi:10.1016/j.neulet.2008.12.059
101. Ye JC, Tak S, Jang KE, Jung J, Jang J. NIRS-SPM: statistical parametric mapping for near-infrared spectroscopy. *Neuroimage* (2009) **44**:428–47. doi:10.1016/j.neuroimage.2008.08.036
102. Cristia A, Dupoux E, Hakuno Y, Lloyd-Fox S, Schuetze M, Kivits J, et al. An online database of infant functional near infrared spectroscopy studies: a community-augmented systematic review. *PLoS One* (2013) **8**:e58906. doi:10.1371/journal.pone.0058906

11

Dysfunction and Dysconnection in Cortical–Striatal Networks During Sustained Attention: Genetic Risk for Schizophrenia or Bipolar Disorder and its Impact on Brain Network Function

Vaibhav A. Diwadkar[1]*, Neil Bakshi[1†], Gita Gupta[1], Patrick Pruitt[1†], Richard White[1] and Simon B. Eickhoff[2,3]

[1] *Department of Psychiatry and Behavioral Neurosciences, Wayne State University, Detroit, MI, USA*
[2] *Institute of Clinical Neuroscience and Medical Psychology, Heinrich-Heine University Düsseldorf, Düsseldorf, Germany*
[3] *Institute of Neuroscience and Medicine (INM-1), Research Center Jülich, Jülich, Germany*

Correspondence:
Vaibhav A. Diwadkar, Department of Psychiatry and Behavioral Neurosciences, Wayne State University School of Medicine, Suite 5B, Tolan Park Medical Building, 3901 Chrysler Drive, Detroit, MI 48201 USA
e-mail: vdiwadka@med.wayne.edu

†Present address:
Neil Bakshi, School of Medicine, University of Michigan, Ann Arbor, MI, USA;
Patrick Pruitt, Department of Neuroscience, University of Michigan, Ann Arbor, MI, USA

Abnormalities in the brain's attention network may represent early identifiable neurobiological impairments in individuals at increased risk for schizophrenia or bipolar disorder. Here, we provide evidence of dysfunctional regional and network function in adolescents at higher genetic risk for schizophrenia or bipolar disorder [henceforth higher risk (HGR)]. During fMRI, participants engaged in a sustained attention task with variable demands. The task alternated between attention (120 s), visual control (passive viewing; 120 s), and rest (20 s) epochs. Low and high demand attention conditions were created using the rapid presentation of two- or three-digit numbers. Subjects were required to detect repeated presentation of numbers. We demonstrate that the recruitment of cortical and striatal regions are disordered in HGR: relative to typical controls (TC), HGR showed lower recruitment of the dorsal prefrontal cortex, but higher recruitment of the superior parietal cortex. This imbalance was more dramatic in the basal ganglia. There, a group by task demand interaction was observed, such that increased attention demand led to increased engagement in TC, but disengagement in HGR. These activation studies were complemented by network analyses using dynamic causal modeling. Competing model architectures were assessed across a network of cortical–striatal regions, distinguished at a second level using random-effects Bayesian model selection. In the winning architecture, HGR were characterized by significant reductions in coupling across both frontal–striatal and frontal–parietal pathways. The effective connectivity analyses indicate emergent network dysconnection, consistent with findings in patients with schizophrenia. Emergent patterns of regional dysfunction and dysconnection in cortical–striatal pathways may provide functional biological signatures in the adolescent risk-state for psychiatric illness.

Keywords: attention, brain networks, schizophrenia, bipolar disorder, dynamic causal modeling abstract

INTRODUCTION

Sustained attention or the ability to remain consistently focused on an ongoing task is one of the most basic of cognitive domains (1, 2) and serves as a fundamental process underlying mechanisms of memory and control (3). Attention competence in childhood and adolescence increases through emergence of functional integration within cortical–striatal circuits. The engagement of frontal regions has been documented in children as young as 4–6 years of age (4) and the maturation of the circuit (including the basal ganglia and the parietal lobe) extends through adolescence (3, 5). This multi-node attention network (6) includes executive regions of the frontal lobe (the dorsal prefrontal cortex and the dorsal anterior cingulate), regions such as the basal ganglia (including the caudate and the putamen) that presumably play central roles in relaying information between and linking signals across brain networks (7, 8), and the parietal lobe that is essential for mechanisms of spatial orientation (9). The ascent of attention competence in adolescence corresponds with linear progression in the development of and anatomical connectivity between these key brain structures in the attention network (10, 11).

Deficits in sustained attention deficits are widely implicated in several psychiatric disorders that are adolescent onset or the origins of which lie in adolescence. These include not only core attention-related disorders such as attention deficit hyperactivity disorder (6, 12), but also bipolar disorder (13) and schizophrenia (14). The evidence regarding schizophrenia and bipolar disorder is compelling as studies now suggest attention deficits serve as a prelude in adolescence to the emergence of these late adolescent or adult-onset phenotypes. In this framework, adolescents with known risk-factors for psychiatric illness may present with neuropsychological deficits, which in turn are expressions of emergent dysfunction in critical brain networks (15). Adolescent children of parents with psychiatric diagnoses (mood disorders or schizophrenia) are an important risk group in whom familial risk may impact the integrity of function in attention networks, in turn decreasing the integrity of attention-related processing and subsequently leading to an increase in expressed attention deficits. In fact, adolescent children of parents with major depressive disorder, bipolar disorder, or schizophrenia all show deficits in neuropsychological tasks of attention including continuous performance tasks (CPT) (14, 16, 17) and other tasks with significant attention components (17). These groups are at significantly higher risk (HGR) for the emergence of psychiatric disorders (18–21). Consequently, a better understanding of the neurobiological impairments of attentional networks may provide important insight and potential biomarkers for the emergence of these disorders.

However, understanding of these biological bases remains obscure. Volumetric studies imply cortical–striatal reductions in brain structure (22, 23) that may be associated with impaired attention function (24, 25). However, the relationship between brain structure and function (as measured with structural and functional MRI, respectively) is not straightforward (26). This limits insight into disordered brain function in adolescence and its implication for psychiatric illness. In turn, understanding disordered effective connectivity between brain regions using causal modeling of brain network interactions assumes particular importance for understanding dysregulated networks in psychiatric disorders (27–29).

Effective connectivity mediates the integration of information between brain regions and refers to the "the influence that one neural system exerts over another, either at a synaptic (i.e., synaptic efficacy) or population level" (27, 30). Assessing brain activations and effective connectivity respectively permit exploration of relative specialization and functional integration of information in the brain (27). The temporal properties of the BOLD response, and the relationship of this to biophysical forward models of the neuronal response (31) permit the modeling of and inference on parameters of effective connectivity estimated from fMRI (32). While different methods for analyzing effective connectivity exist, dynamic causal modeling (DCM) is the currently best evaluated and most widely used approach toward this endeavor (32–35).

Our aims in this investigation were twofold. First, we assessed differences in regional responses across the extended cortical–striatal attention network (36, 37) including frontal, striatal, and parietal cortices. These differences in part constitute differences in the regional specialization of function between groups. Next, using DCM (33), we investigated differences between cortical–striatal network interactions using a competitive network identification framework based on Bayesian model selection (BMS) (38) and comparisons of Bayesian parameter averages (34, 39). fMRI data were collected in children and adolescents (8 years ≤ Age < 20 years) with a family history of psychiatric illness (bipolar disorder or schizophrenia) (henceforth HGR) and controls free of such history to the second degree [henceforth typical controls (TC)]. During the fMRI task, extended attention blocks (120 s) were employed using a variant of the well-established CPT (identical pairs version, CPT-IP) (40) in which subjects must monitor rapidly presented stimuli (in the current context numbers were used) and indicate repetitions in the sequence.

MATERIALS AND METHODS

SUBJECTS

A total of 46 children and adolescents provided informed consent or assent for the fMRI studies approved by the institutional review board at Wayne State University. Of these 46, 24 were TC, with no family history of schizophrenia or mood disorder to the second degree and remaining 22 had a parent with schizophrenia or bipolar disorder and hence at HGR. Subjects were recruited from the greater Detroit area through advertisements and through in patient services at Wayne State University School of Medicine. Screening questionnaires administered using both telephone and personal interviews were used for both rule-outs and to ascertain if subjects had a history of psychotic illness in first-degree relatives. Diagnoses for parents of HGR were reached using the Structured Clinical Interview for DSM-IV schizophrenia (41). Subjects younger than 15 years were clinically characterized using the Schedule for Affective Disorders and Schizophrenia-Child Version (K-SADS) (42); those aged 15 years or above were assessed using the SCID. **Table 1** provides information on subject demographics and characteristics.

fMRI

Functional data were acquired using a full body Bruker MedSpec 4.0 T system running the Siemens Syngo console. Gradient echo planar images (EPI) were collected using an eight-channel head coil (TR = 2000 ms; TE = 30 ms; matrix size = 64 × 64; field of view (FOV) = 240 mm; voxel size = 3.75 mm × 3.75 mm × 4 mm). Images were axially acquired in 24 continuous 4 mm slices positioned parallel to the anterior commissure/posterior commissure (AC–PC) line.

TASK

During fMRI, all subjects performed a modified version of a CPT (Identical Pairs version) previously employed in studying illnesses including schizophrenia and bipolar disorder, and children and adolescents at risk for psychiatric illness (14, 16, 40). Numbers were presented in rapid sequence (50 ms, 250 ms SOA in each condition) and subjects were required to detect the repeated presentation of a number. Attention demands of the task were maintained by manipulating figure-ground contrast (white characters, RGB: 255, 255, 255; Off-white background, RGB: 225, 225, 225) in order to preempt attention gain under maximal contrast (43). Attention load was manipulated across epochs utilizing sequences of two-digit numbers ("low" load) or three-digit numbers ("high" load), motivated by evidence suggesting that access to numerosity

Table 1 | Demographic information for the investigate sample is shown.

	Mean age (SD)	Full scale IQ (SD)
Typical controls (TC, $n = 24$)	15.4 (2.7)	93.1 (15.9)
High genetic risk (HGR, $n = 22$)	14.1 (3.1)	94.2 (14.5)

HGR were healthy apart from the following co-morbidities: separation anxiety (n = 1), attention deficit hyperactivity disorder (n = 3), and social phobia (n = 1). TC by definition were healthy and free of diagnosis.

though rapid (44) interacts with attention systems in the frontal, striatal, and parietal regions (45–47). A goal of manipulating load was to investigate separable load-related effects on region-specific interactions in each experimental group, particularly as parametric variations in load have proven useful in assessing differential regional specialization in risk and disease (48, 49).

To ensure large effect sizes of continuous or sustained attention, we used very long blocks of 120 s (therefore in removing low frequency drifts and fluctuations in subsequent analyses, we used a lenient high pass filter to preserve attention-related responses in the fMRI signals further noted in the fMRI analyses section below). Target frequency during the 120 s experimental epochs was 25%. In addition to experimental epochs, we also employed corresponding two- or three-digit control epochs (for each corresponding level of demand). During these epochs subjects passively observed two- or three-digit strings (“00” or “11”; “000” or “111”). Pure rest epochs (20 s) were also interspersed throughout the experimental run. Subjects signaled responses by button press on a standard response box. A schematic of the task is presented in **Figure 1**.

fMRI PROCESSING (ACTIVATION ANALYSES)

Data were processed with Statistical Parametric Mapping (SPM8). Realignment was performed to correct for head motion artifact during the scan. Realigned images were normalized to the Montreal Neurological Institute (MNI) EPI template and voxels resliced (2 mm × 2 mm × 2 mm). Normalized images were smoothed using an 8 mm FWHM Gaussian kernel. Images where estimated motion exceeded 4 mm were discarded from the analyses (<1% of all images).

In the first (within-subject) level analyses, rest, control, and attention epochs were modeled with boxcar stimulus functions that were convolved with a canonical hemodynamic response function to form regressors. Serial correlations were modeled with an auto-regressive process and low frequency fluctuations were removed with a high pass filter (using a discrete cosine set covering frequencies of 1/256 s or lower). Note that we did not model phasic or event related responses to targets. This was because we were primarily interested in the responses associated with sustained attention.

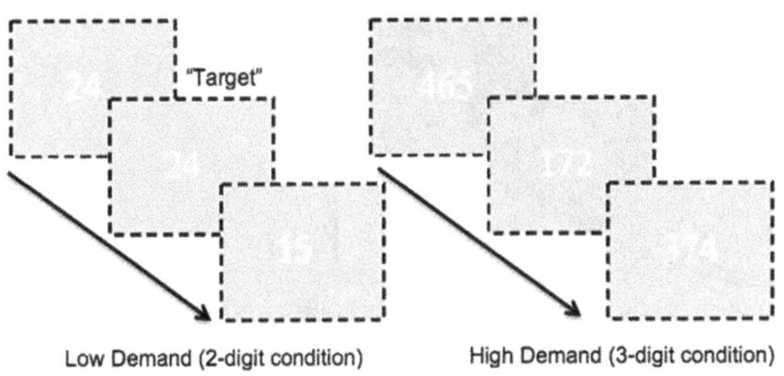

FIGURE 1 | A schematic of the employed CPT-IP task is shown. The task alternated between two- and three-digit extended epochs and subjects were required to detect repeated presentation of numbers. As seen attention demand was modulated by manipulating figure-ground contrast. The numbers in the figure were RGB: 255, 255, 255; the ground was RGB: 225, 225, 225 in order to minimize contrast. In addition, font between successive numbers alternated (arial, times new roman). This ensured a baseline level of "flicker" between successive presentations, pre-empting target detection based on visual cues such as the absence of flicker.

First level contrasts for each level of demand relative to the corresponding control condition (Attention > Control) were computed for each individual subject. That is, we contrasted the beta-estimates for the low-attention condition with those for passively viewing two-digit strings and those for the high attention condition with those for passively viewing three-digit strings. This was performed to identify responses to attention-related (as opposed simply to visual) processing. First level maps were submitted to second level analyses of covariance with Group (HGR, TC) as the independent factor, demand (two-digit vs. three-digit) as non-independent factor, and age, gender, and task performance (assessed with d')(50) as covariates. Clusters of activation ($p < 0.05$, cluster level corrected for multiple comparisons) (51) were employed to identify significant brain regions for each of the effects.

fMRI PROCESSING (LINEAR DCM ANALYSES)

More formal coverage of DCM can be found elsewhere (33, 52, 53). Briefly, DCM allows the interpretation of causal interaction between hidden state variables (32). The brain is viewed as a bilinear input (experimental conditions) – output (fMRI measured hemodynamic response) system. Changes in the neural responses are modeled using the following state differential equation:

$$\frac{dx}{dt} = \left(A + \sum_{j=1}^{m} u_j B^{(j)} \right) x + Cu.$$

where, A represents task-independent endogenous coupling between regions, $B^{(j)}$ represents putative modulation of endogenous connections by experimental manipulations (e.g., Attention, u_j), and C represents sensorimotor driving inputs on (typically) unimodal cortical regions.

A goal of DCM is to identify model(s) with the highest evidence given the observed fMRI data by testing competing hypotheses on a model space (54). Therefore, assessment of effective connectivity using DCM requires evaluation and comparison of neurobiologically plausible competing models, each representing hypotheses on the connective-architecture of the investigated neural system.

The *a priori* attention network of interest included regions both within the executive network (dACC, dPFC, and caudate nucleus) and sensory and spatial attention-related regions (parietal cortex and visual cortex) (6, 36, 37, 55). The particular focus of the modeling space (competing hypothesis) was the role of the dorsal anterior cingulate cortex and the contextual modulation of its efferent connections to other regions of the attention network. This approach was motivated in large part by the significant role played by the dACC in cognitive and resource control as it relates to attention and conflict (56), and its particular place in the control-related hierarchy of the forebrain (57, 58). Notably, disordered cognitive control has emerged as a general framework for understanding the schizophrenia and bipolar diathesis which the at-risk participants in our sample fall under (29, 59–61). DCM was implemented using DCM8 in SPM8. An *a priori* network of nodes was derived using regions of interests in stereotactic space (62). Within each structurally defined node of this network, we summarized regional activity on a subject-specific basis employing the principal eigenvariate of voxels within a 5 mm radius of the peak. **Figure 2** shows the resulting architecture.

MODEL ESTIMATION

Prior to modeling, time series were extracted from each region of interest (ROI) according to established procedures (63, 64) using spheres (5 mm radius) centered on the peak of the "effects of interest" F-contrast ($p_{\text{FWE}} < 0.05$, adjusted for "effects of no interest"). Each of the 72 models was estimated across subjects. To determine the most likely generative model, a random-effects (RFX) BMS procedure was applied. In particular, we used the variational Bayes method to estimate posterior probabilities of competing models. Bayesian parameter averages of coupling estimates (with a focus on modulatory coupling) were analyzed to determine potential differences in modulation as a function of attention and statistical significance was assessed using Bonferroni correction ($p < 0.05$)(32, 34).

RESULTS

BEHAVIORAL RESULTS

Behavioral performance, which is the sensitivity to distinguish targets from distracters was assessed using d' (65), an established metric in Signal Detection theory (50,66). The metric incorporates the hit-rate (e.g., the rate of responding "same" to successively presented stimuli in the same valence category) and the false alarm rate (e.g., the rate of responding "different" to successively presented stimuli in difference valence categories), and is based on the difference between the inverse function of the cumulative Gaussian distribution applied to each, with a higher d' reflecting greater sensitivity to the task.

Behavioral data were analyzed in a repeated measures analysis of variance with Group (HGR vs. TC) as between subjects' factor and attention demand (two-digit vs. three-digit) as within-subjects factor. The main effect of load was significant indicating that attention load reduced the sensitivity of observers, $F_{1,45} = 11.67$, $p < 0.001$, MSe $= 0.25$. A main effect of group was marginally significant, $F_{1,45} = 2.86$, $p < 0.05$, one-tailed, MSe $= 1.71$ suggesting that subjects with a family history of psychiatric illness were marginally less sensitive than controls. No other effects reached significance. **Figure 3** depicts performance data across conditions and groups.

ACTIVATION ANALYSES WITH fMRI (DIFFERENCES IN REGIONAL SPECIALIZATION OF FUNCTION)

A significant main effect of Group (HGR $\neq$ TC) and Group $\times$ Demand interaction was investigated in the constituent regions across the network of interest. Significant clusters under the main effect were observed in both the dorsal prefrontal cortex and the parietal lobe ($p < 0.05$, cluster level) and significant clusters under the interaction term were observed in the basal ganglia. Directionality (HGR $\neq$ TC) of the statistical effects and the interaction terms were inferred based on estimates of the modeled responses extracted under the overall peak within the cluster of significance.

First, relative to TC, HGR subjects evinced reduced engagement of the dorsal prefrontal cortex irrespective of the degree of attention demand. **Figure 4** depicts significant clusters rendered on lateral and medial surfaces of the cortex. By comparison, HGR evinced increased engagement of the parietal cortex irrespective of the degree of attention demand (**Figure 5**).

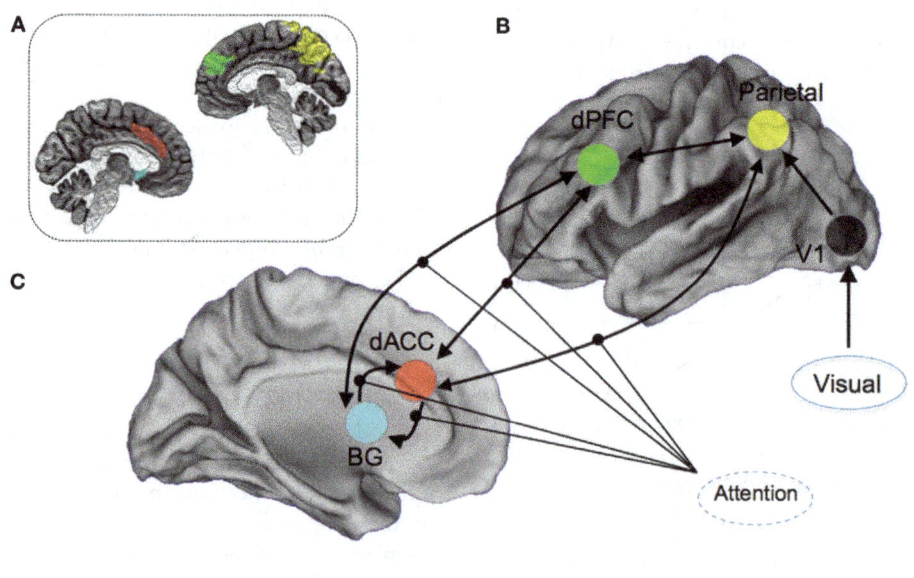

FIGURE 2 | Overview of the DCM model space. Seventy-two competing models were constructed by permuting the modulation of attention on **(A)** dorsal anterior cingulate (dACC) efferent pathways to the Basal Ganglia (BG), the dorsal prefrontal cortex (dPFC), and the parietal lobe, **(B)** dPFC and BG, and **(C)** BG and the dACC. Visual inputs to the system were modeled through the primary visual cortex. For the dACC–BG pathway, the bilateral endogenous connection itself was permuted. The inset image provides a schematic depiction (on a mid-sagittal slices) of the anatomical definitions used in summarizing regional activity for the DCM modeling. The color-coding of the regions of interest is approximately maintained.

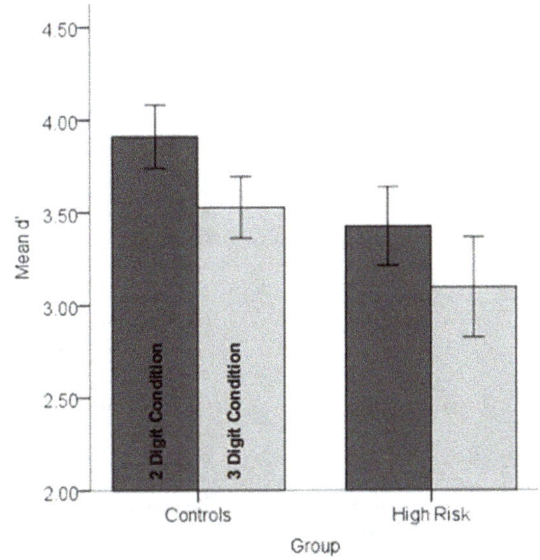

FIGURE 3 | Performance data (d') in each of the controls and high-risk groups are depicted for each of the conditions. Note that there was a marginally significant decrement in performance in the high-risk group and a highly significant effect of load (see text for statistical details). Error bars are ±SEM.

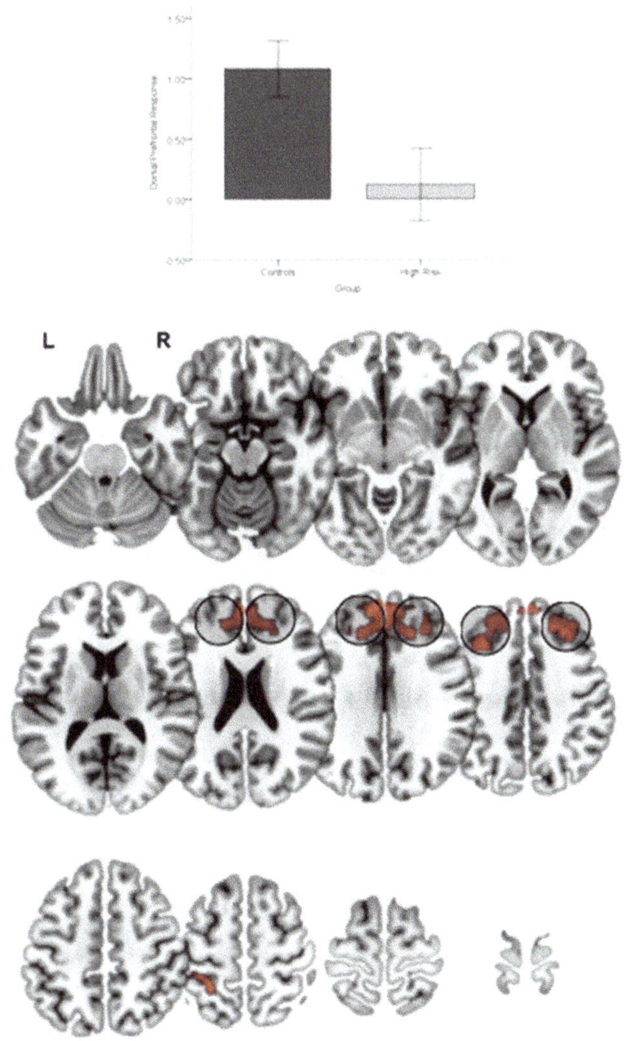

FIGURE 4 | Significant ($p < 0.05$, cluster level) bilateral clusters in the dlPFC and dmPFC (insets) under the overall main effect of group in the activation analyses represent significant hypo-engagement of the structure in HGR compared to TC (graph of parameter estimates from the peak in the dlPFC). The clusters are rendered on an ascending mosaic of axial surfaces. These results imply significant hypo-engagement of the prefrontal cortex in HGR during sustained attention.

In addition to the main effect of group a significant Group × Demand interaction in the basal ganglia (**Figure 6**). As seen in the accompanying graph of the modeled responses, the interaction resulted from an increase in BG engagement with increases in load with a corresponding decrease in engagement in HGR. These activation results suggest that genetic risk confers an imbalance in the patterns of *relative specialization* of attention-related function in adolescence, in particular with diminished engagement on executive regions of the network including the dPFC and the BG, but aberrantly increased reliance on the parietal cortex. The DCM results provide a notable complement for these activation-based analyses by demonstrating the effects of genetic risk in adolescence on the *functional integration* of information across regional networks for attention.

DCM ANALYSES OF fMRI DATA (DIFFERENCES IN FUNCTIONAL INTEGRATION)

Random-effects analyses and BMS revealed a single winning model in each of TC and HGR. **Figure 7** depicts model structure (specifically the pathways modulated by attention) and the observed exceedance probabilities for each of the TC and HGR groups. Notably, these results suggest that the likeliest generative models of the data did not differ across groups, with attention modulating the dACC efferents to the BG and the Parietal cortex. This convergence of model structure implies that any differences in effective connectivity between TC and HGR were to be expected in the parameter estimates of endogenous coupling, or contextual modulation of that coupling by attention (32).

To test for group differences we used the Bayesian parameter average over subjects within each group. This is appropriate because the best model was the same for both groups and therefore a comparison of the group-specific Bayesian parameter averages is unbiased by differences in Bayesian selection. This procedure provides posterior densities over the effective connectivity parameters for both groups, enabling one to estimate the difference between group means and posterior confidence in those differences (shown in terms of a posterior standard error in the figures). Group differences significant at a corrected level of $p < 0.05$, Bonferroni corrected (constituting, $p < 0.003$ for each of the 13 tests) are indicated (*). These P values were based upon the posterior differences in group-specific Bayesian parameter averages – and their significance can be visualized in terms of posterior standard errors in the **Figures 8** and **9** below.

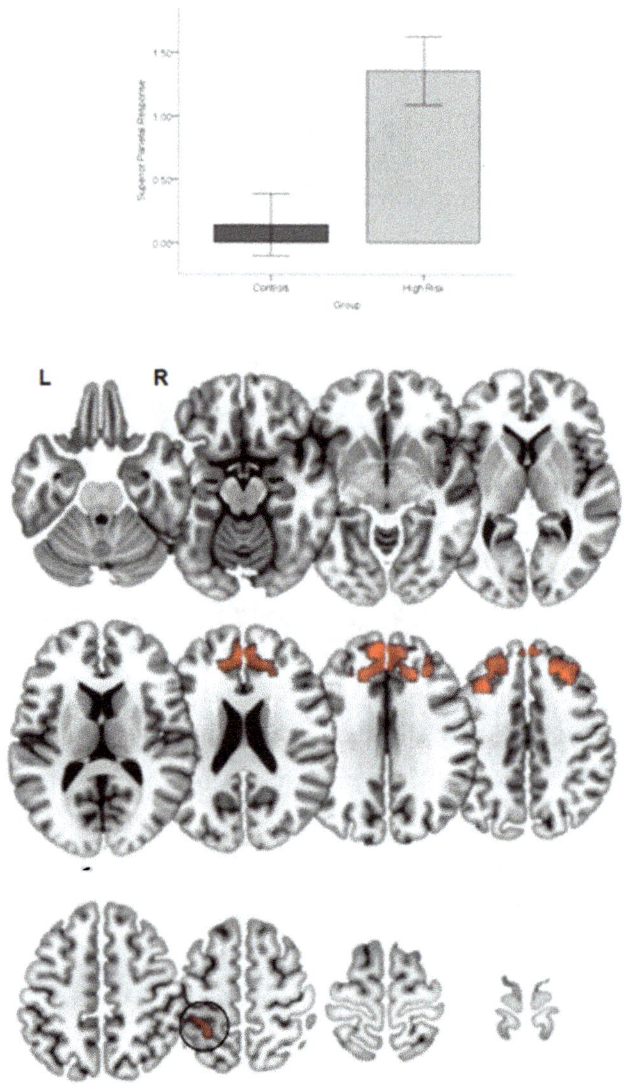

FIGURE 5 | Significant clusters ($p < 0.05$, cluster level) under the overall main effect of group in the activation analyses represent significant hyper-engagement of the parietal cortex (inset) in HGR compared to TC (see graph of parameter estimates from the peak in parietal cortex). The clusters are rendered on an ascending mosaic of axial surfaces. These results imply that HGR may inappropriately hyper-activate the parietal cortex during attention, suggesting an imbalance in the relative specialization of function underlying sustained attention.

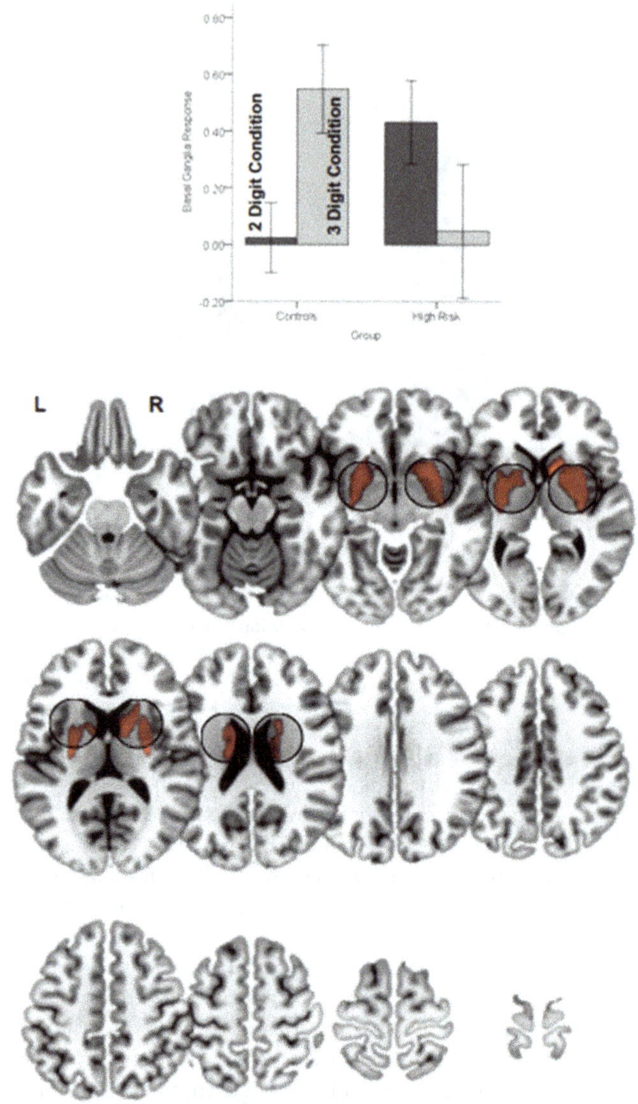

FIGURE 6 | Significant clusters ($p < 0.05$, cluster level) under the group x attention demand interaction term are rendered on an ascending mosaic of axial views. As seen in the graph, the interaction was driven by increased engagement with demand in controls, but decreased engagement in high-risk subjects. By implication, the BG, a core region in the executive attention circuit, appears to "turn off" in risk subjects with an increase in attention-related demand.

Figure 8 depicts observed estimates of endogenous coupling for each of the pairwise connections modeled across the endogenous network. As seen, the results provide an admixture of excitatory and inhibitory coupling across network pairs across the task. The most notable and symmetric finding was the bi-directional hypo-connectivity in the dACC ↔ BG pathway observed in HGR compared to TC (matched shaded insets). Notably, relative to TC, in HGR virtually every dACC efferent pathway was characterized by hypo-connectivity, suggesting convergence with hypothesis on the dysfunctional role of the dACC in schizophrenia and mood disorders. In addition, we also observed a difference between TC and HGR on dPFC ↔ dACC and the dACC ↔ Parietal pathways, with TC characterized by inhibitory coupling but HGR characterized by excitatory coupling (former) and decreased inhibitory coupling (latter).

We also observed notably differences in the attention-related contextual modulation of the efferent pathways from the dACC to the BG and the parietal lobe (**Figure 9**). In both cases, HGR were characterized by attention-related dysmodulation, albeit differing in character. Firstly, during attention epochs the dACC ↔ BG pathway was inhibited in HGR but increased in TC. Secondly, the dACC ↔ Parietal pathway was increase during attention in both

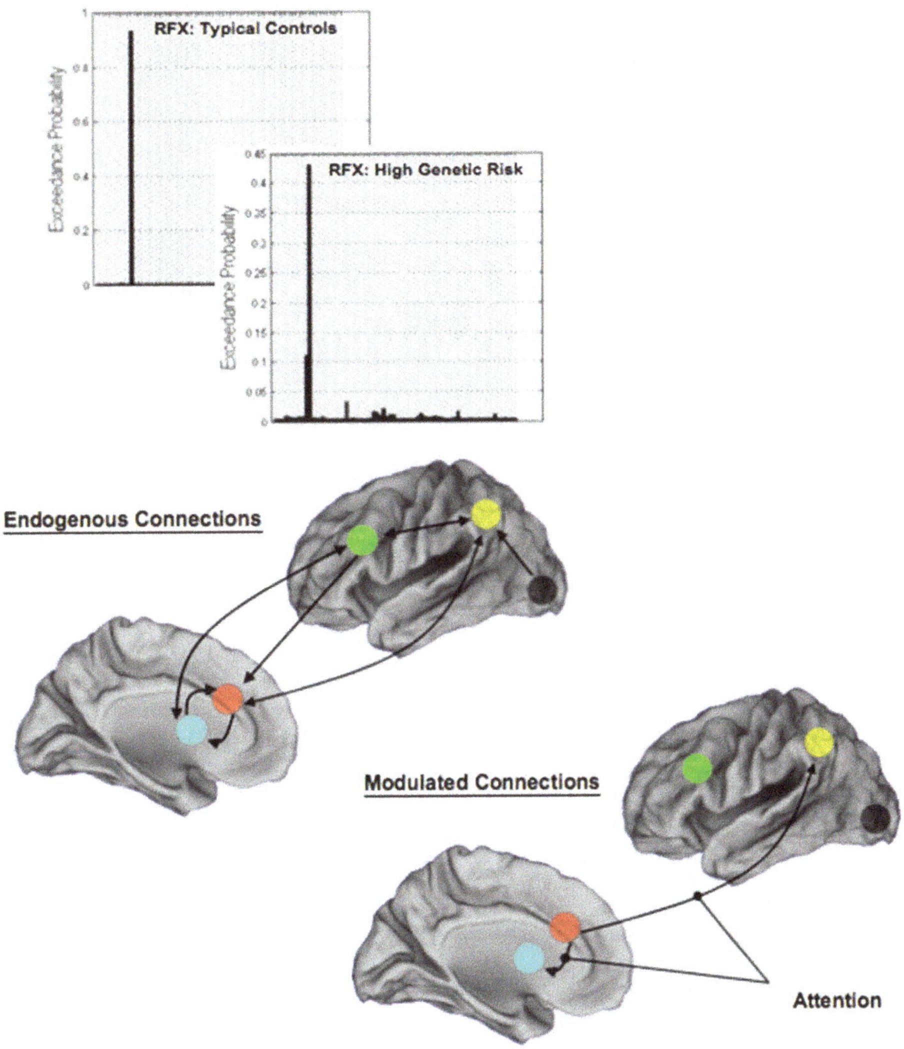

FIGURE 7 | The results of BMS are depicted in each of the TC and the HGR groups, and resulted in the identical model with the highest evidence. Model evidence is more heterogeneous in HGR than TC (see Discussion), evidence of intrinsic heterogeneity in this group. The endogenous connectivity of the winning model and the modulation of connections by attention are shown. Note that the primary modulated connections both originated in the dACC, terminating in the BG and the parietal cortex, respectively. The results of modulation suggest that dACC efferents may be particularly relevant in the implementation of attention in the modeled network of regions.

groups, but the degree of modulation was reduced in HGR. In the remainder of the paper, we discuss the import of these results in inferring the role of genetic risk on brain networks for attention, and the interpretation of the relationships between the analyses of relative specialization differences (activation) and functional integration differences (effective connectivity). We also reflect on the import role of network analyses of fMRI data in inferring accurate profiles of psychiatric risk in brain networks.

DISCUSSION

Assessing activation and effective connectivity differences between TC and HGR revealed striking differences in (a) the regional brain responses and interactive effects of attention demand, and (b) patterns of estimated endogenous and contextual effective connectivity between specific sub-networks, particularly related to dACC efferents. Activation analyses revealed an imbalance in regional brain function in HGR: the degree of dPFC engagement was reduced, with an apparent shifting in the relative degree of engagement to the parietal cortex. Furthermore, the BG in TC was responsive to variations in attention load, but disengaged in HGR. These activation-derived imbalances in regional recruitment in HGR suggest a relative shift away from relying on the dPFC and the BG core regions of the executive attention network (37, 67, 68), and toward regions such as the parietal lobe that may be more associated with spatial attention and orientation (69). These activation-based analyses provide a degree of convergence with fMRI patterns observed in adult patients with frank phenotypes of psychosis or mood disorders. For example, forebrain areas in

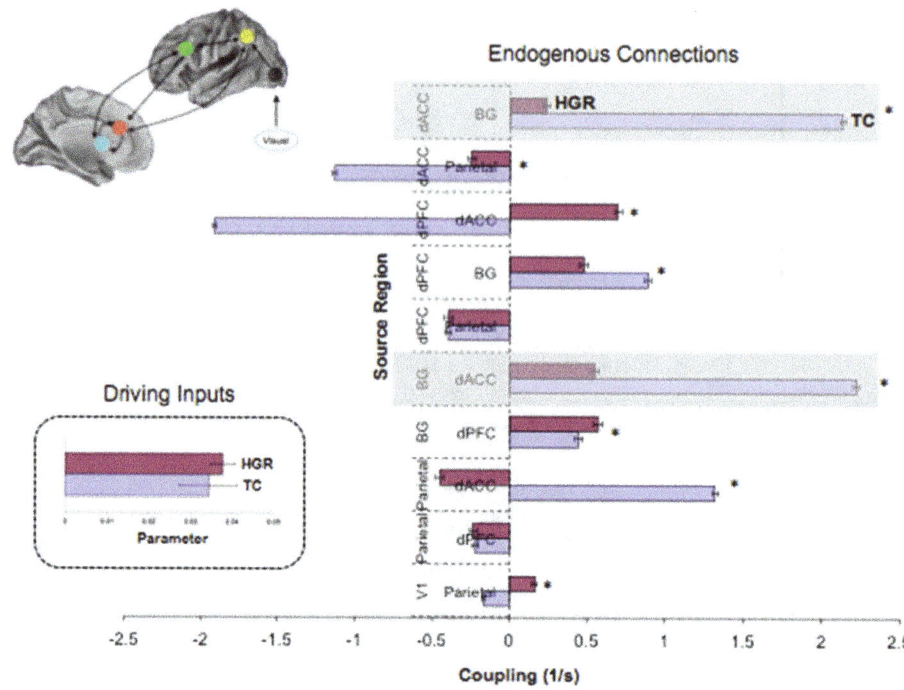

FIGURE 8 | Endogenous connections and driving inputs in TC and HGR. Bayesian parameter averages over all subjects in the winning model (**Figure 7** reproduced here) are depicted for each connection and for each of TC and HGR (± posterior standard errors). For the graph depicting endogenous connections, the source regions are vertically labeled and the target regions are horizontally labeled. TC and HGR reveal a mixture of positive and negative coupling across the modeled network. The shaded areas draw attention to highly significant hypo-connectivity in the bilateral dACC–BG sub-circuit in HGR subjects. The negative/inhibitory dPFC coupling in TC may reflect competitive inhibition between frontal regions most associated with cognitive control, and is absent in HGR. The inset depicts driving inputs to the primary visual cortex (not different between TC and HGR). Despite model evidence suggestive of identical model structures, these data suggest that HGR are characterized by disordered effective connectivity in the modeled sustained attention network.

schizophrenia appear hypo-active during conscious and rapid (as opposed to deliberative) processing tasks that engage attention (40, 70, 71). Moreover, in stimulus-response integration tasks with significant attentional demand, regional profiles of engagement are shifted in schizophrenia toward the parietal cortex (72). Similarly, adult bipolar patients are characterized by decreased basal ganglia activity during sustained attention and thalamus during a sustained attention task (73). Given the unique and integrative role of regions such as the dPFC and the basal ganglia in corticostriatal loops subserving attention and memory (74), this disengagement may reflect the role of genetic risk in creating a latent functional deficit in adolescence that alters the relative specialization of function of attention-related regions. This latent deficit is an important vulnerability marker of predisposition to disorders of psychosis or mood (75–77).

Whereas the observed activation-related in HGR appear to foreshadow adult studies in schizophrenia and bipolar disorder, evidence of disordered effective connectivity in HGR constitutes an entirely novel line of inquiry into the functional network biology attention networks and their relationship to risk (29). In general, applications of effective connectivity analyses of fMRI data in adult schizophrenia or bipolar patients has been fruitful in revealing disordered connectivity in tasks of learning (78), sentence completion tasks (79), emotion processing (80), and working memory (81). Perhaps the closest predecessor related to the current set of results is recent work investigating working memory related disordered effective connectivity in young individuals in the prodromal state for schizophrenia (35). In these subjects, reduced frontal–parietal connectivity during working memory (and intermediate between TC and schizophrenia patients) and the implied reduction in functional integration within these critical brain circuits may be predictive of the eventual transition to psychosis. We note that the prodromal state is itself a unique risk-state, constituting an advanced stage of (non-specific) clinical symptoms, and therefore distinct from the HGR group assessed herein. Nevertheless a significant proportion of HGR subjects are likely to transition toward frank phenotypes by way of prodromal symptoms. In this clinical/sub-clinical context, we highlight two points of plausible convergence. Firstly, reduced dACC ↔ BG endogenous connectivity in HGR may reflect a latent dyscoupling in the dormant risk-state that may impair the scaling up of cortical networks to implement higher order tasks. Given the important role of this sub-network in tasks as diverse as memory, attention, motor and cognitive control, and skill learning (82–86), it is likely that a connectivity deficit in this sub-circuit will foreshadow likely deficits in a slew of psychological domains. Indeed, it is unsurprising that in general large neuropsychological assessments of HGR indicate widespread impairments in

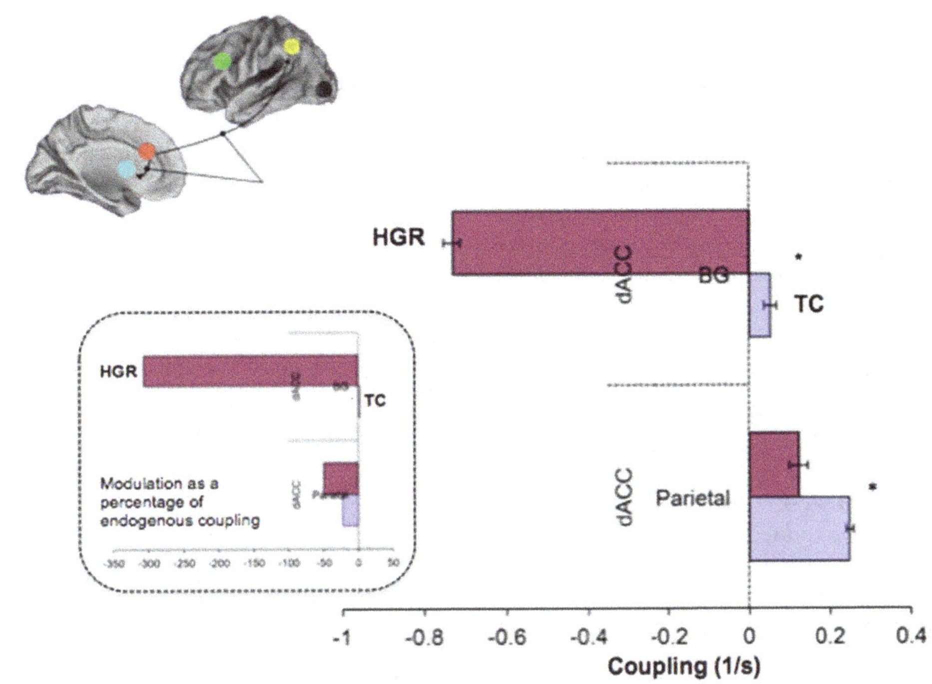

FIGURE 9 | Contextually modulated connections in the winning model in TC and HGR. Bayesian parameter averages over all subjects for the winning model (**Figure 7** reproduced here) are depicted for each modulated connection (± posterior standard errors). The source regions are vertically labeled and the target regions are horizontally labeled. For both dACC efferent pathways, attention has different patterns of modulation in HGR. The degree of positive modulation (excitatory) on the dACC–Parietal pathway is reduced in HGR, suggesting that the gain in connection strength is lower when implementing attention processing. Moreover, the dACC–BG pathway in HGR is significantly inhibited during attention processing. The inset depicts contextual modulation expressed as a percentage of the endogenous coupling values (**Figure 8**). This turning down may reflect critical sub-network disengagement in HGR during attention processing and may encode particular vulnerability for impaired attention, cognition, and control that has been documented in HGR groups.

neurocognitive domains, most of which rely in some form on attention processing (21, 23, 87, 88).

Disordered contextual modulation of dACC ↔ BG and dACC ↔ Parietal efferent pathways provides a parallel and likewise intriguing aspect of network-related dysfunction, particularly as assessments of contextual modulation provide a highly unique contribution of DCM to the study of brain network dynamics and systems theory (33, 89). In this regard, reduced (positive) modulation of the dACC ↔ Parietal pathway and strong inhibition of the dACC ↔ BG pathway in HGR are suggestive of differences of attention-related implementation in the same network. Given that these parameters represent an increase or decrease in connection strength as a function of the implemented task, the inhibition of the dACC ↔ BG pathway indicates the disengagement of this interaction in response to attention processing. As this disengagement is contrary to the expected excitation in TC, it suggests that in addition to being hypo-connected, the dACC ↔ BG sub-network is also "turned down" during attention processing. This turning down (and the disordered response to load) suggests that frontal–striatal network function is suboptimal in the risk-state. This is consistent with the relationship between dopamine and frontal–striatal function (90), the developmental tuning of the dopamine response, and the relevance of frontal–striatal dopamine dysfunction for schizophrenia and risk for schizophrenia (91).

RELATIVE SPECIALIZATION AND FUNCTIONAL INTEGRATION IN HGR

Both the more conventional assessment of regional activation strength and the more advanced analysis of effective connectivity revealed impaired cortical–striatal signals in HGR. Both of them, however, provide unique insight. Activation-based approaches with a general linear model framework do not explicit distinguish between network and/or task constituents (e.g., endogenous connections, modulation by task, sensory inputs) and from the perspective of system's theory, these approaches are slightly incomplete (89). Thus, the observed disordered activations in HGR are neutral in revealing network-based dysfunction underlying genetic risk and provide more general assessments of differences in the relative engagement of brain regions. We also note that activation-based approaches did not identify HGR-TC differences in regions such as the dACC, perhaps reflecting a limitation in classical statistical approaches to fMRI.

By comparison, DCM is limited by *a priori* assumptions in the assessed network and the structure of the model space. It nevertheless has proven to be more sensitive in identifying abnormal biological signatures in risk-groups, where activation analyses were not. For example, using DCM we recently documented disordered cortical–limbic endogenous connectivity and contextual modulation during an emotional appraisal task in children of schizophrenia parents (34). Notably, this finding emerged despite widespread overlap in activation networks across risk and control groups. DCM thus proved to be highly sensitive in uncovering emergent impairments in functional brain organization, not apparent in regional brain activation patterns or behavioral. It has hence repeatedly been proposed that effective connectivity is an important aspect of research on high-risk samples, not only because of its more realistic interactional model but also because of its reliance on Bayesian statistics (38, 92). By contrast, the absence or restriction of significant regional effects in classical statistics may partly be related to its premises of minimizing the type I error (while Bayesian statistics rely on the highest posterior probability) (28, 32).

LIMITATIONS AND PROSPECTUS

We conclude with a brief note on the limitations of the study, and a brief note on the prospective role of fMRI in high-risk research. The present study is limited by the relatively small sample size, though this limitation is slightly offset by the robustness of the results, particularly the effective connectivity analyses. Moreover, we acknowledge that HGR is a heterogeneous group, which may explain the more heterogeneous pattern of model evidence for HGR (**Figure 7**) compared to TC. This heterogeneity is well known and has been characterized before with MRI (25, 36, 93). Moreover, even though children of schizophrenia and bipolar patients are not distinct in terms of attention impairment (assessed with neuropsychological measures) (14), it is plausible that implementation of attention in brain networks may differ. We acknowledge that these differences are not knowable in the current analyses on account of sample size limitations. Also, in assessing effective connectivity, in this first approach, we did not explicitly model effects of attention load (providing a point of asymmetry with the activation-based analyses), though we are currently augmenting our analyses to investigate these effects.

The study of adolescents at genetic risk for schizophrenia or bipolar disorder offers opportunities and challenges. As indicated previously, HGR constitute a unique risk group, distinct from prodromal or clinical high-risk samples (94–97). Studying HGR in the medication naïve state can provide interesting insights into the intersection of genetic risk and abnormal neurodevelopment (98, 99). By focusing on a *profile of cumulative genetic risk*, rather than on *individual genes*, such approaches are important given the polygenic and non-specific genetic bases of psychiatric disorders (100, 101). However, the emergence of frank phenotypes (typically in early adulthood) is mediated by a host of unknown and uncontrolled factors (102), and neurobiological signatures in HGR may be non-specific and carry uncertain predictive value. Nevertheless, we suggest that a focus on critical domains such as sustained attention, and understanding of brain network dysfunction underlying these domains in HGR may provide a particularly fruitful path forward in understanding how genetically mediated vulnerability is encoded in disordered brain network interactions.

AUTHOR CONTRIBUTIONS

Vaibhav A. Diwadkar designed and supervised the project, data acquisition and all analyses and interpretation. Neil Bakshi conducted DCM analysis. Gita Gupta conducted activation bases analysis. Patrick Pruitt and Richard White assisted in data collection and analyses. Simon B. Eickhoff collaborated with Vaibhav A. Diwadkar in design, analyses, and interpretation.

ACKNOWLEDGMENTS

Vaibhav A. Diwadkar acknowledges support from the National Institute of Mental Health (MH6860), the National Alliance for Research on Schizophrenia and Depression (NARSAD), the Children's Research Center of Michigan (CRCM), the Children's Hospital Foundation, the Prechter Pediatric Bipolar Program World Heritage Foundation, and the Lyckaki-Young Fund from the State of Michigan. Additional support was provided by a Career Development Chair from the Office of the President, Wayne State University. We thank Jacqueline Radwan and Eric Murphy for assistance in data analyses and collection, Dalal Khatib for assistance in data collection, and R. Rajarathinam, Al Pizzuti, Caroline Zajac-Benitez, Usha Rajan, and M. S. Keshavan for assistance in recruitment and characterization.

REFERENCES

1. Lawrence NS, Ross TJ, Hoffmann R, Garavan H, Stein EA. Multiple neuronal networks mediate sustained attention. *J Cogn Neurosci* (2003) **15**:1028–38. doi:10.1162/089892903770007416
2. Langner R, Eickhoff SB. Sustaining attention to simple tasks: a meta-analytic review of the neural mechanisms of vigilant attention. *Psychol Bull* (2013) **139**:870–900. doi:10.1037/a0030694
3. Rubia K, Smith AB, Woolley J, Nosarti C, Heyman I, Taylor E, et al. Progressive increase of frontostriatal brain activation from childhood to adulthood during event-related tasks of cognitive control. *Hum Brain Mapp* (2006) **27**:973–93. doi:10.1002/hbm.20237
4. Rueda MR, Rothbart MK, Mccandliss BD, Saccomanno L, Posner MI. Training, maturation, and genetic influences on the development of executive attention. *Proc Natl Acad Sci U S A* (2005) **102**:14931–6. doi:10.1073/pnas.0506897102
5. Posner MI, Rothbart MK. Attention, self-regulation and consciousness. *Philos Trans R Soc Lond B Biol Sci* (1998) **353**:1915–27. doi:10.1098/rstb.1998.0344
6. Fan J, Mccandliss BD, Fossella J, Flombaum JI, Posner MI. The activation of attentional networks. *Neuroimage* (2005) **26**:471–9. doi:10.1016/j.neuroimage.2005.02.004
7. Calzavara R, Mailly P, Haber SN. Relationship between the corticostriatal terminals from areas 9 and 46, and those from area 8A, dorsal and rostral premotor cortex and area 24c: an anatomical substrate for cognition to action. *Eur J Neurosci* (2007) **26**:2005–24. doi:10.1111/j.1460-9568.2007.05825.x
8. Chang C, Crottaz-Herbette S, Menon V. Temporal dynamics of basal ganglia response and connectivity during verbal working memory. *Neuroimage* (2007) **34**:1253–69. doi:10.1016/j.neuroimage.2006.08.056
9. Corbetta M, Shulman GL, Miezin FM, Petersen SE. Superior parietal cortex activation during spatial attention shifts and visual feature conjunction. *Science* (1995) **270**:802–5. doi:10.1126/science.270.5237.802
10. Gogtay N, Giedd JN, Lusk L, Hayashi KM, Greenstein D, Vaituzis AC, et al. Dynamic mapping of human cortical development during childhood through early adulthood. *Proc Natl Acad Sci U S A* (2004) **101**:8174–9. doi:10.1073/pnas.0402680101
11. Barnea-Goraly N, Menon V, Eckert M, Tamm L, Bammer R, Karchemskiy A, et al. White matter development during childhood and adolescence: a cross-sectional diffusion tensor imaging study. *Cereb Cortex* (2005) **15**:1848–54. doi:10.1093/cercor/bhi062
12. March J, Silva S, Curry J, Wells K, Fairbank J, Burns B, et al. The Treatment for Adolescents with Depression Study (TADS): outcomes over 1 year of naturalistic follow-up. *Am J Psychiatry* (2009) **166**:1141–9. doi:10.1176/appi.ajp.2009.08111620
13. Ancin I, Santos JL, Teijeira C, Sanchez-Morla EM, Bescos MJ, Argudo I, et al. Sustained attention as a potential endophenotype for bipolar disorder. *Acta Psychiatr Scand* (2010) **122**:235–45. doi:10.1111/j.1600-0447.2009.01532.x
14. Diwadkar VA, Goradia D, Hosanagar A, Mermon D, Montrose DM, Birmaher B, et al. Working memory and attention deficits in adolescent offspring of schizophrenia or bipolar patients: comparing vulnerability markers.

Prog Neuropsychopharmacol Biol Psychiatry (2011) **35**:1349–54. doi:10.1016/j.pnpbp.2011.04.009
15. Shaw P, Gogtay N, Rapoport J. Childhood psychiatric disorders as anomalies in neurodevelopmental trajectories. *Hum Brain Mapp* (2011) **31**:917–25. doi:10.1002/hbm.21028
16. Erlenmeyer-Kimling L. Neurobehavioral deficits in offspring of schizophrenic parents: liability indicators and predictors of illness. *Am J Med Genet* (2000) **97**:65–71. doi:10.1002/(SICI)1096-8628(200021)97:1<65::AID-AJMG9>3.3.CO;2-M
17. Klimes-Dougan B, Ronsaville D, Wiggs EA, Martinez PE. Neuropsychological functioning in adolescent children of mothers with a history of bipolar or major depressive disorders. *Biol Psychiatry* (2006) **60**:957–65. doi:10.1016/j.biopsych.2006.03.031
18. DelBello MP, Geller B. Review of studies of child and adolescent offspring of bipolar parents. *Bipolar Disord* (2001) **3**:325–34. doi:10.1034/j.1399-5618.2001.30607.x
19. Cornblatt BA. The New York high risk project to the Hillside recognition and prevention (RAP) program. *Am J Med Genet* (2002) **114**:956–66. doi:10.1002/ajmg.b.10520
20. Hillegers MH, Reichart CG, Wals M, Verhulst FC, Ormel J, Nolen WA. Five-year prospective outcome of psychopathology in the adolescent offspring of bipolar parents. *Bipolar Disord* (2005) **7**:344–50. doi:10.1111/j.1399-5618.2005.00215.x
21. Birmaher B, Axelson D, Goldstein B, Monk K, Kalas C, Obreja M, et al. Psychiatric disorders in preschool offspring of parents with bipolar disorder: the Pittsburgh Bipolar Offspring Study (BIOS). *Am J Psychiatry* (2010) **167**:321–30. doi:10.1176/appi.ajp.2009.09070977
22. Bearden CE, Hoffman KM, Cannon TD. The neuropsychology and neuroanatomy of bipolar affective disorder: a critical review. *Bipolar Disord* (2001) **3**:106–50. doi:10.1034/j.1399-5618.2001.030302.x discussion 151-103,
23. Keshavan MS, Diwadkar VA, Montrose DM, Stanley JA, Pettegrew JW. Premorbid characterization in schizophrenia: lessons from the Pittsburgh High Risk Study. *World Psychiatry* (2004) **3**:163–8.
24. Diwadkar V, Sweeney J, Boarts D, Montrose D, Keshavan M. Oculomotor delayed response abnormalities in young offspring and siblings at risk for schizophrenia. *CNS Spectr* (2001) **6**(11):899–903.
25. Diwadkar VA, Montrose DM, Dworakowski D, Sweeney JA, Keshavan MS. Genetically predisposed offspring with schizotypal features: an ultra high-risk group for schizophrenia? *Prog Neuropsychopharmacol Biol Psychiatry* (2006) **30**:230–8. doi:10.1016/j.pnpbp.2005.10.019
26. Diwadkar VA, Pruitt P, Goradia D, Murphy E, Bakshi N, Keshavan MS, et al. Fronto-parietal hypo-activation during working memory independent of structural abnormalities: conjoint fMRI and sMRI analyses in adolescent offspring of schizophrenia patients. *Neuroimage* (2011) **58**:234–41. doi:10.1016/j.neuroimage.2011.06.033
27. Friston KJ. Models of brain function in neuroimaging. *Annu Rev Psychol* (2005) **56**:57–87. doi:10.1146/annurev.psych.56.091103.070311
28. Stephan KE, Roebroeck A. A short history of causal modeling of fMRI data. *Neuroimage* (2012) **62**:856–63. doi:10.1016/j.neuroimage.2012.01.034
29. Diwadkar VA, Ofen N. Disordered brain network function in adolescence: impact on thought, language and vulnerability for schizophrenia. In: Brambilla P, Marini A editors. *Brain Evolution, Language and Psychopathology in Schizophrenia*. Oxford, UK: Taylor and Francis Group (2014). p. 73–95.
30. Aersten A, Preisl H. Dynamics of activity and connectivity in physiological neuronal networks. In: Schuster HG editor. *Non-Linear Dynamics and Neuronal Networks*. New York: VCH Publishing (1991). p. 281–302.
31. Buxton RB. Dynamic models of BOLD contrast. *Neuroimage* (2012) **62**(2):953–61. doi:10.1016/j.neuroimage.2012.01.012
32. Stephan KE, Penny WD, Moran RJ, Den Ouden HE, Daunizeau J, Friston KJ. Ten simple rules for dynamic causal modeling. *Neuroimage* (2010) **49**:3099–109. doi:10.1016/j.neuroimage.2009.11.015
33. Friston KJ, Harrison L, Penny W. Dynamic causal modelling. *Neuroimage* (2003) **19**:1273–302. doi:10.1016/S1053-8119(03)00202-7
34. Diwadkar VA, Wadehra S, Pruitt P, Keshavan MS, Rajan U, Zajac-Benitez C, et al. Disordered cortico-limbic interactions during affective processing in children and adolescents at risk for schizophrenia revealed by fMRI and dynamic causal modeling. *Arch Gen Psychiatry* (2012) **69**:231–42. doi:10.1001/archgenpsychiatry.2011.1349
35. Schmidt A, Smieskova R, Aston J, Simon A, Allen P, Fusar-Poli P, et al. Brain connectivity abnormalities predating the onset of psychosis: correlation with the effect of medication. *JAMA Psychiatry* (2013) **70**:903–12. doi:10.1001/jamapsychiatry.2013.117
36. Diwadkar VA, Segel J, Pruitt P, Murphy ER, Keshavan MS, Radwan J, et al. Hypo-activation in the executive core of the sustained attention network in adolescent offspring of schizophrenia patients mediated by pre-morbid functional deficits. *Psychiatry Res* (2011) **192**:91–9. doi:10.1016/j.pscychresns.2010.12.005
37. Posner MI. Imaging attention networks. *Neuroimage* (2012) **61**:450–6. doi:10.1016/j.neuroimage.2011.12.040
38. Stephan KE, Penny WD, Daunizeau J, Moran RJ, Friston KJ. Bayesian model selection for group studies. *Neuroimage* (2009) **46**:1004–17. doi:10.1016/j.neuroimage.2009.03.025
39. Penny WD, Stephan KE, Daunizeau J, Rosa MJ, Friston KJ, Schofield TM, et al. Comparing families of dynamic causal models. *PLoS Comput Biol* (2011) **6**:e1000709. doi:10.1371/journal.pcbi.1000709
40. Salgado-Pineda P, Junque C, Vendrell P, Baeza I, Bargallo N, Falcon C, et al. Decreased cerebral activation during CPT performance: structural and functional deficits in schizophrenic patients. *Neuroimage* (2004) **21**:840–7. doi:10.1016/j.neuroimage.2003.10.027
41. First MD, Gibbon M, Spitzer RL, Williams JBW, Benjamin LS. *Structured Clinical Interview for DSM-IV Axis II Personality Disorders*. New York: Biometrics Research Department, NYSPI (1997).
42. Kaufman J, Birmaher B, Brent D, Rao U, Flynn C, Moreci P, et al. Schedule for affective disorders and schizophrenia for school-age children-present and lifetime version (K-SADS-PL): initial reliability and validity data. *J Am Acad Child Adolesc Psychiatry* (1997) **36**:980–8. doi:10.1097/00004583-199707000-00021
43. Dresp B, Grossberg S. Spatial facilitation by color and luminance edges: boundary, surface, and attentional factors. *Vision Res* (1999) **39**:3431–43. doi:10.1016/S0042-6989(99)00026-7
44. Butterworth B. The development of arithmetical abilities. *J Child Psychol Psychiatry* (2005) **46**:3–18. doi:10.1111/j.1469-7610.2004.00374.x
45. Rosso IM, Bearden CE, Hollister JM, Gasperoni TL, Sanchez LE, Hadley T, et al. Childhood neuromotor dysfunction in schizophrenia patients and their unaffected siblings: a prospective cohort study. *Schizophr Bull* (2000) **26**:367–78. doi:10.1093/oxfordjournals.schbul.a033459
46. Cannon TD, Hennah W, Van Erp TG, Thompson PM, Lonnqvist J, Huttunen M, et al. Association of DISC1/TRAX haplotypes with schizophrenia, reduced prefrontal gray matter, and impaired short- and long-term memory. *Arch Gen Psychiatry* (2005) **62**:1205–13. doi:10.1001/archpsyc.62.11.1205
47. Cohen Kadosh R, Henik A, Rubinsten O, Mohr H, Dori H, Van De Ven V, et al. Are numbers special? The comparison systems of the human brain investigated by fMRI. *Neuropsychologia* (2005) **43**:1238–48. doi:10.1016/j.neuropsychologia.2004.12.017
48. Callicott JH, Bertolino A, Mattay VS, Langheim FJ, Duyn J, Coppola R, et al. Physiological dysfunction of the dorsolateral prefrontal cortex in schizophrenia revisited. *Cereb Cortex* (2000) **10**:1078–92. doi:10.1093/cercor/10.11.1078
49. Bakshi N, Pruitt P, Radwan J, Keshavan MS, Rajan U, Zajac-Benitez C, et al. Inefficiently increased anterior cingulate modulation of cortical systems during working memory in young offspring of schizophrenia patients. *J Psychiatr Res* (2011) **45**:1067–76. doi:10.1016/j.jpsychires.2011.01.002
50. Wickens TD. *Elementary Signal Detection Theory*. Oxford, UK: Oxford University Press (2001).
51. Ward BD. *Simultaneous Inference for fMRI Data*. Milwaukee, WI: Medical College of Wisconsin (2000).
52. Stephan KE, Harrison LM, Kiebel SJ, David O, Penny WD, Friston KJ. Dynamic causal models of neural system dynamics: current state and future extensions. *J Biosci* (2007) **32**:129–44. doi:10.1007/s12038-007-0012-5
53. Friston KJ, Li B, Daunizeau J, Stephan KE. Network discovery with DCM. *Neuroimage* (2012) **56**:1202–21. doi:10.1016/j.neuroimage.2010.12.039
54. Friston KJ. Functional and effective connectivity: a review. *Brain Connect* (2011) **1**:13–36. doi:10.1089/brain.2011.0008
55. Corbetta M, Akbudak E, Conturo TE, Snyder AZ, Ollinger JM, Drury HA, et al. A common network of functional areas for attention and eye movements. *Neuron* (1998) **21**:761–73. doi:10.1016/S0896-6273(00)80593-0

56. Fan J, Hof PR, Guise KG, Fossella JA, Posner MI. The functional integration of the anterior cingulate cortex during conflict processing. *Cereb Cortex* (2008) **18**:796–805. doi:10.1093/cercor/bhm125
57. Paus T. Primate anterior cingulate cortex: where motor control, drive and cognition interface. *Nat Rev Neurosci* (2001) **2**:417–24. doi:10.1038/35077500
58. Botvinick MM, Cohen JD, Carter CS. Conflict monitoring and anterior cingulate cortex: an update. *Trends Cogn Sci* (2004) **8**:539–46. doi:10.1016/j.tics.2004.10.003
59. Serene JA, Ashtari M, Szeszko PR, Kumra S. Neuroimaging studies of children with serious emotional disturbances: a selective review. *Can J Psychiatry* (2007) **52**:135–45.
60. Barbalat G, Chambon V, Franck N, Koechlin E, Farrer C. Organization of cognitive control within the lateral prefrontal cortex in schizophrenia. *Arch Gen Psychiatry* (2009) **66**:377–86. doi:10.1001/archgenpsychiatry.2009.10
61. Fornito A, Yoon J, Zalesky A, Bullmore ET, Carter CS. General and specific functional connectivity disturbances in first-episode schizophrenia during cognitive control performance. *Biol Psychiatry* (2011) **70**:64–72. doi:10.1016/j.biopsych.2011.02.019
62. Maldjian JA, Laurienti PJ, Kraft RA, Burdette JH. An automated method for neuroanatomic and cytoarchitectonic atlas-based interrogation of fMRI data sets. *NeuroImage* (2003) **19**:1233–39. doi:10.1016/S1053-8119(03)00169-1
63. Eickhoff SB, Grefkes C, Fink GR, Zilles K. Functional lateralization of face, hand, and trunk representation in anatomically defined human somatosensory areas. *Cereb Cortex* (2008) **18**:2820–30. doi:10.1093/cercor/bhn039
64. Muller VI, Cieslik EC, Turetsky BI, Eickhoff SB. Crossmodal interactions in audiovisual emotion processing. *Neuroimage* (2012) **60**:553–61. doi:10.1016/j.neuroimage.2011.12.007
65. Macmillan NA, Creelman CD. *Detection Theory: A Users Guide.* Mahwah, NJ: Lawrence Erlbaum Associates (2005).
66. Green DM, Swets JA. *Signal detection theory and psychophysics.* New York: Wiley (1966).
67. Rubia K, Overmeyer S, Taylor E, Brammer M, Williams SC, Simmons A, et al. Functional frontalisation with age: mapping neurodevelopmental trajectories with fMRI. *Neurosci Biobehav Rev* (2000) **24**:13–9. doi:10.1016/S0149-7634(99)00055-X
68. Posner MI. Attentional networks and consciousness. *Front Psychol* (2012) **3**:64. doi:10.3389/fpsyg.2012.00064
69. Corbetta M, Kincade JM, Shulman GL. Neural systems for visual orienting and their relationships to spatial working memory. *J Cogn Neurosci* (2002) **14**:508–23. doi:10.1162/089892902317362029
70. Dehaene S, Artiges E, Naccache L, Martelli C, Viard A, Schurhoff F, et al. Conscious and subliminal conflicts in normal subjects and patients with schizophrenia: the role of the anterior cingulate. *Proc Natl Acad Sci U S A* (2003) **100**:13722–7. doi:10.1073/pnas.2235214100
71. Filbey FM, Russell T, Morris RG, Murray RM, Mcdonald C. Functional magnetic resonance imaging (fMRI) of attention processes in presumed obligate carriers of schizophrenia: preliminary findings. *Ann Gen Psychiatry* (2008) **7**:18. doi:10.1186/1744-859X-7-18
72. Cieslik EC, Muller VI, Kellermann TS, Grefkes C, Halfter S, Eickhoff SB. Shifted neuronal balance during stimulus-response integration in schizophrenia: an fMRI study. *Brain Struct Funct* (2013). doi:10.1007/s00429-013-0652-1
73. Fleck DE, Eliassen JC, Durling M, Lamy M, Adler CM, Delbello MP, et al. Functional MRI of sustained attention in bipolar mania. *Mol Psychiatry* (2012) **17**:325–36. doi:10.1038/mp.2010.108
74. Haber SN, Calzavara R. The cortico-basal ganglia integrative network: the role of the thalamus. *Brain Res Bull* (2009) **78**:69–74. doi:10.1016/j.brainresbull.2008.09.013
75. Murray RM, Fearon P. The developmental 'risk factor' model of schizophrenia. *J Psychiatr Res* (1999) **33**:497–9. doi:10.1016/S0022-3956(99)00032-1
76. Murray RM, Sham P, Van Os J, Zanelli J, Cannon M, Mcdonald C. A developmental model for similarities and dissimilarities between schizophrenia and bipolar disorder. *Schizophr Res* (2004) **71**:405–16. doi:10.1016/j.schres.2004.03.002
77. Keshavan MS, Diwadkar V, Rosenberg DR. Developmental biomarkers in schizophrenia and other psychiatric disorders: common origins, different trajectories? *Epidemiol Psichiatr Soc* (2005) **14**:188–93. doi:10.1017/S1121189X00007934
78. Banyai M, Diwadkar VA, Erdi P. Model-based dynamical analysis of functional disconnection in schizophrenia. *Neuroimage* (2011) **58**:870–7. doi:10.1016/j.neuroimage.2011.06.046
79. Allen P, Stephan KE, Mechelli A, Day F, Ward N, Dalton J, et al. Cingulate activity and fronto-temporal connectivity in people with prodromal signs of psychosis. *Neuroimage* (2010) **49**:947–55. doi:10.1016/j.neuroimage.2009.08.038
80. Almeida JR, Mechelli A, Hassel S, Versace A, Kupfer DJ, Phillips ML. Abnormally increased effective connectivity between parahippocampal gyrus and ventromedial prefrontal regions during emotion labeling in bipolar disorder. *Psychiatry Res* (2009) **174**:195–201. doi:10.1016/j.pscychresns.2009.04.015
81. Crossley NA, Mechelli A, Fusar-Poli P, Broome MR, Matthiasson P, Johns LC, et al. Superior temporal lobe dysfunction and frontotemporal dysconnectivity in subjects at risk of psychosis and in first-episode psychosis. *Hum Brain Mapp* (2009) **30**:4129–37. doi:10.1002/hbm.20834
82. Rao SM, Mayer AR, Harrington DL. The evolution of brain activation during temporal processing. *Nat Neurosci* (2001) **4**:317–23. doi:10.1038/85191
83. Owen AM, Mcmillan KM, Laird AR, Bullmore E. N-back working memory paradigm: a meta-analysis of normative functional neuroimaging studies. *Hum Brain Mapp* (2005) **25**:46–59. doi:10.1002/hbm.20131
84. Witt ST, Laird AR, Meyerand ME. Functional neuroimaging correlates of finger-tapping task variations: an ALE meta-analysis. *Neuroimage* (2008) **42**:343–56. doi:10.1016/j.neuroimage.2008.04.025
85. Voytek B, Knight RT. Prefrontal cortex and basal ganglia contributions to visual working memory. *Proc Natl Acad Sci U S A* (2010) **107**:18167–72. doi:10.1073/pnas.1007277107
86. Rottschy C, Langner R, Dogan I, Reetz K, Laird AR, Schulz JB, et al. Modelling neural correlates of working memory: a coordinate-based meta-analysis. *Neuroimage* (2012) **60**:830–46. doi:10.1016/j.neuroimage.2011.11.050
87. Cornblatt B, Obuchowski M, Roberts S, Pollack S, Erlenmeyer-Kimling L. Cognitive and behavioral precursors of schizophrenia. *Dev Psychopathol* (1999) **11**:487–508. doi:10.1017/S0954579499002175
88. Keshavan MS, Diwadkar VA, Montrose DM, Rajarathinam R, Sweeney JA. Premorbid indicators of risk for schizophrenia: a selective review and update. *Schizophr Res* (2005) **79**:45–57. doi:10.1016/j.schres.2005.07.004
89. Stephan KE. On the role of general system theory for functional neuroimaging. *J Anat* (2004) **205**:443–70. doi:10.1111/j.0021-8782.2004.00359.x
90. Cools R, D'Esposito M. Inverted-U-shaped dopamine actions on human working memory and cognitive control. *Biol Psychiatry* (2011) **69**:e113–25. doi:10.1016/j.biopsych.2011.03.028
91. Howes OD, Montgomery AJ, Asselin MC, Murray RM, Valli I, Tabraham P, et al. Elevated striatal dopamine function linked to prodromal signs of schizophrenia. *Arch Gen Psychiatry* (2009) **66**:13–20. doi:10.1001/archgenpsychiatry.2008.514
92. Moran RJ, Jung F, Kumagai T, Endepols H, Graf R, Dolan RJ, et al. Dynamic causal models and physiological inference: a validation study using isoflurane anaesthesia in rodents. *PLoS One* (2011) **6**:e22790. doi:10.1371/journal.pone.0022790
93. Barbour T, Pruitt P, Diwadkar VA. fMRI responses to emotional faces in children and adolescents at genetic risk for psychiatric illness share some of the features of depression. *J Affect Disord* (2012) **136**:276–85. doi:10.1016/j.jad.2011.11.036
94. McGorry PD, Yung AR, Phillips LJ. The "close-in" or ultra high-risk model: a safe and effective strategy for research and clinical intervention in prepsychotic mental disorder. *Schizophr Bull* (2003) **29**:771–90. doi:10.1093/oxfordjournals.schbul.a007046
95. Fusar-Poli P, Borgwardt S. Integrating the negative psychotic symptoms in the high risk criteria for the prediction of psychosis. *Med Hypotheses* (2007) **69**:959–60. doi:10.1016/j.mehy.2006.12.044
96. Cannon TD, Cadenhead K, Cornblatt B, Woods SW, Addington J, Walker E, et al. Prediction of psychosis in youth at high clinical risk: a multisite longitudinal study in North America. *Arch Gen Psychiatry* (2008) **65**:28–37. doi:10.1001/archgenpsychiatry.2007.3
97. Fusar-Poli P, Borgwardt S, Bechdolf A, Addington J, Riecher-Rossler A, Schultze-Lutter F, et al. The psychosis high-risk state: a comprehensive state-of-the-art review. *JAMA Psychiatry* (2013) **70**:107–20. doi:10.1001/jamapsychiatry.2013.269
98. Weinberger DR. Implications of normal brain development for the pathogenesis of schizophrenia. *Arch Gen Psychiatry* (1987) **44**:660–9. doi:10.1001/archpsyc.1987.01800190080012
99. Diwadkar VA, Prasad KM, Keshavan MS. Approaches for adolescents with an affected family member with schizophrenia. *Curr Psychiatry Rep* (2004) **6**:296–302. doi:10.1007/s11920-004-0080-2

100. Cross-Disorder Group of the Psychiatric Genomics Consortium; Lee SH, Ripke S, Neale BM, Faraone SV, Purcell SM, et al. Genetic relationship between five psychiatric disorders estimated from genome-wide SNPs. *Nat Genet* (2013) **45**:984–94. doi:10.1038/ng.2711
101. Millan MJ. An epigenetic framework for neurodevelopmental disorders: from pathogenesis to potential therapy. *Neuropharmacology* (2013) **68**:2–82. doi:10.1016/j.neuropharm.2012.11.015
102. Lewis DA, Levitt P. Schizophrenia as a disorder of neurodevelopment. *Annu Rev Neurosci* (2002) **25**:409–32. doi:10.1146/annurev.neuro.25.112701.142754

12

Working Memory Capacity and Psychotic-Like Experiences in a General Population Sample of Adolescents and Young Adults

Tim B. Ziermans[1,2] *

[1] Department of Clinical Child and Adolescent Studies, Leiden University, Leiden, Netherlands
[2] Department of Neuroscience, Karolinska Institutet, Stockholm Brain Institute, Stockholm, Sweden

Correspondence:
Tim B. Ziermans, Department of Clinical Child and Adolescent Studies, Leiden University, Postbus 9555, 2300 RB Leiden, Netherlands
e-mail: t.b.ziermans@fsw.leidenuniv.nl

Working memory (WM) impairment is a common feature in individuals with schizophrenia and high-risk for psychosis and a promising target for early intervention strategies. However, it is unclear to what extent WM impairment parallels specific behavioral symptoms along the psychosis continuum. To address this issue, the current study investigated the relation of WM capacity with psychotic-like experiences (PLEs) in a large Swedish population sample ($N = 1012$) of adolescents and young adults ($M = 24.4$ years, range 12–35). WM was assessed with two online computer tasks: a task where participants had to identify and remember the location of an odd shape and a task of remembering and following instructions. PLE scores were derived from a translated symptom questionnaire (Community Assessment of Psychic Experiences), which includes positive, negative, and depressive symptom scales. Positive and negative symptom scales were further subdivided into symptom clusters based on factor analyses. The results showed that low WM capacity was modestly associated with increased reports of bizarre experiences (BE) and depressive symptoms, after controlling for age, gender, and global symptom scores. Interestingly, when analyses were repeated for separate age groups, low WM was exclusively associated with a higher frequency of BE for young adults (20–27 years) and with depressive symptoms for older adults (28–35 years). These findings suggest that specific PLEs can be indicative of reduced WM capacity in early adulthood, which in turn may reflect an increased risk for psychosis and a greater need for targeted intervention. In contrast, during adolescence individual differences in cognitive development may influence the strength of the relationships and thereby mask potential vulnerabilities for psychopathology.

Keywords: working memory, PLEs, schizotypy, psychosis proneness, CAPE, adolescence, internet

INTRODUCTION

Working memory (WM) refers to the cognitive function to retain and manipulate information over a brief period of time. Intact WM relies heavily on the dopaminergic regulation of neuronal networks, particularly in the prefrontal cortex [e.g., Ref. (1–3)]. Disrupted regulation has commonly been associated with behavioral expressions observed in a variety of neuropsychiatric disorders, including schizophrenia. Since the groundbreaking work of Goldman-Rakic and colleagues on prefrontal lobe function and the cellular mechanisms of WM (4, 5) the scientific community has largely embraced the notion that WM dysfunction constitutes a fundamental neurocognitive impairment pivotal to the pathogenesis of schizophrenia.

Indeed, meta-analytic evidence supports that impairments in WM, as well as in a wide range of other neurocognitive domains, are a common feature among individuals suffering from schizophrenia (6), schizoaffective disorders (7) and, to a lesser extent, young individuals at clinical high-risk for developing a psychotic disorder (8). The latter findings suggest that WM impairments may already be present during the earliest stages of the disorder when the first symptoms are starting to appear. However, most high-risk studies only recruit help-seeking individuals and rely on categorical group comparisons defined by clinical cut-off scores. These strategies are unfit to address whether WM is associated with sub-clinical symptomatology in the population at large as well. Given the recent surge of interest in WM training programs as an intervention aid in early schizophrenia and high-risk populations (9, 10), it is critical to improve our understanding of the putative relationship between WM performance and psychotic-like symptomatology in order to optimize their use and efficacy.

The extended psychosis phenotype refers to the observation that psychotic symptoms or "psychotic-like experiences" (PLEs) exist on a continuum in the general population with clinical schizophrenia on one end and mild, non-clinical schizotypy on the other (11, 12). A recent estimate indicates that the prevalence of PLEs is 7.2% in the general population and for approximately 20% of these individuals the symptoms will persist over time (13). Although PLEs do not necessarily cause distress or affect daily functioning for a majority of individuals, epidemiological studies do indicate that a high intensity of PLEs is associated with an increased risk for psychosis (14–16). Interestingly, prevalence of symptoms may differ across genders and appears to be higher in adolescence than in adulthood (17, 18), a period when the first PLEs typically begin to appear and WM skills are still under maturation (19). Both gender and age may therefore represent moderating variables of the relation between WM and PLEs.

Very few large-scale studies have examined the relationship between WM and PLEs in non-clinical populations, in part due to the time- and resource-consuming aspects of on-site neurocognitive assessments. In addition, available studies have typically focused on one of three classical schizophrenia symptom groups: positive (e.g., hallucinations, delusions), negative [e.g., blunted affect, social withdrawal (SW)], or disorganized (e.g., odd speech and behavior) symptoms. While most findings indicate that reduced WM capacity is associated with increased symptoms, results are mixed for positive and negative symptoms (20–22). This could partly be due to use of different WM measures and clinical instruments, insufficient differentiation of symptoms clusters or sample bias (most studies recruited students). Consequently, it remains unclear whether WM is more commonly associated with specific schizotypal features.

In the current study the relationship between WM capacity and PLEs was further investigated with a fully automated online assessment procedure in a general population sample of Swedish adolescents and young adults. Previous population studies have demonstrated that PLEs do not represent a homogenous entity and can be divided into different subtypes for both positive and negative symptom dimensions (23, 24). These subtypes may convey a different level of risk for psychotic disorders and therefore also exhibit a different interplay with cognitive functions such as WM. It was expected that positive and negative PLEs would be best represented by previously established subdivisions of symptom clusters (18, 24–26) and that clusters associated most with an elevated risk of psychosis [bizarre experiences, persecutory ideas, perceptual abnormalities] (27) would show the strongest negative association with WM capacity.

MATERIALS AND METHODS

PARTICIPANTS

The study was carried out in a sample of 1087 Swedish citizens between 12 and 35 years of age. Participants were recruited via a company specialized in online data collection and population surveys (http://www.norstat.se). Individuals aged 15 years or older provided their informed consent via an online consent form. For individuals younger than 15 years one of their parents provided consent. The study was approved by the Central Ethical Review Board on Research Involving Humans at Karolinska Institutet. The role of the recruitment company was restricted to generating a study sample representative of the Swedish population and it was not involved in the design or execution of the study. Participants were drawn randomly from a voluntarily registered panel of over 100,000 Swedish citizens. A total of 9582 adult individuals received an invitation to participate and an additional 4652 parents of children between 12 and 18 years received an invitation for participation of their child (total response rate = 7.3%). In addition to meeting the age criterion, participants were required to be fluent in Swedish and to have access to a computer with internet connectivity and an operational sound system.

INSTRUMENTS AND TEST PROCEDURE

Psychotic-like experiences

Psychotic-like experiences were assessed with a Swedish version of the Community Assessment of Psychic Experiences (CAPE) (28). This self-report scale measures the lifetime prevalence of positive, negative, and depressive symptoms on both a frequency scale (0 = never to 3 = nearly always) and a distress scale (1 = not distressed to 4 = very distressed). The CAPE questions were translated from English into Swedish and back-translated to increase reliability. Three qualified Swedish researchers with a clinical background carried out the translation. An independent professional translator completed the back-translation, after which a consensus version was drawn up for implementation as an online survey. Frequency scores were transformed to range from 1 to 4 for further analysis and internal consistency of the total CAPE was high ($\alpha = 0.91$). The translated questionnaire is freely available online at http://cape42.homestead.com/.

Working memory

Two tasks of the Cogmed Progress Indicator (CPI) developed by Cogmed, Pearson Assessment, were used to assess WM capacity. The CPI tasks were originally designed to measure WM training improvements with non-trained tasks. The first WM task was the "Odd One Out" [based on a similar task in the Automated Working Memory Assessment (29)] and the second a digital variant of the "Following Instructions" task (30). **Figure 1** shows a single frame taken from both tasks.

In the Odd One Out, the participant is prompted to identify which shape out of three is the odd one and then remember its location. The procedure is then repeated with three new shapes after which three empty slots appear. The participant is required to respond by indicating *where* the odd shapes had appeared, in the correct order of appearance. Once the participant has successfully completed the practice trials with two items, the task begins with two items. Two correct trials on each level will lead to progression to the next level where the item load is increased by one. The test is completed when two trials on the same level are incorrect. The final score is calculated based on performance on the highest level achieved where at least one trial was passed, after which 0.3 would be subtracted for each incorrect answer on that level along with 0.15 subtraction for each incorrect answer on levels below the highest level achieved.

The Following Instructions task consists of common classroom items laid out on a table (e.g., eraser, crayon, box) and the task is to follow the verbal instructions given as accurately as possible. The instruction could for instance be "Click on the green eraser, then drag the black crayon to the yellow box," which would be a trial on span level three (because there are three items to remember what to do with). Practice trials with one and then two items are presented. The task has the same progression, stopping and scoring rules as described for the Odd One Out task above. Subjects exhibiting signs of floor effects (below a cut-off score of 2) were excluded from further data analysis. Finally, scores on both WM tasks were transformed into z-scores and an average z-score was calculated for each individual as a proxy for WM capacity.

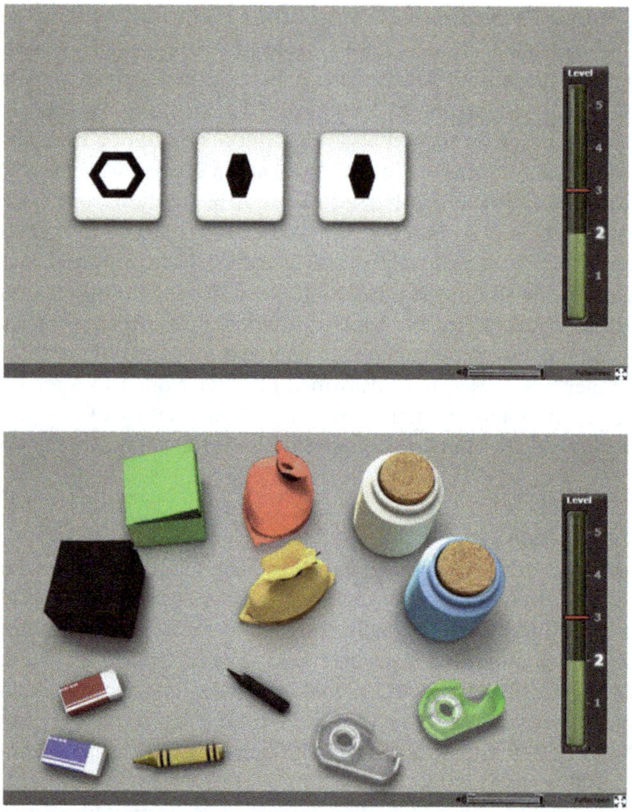

FIGURE 1 | Screen images of the online working memory tasks: Odd One Out (top) and Following Instructions (bottom).

Test procedure

After consent was provided, participants received a link to the online assessment together with a unique username and password combination, valid for one assessment only. Participants were strongly advised to complete the assessment in a quiet environment. The order of the WM tasks was always the same [(1) Odd One Out, (2) Following Instructions]. After completion participants were automatically redirected to the web-based CAPE questionnaire. In order to progress each question required an answer, thereby preventing the occurrence of missing values. Participants that completed the assessment received a cinema voucher as a reward. The total duration of the recruitment period was 6 weeks.

DATA ANALYSIS

Statistical analyses were performed with IBM SPSS version 20.0. All data were checked for normality, homogeneity, duplicate cases, and outliers. To establish the presence of subtypes of PLEs in the present sample, it was first tested whether the positive symptoms scale contained a similar factor structure as reported in previous studies (18, 25, 26). For this purpose, a confirmatory factor analysis was conducted with IBM Amos 21 and three different models with a four-factor structure were compared. To determine the factor structure of negative symptoms an exploratory factor analysis was preferred, since only one known study (24) has previously reported on this for the CAPE. Frequency scores were entered in a principal component analysis (PCA) with direct oblimin rotation. Three factors had an Eigenvalue ≥ 1 and the scree plot also indicated a cut-off of three factors. Subsequent parallel analysis with Monte Carlo simulation (31) confirmed that the three-factor structure best represented the data. Kaiser–Meyer–Olkin (KMO) measure of sampling adequacy and Bartlett's test of sphericity were used to assess whether the factor model was appropriate. KMO was 0.91 and Bartlett's test significant ($p < 0.001$), which suggested that data properties were excellent for factor analysis (32).

Next, sum scores for all subscales (four positive, three negative) were generated. An additional subscale for depressive symptoms (eight items) was also added for explorative reasons. All subscales were first checked for gender and age differences with non-parametric Mann–Whitney U and Kruskal–Wallis tests. For age comparisons participants were divided into three groups with a total age span of 8 years each: "adolescents" (12–19 years), "young adults" (20–27 years), and "adults" (28–35 years). *Post hoc* testing was based on the assumption of unequal sample sizes and variances and checked with Tamhane's T2 tests. Next, it was assessed whether there were any linear associations between WM and CAPE subscale scores. Spearman's rho was used for bivariate correlations and the p-value was Bonferroni corrected for multiple comparisons ($p < 0.0063$). Multiple hierarchical regression models were used to further investigate the association of WM with symptom scores. For regression analyses p-values < 0.05 were considered to be statistically significant.

RESULTS

PARTICIPANTS

A total of 1087 assessments were completed. Fifty-one duplicate cases were identified and excluded. Fourteen participants did not meet the age criterion and 10 additional adolescents were excluded after verification that a parent had either partially or completely filled out the CAPE on their behalf. This resulted in 1012 subjects for factor analysis of the CAPE, consisting of 547 female (54%) and 465 male (46%) individuals between 12 and 35 years ($M = 24.4$ years $\pm$ 6.6). The geographic distribution of participants was spread over all 21 counties (*län*) of Sweden and central tendency scores (mean, mode, median) for "highest education completed" indicated that a secondary education was the most common and average level of completed education in the sample.

CONFIRMATORY FACTOR ANALYSIS AND POSITIVE SYMPTOM SUBSCALES

Model-fitting statistics are provided in **Table 1**. In sum, the results show that a four-factor solution for the positive symptoms dimension is plausible for our sample. Comparison of the three models indicates that the base model derived from Ref. (18), is the single model that would meet broadly used cut-off criteria for model-fitting indices (33). The model slightly improved when error terms of three item-pairs were correlated. The models based on the factor structure by Yung et al. (25) and Armando et al. (26), required an additional number of correlated error terms to obtain an adequate fit. Based on the comparison, the model of Ref. (18) was adopted in this study to generate sum scores for the subtypes: bizarre experiences (BE), persecutory ideas (PI), perceptual abnormalities

Table 1 | Confirmatory factor analysis: fitting of three different models for the Community Assessment of Psychic Experiences – positive symptoms dimension.

Models	χ^2	df	χ^2/df	CFI	RMSEA	RMSEA interval	AIC
(25) – four-factor model (BE, PI, PA, MT)							
Base	729.8	164	4.45	0.85	0.06	0.05–0.06	821.8
+ *r* (q: 2–6, 2–22, 11–13, 15–20, 33–34)	470.9	159	2.96	0.92	0.04	0.04–0.05	573.0
– PI → q41	416.2	141	2.95	0.93	0.04	0.04–0.05	514.2
(18) – four-factor model (BE, PI, PA, GR)							
Base	478.1	129	3.71	0.90	0.05	0.05–0.06	562.1
+ *r* (q: 2–6, 2–22, 33–34)	371.1	126	2.95	0.93	0.04	0.04–0.05	461.1
(26) – four-factor model (BE, PI, PA, MT)							
Base	735.2	164	4.48	0.85	0.06	0.05–0.06	827.2
+ *r* (q: 2–6, 2–22, 11–13, 33–34)	491.3	160	3.10	0.91	0.05	0.04–0.05	591.3
+ BE → q5, q7 and PA → q31	549.0	163	3.43	0.90	0.05	0.04–0.05	649.0

CFI, comparative fit index; RMSEA, root mean square error of approximation; AIC, akaike information criterion; BE, bizarre experiences; PA, perceptual abnormalities; PI, persecutory ideas; MT, magical thinking; GR, Grandiosity; +/– = added/removed; r, correlated error terms; q, question; → = model pathway.

(PA), and grandiosity (GR). The factor loadings for both studies are displayed in **Table 2**.

EXPLORATORY FACTOR ANALYSIS AND NEGATIVE SYMPTOM SUBSCALES

The three-factor solution explained 54% of the variance and all items loaded high (>0.4) on one factor variable and only one item (item 29) had a cross-loading ≥0.25 (**Table 3**). The first factor was related to avolition (AV) and consisted of seven items, three items loaded on a second factor related to affective flattening (AF) and the last factor consisted of four items related to social withdrawal (SW). Compared to the only available factor structure of CAPE negative symptoms (24) loadings were in high agreement (**Table 3**). One item (16; "Do you ever feel you have no interest to be with other people?") loaded highest on SW in the current study as opposed to AV in the previous study and was therefore included in the SW sum score only.

FREQUENCY OF PSYCHOTIC-LIKE EXPERIENCES

Average prevalence of positive symptoms, determined by individuals reporting ≥2 on the frequency scales (=sometimes or more), was relatively high for PI and GR items (respectively 45 and 62%). Fewer individuals reported having experienced BE or PA (respectively 20 and 5%). All prevalence rates substantially decreased as the frequency rate increased (see **Table 2**). For negative symptoms the average prevalence rate was highest for SW (75%), then AV (70%), and lowest for AF (47%). In concordance with positive symptoms there was a steep decline in prevalence rates of negative symptoms with increased frequency (see **Table 3**). Depressive symptoms were also relatively common ($M = 63\%$; range: 28–93%), with an average of 3% (range: 1–6%) of respondents indicating that the symptoms were almost always present.

PSYCHOTIC-LIKE EXPERIENCES BY GENDER AND AGE

Average CAPE scores divided by gender and age groups are available in **Table 4**. There was no overall pattern of gender differences. Female individuals reported higher scores on PI ($U = 115{,}642$, $p = 0.011$) and depression ($U = 102{,}606.5$, $p < 0.001$) than males and there was a trend for higher PA in females as well ($p = 0.053$). In contrast, males reported higher frequencies of GR ($U = 137{,}215$, $p < 0.026$) and AF ($U = 115{,}642$, $p = 0.011$). Comparisons between age-groups showed that the reported frequency of all symptom scales differed significantly with age (all $p < 0.05$). *Post hoc* testing suggested that positive symptoms were more common in adolescents, while the highest frequency of negative and depressive symptoms was found in the young adult group (**Table 4**).

WORKING MEMORY CAPACITY

Data of the WM assessment was missing for 16 subjects due to registration errors. Another 92 subjects were excluded based on suspected floor effects on at least one of both WM variables, leaving 904 remaining subjects for WM analysis ($M_{age} = 24.7$ years ± 6.4; 420 males, 484 females). Average performance level was higher for the Odd One Out task ($M = 5.81$, SD = 1.21, range = 2.4–11.0) than for the Following Instructions task ($M = 4.89$, SD = 1.02, range = 2.0–8.4). The Pearson correlation coefficient between tasks was $r = 0.31$, $p < 0.001$. Correlations of both tasks with overall WM capacity (average *z*-score) was $r = 0.81$, $p < 0.001$. When checked, there was no gender difference in WM capacity ($t_{902} = 0.70$, $p = 0.48$).

CORRELATIONS BETWEEN WORKING MEMORY AND PSYCHOTIC-LIKE EXPERIENCES

Correlations of CAPE subscale frequency scores with WM capacity were calculated for 904 participants. After correction for multiple comparisons WM showed a negative association with positive symptom subtypes (BE: $r = -0.13$, $p = 0.00005$; PI: $r = -0.10$, $p = 0.003$) and depression ($r = -0.10$, $p = 0.003$). Partial correlations controlled for age and gender gave similar results (BE: $r = -0.10$, $p = 0.004$; PI: $r = -0.09$, $p = 0.006$; depression: $r = -0.11$, $p = 0.001$).

MULTIPLE REGRESSION WITH WORKING MEMORY AND PSYCHOTIC-LIKE EXPERIENCES

Subscales correlating with WM capacity (BE, PI, and depression) were entered as dependent variables in hierarchical multiple

Table 2 | Community assessment of psychic experiences: positive symptoms frequency scores and factor analysis.

	Frequencies (%)		CFA current study				EFA (18)			
	≥ Sometimes	Almost always	F1	F2	F3	F4	F1	F2	F3	F4
BIZARRE EXPERIENCES (BE)										
26 Do you ever feel as if the thoughts in your head were not your own?	13.3	0.5	0.61				0.68			
28 Have your thoughts ever been so vivid that you were worried other people would hear them?	17.3	0.5	0.58				0.55			
31 Do you ever feel as if you are under the control of some force or power other than yourself?	12.8	0.6	0.58				0.47			
24 Do you ever feel as if the thoughts in your head are being taken away from you?	19.3	0.4	0.51				0.67			
30 Do you ever hear your own thoughts being echoed back to you?	14.9	0.9	0.56				0.49			
17 Do you ever feel as if electrical devices such as computers can influence the way you think?	34.2	1.6	0.47				0.47			
5 Do you ever feel as if things in magazines or on TV were written especially for you?	30.0	0.1	0.33				0.48			
PERCEPTUAL ABNORMALITIES (PA)										
42 Do you ever see objects, people or animals that other people can't see?	6.0	0.6		0.60					−0.76	
34 Do you ever hear voices talking to each other when you were alone?	2.5	0.3		0.56					−0.83	
41 Do you ever feel as if a double has taken the place of a family member, friend or acquaintance?	4.0	0.4		0.48					−0.36	
33 Do you ever hear voices when you were alone?	7.7	0.7		0.47					−0.76	
PERSECUTORY IDEAS (PI)										
10 Do you ever feel as if there is a conspiracy against you?	14.7	0.5				0.60				0.49
7 Do you ever feel that you are being persecuted in some way?	16.5	0.2				0.58				0.40
22 Do you ever feel that people look at you oddly because of your appearance?	45.1	1.2				0.54				0.69
6 Do you ever feel as if some people are not what they seem to be?	88.8	1.8				0.39				0.58
2 Do you ever feel as if people seem to drop hints about you or say things with a double meaning?	62.3	3.6				0.32				0.81
GRANDIOSITY (GR)										
13 Do you ever feel that you are a very special or unusual person?	69.4	6.7			0.85			0.81		
11 Do you ever feel as if you are destined to be someone very important?	54.2	3.1			0.53			0.82		
CORRELATION MATRIX										
F1–BE			1	0.83	0.37	0.75	Correlations not available			
F2–PA				1	0.28	0.65				
F3–GR					1	0.49				
F4–PI						1				

CFA, confirmatory factor analysis; EFA, exploratory factor analysis.

Table 3 | Community assessment of psychic experiences: negative symptoms frequency scores and factor analysis.

	Frequencies (%)		EFA current study			EFA (24)		
	≥Sometimes	Almost always	F1	F2	F3	F1	F2	F3
AVOLITION (AV)								
25 Do you ever feel that you are spending all your days doing nothing?	59.7	4.3	0.73			0.59		
36 Do you ever feel that you can never get things done?	88.4	4.8	0.73			0.71		
23 Do you ever feel that your mind is empty?	57.2	1.0	0.69			0.46		
21 Do you ever feel that you are lacking in energy?	91.0	4.7	0.68			0.59		
18 Do you ever feel that you are lacking in motivation to do things?	91.8	4.7	0.66			0.60		
37 Do you ever feel that you have only few hobbies or interests?	59.1	7.9	0.54			0.40		
35 Do you ever feel that you are neglecting your appearance or personal hygiene?	45.5	1.5	0.51			0.62		
AFFECTIVE FLATTENING (AF)								
8 Do you ever feel that you experience few or no emotions at important events?	49.3	3.0		0.87			0.70	
27 Do you ever feel that your feelings are lacking in intensity?	40.7	1.8		0.79			0.74	
32 Do you ever feel that your emotions are blunted?	50.4	1.9		0.75			0.72	
SOCIAL WITHDRAWAL (SW)								
4 Do you ever feel that you are not much of a talker when you are conversing with other people?	78.6	6.2			0.84			0.71
3 Do you ever feel that you are not a very animated person?	73.5	3.5			0.74			0.69
29 Do you ever feel that you are lacking in spontaneity?	72.1	3.6	0.33		0.50			0.42
16 Do you ever feel you have no interest to be with other people?	76.9	1.7			0.42	0.33		
CORRELATION MATRIX								
F1–AV			1	0.36	0.36	1	0.46	0.43
F2–AF				1	0.29		1	0.32
F3–SW					1			1

EFA, exploratory factor analysis.

regression models. Age (z-score) and gender were entered first, next WM capacity, and finally the models were checked for interactions with age and gender. For BE the procedure was followed without inclusion of gender terms in the model. An overview of the regression outcomes is provided in **Table 5**. All models were highly significant ($p < 0.001$) and WM was negatively associated with BE, PI, and depression, regardless of age_z (BE, PI) or gender (PI, depression) effects (all $p < 0.01$). For depression there was an additional interaction effect of $age_z \times$ WM ($t = -2.18$, $p = 0.03$). All effect sizes (β) of significant predictors were considered small. To investigate the specificity of the association between WM and the symptom subscales, regression analyses were repeated with total CAPE score entered as an additional covariate. WM remained a significant predictor for BE and depression (both $p < 0.05$) and at trend-level for PI ($p < 0.06$). To further explore the presence of more specific age-effects, the sample was split into the three age-groups described above and regression analyses were repeated. WM significantly predicted BE in the young adult group [$\beta = -0.12$, $t(419) = -2.43$, $p = 0.016$] and depression in the adult group [$\beta = -0.11$, $t(321) = -2.04$, $p = 0.046$]. There were no significant associations between WM and symptom scores in the adolescent group.

DISCUSSION

Understanding how cognitive functions relate to behavioral symptoms in the general population can provide further insight into underlying mechanisms of emerging psychopathology and lead to identification of early intervention targets. WM represents a cognitive function that is commonly compromised in schizophrenia spectrum disorders and in individuals at-risk for psychosis, though little is known about specific contributions of WM impairments to schizotypal symptomatology. This study aimed to investigate whether WM capacity was related to presence of PLEs in a large population sample of adolescents and young adults. WM was negatively associated with subtypes of positive (BE and persecutory ideas) and depressive symptoms, also after adjusting for age, gender, and global symptom scores (trend-level for persecutory ideas). However, effect sizes were small and when divided into different age groups, WM was exclusively associated with BE in young

Table 4 | Community assessment of psychic experiences (CAPE) scores divided by gender and age group.

Symptom scales	Gender		Statistic	*p*	Age groups			Statistic	*p*
	Female ($n = 547$)	Male ($n = 465$)			Adolescents (12–19 years; $n = 252$)	Young adults (20–27 years; $n = 429$)	Adults (28–35 years; $n = 331$)		
Total CAPE	68.2 ± 12.6	66.1 ± 12.4	$U = 121{,}073$	0.204	69.0 ± 13.6	68.8 ± 12.4	65.4 ± 11.5	$H = 17.26$	<0.001[a]
Positive	27.0 ± 5.6	26.7 ± 5.4	$U = 123{,}427$	0.446	29.8 ± 5.9	27.3 ± 5.2	25.8 ± 4.4	$H = 65.14$	<0.001[b]
BE	8.6 ± 2.0	8.8 ± 2.4	$U = 133{,}381$	0.166	9.5 ± 2.7	8.7 ± 2.1	8.1 ± 1.7	$H = 81.28$	<0.001[b]
PA	4.3 ± 0.7	4.3 ± 1.0	$U = 121{,}874$	0.053	4.5 ± 1.1	4.2 ± 0.8	4.2 ± 0.7	$H = 22.73$	<0.001[b]
PI	7.9 ± 1.9	7.6 ± 1.8	$U = 115{,}642$	0.011	8.2 ± 2.3	7.8 ± 1.8	7.4 ± 1.5	$H = 24.57$	<0.001[b]
GR	3.6 ± 1.3	3.8 ± 1.4	$U = 137{,}215$	0.026	4.0 ± 1.5	3.8 ± 1.4	3.3 ± 1.2	$H = 38.70$	<0.001[a]
Negative	25.9 ± 5.9	26.3 ± 6.3	$U = 131{,}296$	0.346	25.6 ± 6.4	26.8 ± 6.1	25.5 ± 5.8	$H = 10.54$	0.005[c]
AV	13.5 ± 3.5	13.3 ± 3.6	$U = 121{,}441$	0.214	13.4 ± 3.6	13.8 ± 3.6	12.9 ± 3.2	$H = 9.22$	0.010[c]
AF	4.4 ± 1.6	5.1 ± 1.9	$U = 155{,}342.5$	<0.001	4.6 ± 1.8	4.9 ± 1.8	4.7 ± 1.7	$H = 8.74$	0.013[d]
SW	7.9 ± 2.1	7.9 ± 2.1	$U = 127{,}192$	0.997	7.6 ± 2.3	8.1 ± 2.0	7.9 ± 2.1	$H = 16.12$	<0.001[e]
Depression	14.9 ± 3.8	13.5 ± 3.4	$U = 102{,}606.5$	<0.001	14.3 ± 3.9	14.7 ± 3.7	14.4 ± 3.4	$H = 7.08$	0.029[c]

BE, bizarre experiences; PA, perceptual abnormalities; PI, paranoid ideations; GR, grandiosity; social withdrawal; affective flattening; avolition; Post hoc results ($p < 0.05$).

[a]Adolescents and young adults > adults.

[b]Adolescents > young adults > adults.

[c]Young adults > adults.

[d]Young adults > adolescents (trend: $p = 0.08$).

[e]Young adults > adolescents.

Table 5 | Regression models of symptom scores with working memory, age, and sex as predictors.

Dependent variable		Block 1			Block 2			Block 3		
		B	SE *B*	β	*B*	SE *B*	β	*B*	SE *B*	β
Bizarre experiences	(Constant)	8.68	0.07		8.68	0.07		8.69	0.07	
	Age_z	−0.54	0.07	−0.25**	−0.52	0.07	−0.24**	−0.53	0.07	−0.25**
	Working $memory_z$				−0.25	0.09	−0.09**	−0.52	0.09	−0.09**
	Age_z × working $memory_z$							−0.07	0.09	−0.03
	R^2			0.06			0.07			0.07
	ΔR^2						0.01**			0.01
Persecutory ideas	(Constant)	7.88	0.08		7.88	0.08		7.89	0.08	
	Age_z	−0.33	0.06	−0.18**	−0.31	0.06	−0.17**	−0.31	0.06	−0.17**
	Gender	−0.24	0.12	−0.07*	−0.25	0.12	−0.07*	−0.25	0.12	−0.07*
	Working $memory_z$				−0.20	0.08	−0.09**	−0.33	0.10	−0.15**
	Age_z × working $memory_z$							0.02	0.08	0.01
	Gender × working $memory_z$							0.26	0.15	0.08
	R^2			0.04			0.04			0.04
	ΔR^2						0.01**			0.00
Depressive symptoms	(Constant)	14.92	0.16		14.94	0.16		14.94	0.16	
	Age_z	−0.05	0.12	−0.01	−0.01	0.12	−0.00	−0.06	0.12	−0.01
	Gender	−1.11	0.24	−0.15**	−1.14	0.24	−0.16**	−1.09	0.24	−0.15**
	Working $memory_z$				−0.49	0.15	−0.11**	−0.62	0.21	−0.14**
	Age_z × working $memory_z$							−0.32	0.15	−0.07*
	Gender × working $memory_z$							0.29	0.29	0.05
	R^2			0.04			0.05			0.05
	ΔR^2						0.01**			0.01

SE, Standard Error; β = standardized beta values.

$*p < 0.05$; $**p < 0.01$.

adults (20–27 years) and with depression in the adult group (28–35 years).

Negative associations between WM and PLEs have previously been reported for clinical (34–36) and non-clinical samples (37, 38), but relatively few studies have assessed these relations for multiple schizotypal dimensions and simultaneously accounted for their shared variance in the analyses. Two studies that did apply this approach found that reduced WM is associated with more positive symptoms, which was confirmed by the current study. Schmidt-Hansen and Honey (20) reported a strong association for three out of four WM parameters derived from an *n*-back task ($N = 289$). Likewise, Matheson and Langdon (21) reported a negative association for performance on a Letter-Number sequencing task ($N = 97$). However, both studies also found evidence for a link between WM and negative symptoms. This discrepancy with the current findings may partially be caused by differences in study sample, as both previous studies were conducted in student populations. Furthermore, all three studies used different WM assessments and symptom questionnaires, which restricts direct comparisons. Here, performance on two computerized WM tasks was averaged to create a global estimate of each individual's WM capacity. For future studies the use of multiple parameters delineating different aspects of WM function could provide further detail about specific contributions to the underlying associations with PLEs.

Several additional findings in this study require further emphasis. First, the presented data confirm the presence of underlying subtypes of CAPE positive and negative symptom dimensions, corroborating earlier findings in clinical (23) and non-clinical (17, 18, 24–26) study cohorts. This strengthens the idea that the classical schizophrenia dimensions do not represent homogenous entities and can be subdivided into meaningful symptom clusters. Second, associations with low WM capacity complement previous observations of increased distress and decreased global functioning for high intensity of bizarre experiences and persecutory ideas (17, 18). It also supports the notion that high frequencies of these types of positive symptoms may reflect an increased vulnerability for psychosis (27). Third, there were marked age differences in symptom frequency, which also affected the strength of associations with WM capacity. Perhaps most surprising was the absence of significant WM associations for adolescent participants. This suggests that although PLEs are more frequent in adolescents (39) they are not necessarily a marker of decreased cognitive capacity. Speculatively, for some adolescents low WM capacity may simply reflect delayed cognitive maturation instead of underlying psychopathology. Fourth, the finding that depressive symptoms were uniquely associated with WM capacity was somewhat unexpected, although these scores tend to correlate highly with bizarre experiences and persecutory ideas on the CAPE questionnaire (18, 23) and may therefore share some overlap in associated cognitive dispositions. However, the association with WM was strongest in adult individuals, which could suggest an age-related shift in the idiosyncratic nature of WM impairment as a vulnerability marker for different types of psychopathology. Although this finding awaits replication, it underlines the divergent validity of the CAPE depression scale, which can be used independently to explore unique relations with cognitive factors of interest in future studies.

The computerized WM tasks used for this study were originally designed to measure WM training improvements or "transfer effects" on non-trained tasks, based on previous findings (40, 41). Despite ongoing debate regarding the actual extent of transfer effects, there is overall agreement that WM training can enhance performance on more complex cognitive tasks in addition to improved WM capacity (42–45). This apparent display of cognitive plasticity is accompanied by underlying functional brain changes, for example in the (striatal) dopamine system (46–48), dysregulation of which is particularly associated with presence of positive symptoms (49). Furthermore, cognitive remediation strategies that target WM and other cognitive functions have proven successful with regard to cognitive and functional outcome in chronic schizophrenia (50, 51), and bear promise for individuals at-risk for psychosis (52). However, cognitive training can be costly, labor intensive, and its efficacy may vary across individuals. Therefore it would be advantageous to select more narrowly defined participant groups with an increased chance of clinical improvement. Based on the current study results it is tempting to speculate that individuals with high expression of specific positive and depressive symptoms can potentially accomplish the greatest clinical gain from WM training. However, in this study WM only explained a very small proportion of variance in CAPE scores (1%). As such, it is deemed unlikely that stand-alone WM training could directly influence the presence of PLEs for most individuals. Notwithstanding, it is possible that WM training can channel its efficacy in a more indirect manner, e.g., by creating more optimal neurocognitive properties to benefit from other types of treatment. Additional research on actual training interventions is needed to further address this issue.

The current study has multiple methodological strengths and limitations that merit additional commenting. By implementing a fully automated online assessment procedure it was possible to reach a large number of participants within a relatively short time period. Moreover, it allowed for recruitment of a study sample that is considered more or less representative of the general Swedish population between 12 and 35 years. Although the sample may not be completely devoid of any selection bias, it contains, for example, more regional and occupational diversity than community or student populations, which are typically used for this type of large-scale studies. In addition, it has been demonstrated that online assessment of CAPE symptoms is robust against symptom simulation (53) and by requiring individuals to answer each individual question in order to proceed, the problem of dealing with missing data was omitted. Regardless, the assessment could have benefited from adding several items to help detect any malingering participants. Furthermore, the monetary incentive (cinema voucher) may have encouraged participants to register more than once. Although extra precaution was taken to prevent this from happening and data were carefully screened for double entries, it could not be verified completely that all registered participants represented unique individuals. Future studies using a similar approach are advised to apply more rigorous personal identification methods (e.g., via social security number) and to refrain from using a monetary incentive, which would circumstantially further reduce the study costs as well. Finally, even though the online cognitive assessments had considerable logistic advantages over on-site assessments, they did not allow for a fully controlled study environment, which may have influenced the outcome. In general, the adopted online assessment strategy has multiple caveats, though more traditional assessment procedures are by no means less prone to measurement error or sample bias. Furthermore, there are substantial advantages of online recruitment and assessment procedures regarding data completion, project duration, and costs.

To sum up, the current study has provided further evidence for the presence of discernible subtypes of positive and negative PLEs in a large population sample of Swedish adolescents and young adults. There was an inverse relation of WM capacity with presence of positive symptom subtypes (bizarre experiences and persecutory ideas) as well as depressive symptoms, which was moderated by age. However, these relations should be interpreted in light of small effect sizes and marginal impact of WM capacity on symptom variability. Together these findings suggest that specific schizotypal traits may be indicative of reduced WM capacity in different age groups and potentially harbor a greater need for targeted intervention.

AUTHOR CONTRIBUTIONS

Tim B. Ziermans conceived the idea and methodology of this study, organized participant recruitment and data processing, conducted the statistical analyses, and wrote the final manuscript.

ACKNOWLEDGMENTS

The author would like to thank the following people for their respective contributions: Torkel Klingberg, Megan Spencer-Smith, Henrik Ullman, Elin Lidman, Elin Helander, Henrik Malmqvist, Annie Möller, Maria Kareliusson, and Pedro Ribeiro (Klingberg lab); Jonas Beckeman, Sissela Bergman-Nutley, Lars Blåsjö, Michael Smietana, and Stina Söderqvist (Cogmed, Pearson Assessment); Per-Tomas Brettell, Johan Hermansson, and Jonas Horn (Norstat); Ida Enqvist, Rebecca Ahlfeldt. Dr. Ziermans was supported by a COFAS Marie Curie Fellowship.

REFERENCES

1. Sawaguchi T, Goldman-Rakic PS. D1 dopamine receptors in prefrontal cortex: involvement in working memory. *Science* (1991) **251**(4996):947–50. doi:10.1126/science.1825731
2. Arnsten AF. Catecholamine modulation of prefrontal cortical cognitive function. *Trends Cogn Sci* (1998) **2**(11):436–47. doi:10.1016/S1364-6613(98)01240-6
3. Goldman-Rakic PS. Regional and cellular fractionation of working memory. *Proc Natl Acad Sci U S A* (1996) **93**(24):13473–80. doi:10.1073/pnas.93.24.13473
4. Goldman-Rakic PS. Working memory dysfunction in schizophrenia. *J Neuropsychiatry Clin Neurosci* (1994) **6**(4):348–57.
5. Arnsten AFT. The neurobiology of thought: the groundbreaking discoveries of Patricia Goldman-Rakic 1937–2003. *Cereb Cortex* (2013) **23**(10):2269–81. doi:10.1093/cercor/bht195
6. Forbes NF, Carrick LA, McIntosh AM, Lawrie SM. Working memory in schizophrenia: a meta-analysis. *Psychol Med* (2009) **39**(6):889–905. doi:10.1017/S0033291708004558
7. Bora E, Yucel M, Pantelis C. Cognitive impairment in schizophrenia and affective psychoses: implications for DSM-V criteria and beyond. *Schizophr Bull* (2010) **36**(1):36–42. doi:10.1093/schbul/sbp094
8. Fusar-Poli P, Deste G, Smieskova R, Barlati S, Yung AR, Howes O, et al. Cognitive functioning in prodromal psychosis: a meta-analysis. *Arch Gen Psychiatry* (2012) **69**(6):562–71. doi:10.1001/archgenpsychiatry.2011.1592
9. Fisher M, Loewy R, Hardy K, Schlosser D, Vinogradov S. Cognitive interventions targeting brain plasticity in the prodromal and early phases of schizophrenia. *Annu Rev Clin Psychol* (2013) **9**:435–63. doi:10.1146/annurev-clinpsy-032511-143134
10. Barlati S, De Peri L, Deste G, Fusar-Poli P, Vita A. Cognitive remediation in the early course of schizophrenia: a critical review. *Curr Pharm Des* (2012) **18**(4):534–41. doi:10.2174/138161212799316091
11. van Os J, Linscott RJ, Myin-Germeys I, Delespaul P, Krabbendam L. A systematic review and meta-analysis of the psychosis continuum: evidence for a psychosis proneness-persistence-impairment model of psychotic disorder. *Psychol Med* (2009) **39**(2):179–95. doi:10.1017/S0033291708003814
12. Meehl PE. Schizotaxia revisited. *Arch Gen Psychiatry* (1989) **46**(10):935–44. doi:10.1001/archpsyc.1989.01810100077015
13. Linscott RJ, van Os J. An updated and conservative systematic review and meta-analysis of epidemiological evidence on psychotic experiences in children and adults: on the pathway from proneness to persistence to dimensional expression across mental disorders. *Psychol Med* (2013) **43**(6):1133–49. doi:10.1017/S0033291712001626
14. Mossaheb N, Becker J, Schaefer MR, Klier CM, Schloegelhofer M, Papageorgiou K, et al. The Community Assessment of Psychic Experience (CAPE) questionnaire as a screening-instrument in the detection of individuals at ultra-high risk for psychosis. *Schizophr Res* (2012) **141**(2–3):210–4. doi:10.1016/j.schres.2012.08.008
15. Dominguez MD, Wichers M, Lieb R, Wittchen HU, van Os J. Evidence that onset of clinical psychosis is an outcome of progressively more persistent subclinical psychotic experiences: an 8-year cohort study. *Schizophr Bull* (2011) **37**(1):84–93. doi:10.1093/schbul/sbp022
16. Kaymaz N, Drukker M, Lieb R, Wittchen HU, Werbeloff N, Weiser M, et al. Do subthreshold psychotic experiences predict clinical outcomes in unselected non-help-seeking population-based samples? A systematic review and meta-analysis, enriched with new results. *Psychol Med* (2012) **42**(11):2239–53. doi:10.1017/S0033291711002911
17. Wigman JT, Vollebergh WA, Raaijmakers QA, Iedema J, van Dorsselaer S, Ormel J, et al. The structure of the extended psychosis phenotype in early adolescence – a cross-sample replication. *Schizophr Bull* (2011) **37**(4):850–60. doi:10.1093/schbul/sbp154
18. Armando M, Nelson B, Yung AR, Ross M, Birchwood M, Girardi P, et al. Psychotic-like experiences and correlation with distress and depressive symptoms in a community sample of adolescents and young adults. *Schizophr Res* (2010) **119**(1–3):258–65. doi:10.1016/j.schres.2010.03.001
19. Thaler NS, Goldstein G, Pettegrew JW, Luther JF, Reynolds CR, Allen DN. Developmental aspects of working and associative memory. *Arch Clin Neuropsychol* (2013) **28**(4):348–55. doi:10.1093/arclin/acs114
20. Schmidt-Hansen M, Honey RC. Working memory and multidimensional schizotypy: dissociable influences of the different dimensions. *Cogn Neuropsychol* (2009) **26**(7):655–70. doi:10.1080/02643291003644501
21. Matheson S, Langdon R. Schizotypal traits impact upon executive working memory and aspects of IQ. *Psychiatry Res* (2008) **159**(1–2):207–14. doi:10.1016/j.psychres.2007.04.006
22. Noguchi H, Hori H, Kunugi H. Schizotypal traits and cognitive function in healthy adults. *Psychiatry Res* (2008) **161**(2):162–9. doi:10.1016/j.psychres.2007.07.023
23. Yung AR, Buckby JA, Cotton SM, Cosgrave EM, Killackey EJ, Stanford C, et al. Psychotic-like experiences in nonpsychotic help-seekers: associations with distress, depression, and disability. *Schizophr Bull* (2006) **32**(2):352–9. doi:10.1093/schbul/sbj018
24. Barragan M, Laurens KR, Navarro JB, Obiols JE. Psychotic-like experiences and depressive symptoms in a community sample of adolescents. *Eur Psychiatry* (2011) **26**(6):396–401. doi:10.1016/j.eurpsy.2010.12.007
25. Yung AR, Nelson B, Baker K, Buckby JA, Baksheev G, Cosgrave EM. Psychotic-like experiences in a community sample of adolescents: implications for the continuum model of psychosis and prediction of schizophrenia. *Aust N Z J Psychiatry* (2009) **43**(2):118–28. doi:10.1080/00048670802607188
26. Armando M, Nelson B, Yung AR, Saba R, Monducci E, Dario C, et al. Psychotic experience subtypes, poor mental health status and help-seeking behaviour in a community sample of young adults. *Early Interv Psychiatry* (2012) **6**(3):300–8. doi:10.1111/j.1751-7893.2011.00303.x

27. Nelson B, Fusar-Poli P, Yung AR. Can we detect psychotic-like experiences in the general population? *Curr Pharm Des* (2012) **18**(4):376–85. doi:10.2174/138161212799316136
28. Stefanis NC, Hanssen M, Smirnis NK, Avramopoulos DA, Evdokimidis IK, Stefanis CN, et al. Evidence that three dimensions of psychosis have a distribution in the general population. *Psychol Med* (2002) **32**(2):347–58. doi:10.1017/S0033291701005141
29. Alloway TP. *Automated Working Memory Assessment Manual.* Oxford: Harcourt (2007).
30. Gathercole SE, Durling E, Evans M, Jeffcock S, Stone S. Working memory abilities and children's performance in laboratory analogues of classroom activities. *Appl Cogn Psychol* (2008) **22**(8):1019–37. doi:10.1002/acp.1407
31. O'Connor BP. SPSS and SAS programs for determining the number of components using parallel analysis and Velicer's MAP test. *Behav Res Methods Instrum Comput* (2000) **32**(3):396–402. doi:10.3758/BF03200807
32. Tabachnick BG, Fidell LS. *Using Multivariate Statistics.* Boston: Pearson Education, Limited (2007).
33. Hu L-t, Bentler PM. Cutoff criteria for fit indexes in covariance structure analysis: conventional criteria versus new alternatives. *Struct Equ Modeling* (1999) **6**(1):1–55. doi:10.1080/10705519909540118
34. Carter CS, Robertson LC, Nordahl TE, Chaderjian M, Kraft L, Oshoracelaya L. Spatial working-memory deficits and negative symptoms in schizophrenia. *Schizophr Res* (1995) **15**(1–2):111. doi:10.1016/0920-9964(95)95341-6
35. Gooding DC, Tallent KA. Nonverbal working memory deficits in schizophrenia patients: evidence of a supramodal executive processing deficit. *Schizophr Res* (2004) **68**(2–3):189–201. doi:10.1016/j.schres.2003.07.007
36. Perlstein WM, Carter CS, Noll DC, Cohen JD. Relation of prefrontal cortex dysfunction to working memory and symptoms in schizophrenia. *Am J Psychiatry* (2001) **158**(7):1105–13. doi:10.1176/appi.ajp.158.7.1105
37. Tallent KA, Gooding DC. Working memory and Wisconsin Card Sorting Test performance in schizotypic individuals: a replication and extension. *Psychiatry Res* (1999) **89**(3):161–70. doi:10.1016/S0165-1781(99)00101-8
38. Lenzenweger MF, Gold JM. Auditory working memory and verbal recall memory in schizotypy. *Schizophr Res* (2000) **42**(2):101–10. doi:10.1016/S0920-9964(99)00121-8
39. Rossler W, Riecher-Rossler A, Angst J, Murray R, Gamma A, Eich D, et al. Psychotic experiences in the general population: a twenty-year prospective community study. *Schizophr Res* (2007) **92**(1–3):1–14. doi:10.1016/j.schres.2007.01.002
40. Bergman Nutley S, Soderqvist S, Bryde S, Thorell LB, Humphreys K, Klingberg T. Gains in fluid intelligence after training non-verbal reasoning in 4-year-old children: a controlled, randomized study. *Dev Sci* (2011) **14**(3):591–601. doi:10.1111/j.1467-7687.2010.01022.x
41. Holmes J, Gathercole SE, Dunning DL. Adaptive training leads to sustained enhancement of poor working memory in children. *Dev Sci* (2009) **12**(4):F9–15. doi:10.1111/j.1467-7687.2009.00848.x
42. Morrison AB, Chein JM. Does working memory training work? The promise and challenges of enhancing cognition by training working memory. *Psychon Bull Rev* (2011) **18**(1):46–60. doi:10.3758/s13423-010-0034-0
43. Klingberg T. Training and plasticity of working memory. *Trends Cogn Sci* (2010) **14**(7):317–24. doi:10.1016/j.tics.2010.05.002
44. Jaeggi SM, Buschkuehl M, Shah P, Jonides J. The role of individual differences in cognitive training and transfer. *Mem Cognit* (2013). doi:10.3758/s13421-013-0364-z
45. Harrison TL, Shipstead Z, Hicks KL, Hambrick DZ, Redick TS, Engle RW. Working memory training may increase working memory capacity but not fluid intelligence. *Psychol Sci* (2013). doi:10.1177/0956797613492984
46. Báckman L, Nyberg L. Dopamine and training-related working-memory improvement. *Neurosci Biobehav Rev* (2013). doi:10.1016/j.neubiorev.2013.01.014
47. Backman L, Nyberg L, Soveri A, Johansson J, Andersson M, Dahlin E, et al. Effects of working-memory training on striatal dopamine release. *Science* (2011) **333**(6043):718. doi:10.1126/science.1204978
48. McNab F, Varrone A, Farde L, Jucaite A, Bystritsky P, Forssberg H, et al. Changes in cortical dopamine D1 receptor binding associated with cognitive training. *Science* (2009) **323**(5915):800–2. doi:10.1126/science.1166102
49. Keshavan MS, Tandon R, Boutros NN, Nasrallah HA. Schizophrenia, "just the facts": what we know in 2008 Part 3: neurobiology. *Schizophr Res* (2008) **106**(2–3):89–107. doi:10.1016/j.schres.2008.07.020
50. Wykes T, Huddy V, Cellard C, McGurk SR, Czobor P. A meta-analysis of cognitive remediation for schizophrenia: methodology and effect sizes. *Am J Psychiatry* (2011) **168**(5):472–85. doi:10.1176/appi.ajp.2010.10060855
51. McGurk SR, Twamley EW, Sitzer DI, McHugo GJ, Mueser KT. A meta-analysis of cognitive remediation in schizophrenia. *Am J Psychiatry* (2007) **164**(12):1791–802. doi:10.1176/appi.ajp.2007.07060906
52. Bechdolf A, Wagner M, Ruhrmann S, Harrigan S, Putzfeld V, Pukrop R, et al. Preventing progression to first-episode psychosis in early initial prodromal states. *Br J Psychiatry* (2012) **200**(1):22–9. doi:10.1192/bjp.bp.109.066357
53. Moritz S, Van Quaquebeke N, Lincoln TM, Kother U, Andreou C. Can we trust the internet to measure psychotic symptoms? *Schizophr Res Treatment* (2013) **2013**:457010. doi:10.1155/2013/457010

13

Mismatch Negativity: Translating the Potential

Juanita Todd[1,2,3,4]*, *Lauren Harms*[1,2,3,4], *Ulrich Schall*[2,3,4,5] *and Patricia T. Michie*[1,2,3,4]

[1] School of Psychology, University of Newcastle, Callaghan, NSW, Australia
[2] Priority Research Centre for Brain and Mental Health, University of Newcastle, Callaghan, NSW, Australia
[3] Schizophrenia Research Institute, Darlinghurst, NSW, Australia
[4] Hunter Medical Research Institute, Newcastle, NSW, Australia
[5] School of Medicine and Public Health, University of Newcastle, Callaghan, NSW, Australia

The mismatch negativity (MMN) component of the auditory event-related potential has become a valuable tool in cognitive neuroscience. Its reduced size in persons with schizophrenia is of unknown origin but theories proposed include links to problems in experience-dependent plasticity reliant on *N*-methyl-d-aspartate glutamate receptors. In this review we address the utility of this tool in revealing the nature and time course of problems in perceptual inference in this illness together with its potential for use in translational research testing animal models of schizophrenia-related phenotypes. Specifically, we review the reasons for interest in MMN in schizophrenia, issues pertaining to the measurement of MMN, its use as a vulnerability index for the development of schizophrenia, the pharmacological sensitivity of MMN and the progress in developing animal models of MMN. Within this process we highlight the challenges posed by knowledge gaps pertaining to the tool and the pharmacology of the underlying system.

Correspondence:
Juanita Todd, School of Psychology, University of Newcastle, University Drive, Callaghan, NSW 2308, Australia
e-mail: juanita.todd@newcastle.edu.au

Keywords: mismatch negativity, auditory event-related potential, schizophrenia, NMDA, synaptic plasticity, NMDAR

With more than 150 papers discussing or reporting smaller mismatch negativity (MMN) amplitude in schizophrenia, changes in this component of the auditory event-related potential (ERP) are now recognized as one of the most replicable electrophysiological abnormalities in this group. This review begins with an explanation of why this finding holds so much potential as a tool in the study of biological changes associated with the schizophrenia illness. However, the sections that follow expose the many challenges to the endeavor to translate this research – both in terms of understanding the meaning, relevance, and cause of smaller MMN amplitude and in terms of building animal models that can provide insight into etiology.

THE POTENTIAL – WHY IS THERE SO MUCH INTEREST IN MMN IN SCHIZOPHRENIA?

Auditory MMN is evident in scalp-recorded evoked potentials when an unexpected event or sound transition occurs in a regular repeating pattern (1). MMN is not a response to novelty *per se* but rather to how unlikely a particular sound transition is given a preceding sequence (2). It is therefore a very context-dependent evoked potential that only occurs when a pre-existing *prediction-model* exists specifying the most likely sound transitions in the present environment.

The nature of sound sequences used to elicit and study MMN range from very simple to highly complex. The vast majority of studies in schizophrenia employ the former in which a regular repeating identical sound occurs with high probability (the *standard*) and a physically deviant sound (the *deviant*) interrupts these repetitious trains on rare occasions (estimates suggest max $p \leq 0.30$) (3). Sequences of this kind, known as oddball sequences, promote the formation of a prediction-model specifying that acoustic input is best explained by standard-to-standard transitions and the rare occurrence of a standard-to-deviant transition is generally used to index MMN (although note that deviant-to-standard transitions also elicit a smaller MMN-like response). Regularities are implicitly learned as MMN does not require attention to sounds: sound sequences are usually presented via headphones to participants who are asked to ignore sounds and direct attention to an alternate task (3).

The classical derivation of MMN involves a deviant-minus-standard difference waveform with MMN quantified as the most negative peak evident between ~100 and 250 ms following the point of deviance (4). The quintessential finding in studies of this kind is that the averaged response to standard stimuli is similar in schizophrenia and matched control groups but the response to the deviant is significantly smaller resulting in smaller MMN in the difference waveform (5).

The major cortical sources contributing to scalp-recorded MMN are located bilaterally in primary and secondary auditory cortices with the precise locations dependent upon the sound characteristics (6). Intra-cortical recordings in primates suggest that the additional negativity in scalp-recorded response to deviations has its origin in lamina II/III of the auditory cortex (7). The neural mechanisms contributing to the difference in response to predicted versus deviating sound are the topic of considerable debate. There is general acceptance that processes such as neuronal adaptation make an important contribution; that is, the regular stimulation of the same afferent pathways will result in adaptation which reduces the response to sounds matching these properties, while in contrast deviating tones that are physically different will stimulate new afferent pathways (8–10). However, both sophisticated sequence designs and computational modeling support the existence of additional processes subserving prediction. Although some of these will be reviewed in more detail below (see The Measurement of MMN – Is there an Optimal Paradigm with Which to Study MMN in Schizophrenia?), extensive discussions can be found elsewhere (2, 3, 11–13). In summary, there is accumulating evidence that the altered responsiveness to sounds (reduced to expected and sensitized to deviant) cannot be explained by neuronal adaptation alone. Computational models suggest that predictions are expressed in the input from higher to lower levels within a hierarchical network (11, 12, 14). Changed response to sound therefore becomes a function of both neuronal adaptation and top-down inputs to auditory cortex (e.g., from secondary to primary cortex and from prefrontal to secondary cortex) that modify responsiveness to sound reflecting the predicted continuation of a learned pattern.

A network-level appreciation of MMN generation is valuable because it emphasizes that understanding the smaller MMN amplitude in schizophrenia could require consideration of both cause and consequence, acknowledging the functional role of the signal. According to free-energy conceptualizations of brain function, prediction-modeling (the use of regularity to extrapolate patterns) provides a regulatory service allowing the brain to conserve energy (15). Reduced response to the predicted causes of sensory stimulation, such as diminished response to standard input, reserves resources for events that contradict expectations and that may signal important changes in the environment prompting new learning. MMN signals a *prediction-error* indicating that the model presently influencing cortical response has failed to account for the current sensory event. The error communicates a need to adjust the current model to facilitate more accurate predictions, and simultaneously alerts the system to the possible importance of the eliciting event (15, 16). The error is communicated upward (via feed-forward connections) within a hierarchical network which enables future predictions to be weighted by error frequency (17). When a model is highly reinforced (low error frequency) predictions specified in top-down connections are weighted strongly and errors elicit large MMN. Conversely, when error frequency is higher the weighting on top-down predictions is reduced and MMN elicited by errors is smaller in amplitude. This concept has elsewhere been described as *predictive confidence* in a model which is of course inversely related to the probability of deviations (2). MMN amplitude therefore reflects quantification of confidence that the eliciting event violates a contextual regularity. Large MMN can trigger an orienting response with consequences for performance of concurrent tasks (18–23). These observations demonstrate the way in which a deviation from predictions can draw upon resources engaged in other activities.

In schizophrenia, MMN as a process appears to be largely intact in that it obeys similar principles to those evident in healthy comparison groups – MMN is larger for deviations that are rarer and/or more physically different from the current prediction-model (24). However, MMN amplitude reaches asymptote at a lower amplitude resulting in the most pronounced group differences generally being observed where MMN is very large in controls (25–27). Understanding the functional relevance of MMN amplitude is pivotal to understanding the potential impact of smaller MMN in schizophrenia. It has been proposed that MMN amplitude in part communicates the change in cortical responsiveness required to accommodate the new event into prediction-models (16). To the extent that this is true, the lower plateau in MMN amplitude in schizophrenia means that the adjustment to predictions prompted by larger or rare deviations may be equivalent to that for smaller or more frequent deviations. So if the size of the error-signal itself influences the adjustment in predictions, then equivalence of error signals across a range of deviant probabilities or physical differences (25–27) would perpetuate insensitivity to these different contexts.

This circular challenge becomes particularly relevant when considering how smaller MMN is related to biological changes associated with the illness, such as gray matter changes and involvement of the *N*-methyl-D-aspartate (NMDA) glutamate receptor (NMDAGluR) system. A key biological change observed in schizophrenia is loss of cortical gray matter volume (28–35). Within the auditory system this volume loss is due to a combination of reduced pyramidal somal cell size, reduced dendritic spine density, and (a correlated) reduction in axon terminal density in lamina III (36–39). Molecular-level studies in schizophrenia therefore place a core pathological process in the very same cortical layer implicated in the generation of MMN. The projected functional consequence of reduced volume in this cell layer is a net "diminished excitatory synaptic connectivity" consistent with an impact on the spread of activation [(36), p. 384]. The generation of MMN includes spreading activation across lamina III within A1 (Heschyl's gyrus or primary auditory cortex) but also importantly from A1 to STG [superior temporal gyrus or auditory association cortex (11, 17)]. So in terms of MMN generation, this pathology in auditory cortical regions is expected to lead to smaller MMN generated in response to error and/or a lower limit to MMN size [consistent with experimental observations reviewed (36, 38)]. This predicted consequence is also consistent with observations that in schizophrenia (but not in matched controls) limited MMN size correlates with reduced gray matter volume in auditory regions (35, 40) and in the only published longitudinal study, progressive loss of gray matter in auditory cortices correlated with progressive reduction in MMN (40).

The etiology of this auditory cortical pathology in schizophrenia is unclear but two hypotheses put forward include a developmental origin and/or failure in sustained support of structural integrity (36). The first supposes that there is an over-elimination of excitatory synapses in lamina III during development. Since this process is very protracted [continuing into the third decade in auditory cortices (41)], it maps well onto data showing progressive reductions in STG gray matter volume in schizophrenia over this period (42). However, experience-dependent plasticity modifies dendritic spine structure throughout life (through long term potentiation and depression) and this activity has a stabilizing effect on these structural elements. The same pathology could therefore also arise (uniquely or in conjunction with developmental over-pruning) through failure in the factors that should support structural integrity.

The second and not unrelated biological factor with relevance for smaller MMN in schizophrenia is the impairment in NMDAGluR system function proposed in glutamatergic models of schizophrenia which have become increasingly accepted as etiopathological models of schizophrenia. These models arose from observations that the drug phencyclidine (PCP) has (i) psychotomimetic effects and (ii) non-competitively blocks NMDAGluRs [for detailed reviews see Ref. (43–45)]. NMDAGluRs have a key role to play in experience-dependent synaptic plasticity, and in particular long term potentiation and depression. Importantly (as reviewed later in Section "How do Pharmacological Manipulations Alter the MMN Process?"), MMN is reduced in healthy individuals administered an NMDAGluR antagonist, such as ketamine. So the question that emerges is this: is smaller MMN in schizophrenia a consequence of gray matter reduction and/or NMDAGluR hypofunction in auditory cortex, or could the process of prediction-modeling in audition provide clues as to why structural integrity in this region is inadequately supported? In summary, the reasons to suppose that MMN can be used as tool to provide insights into schizophrenia-related brain changes are many and derive from both empirical and theoretical origins. In the following sections we review MMN research from several perspectives to identify some important challenges to realizing its potential in the study of biological processes linked to schizophrenia.

THE MEASUREMENT OF MMN – IS THERE AN OPTIMAL PARADIGM WITH WHICH TO STUDY MMN IN SCHIZOPHRENIA?

Smaller MMN in schizophrenia has been observed over a number of different experimental paradigms so the underlying reasons for MMN-reduction are likely to reflect the common demands inherent in processing the various sound sequence types. Different paradigms each have advantages and disadvantages (reviewed below) and it is the authors' opinion that there is no ideal paradigm. In fact, to nominate an ideal could be detrimental to the field – the advantage in doing so (increased comparability between studies) is outweighed by the disadvantage which is neglect of the opportunities to use this tool to address specific questions about the integrity of the underlying system.

CONSIDERATIONS IN MEASURING A DIFFERENCE WAVEFORM

There are at least three contributing factors to MMN obtained in the classical deviant-minus-standard waveform: (i) differences in physical attributes of the deviant and standard sounds (this is particularly likely when the deviant contains physical features that vary in acoustic energy such duration or intensity), (ii) differences in refractoriness (or more properly called adaptation) of the neural generators of responses to the more frequently presented standard versus rare deviant stimulus and (iii) a genuine deviance-detection process or the *true MMN* resulting from the deviant violating predictions derived from contextual regularities. This means that a group difference in classically derived MMN could arise from any one or a combination of these factors. A number of experimental control protocols have been developed to refine a measure of *true MMN* – the primary motivation for these studies being to determine whether a true MMN exists or whether what is measured as MMN could be accounted for entirely by adaptation effects on other components of the ERP. In a series of papers, Schröger and his colleagues devised a random control stimulus sequence, the *many-standards* sequence. For example in the case of a frequency deviant, a many-standards control would involve random presentations of tones of different frequencies (including tones with the frequencies of the deviant and standard tone) each having the same probability as the deviant in the oddball sequence [Frequency/pitch: (46–48); Duration: (49); Location: (50)]. A comparison of responses to the deviant from an oddball sequence and to the same sound in a many-standards sequence controls for physical differences and adaptation contributions to the classically derived MMN. In this way the resultant difference waveform can be attributed to a novel event violating a *stored neural representation* of regularity in recent stimulation. This is because the random presentation order of the many-standards sequence *prevents the development of a representation of regularity in recent stimulation* but preserves the rate of occurrence and therefore some level of equivalence in terms of adaptation effects.

To our knowledge there are no studies that have implemented conservative control procedures to extract true MMN in schizophrenia. As noted above, the vast majority of the published literature in schizophrenia has employed MMN derived using the classical oddball derivation. The common finding of similar responses to standards in schizophrenia and matched control groups is reassuring in that it suggests that adaptation effects on the standard response at least are not detectably impaired in patients and implies that the major group differences are in how the brain responds to deviations. However whether there are group differences in the extent of cross adaptation to other frequencies (or durations/intensities, etc., in the case of simple deviance paradigms) is unknown and this could impact on the response to a physically different deviant tone. It is also reassuring to note that in healthy individuals, even when stringent controls such as the many-standards control are implemented, the classical derivation gives a reasonable approximation of the true MMN (49). But once again – whether this is equally true in patients is unknown. Below we review some of the literature employing non-classical MMN derivations indicating that there may indeed be some group differences in response to repetitive sound as well as the response to deviations.

EXAMPLES OF PARADIGMS USED IN SCHIZOPHRENIA

A few patient studies have employed methods that can differentiate components of the MMN process and these have yielded mixed findings. Some have controlled for the physical differences between standard and deviants sounds, either by presenting two oddball sequences with the roles of deviant and standard sounds reversed [a flip-flop design: (51, 52)] or by presenting a sequence consisting of repeated presentations of deviant sounds only (53), referred to as a deviant-as-standard sequence. In both instances, it is possible to derive difference waveforms from comparing responses to the *same sound* as a repetitive standard and a deviant event. While these studies report no group difference in response to the repetitive oddball standard presentations, Todd et al. (54) recently found evidence of clear group differences in the morphology of ERPs to the repetitious presentation of deviants and these differences had a significant impact on computation of the MMN. The group difference appeared in a negative component of the ERP to repetitive sounds occurring ~200–300 ms post-stimulus. While its origin and functional role are unknown, it suggests that such differences in cortical response to a repetitive sound more generally warrant further investigation. However, neither the flip-flop control nor the deviant-as-standard sequence removes the contribution of adaptation effects to the difference waveform. Nor does it ensure that the computed MMN represents true deviance detection of a violation of contextual regularity. That is, these procedures do not allow the extraction of the *true MMN.*

The roving paradigm is another method that can partially address group differences in various contributions to MMN. In a typical roving paradigm a string of sounds of the same pitch are eventually interrupted by a sound with a higher or lower pitch which then continues to repeat. Predictive processing is highly dynamic so within two to three repetitions, the new sound becomes a standard and deviations from its properties will now elicit MMN (55–57). In the roving paradigm, it is possible to study the way the response to a new standard changes after incremental repetitions (e.g., 6 vs. 12 vs. 24, etc.). An increasing positivity as a function of repetition length, termed "repetition positivity," is apparent in the ERP to standards approximately 50–200 ms post-stimulus. The increase in MMN amplitude with the length of repetition is referred to as a memory trace effect and is a function of both this apparent increased positivity (which is in fact a decrease in negativity) to the standard and increased negativity to a subsequent deviant [although see Ref. (58)]. In schizophrenia, the increment in both components is smaller than that in controls (59), but more notably in this study, the positivity in response to standard repetitions failed to increment at all. So in this paradigm smaller MMN in schizophrenia appears to indicate less change in responsiveness to sound generally.

In a recent magnetoencephalographic (MEG) study in schizophrenia (60), the MMN_m data in a similar roving paradigm was explored using a technique called dynamic causal modeling (DCM). DCM differs from conventional source modeling and brain connectivity methods by utilizing a biologically informed causal model placing constraints on model inversion such that the parameters of reconstruction describe specific processes like change in synaptic coupling strength between source locations and postsynaptic gain. Rather than estimating dipole activity at a particular point in time; it models dipole activity over a period of time to identify parameters that change (11). When applied to the roving paradigm, DCM has provided evidence supporting the conceptualization of MMN as an active contextual perceptual inference process. The "best fit" to experimental data is achieved by a model that incorporates both local intrinsic adaptation effects as well as plastic changes in extrinsic inputs to auditory cortex (i.e., from STG to A1 and also from areas of the prefrontal cortex to STG). When applied to schizophrenia data, DCM has provided evidence for problems in two of three components: the largest effect size for group differences was for reduced change in intrinsic connections within primary auditory cortex A1. Such changes are considered evidence of impaired feature specific adaptation. There was also a reversed polarity in changes to connectivity between prefrontal and auditory areas which was interpreted as a failure in the normal influence of these top-down inputs in modifying auditory cortical response. The authors also comment on reduced modulation of the forward connection from the A1 to the STG (but this was not significant according to **Table 2**, p. 26). Although this is the first study of its kind in schizophrenia, the results conform to the view that impaired signaling of error (smaller MMN) could be indicative of impairment in encoding the contextual memory against which deviance is registered (potentially including impaired adaptation), but also consequently impaired ongoing modification of cortical responsiveness by feedback projections. It is therefore possible that the roving standard paradigm is more sensitive to any problems in forming a contextual memory based on tone repetitions. However, when interpreting results it is important to consider the assumptions of the roving paradigm carefully before drawing this conclusion. The MMN elicited to a change in frequency in a roving paradigm signals that the current prediction-model failed to account for the present stimulus properties and the model may require updating. With repetition of the new frequency, an updated prediction-model is built. The degree to which the model requires updating will be a function of the difference between the representation of the new and former standard frequencies. Given that the changes in frequency can be quite subtle and that frequency discrimination is impaired in schizophrenia (53, 61, 62), it is possible that less evidence of updating after a new standard (repetition positivity) could in part reflect less distinct representations of the new and former frequency. So the roving paradigm places considerable weight on stimulus-specific adaptation to a new frequency, which therefore may augment the importance of intrinsic adaptation in A1. Whether DCM of a classic oddball paradigm would replicate major group differences in intrinsic A1 connections remains to be determined.

At present the literature certainly suggests that altered (smaller) response to sequence deviations is a major contributor to smaller MMN in schizophrenia. It is clear that the reduction in classical MMN is not only robust across many different cohorts, laboratories, ethnic groups, etc. (5), but also exhibits substantial stability over time (63). However there is reason to suppose that there may also be differences in responding to repetitive sound more generally that could be contributing to problems in prediction-modeling and/or MMN computation. Novel paradigms and novel data processing approaches are likely to provide valuable data with which to address these contributions. Despite these differences it should be noted that many elements of the predictive process underlying MMN remain intact in schizophrenia. In addition to those covered above we recently demonstrated that persons with schizophrenia, despite producing smaller MMN amplitude to deviants, are equally able to *reduce* MMN size to a deviant if the occurrence of that deviant could be inferred from the identity of the prior tone. The equivalent use of this predictive information in both schizophrenia and control group reinforces the position that abnormalities in the MMN process in schizophrenia primarily involve limited gain in the differential response to a very rare versus common event. So while the choice of paradigm used to study MMN in schizophrenia will depend not only on the questions driving your research but also the time you have available, the one principal recommendation that we do put forward is to ensure that you adopt a very rare deviant event (<15%) to maximize your power to expose group differences.

DOES MMN-REDUCTION INDICATE VULNERABILITY TO SCHIZOPHRENIA?

In this section we review studies addressing whether small MMN may be a vulnerability index for schizophrenia. It should be noted that research into schizophrenia has always been limited by its diagnostic heterogeneity and phenomenological overlap with related developmental, affective, or personality disorders which all can share some of the clinical features of schizophrenia, such as psychosis, cognitive impairment, or therapeutic response to certain classes of pharmacological agents (64). Not surprisingly, attempts to find a diagnostic marker for schizophrenia – that not only represents an *endophenotype* of the disorder but can also serve as a tool helping to unveil its pathology – continues to be limited by the lack of a pathogenomic definition of the condition. Diagnostic limitations notwithstanding, a number of groups have indeed investigated MMN's status as an endophenotype for schizophrenia as defined by current diagnostics tools and this research is pertinent to evaluating the translational potential of MMN in schizophrenia. The definition upon which the evaluation is based is that proposed by Gottesman and Gould (65) where an endophenotype is defined as an intermediate phenotype along the pathway between genotype and the observable established aspects of the illness. Specific criteria to be met include: (i) it is associated with illness in the population; (ii) it is heritable; (iii) it is primarily state-independent (manifests in an individual whether or not illness is active); (iv) within families, small MMN and the illness co-segregate; and (v) smaller MMN is evident in non-affected family members at a higher rate than in the general population (65).

CRITERION (I) AND (II)

Mismatch negativity amplitude reduction in schizophrenia is a very robust finding with an effect size of 0.99 observed by Umbricht and Krljes (5) in their meta-analysis of 32 studies published prior to 2004. Reduced MMN is less prevalent in related conditions, such as bipolar affective disorder independent of the presence of psychotic symptoms (52, 66–68) and in major depression (66) but see (69–71). That is, there is considerable evidence that criterion (i) is met in terms of its association with the illness, although its specificity to schizophrenia is less clear than initially thought. MMN appears to be heritable based on twin studies with heritability estimates ranging from 0.48 to 0.68 when using a duration increment deviant (67, 72) but not for a frequency deviant (73). However, even duration MMN shows only weak phenotypic association (0.39) with schizophrenia (67). Nonetheless, there is preliminary evidence supporting criterion (ii) for endophenotypic status of MMN.

CRITERION (III)

Across the large number of studies on MMN in schizophrenia there are no consistent relationships between MMN size and the severity of symptoms of psychosis. Although impaired prediction-error signaling is implicated in the genesis of delusions (74) and although there is preliminary but consistent evidence from one group of a relationship with auditory hallucinations (75–77), the literature fails to demonstrate consistent relationships across studies. The meta-analysis by Umbricht and Krljes (5) emphasized that the majority of studies did not find correlations (either with positive or negative symptoms) and observed no change in MMN when symptoms improved. Further (63), found duration MMN in very large sample of patients ($N = 163$) exhibited substantial stability across a 1 year retest interval, and to be independent of fluctuations in clinical symptoms, positive or negative. So at face-value, these results from cross-sectional designs seem to support state-independence of presence of smaller MMN [criterion (iii)]. However, the evidence about state-independence of degree to which MMN is reduced in patients in an acute phase vs. a post-acute phase is mixed (78, 79) although differences due to medication changes cannot be eliminated (see later Section "How do Pharmacological Manipulations Alter the MMN Process?" for further discussion of state vs. trait effects on MMN as a vulnerability marker).

The failure to demonstrate state-dependence is paralleled by more consistent relationships between MMN amplitude and relatively stable features of the illness such as level of functioning (80) and cognitive impairments (81) despite substantial changes in negative and positive symptom severity. Various measures of current functioning have been shown to be associated with MMN amplitude in patients: global assessment of function [GAF: (82–84)], social and occupational functioning assessment scale [SOFAS; (35) but not in first episode patients (85)], the independent living scales [ILS: (86)], and work functioning and independent living ratings from the role functioning scale (87). It has been suggested that the relationship between reduced MMN and impaired functioning might be mediated by anatomical changes such as gray matter loss in relevant brain regions (35). Impaired cognition (whether independent of gray matter declines or consequential) could also mediate the relationship between MMN and functional status since there is a wealth of evidence now that the strongest predictor of functional outcomes in patients is cognition [also often called neurocognition: (88)]. However, the number of published MMN studies in schizophrenia that examine not only cognition in the same sample but correlations between MMN and cognitive performance as well, is quite limited. This is despite reasonable expectations that the reliance of MMN generation on the the NMDAGluR system (see How do Pharmacological Manipulations Alter the MMN Process? and Translation to Animal Models below for further discussion) should lead to relationships with those aspects of cognition that are also reliant on the unique characteristics of the NMDAGluR, such as context-dependent effects, integration of information over time and new learning (44). However, there are some data that suggest such relationships do exist at least in patients (but not necessarily in healthy controls).

NMDAGluRs have a number of unique features. Firstly, activation of NMDAGluRs currents is conditional in that channels only gate following presynaptic release of glutamate and concurrent postsynaptic membrane depolarization which relieves Mg^{2+} blockade. This conditional characteristic of the NMDAGluR is likely to be particularly important where responses are determined by context, as is the case for MMN, but also in situations where flexibility of response is required dependent on context. One specific example of contextual processing is the AX version of the continuous performance (AX-CPT) task where a response to the letter X on screen should only executed when the X is preceded by the letter A. It is well established that patients are impaired on the AX-CPT task, producing often fewer correct responses to AX sequences (impaired priming of response by a target-consistent cue) and higher rates of false alarms to BX sequences [impaired inhibition of a response prompted by a target-inconsistent cue (89)]. However, despite reports of concurrent smaller MMN and AX-CPT impairments, there appear to be no reports of a correlation between the two (90) and one explicit report of no association between the two (54).

Secondly, although NMDGluRs exhibit complex kinetics with evidence of multiple gating modes characterized by different mean open times (91–93), it is generally accepted that they mediate long duration excitatory postsynaptic currents in the brain and participate in synaptic integration and certain forms of synaptic plasticity (92). Prefrontal cortex NMDAGluRs in particular have slower kinetics than sensory regions (94) and therefore are potentially involved in maintaining activity in prefrontal neurons (95), for example during the delay periods of working memory tasks. There are reports of co-occurrence of working memory deficits and reduced MMN in patients with schizophrenia (63, 90) but to our knowledge, only one report of a correlation between working memory (measured using the digit sequencing task from the Japanese version of the brief assessment of cognition) and (duration) MMN in patients (96). Both classic oddball MMN amplitude (97) and longer term effects on growth in MMN amplitude (98) have been shown to correlate with digit span (the ability to maintain and or manipulate acoustic presentation of digits) in a healthy control group consistent with the requirement to store auditory information over time for both indices.

Thirdly, NMDAGluR activation leads to a cascade of events that initiate long term potentiation and depression, the primary processes responsible for new memory formation and learning in hippocampus and cortex. Retention or storage of information is less reliant on NMDAGluR. One of the most robust cognitive deficits exhibited by patients are deficits in memory (verbal declarative memory in particular) with the majority of evidence suggesting that the largest deficit, as measured by effect size, occurs for encoding or new learning of material in comparison to retention [although there is still a small deficit in retention even when initial learning differences are taken into account (99)]. Four studies report relationships between MMN and memory performance but in patients only. Baldeweg et al. (59) using a roving oddball paradigm found that the MMN trace effect (the increase in MMN that occurs with increasing repetition of prior standards) correlated with performance on an everyday memory test (Rivermead behavioral memory test). Kawakubo et al. (100) in a study that reports data on patients only found that MMN elicited by a phoneme duration deviant (but not a tone duration deviant) was correlated with immediate free recall (initial learning or encoding measure) from a list learning task, the Rey auditor verbal learning task (RAVLT). In contrast, Kaur et al. (101) found that tone duration MMN correlated with verbal memory assessed using the RAVLT in first episode psychosis patients with a schizophrenia spectrum diagnosis of either schizophrenia, schizoaffective, and schizophreniform illness. No correlations were reported for controls. Kiang et al. (84) in a standard oddball paradigm found duration MMN was correlated in patients only with short-delay as well as long delay free recall but not (significantly) with immediate free recall on another list learning task, the California verbal learning task, but neither of the free recall measures was adjusted for initial or prior learning differences. So while there is evidence of MMN correlations with memory, these correlations may not be restricted to initial learning or encoding phase.

In addition, there is evidence of relationships between MMN amplitude and other cognitive domains that are commonly shown to be impaired in patients but are less clearly dependent on NMDAGluR properties, such as executive functions [anti-saccade performance: (102); proverb interpretation: (84); perseverative errors on the Wisconsin Card Sorting Task: (103); mental control subtest of WMS-III: (85)].

In summary – MMN does not appear to be consistently related to the severity of either positive or negative symptoms experienced by the patient at the time of recording (either examined across patients or assessed within patients at different time points), consistent with (symptom) state-independence of MMN. However, MMN amplitude does appear to vary across individuals as a function of more stable features of their illness. The relationship of MMN to functional measures is relatively robust and there is growing evidence of correlations not only between MMN amplitude and those aspects of cognition that are likely to be reliant on unique aspects of NMDAGluR but other domains of cognition that are reliably impaired in patients such as executive functions. However, these are issues that deserve more attention and in particular, more systematic investigations are required before any strong assertions can be made about contributions from a common mechanism of NMDAGluR-dysfunction to MMN-reduction and cognitive deficits in schizophrenia.

CRITERION (IV) AND (V)

Mismatch negativity has also been investigated as a potential predictor of developing psychosis or schizophrenia in populations considered at-risk mental state (ARMS). For instance, the comprehensive assessment of at-risk mental state (CAARMS) criteria (104) defines ARMS as (1) a significant drop of global functioning over a period of 12 months and having a close biological relative with a psychotic disorder and/or (2) experiencing attenuated or very brief episodes of psychotic symptoms in combination with functional decline. MMN has been investigated in both groups; however, to date there appear to have been no MMN longitudinal studies of transition to psychosis specifically within a clinically unaffected genetic group.

Whether MMN is reduced in unaffected first-degree biological relatives of patients with schizophrenia is controversial. The initial studies by Jessen et al. (105)[1] and Michie et al. (106) reported reduced oddball frequency and duration MMN respectively in first-degree relatives when compared to healthy controls, but these results with one exception were not replicated in later publications, neither for duration deviants – (72, 107–109) and (102), [based on a larger sample from the same source as (106)], nor frequency deviants – (73, 108, 109). The one exception is (110) which interestingly used an identical MMN duration deviant paradigm as (106). While there are design and other methodological

[1] A somewhat puzzling result in the Jessen et al. study, is that patient MMN amplitude was not significantly reduced in contrast to relatives.

differences between those studies (three in total) that show significant MMN-reductions in first-degree relatives and those that do not (six in total), the bulk of the evidence suggests that at-risk but clinically unaffected family members do not exhibit reduced MMN (minimal support for criterion (iv) and (v) of endophenotype criteria).

The evidence that MMN is reduced in the ARMS group, is more consistent, although data on whether reduced MMN predicts transition to psychosis is still preliminary. It is important to note that while the term *prodromal* is sometimes used to describe those clinically defined at-risk groups (111), strictly speaking whether they are prodromal or not at the time of assessment can only be determined subsequently by whether they develop a schizophrenia spectrum disorder within the follow-up period (usually 12–24 months). All of the MMN investigations in ARMS have used duration deviants, either a duration increment (112–117), or a duration decrement (111, 118) or both (112) but some also report data on frequency deviants in the same sample (111, 116–118) or a double deviant [deviant on both frequency and duration (117)]. Of these eight papers, five found that duration increment MMN was significantly reduced in the ARMS group (112–114, 116, 117) whereas duration decrement MMN was either not significant (111, 118) or showed a smaller effect size (112). The findings for frequency MMN are mixed: (117) found that frequency MMN was reduced (as was the double deviant) but (116) did not. To date therefore, the evidence seems to suggest that deviants that differ from standards by being longer in duration are more sensitive to the at-risk mental state that other deviant types. It seems unlikely that these findings are due to the effects of medication since in each sample the numbers of ARMS individuals who were medicated with anti-psychotics at the time of testing was small as were the dosages.

Most investigations of clinical high risk groups also report transition data and examine whether MMN predicts those who will subsequently develop a schizophrenia disorder – although in two cases, the number of transitions was too small for statistical analysis (112, 113). Bodatsch et al. (118) were the first to report transition data. Interestingly they found that duration (decrement) MMN predicted those who converted to schizophrenia within a 24 month period of the assessment date whereas frequency MMN did not. Higuchi et al. (115) and Shaikh et al. (114) observed similar results for duration (increment) MMN. Neither included a frequency MMN deviant. However (117), found that the best predictor of later transition to schizophrenia was MMN to their double deviant. Neither duration alone nor frequency alone was significant. Perhaps importantly, the double deviant elicited the largest MMN (larger than that to frequency or duration alone) which perhaps reflects the importance of challenging the upper limits on MMN size in at-risk groups as well as patients with an established illness. In summary, evidence for smaller MMN within families in general is not strong but the evidence for smaller MMN in clinical high risk groups is quite compelling. Therefore endophenotype criterion (iv) and (v) are only partially met at best. It remains to be seen whether the reduction in the at-risk groupings is really about risk status *per se* or a reflection of schizophrenia-related pathology that has begun to impact on brain function.

HOW DO PHARMACOLOGICAL MANIPULATIONS ALTER THE MMN PROCESS?

Pharmacology as a field of research offers a unique avenue to study MMN both in terms of how different chemicals can perturb the perceptual inference process and how they may relate to schizophrenia pathology. When considering the pharmacological sensitivity of MMN, it is clear that a change in MMN could reflect an effect on any one of a number of constituent processes described in Section "The Measurement of MMN – Is there an Optimal Paradigm with Which to Study MMN in Schizophrenia?" Surprisingly few studies provide details on how a substance affected response to standard repetitious sounds with the majority reporting on the difference waveforms only (16/27 studies, see **Tables 1–3**). For the purpose of this review we have restricted Tables to acute drug effects on healthy adult populations. One of the key foci in pharmacological research on MMN is how it is affected by alterations to NMDAGluR activity (**Table 1**).

Several groups have argued that impaired plasticity linked to NMDAGluRs is a core feature of the schizophrenia illness (45, 128, 129). The first study to demonstrate this link was actually in the macaque where Javitt and colleagues demonstrated a dose-dependent reduction in MMN following local infusion of the NMDAgluR antagonist, PCP (130). Using a flip-flop control design (see The Measurement of MMN – Is there an Optimal Paradigm with Which to Study MMN in Schizophrenia? above for description and Translation to Animal Models below for additional detail) the authors report no significant effect of phencyclidine on response to the repetitive sound (at least in these local field potentials, see Translation to Animal Models for further discussion) but a pronounced dose-dependent effect on the response to the deviant. The authors conclude that NMDAGluR activity is critical to forming the associative links between stimuli (i.e., accumulating information about transition statistics) that define the context against which a rare deviant sound is recognized as an aberrant event. Studies in humans are largely consistent with this initial study. Of eight published studies, seven report significant dose-dependent reduction of MMN amplitude after ketamine [although one only in combination with the CB1 inverse agonist rimonabant (125)]. The one exception (a low-dose study) used a selective attention paradigm in which participants were asked to attend and respond to stimuli in one ear while simultaneously hearing stimuli in the other ear (unattended) from which MMN was derived (119). Of the studies showing an effect of ketamine on MMN, four explicitly picture and/or discuss response to the repetitive standard tones with only one (120) reporting a slight but significant increase in the obligatory N1 component to repetitive sounds in the presence of the drug. The low-dose ketamine study by Oranje and colleagues also show enhanced N1. The most recent study reports on a roving standard paradigm demonstrating that, although MMN was reduced under ketamine overall, the effect of ketamine was more pronounced with increased repetition of the standard [i.e., when predictive confidence was highest (126)]. The paper, however, did not report on whether this pattern was due to effects on the positivity to repetitive standards or increased negativity to deviants or both. The grand-averaged (i.e., across repetitions) ERP to standards is presented in a subsequent paper reporting a DCM analysis of the same data (14). A visual

Table 1 | *N*-methyl-d-aspartate receptor studies.

Reference	Study design	Main findings	Comments
Oranje et al. (119)	Double-blind, placebo-controlled randomized ketamine challenge (0.3 mg/kg) in 18 healthy male volunteers	Processing negativity (PN) and P3 amplitude reduced and N1 amplitude increased with ketamine; no effects observed on MMN (frequency deviants)	Ketamine did not affect error rate and reaction time in selective attention task; dose lower than in studies showing an effect on MMN; study reported ERPs in response to standard stimuli
Umbricht et al. (120)	Single-blind placebo-controlled ketamine challenge (0.9 mg/kg/h) in 20 healthy volunteers whilst performing a continuous performance task	N1 peak amplitude increase with ketamine; MMN (i.e., frequency and duration deviants) amplitude reduction with ketamine; MMN (i.e., duration deviants) peak amplitude latency increase with ketamine	MMN topography was not altered by ketamine; study did not report ERPs in response to standard stimuli
Kreitschmann-Andermahr et al. (121)	On-off ketamine (0.3 mg/kg) single-session MEG trial in 13 healthy volunteers (final sample size $N = 10$ with sufficient data quality)	Ketamine affected MMF latency and dipole moment due to effects on deviants (frequency, duration, and intensity); no effect on N1	Ketamine reduced mean global field power for MMF; study reported ERPs in response to standard stimuli
Umbricht et al. (122)	Single-blind, placebo-controlled psilocybin challenge (0.28 mg/kg) over two sessions; ERP recorded 70 min after drug administration in 18 healthy volunteers	N1 peak amplitude reduction with psilocybin; no effect on P2	Non-significant trend toward smaller MMN amplitudes for frequency deviants with psilocybin; study did not report ERPs in response to standard stimuli
Korostenskaja et al. (123)	Randomized, double-blind, placebo-controlled crossover challenge of memantine (30 mg) in 13 healthy volunteers	Trend of MMN amplitude increase in response to frequency deviants with memantine	No effect on MEG derived measures of MMN, P1 and N1; study did not report ERPs in response to standard stimuli
Heekeren et al. (124)	Randomized, double-blind, crossover ketamine of 0.007–0.2 mg/kg and dimethyltryptamine of 0.011–0.3 mg/kg challenges, with same-day (after 2 h break) single-blind low and a high-dose drug administration, respectively, in 15 healthy volunteers (9 study participants completed both drug challenges)	Reduced MMN amplitude with ketamine; no effect with dimethyltryptamine	Subjects performed a continuous performance task was performed whilst EEG was recorded; study reported ERPs in response to standard stimuli
Roser et al. (125)	Randomized, double-blind, placebo-controlled, crossover ketamine (0.5 mg/kg/h following bolus of 0.24 mg/kg) and rimonambant (20 mg) challenge in 24 healthy male volunteers	No effect of ketamine alone on MMN amplitudes (i.e., frequency and duration deviants); addition of rimonambant resulted in MMN amplitude reduction	Ketamine dose lower than in studies showing an effect on MMN; study did not report ERPs in response to standard stimuli
Schmidt et al. (126)	Double-blind, placebo-controlled ketamine challenge (0.006 mg/kg/min following bolus of 10 mg) in 19 healthy volunteers and psilocybin challenge of 0.115 mg/kg in 20 healthy volunteers	Reduced frontal MMN with ketamine with increasing number of standards (roving paradigm); no effect on MMN with psilocybin	Placebo MMN amplitudes correlated with severity of cognitive impairment induced by ketamine; study did not report ERPs in response to standard stimuli
Gunduz-Bruce et al. (127)	Double-blind, placebo-controlled ketamine challenge (a bolus of 0.23 mg/kg over 1 min followed by 0.58 mg/kg for 30 min and then 0.29 mg/kg for 40 min) with and without *N*-acetylcystein co-administration (oral doses of 2000 mg followed by 1000 mg 2 h later) in 16 healthy volunteers	MMN amplitude reduced for intensity and frequency deviants but not duration deviants; *N*-acetylcystein did not alter the impact of ketamine on MMN	MMN recorded with multi-deviant paradigm; study did not report ERPs in response to standard stimuli
Schmidt et al. (14)	Double-blind, placebo-controlled ketamine challenge (0.006 mg/kg/min following bolus of 10 mg) in 19 healthy volunteers (17 subjects entered the final dynamic causal modeling analysis)	Ketamine selectively reduced synaptic plasticity in the forward connection from the left primary auditory cortex (A1) to the left superior temporal gyrus along with MMN amplitude reduction	Ketamine effects on synaptic plasticity correlated significantly with ratings of ketamine-induced cognitive impairments; study reported ERPs in response to standard stimuli

Table 2 | Nicotine receptor studies.

Reference	Study design	Main findings	Comments
Harkrider and Hedrick (137)	Single-blind placebo-controlled nicotine challenge in 10 smokers (21 mg/day) and 4 non-smokers (7 mg/day)	Larger MMN area and steeper slope in response to deviant stimuli	Small and heterogeneous sample; study reported ERPs in response to standard stimuli
Inami et al. (142)	Counterbalanced placebo versus nicotine administration (equivalent to 16.1 ± 2.7 mg/day) 10 healthy non-smokers (5 males)	Nicotine shortened MMN peak latency	Small sample size; study reported ERPs in response to standard stimuli
Baldeweg et al. (138)	Randomized placebo-controlled nicotine challenge (2 mg) in 20 healthy smokers	Nicotine increased MMN amplitude mainly by affecting response to standard stimuli (no change in response to deviant stimuli)	Nicotine enhanced repetition positivity; study reported ERPs in response to standard stimuli
Knott et al. (143)	Nicotine challenge (6 mg single dose) in 14 healthy non-smokers	No effect on MMN (frequency deviants)	Study did not report ERPs in response to standard stimuli
Dunbar et al. (139)	Randomized and placebo-controlled challenge with oral nicotine agonist AZD3480 (ascending doses from 2 to 320 mg) in 48 healthy subject and in 24 subject receiving repeatedly constant oral dose or placebo	Increased MMN amplitude with reduced latency after 10 days of consecutive agonist administration and/or single dose of 200 mg	Study did not report ERPs in response to standard stimuli
Martin et al. (141)	Single-blind, placebo-controlled nicotine challenge (4 mg) in 11 non-smokers and 9 smokers (following 2 h nicotine abstinence)	Increased MMN amplitude in response to nicotine without affecting N1 and ERPs in response to standard stimuli	Study reported ERPs in response to standard stimuli
Knott et al. (140)	Randomized double-blind, placebo-controlled crossover nicotine challenge (6 mg) in 21 non-smokers (11 males)	Drug by gender interaction of non-significant MMN amplitude increase in females and non-significant MMN amplitude decrease in males	Study reported ERPs in response to standard stimuli

comparison of Figure 1 (placebo) and Figure 2 (ketamine) from the paper suggests that the effect of ketamine on MMN was perhaps a combination of reduced positivity in the standard waveform and reduced negativity in response to the deviant. However, DCM analyses applied to the data indicated the ketamine had a selective effect on parameters representing synaptic plasticity with no effect on indices reflecting adaptation. Additionally, analysis indicated that the major effect of ketamine was to reduce the normal increase in synaptic plasticity in the forward connection between left A1 and left STG in response to the deviant tones. Therefore while ketamine administration and schizophrenia are both associated with reduced MMN, the pattern of change (at least for this roving paradigm) is quite distinct. Ketamine-induced a prominent change in feed-forward connections between A1 and STG only (14) while schizophrenia was associated principally with reduced intrinsic connections within A1 and significant alteration in prefrontal-STG connections (60).

In Schmidt et al. (14, 126), and an earlier observation by Umbricht and colleagues (131), MMN measures were associated with the intensity of psychotic-like reactions to ketamine. Schmidt et al. (126) reported that participants with the most restricted growth in MMN with increased standard repetition experienced the most pronounced disturbances noted on a "control and cognition" subscale of the altered state of consciousness questionnaire in the presence of ketamine. Similarly Umbricht and colleagues observed that the participants who produced the smallest MMNs at baseline experienced the highest symptom ratings (on a variety of measures) under ketamine. In the subsequent DCM analysis of Schmidt et al. (14), those who experienced the most pronounced "control and cognition" subscale disturbances in the presence of ketamine also showed the most pronounced decrease in plasticity in the left A1-STG connections under ketamine. Although the measures differ between studies, these observations invite the intriguing conclusion that small MMN amplitude (and/or limited growth in MMN) may indicate a limitation in synaptic plasticity that is linked to vulnerability to psychotic-like phenomena. Interestingly, this vulnerability does not appear to be generic as studies have shown no relationship between MMN amplitude and psychotic-like response to psilocybin and no significant effect of psilocybin on MMN amplitude (122, 126). Furthermore, there is evidence that this effect on NMDAGluR-mediated plasticity shows some specificity to ketamine-induced antagonism. Memantine (also an NMDAGluR antagonist) actually augmented MMN amplitude (123). The downstream effect of ketamine (and MK-801) has recently been demonstrated to be quite different to that of memantine. One interesting observation is that these compounds have opposing effects on postsynaptic density proteins – namely ketamine and MK-801 reliably increased *Homer1a* relative to *Homer1b* expression while memantine has the reverse effect. Authors suggest that the former impacts the expression of genes related to response to neuronal injury and preservation of homeostatic scaling of synaptic response. The latter, in contrast,

Table 3 | Monoamine receptor studies.

Reference	Study design	Main findings	Comments
Mervaala et al. (157)	Noradrenaline challenge with alpha 2-antagonist atipamezole (0.1 mg/kg) in six healthy male volunteers	Reduced P3 amplitude without affecting MMN and Nd; improved digit span and word recognition performance	Small sample size; study did not report ERPs in response to standard stimuli
Schreiber et al. (158)	Double-blind, placebo-controlled crossover administration of ceruletide (0.5 and 2.5 mg) in 13 healthy volunteers	No effect on MMN; PN larger with ceruletide	Study did not report ERPs in response to standard stimuli
Kahkonen et al. (159)	Placebo-controlled haloperidol challenge (2 mg) in 12 healthy volunteers	MMN increased with haloperidol without affecting other ERP components	MEG measures were unaffected; study reported ERPs in response to standard stimuli
Pekkonen et al. (160)	Haloperidol challenge 2 mg in 12 healthy volunteers	No effect on MMN	Study reported ERPs in response to standard stimuli
Ahveninen et al. (161)	5HT challenge using acute tryptophan depletion versus placebo control in 13 healthy volunteers	Delayed MMN latency	Study reported ERPs in response to standard stimuli
Umbricht et al. (131)	Single-blind, placebo-controlled psilocybin challenge (0.28 mg/kg) in 18 healthy volunteers and ketamine (0.9 mg/kg/h) in 20 healthy volunteers whilst performing a continuous performance task	Smaller MMN to frequency and duration deviants was correlated with stronger effects on the brief psychiatric rating scale during ketamine but not psilocybin	Study does not report MMN in the respective placebo conditions and did not report ERPs in response to standard stimuli
Leung et al. (162)	Double-blind, placebo-controlled crossover administration of bromocriptine (2.5 mg) or pergolide (0.1 mg) in 15 healthy volunteers	No effect on MMN, P1, N1, N2, and P3	Study reported ERPs in response to standard stimuli
Korostenskaja et al. (163)	Double-blind, placebo-controlled crossover administration of methylphenidate challenge (40 mg) in 13 healthy volunteers	No effect on MMN or N1; P2 amplitude reduction with methylphenidate	Study reported ERPs in response to standard stimuli
Leung et al. (164)	Double-blind, placebo-controlled crossover design following tyrosine/phenylalanine and/or tyrosine depletion intervention in 16 healthy volunteers	No effects on ERPs	Study reported ERPs in response to standard stimuli

strengthens synaptic transmission. These very different effects on plasticity may go some way to explaining the opposing effects of these NMDAGluR-antagonists on MMN and invite speculation as to whether individual differences in these same ratios may in fact confer differential susceptibility to ketamine-induced psychotic-like experiences (and disruption to the MMN process, however see also discussion of animal research using memantine in Section "Translation to Animal Models"). In summary, antagonism of NMDAGluRs in the presence of ketamine produces quite consistent reduction in MMN amplitudes and continues to hold promise in furthering our understanding of the plasticity underlying MMN as well as vulnerability to psychotic phenomena. Of course it should be remembered that acute disruption under ketamine is unlikely to mirror the full consequences of adjustment to a more chronic compromise in function (if present) in schizophrenia.

Just as there are multiple elements to the MMN process, there are multiple ways to pharmacologically influence NMDAGluR-mediated synaptic plasticity [for a relevant review see Ref. (132)]. NMDAGluR antagonism also occurs under acute exposure to alcohol and consistent with this, acute administration of ethanol has been shown to reduce MMN amplitude (133, 134). Nicotine in contrast enhances synaptic plasticity with mechanisms linked to effects on presynaptic NMDAGluRs (135). Nicotine exerts its effects on the central nervous system via acetylcholine receptors (135). Galantamine has been used to test theories about how augmentation of cholinergic neurotransmission can modulate gain in MMN (136). The results of both an empirical study and a simulation experiment indicate that enhanced cholinergic neurotransmission alters precision in prediction-modeling – i.e., changes confidence in the current inference model. More specifically, under these conditions the system places a greater emphasis on bottom-up input and "boosts" the response to deviants while also attenuating the usual reduction in confidence in a model following the occurrence of a deviance. The authors suggest that acetylcholine plays a key role in modulating gain in superficial pyramidal neurons in early sensory brain areas. Consistent with this action, five of the seven studies listed in **Table 2** support nicotine enhancement of MMN. Significant enhancement of MMN has been demonstrated under both acute (137–141) and more prolonged exposure (139). Of the seven studies listed, five present or report on response to standard tones but only one indicates significant drug effects. Baldeweg et al. employed the roving standard paradigm and revealed that the increase in MMN amplitude with nicotine was due to a selective augmentation of the positivity to repeated standards with no significant effect on response to deviants.

Cannabis use is considered by some to be a risk factor in the development of psychosis. Furthermore, chronic cannabis use has been associated with gray matter volume changes and cognitive deficits reminiscent of those in schizophrenia (144–147). The action of endogenous cannabanoids is also linked to NMDAGluRs in protecting against excessive stimulation at glutamatergic synapses. The cannabanoids are released from postsynaptic neurons and exert their action on CB1 receptors located on presynaptic neurons which transiently decreases neurotransmitter release [(148) for review]. There are currently two published studies on the acute effects of cannabis [in fact the latter is a reanalysis of the former with genetic data included (149, 150)]. The first of these explored the effect of administering Δ9-tetrahydrocannabinol (THC) alone (the psychoactive component of cannabis) versus in combination with the other cannabinoids present in cannabis extract. The results indicated no significant impact of Δ9-THC alone, but significant augmentation of MMN at central sites in the presence of cannabis extract compared to placebo. However the study also demonstrated a significant correlation such that higher concentration of the Δ9-THC-metabolite 11-OH-THC was associated with smaller MMN amplitude ($r = 0.62$, $p = 0.002$). In their later combination with genetic data the same group revealed that susceptibility to MMN-reduction in the presence of Δ9-THC was a function of genotype for neuregulin 1 (MMN reduced in the presence of Δ9-THC for those with NRG1 rs7834206 polymorphism). Neuregulin 1 is a gene implicated in schizophrenia that influences synaptic plasticity via multiple pathways, including those involving NMDAGluRs (128). The possibility that genes confer vulnerability to Δ9-THC effects on cognitive processing also finds support in animal research where heterozygous Neuregulin 1 knockout mice have been observed to show differential sensitivity to the acute effects of Δ9-THC on behavioral phenotypes of schizophrenia (151).

Despite dopamine being a modulator of NMDAGluRs and a central focus of treatment and models of schizophrenia (37, 132), there are no studies supporting a significant effect of altered dopamine levels on MMN amplitude in healthy adults (see **Table 3**). Furthermore, with one recent exception (reviewed below), studies within schizophrenia do not support a significant effect of medication type or dose on MMN [see Ref. (5) for review], and no significant differences in MMN amplitude between medicated and unmedicated patients (52, 152). However, Zhou and colleagues (79) have recently reported a significant progressive increment in MMN in persons with schizophrenia treated with aripiprazole (larger at 4 and 8 weeks of treatment than at baseline). MMN was measured using a traditional oddball paradigm with two deviant types (frequency and duration) and effects are presented and reported for the difference waveforms only. Aripiprazole differs from other second generation anti-psychotics in that its action at dopamine D2 receptors shows *functional selectivity* (153–155). It has been proposed that this selectivity may be related to observations that it has differential effects on the two main dopaminergic pathways, namely a predominant effect on the mesolimbic pathway (156). Although MMN remained significantly smaller than that in matched controls, the authors argue that the effect of the drug treatment on MMN does raise questions about whether MMN amplitude is really a trait or state marker. Finally studies on benzodiazepines, often prescribed to persons with schizophrenia, have consistently failed to demonstrate any effect on MMN amplitude (see **Table 3**).

In summary, the literature to date on the pharmacology of MMN generally reflects its obvious relationship with experience-dependent synaptic plasticity. The observed effects of ketamine, nicotine and cannabis provide support for the NMDAGluR-susceptibility of the system underlying MMN and therefore utility to schizophrenia research on MMN as they offer useful insights into the neurobiological processes that can influence or modulate MMN amplitude. However the memantine studies clearly caution that the relationship between perturbation of NMDAGluRs and MMN amplitude is not a simple one. There is insufficient information within most published studies to determine exactly how the various agents are altering the underlying processes with most reporting on difference waveforms only. Clarity regarding which elements of changed responsiveness are affected by drugs is particularly important to a thorough understanding of the process and these issues are discussed further in Section "Translation to Animal Models" below. Where possible it may be advantageous to add genotyping to pharmacology studies as it is well known that susceptibility to drug effects can be dependent on genetic profiles but of course the cost and sample size requirements are often prohibitive.

TRANSLATION TO ANIMAL MODELS

Animal models have the potential to inform investigation of the physiological basis of MMN and potentially how it is disrupted in persons with schizophrenia. However, the primary issue of debate in animal models of MMN is to determine which components of the MMN process can be observed (and under which conditions they can be observed) in animals, there being some skepticism expressed in the past over whether the rodent brain exhibits "true MMN" (165). Debate over how exactly to measure MMN (see The Measurement of MMN – Is there an Optimal Paradigm with Which to Study MMN in Schizophrenia?) is therefore particularly relevant to animal work. Results from several different control designs are reviewed in this section and for ease of communication they are presented diagrammatically in **Figure 1**.

The presence of adaptation to repeated stimuli (or stimulus-specific adaptation, SSA) in A1 is well-described in the cat (8, 166), rat (167–170), and macaque (171). A1 neuron populations will adapt to repetitive stimuli and will exhibit relatively large responses to a rare deviant compared to a common standard. However, as reviewed in Section "The Measurement of MMN – Is there an Optimal Paradigm with Which to Study MMN in Schizophrenia?" evidence of "true MMN" must include something more than just adaptation effects. Terminology used is not consistent across animal and human studies so for simplicity we adopt the following nomenclature: oddball mismatch response (MMR) is used when referring to the difference between the response to a rare deviation and the regular (usually physically different) repeating sound; and controlled MMR is used to define evidence of contextual deviance detection when a study has included some kind of control for adaptation and physical characteristics of the stimuli (see **Figure 1**).

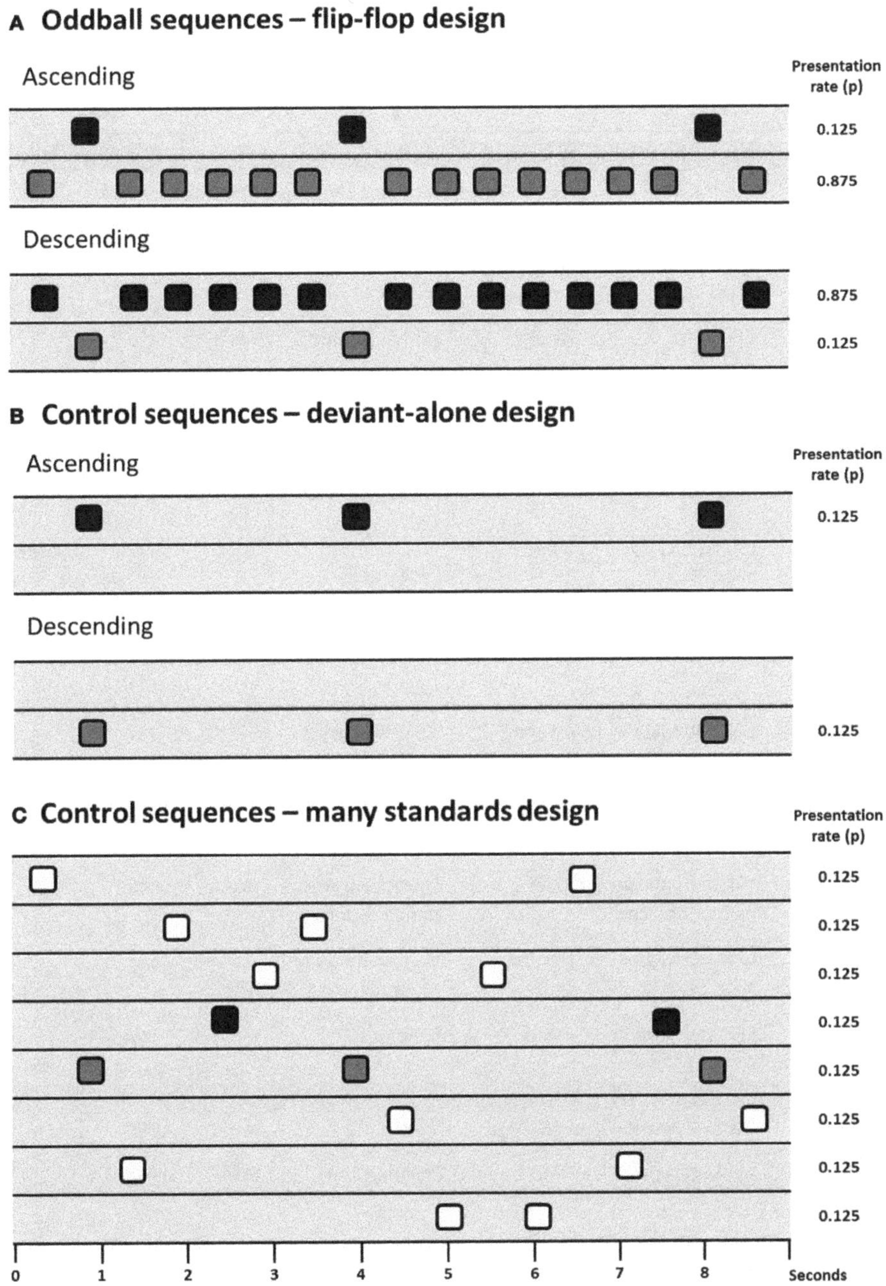

FIGURE 1 | Schematic of sequence design showing sequences with deviants presented at a probability of 0.125 (1/8), two oddball sequences are presented in a flip-flop design (A), controlling for the physical characteristics of the stimuli. Differential adaptation can be controlled for through the use of a deviant-alone control **(B)**, which presents the deviant at the same temporal rate as it is presented in the oddball sequence, but without the intervening standards; or the many-standards control **(C)**, which presents several stimuli (including the deviant) at the same temporal rate as the oddball sequences.

WHAT IS THE EVIDENCE FOR A "CONTROLLED MMR" IN LOCAL FIELD POTENTIALS?

Table 4 summarizes the animal studies that utilize oddball paradigms to test for evidence that a contextually deviant sound has been detected. The location of the recording electrode plays a large role in the findings of these studies, as epidural-placed electrodes receive input from a larger and more distributed network of cortical neurons than local field potential electrodes (LFP; measuring changes in synaptic potentials) or electrodes that register multi- or single-unit spike activity [MUA, SUA; see Ref. (165)]. The majority of studies using LFP recordings have searched for evidence of contextual deviance detection by recording from A1, but some also have recorded from the hippocampus (172–174). The majority of investigations using LFP or MUA

Table 4 | Summary of papers investigating mismatch responses in animal models.

Reference	Species/strain	Recording type/location	Anesthesia	Control type	Oddball MMR finding	Controlled MMR finding	Effects of NMDAGluR antagonism
SUBDURAL RECORDINGS							
Ulanovsky et al. (8)	Cat	MUA in A1 and MGB	Xylazine/ ketamine	None	Yes	N/A	
Ulanovsky et al. (166)	Cat	LFP in A1 and MGB	Xylazine/ ketamine	None	Yes	N/A	
Fishman and Steinschneider (171)	Cat	LFP in A1	Awake	Many-standards	Yes	No	
Javitt et al. (130)	Macaque	LFP in A1	Awake	None	Yes	N/A	Infusions of PCP (5 and 10 μg) into the auditory cortex reduced oddball MMR
Ehrlichman et al. (172)	Mouse (DBA/2Hsd)	LFP in CA3	Awake	None	Yes	N/A	Ketamine (10 mg/kg) reduced oddball MMR
Ehrlichman et al. (173)	Mouse (C57/129Sv background)	LFP in CA3	Awake	None	Yes	N/A	
Farley et al. (169)	Rat (unknown strain)	LFP and MUA in A1	Awake	Many-standards	Yes	No	
Eriksson and Villa (167)	Rat (Long–Evans)	LFP in A1	Awake	Deviant-alone	Yes	No	
Imada et al. (175)	Rat (Long–Evans)	LFP in frontal and parietal cortices	Awake	Deviant-alone, standard-alone	Yes	Yes	
Taaseh et al. (170)	Rat (Sabra)	LFP and MUA in A1	Halothane	Many-standards, deviant-alone	Yes	Yes	
von der Behrens et al. (168)	Rat (Sprague–Dawley)	LFP and MUA in A1	Awake	None	Yes	N/A	
EPIDURAL RECORDINGS							
Pincze et al. (176)	Cat	Epidural above A1	Awake	None	Yes	N/A	
Umbricht et al. (177)	Mouse (C57/129)	Epidural above A1	Awake	Deviant-alone	Yes	No	
Jung et al. (178)	Rat (black hooded)	Epidural above A1	Awake	Many-standards	Yes	Yes	
Tikhonravov et al. (179)	Rat (Hannover–Wistar)	Epidural near A1	Pentobarbital sodium	Deviant-alone	Yes	Yes	High-dose (0.3 mg/kg), but not low-dose (0.1 mg/kg) MK-801 reduced oddball MMR
Tikhonravov et al. (180)	Rat (Hannover–Wistar)	Epidural near A1	Pentobarbital sodium	Deviant-alone	Yes	Yes	Low-dose (3 mg/kg) memantine increased oddball MMR, high-dose (10 mg/kg) reduced oddball MMR
Roger et al. (181)	Rat (Long–Evans)	Epidural above motor, parietal and anterior cingulate cortices	Awake	None	Yes	N/A	

(Continued)

Table 4 | Continued

Reference	Species/strain	Recording type/location	Anesthesia	Control type	Oddball MMR finding	Controlled MMR finding	Effects of NMDAGluR antagonism
Ahmed et al. (182)	Rat (Sprague–Dawley)	Epidural above A1	Urethane	Many-Standards	Yes	Yes	
Astikainen et al. (183)	Rat (Sprague–Dawley)	Epidural above A1	Urethane	Many-Standards	Yes	Yes	
Lazar and Metherate (184)	Rat (Sprague–Dawley)	Epidural above A1	Urethane/ xylazine	Deviant-alone	Yes	No	
Ruusuvirta et al. (174)	Rat (Sprague–Dawley)	Epidural above A1/LFP in subiculum, DG, CA1	Urethane	None	Yes	N/A	
Astikainen et al. (185)	Rat (Wistar)	Epidural above A1	Urethane	None	Yes	N/A	
Nakamura et al. (186)	Rat (Wistar)	Epidural near A1	Awake	Many-Standards	Yes	Yes	
Ruusuvirta et al. (187)	Rat (Wistar)	Epidural above A1	Urethane	Deviant-alone	Yes	Yes	
Ruusuvirta et al. (188)	Rat (Wistar)	Epidural above A1	Urethane	None	Yes	N/A	

A1, primary auditory cortex; CA1, CA1 region of hippocampus; DG, dentate gyrus; LFP, local field potentials; MGB, medial geniculate body of thalamus; MUA, multi-unit activity; SUA, single-unit activity.

(intra-cortical recordings), that also use many-standards or deviant-alone control, have not found any evidence for true MMR in the A1 (8, 167, 169, 171), whereas the majority of studies using *epidural* recordings and appropriate controls *have* found evidence for contextual deviance detection. This indicates that while adaptation to stimulus frequency/pitch does occur in the A1, the deviance-detection component of the MMN has not been identified in this region, and if it is present in the A1, it may be generated by more distributed networks than can only be observed using LFP recordings.

One of the first animal model studies (130) found larger responses to deviant sounds in an oddball paradigm originate in the supragranular layers (II–III) and are dependent upon normal functioning of the NMDAGluR (covered in Section "How do Pharmacological Manipulations Alter the MMN Process?"). However, Javitt et al. did not utilize a many-standard control and in a more recent study that did (171), larger responses *were not* observed to the deviant compared to the same tone in the many-standards sequence (no evidence of true MMR). The many-standards control in this study may have overestimated adaptation, however, as the deviant was presented at a probability of 10% in the oddball sequence, and the tones used for the many-standards control were presented at a maximum rate of 5% (171).

There are, to our knowledge, only two studies thus far utilizing LFP recording that have found some evidence for what might be considered controlled MMR in the rat brain (170, 175). Imada et al. (175), using a frequency deviant paradigm, found that the difference between the ERPs to deviant and standard stimuli was significantly elevated from 0 in an oddball MMR. However as a control they included separate sequences preserving the timing of standard sounds (without deviants) and deviant sounds (without standards) from the original oddball sequence. The ERP to deviant-alone and the standard-alone did not differ (175). According to the authors, this indicates that there was a statistically significant change in the response to the deviant stimuli in the oddball measure, over and above adaptation, which may hint at the presence of true MMR, albeit one that is not large enough to produce a statistically significant difference in responses to the oddball deviant compared to the deviant-alone. Taaseh et al. (170) utilized both LFP and MUA recording and found that the response to the oddball deviant tones did not exceed the response to the same tone in a many-standards control sequence (their *diverse-broad* sequence). However, the response to the deviant sound *was* larger than the many-standards control in some recordings (although not at a population level), indicating that perhaps a subset of neurons do exhibit sensitivity to the contextual deviance of the sound (170). In addition, their thorough characterization of adaptation effects was used to generate a model which predicted that if only adaptation were occurring, the response to the deviant would be smaller than the response to the same tone in the many-standards control. However, these responses did not differ significantly, suggesting (albeit rather indirectly) that contextual deviance detection is occurring in the auditory cortex. There is therefore some evidence that recognition of contextual deviance occurs in the rat A1. Such hints of response to contextual aberrance may represent the first step in a cascade that results in full MMN responses (170). This study, however, did not identify the significantly elevated response to the deviant compared to the control that is similar to the MMN typically seen in humans– a pattern only observed in animal models when recorded from larger brain volumes (165).

WHAT IS THE EVIDENCE FOR A "CONTROLLED MMR" IN EPIDURAL RECORDINGS?

Studies using epidural recordings in animals (mainly rats) use electrodes implanted in the skull or sitting on the dura over the auditory cortex (or close to the auditory cortex) to record ERPs elicited during oddball sequences. **Table 2** summarizes these studies. Of these, four use the many-standards control. Ahmed et al. (182) used speech sounds as stimuli, and found larger responses to the deviant sound/ba/in an oddball sequence compared to the same sound presented at the same rate in a many-standards control in anesthetized rats (182). Nakamura et al. (186) and Jung et al. (178) both investigated responses to frequency/pitch deviants in awake rats, and found larger responses to deviant stimuli compared to those in the many-standards control sequence (178, 186). Astikainen et al. (183) examined responses to frequency deviants in *anesthetized* rats and found evidence of deviance detection when the deviant was a high frequency (4.2 kHz) stimulus, not a low frequency stimulus (3.8 kHz), as was also found in Nakamura et al. (3.6 Vs. 2.5 kHz) (183). Nakamura et al. also investigated the effect of duration deviants and identified larger responses to long (but not short) duration deviants compared to the same tones in the many-standards control sequence (186). Therefore all four studies using the many-standards control have indeed observed a response reminiscent of controlled MMR.

Although all these studies all report deviance detection in the rat brain, the morphology of the ERPs differs between each of the studies, with the most dramatic difference in ERPs being observed between the awake recordings (178, 186) and the anesthetized recordings (182, 183). Awake ERPs comprise 3–4 negative and positive components, and the anesthetized recordings feature only one large positive component. The polarity of the deviance-detection effects is also different, with negative deflections in response to the deviant in the awake animals, and positive deflections in anesthetized animals. Such trends can be similarly observed in other studies (**Table 4**), with the majority differences between the deviant and the standard being positive in anesthetized rats and negative in awake rats. These findings illustrate that deviance-detection need not be a response that exactly mimics the human MMN (insofar as being of the same polarity). Indeed human mismatch responses (MMR) change from negative to positive in polarity when the recording location is moved from fronto-centrally sites to the mastoid when recorded using a nose reference (189).

The remainder of studies examining epidural ERPs in oddball paradigms use either the deviant-alone to control for adaptation, or use no adaptation control at all. Although the deviant-alone sequence may overestimate the contribution of adaptation (165), three of the five studies utilizing this control sequence find evidence for controlled MMR recorded from epidural electrodes (179, 180, 187). Of those epidural studies that did not implement a control for adaptation, several did not use simple frequency deviants (which are highly predisposed to be affected by adaptation mechanisms in the A1), but rather used more complex deviants that presumably elicited responses that would not be so readily perturbed by neural adaptation. For instance, Roger et al. (181) measured responses to duration deviants [which are not affected by adaptation in the A1 to the same degree as frequency deviants; (169)], and found larger responses to duration deviants (181). In addition, Ruusuvirta et al. (174) examined responses to duration deviants in combination with stimulus onset asynchrony deviants, and found evidence for larger deviant responses (compared to standards) only in the condition in which the deviant occurred earlier than expected and deviated in duration, indicating a possible threshold level for deviance that needs to be reached before a deviance-detection-like response iselicited (174). However, without the use of a many-standards (or even a deviant-alone) control, it remains difficult to conclude that such responses are completely independent of adaptation effects. Although tone duration is coded in a different way to the frequency, and previous studies have demonstrated that adaptation mechanisms for duration are not as robust as they are for frequency (169), this was examined in the auditory cortex only, and it cannot be ruled out that another region (or network of regions) adapts to stimulus duration in the same way as the auditory cortex does for frequency. These studies show that when using methods that detect shifts in potential at a network-level (i.e., a large spatial scale), signs of human-like MMR (independent of adaptation) are evident in animals.

HOW DOES ANIMAL RESEARCH AUGMENT HUMAN RESEARCH ON MMN?

Animal models are an ideal tool with which to investigate the underlying neurobiology of MMR because of the ability to perform more invasive and selective neurobiological manipulations (e.g., drug microinjection to specific regions). In addition, the comprehensive genetic toolkit available for mouse models will enable researchers to determine the role of specific genes and neural populations in the generation of MMR using transgenic animals and optogenetics. With a consensus emerging regarding the ideal recording method (epidural) and the current preferred control to use (many-standards) to examine MMR (adaptation and deviance detection) in animal models, the time is ripe for further studies examining the neurobiology of these elements of MMR, using pharmacological, developmental, and genetic manipulations. Unfortunately, few studies implement a control for adaptation effects (or if they do, do not adequately report drug effects on these), and it is therefore difficult to determine whether or not the agents given affect adaptation, deviance-detection, or both. The preferable way to investigate the pharmacology of MMN in animal models would be test different manipulations in a model that exhibits both adaptation and deviance detection [e.g., Ref. (178)], and to compare how different agents affect the responses to standards, deviants, and control stimuli; with the difference between the control and standard representing adaptation and the difference between the deviant and the control representing MMR and the effects of drug interventions on these two separate components can be examined. To our knowledge, no studies have tested such a model thus far.

Studies in rats and mice (like those on the macaque described above) have been used to study the role of the NMDAGluR system in MMN. These studies, in contrast to Javitt et al. (130), suggest that perturbations in NMDAR signaling can also alter responses to standard stimuli. In the absence of a control for adaptation effects, Ehrlichman et al. found that ketamine (a non-competitive NMDAGluR antagonist) concurrently *increased* the response to the standard (which was small to start with) and *reduced* the response to the deviant, albeit not to a significant degree, in awake mice (172). Tikhonravov et al. used a low (0.1 mg/kg) and high (0.3 mg/kg) dose of intraperitoneal MK-801 to examine the effects of NMDAGluR perturbation on responses to oddball stimuli, in addition to a deviant-alone control in pentobarbital-anesthetized rats (179). Responses to the deviant were more positive than the responses to the standard for the saline condition and were relatively unchanged by the low-dose of MK-801. However, the high-dose of MK-801 lowered the response to the deviant and increased the response to the standard, effectively reversing the polarity of the oddball effect. The degree to which MK-801 altered the *magnitude* of the difference between the oddball deviant and the deviant-alone was not reported. However, the period over which the deviant was significantly different from the deviant-alone was reported: there was a positive deflection in response to the deviant (relative to deviant-alone) in saline-treated animals (indicating deviance detection), which was absent after low-dose MK-801 and reversed in polarity after high-dose MK-801 (179). The finding that low-dose MK-801 can reduce the difference between the oddball deviant and deviant-alone, without a change in the differences between deviant and standard could indicate that this dose can preferentially disrupt deviance detection, while sparing adaptation. However, the high-dose of MK-801 not only disrupted both deviance detection and adaptation but reversed the polarity of these changes. Such reversals, caused by an increase in the response to the standard and a decrease in the response to the deviant, are similar to those found after ketamine by Ehrlichman et al.

In a second study, Tikhonravov et al. investigated the effects of a low (3 mg/kg) and a high (10 mg/kg) dose of memantine on responses to oddball stimuli and deviant-alone stimuli in anesthetized rats (180). Like MK-801, memantine is an uncompetitive NMDAGluR antagonist, but unlike MK-801, is a very low-affinity antagonist and has potential as a cognitive enhancer [(190) see also discussion of memantine in Section "How do Pharmacological Manipulations Alter the MMN Process?"]. Similar to previous studies in anesthetized rats, the oddball MMR was positive in saline-treated rats. The low-dose of memantine resulted in a significant increase in the response to the deviant and the oddball MMR was significantly prolonged compared to the saline group. The high-dose of memantine, on the other hand, reduced the time over which the oddball MMR was significantly different from 0 and reversed the late phase of the difference waveform, possibly due to an increase in the response to the standard (180). With regard to deviance-detection-specific changes, the deviant was more positive than the deviant-alone in saline-treated rats, an effect that was prolonged in the low-dose memantine group. In rats treated with the high-dose of memantine, however, no deviance-detection response was observed. These findings indicate that low-dose memantine potentiates the deviance-detection response, with no significant effect on the adaptation response, but that high-dose memantine acts similarly to high-dose MK-801, affecting both adaptation and deviance detection and reversing the polarity of the oddball MMR.

Overall, these pharmacological studies suggest that NMDAGluR-antagonists act in a dose-dependent fashion, with low-dose/low-affinity antagonists facilitating deviance detection (by increasing the response to the deviant), then as NMDAGluR perturbations are increased with low-dose/high affinity antagonists, deviance detection is inhibited while adaptation is spared. However, with high-doses of high affinity blockers (ketamine and MK-801), the response to the standard is increased, thus indicating impaired adaptation. The selective impairment of deviance detection and not adaptation after MK-801 is also highlighted in (169), where it was reported that subcutaneous MK-801 (maximum dose, 0.1 mg/kg) reduced responses to both the deviant and the standard together, while preserving the difference between them, indicating that this dose *did not* affect neural adaptation in A1, similar to findings in the study in which the same drug was given intraperitoneally (179). These studies indicate that the mechanism by which NMDAGluR-antagonists may reduce the MMN may be rather complex, with the dose and affinity of the antagonist interacting with adaptation and deviance-detection resulting in varied effects on these elements of the MMN. This animal work highlights a complexity in the role of NMDAGluRs in the generation of MMRs that was not discovered in human studies using NMDAGluR-antagonists, most likely due to the smaller dose-range, smaller sample size, and lack of consistent reporting of the response to standards seen in the human work. This animal work therefore highlights the need to examine a larger dose-range, as well as the need for consistent reporting of both standard and deviant responses in human pharmacological MMN studies.

Several of the previously mentioned animal pharmacological studies have similar weaknesses highlighted for the human studies. While (179, 180) used a control for adaptation (the deviant-alone control), they did not report directly on the magnitude of responses to the standard, the deviant and the deviant-alone control, thus making the interpretation of the mechanisms affected by pharmacological agents very problematic. While these animal model investigations are still in their infancy, the promise of such models is far-reaching. Future investigations will be able to focus on a range of doses of NMDAGluR-antagonists in paradigms in which adaptation and deviance detection are well-described, to further explore the role of NMDAGluR signaling in both of these components. In addition, NMDAGluR-antagonists can be infused directly into regions of interests [as performed by Javitt et al. (130)], to determine where NMDAGluR signaling is important for MMR. Further, high-doses of muscimol [a Gamma-Amino Butyric Acid (A) agonist] can be infused to completely inactivate regions to determine their contribution to deviance detection. For example (174) found evidence of MMR in rat hippocampus – the degree to which these contribute to epidural-recorded MMR can be determined by infusing muscimol into selected hippocampal regions. In addition, animal models of schizophrenia-like reductions in MMN could possibly be developed. (173) used transgenic mice heterozygous for *neuregulin 1* (*nrg1*; an hypothesized schizophrenia-susceptibility gene) and found a reversal in polarity of the oddball MMR in *nrg1* mutants compared to wild type mice. However, this study did not adopt a control for adaptation effects, so it is unknown in *nrg1* plays a role in adaptation or adaptation-independent deviance-detection. Experiments in our lab are currently underway to determine the effect of maternal immune activation on MMR (both adaptation and deviance detection) in rats. Maternal immune activation is a risk factor for schizophrenia and when modeled in rats and mice, is associated with numerous schizophrenia-like behavioral and neurodevelopmental outcomes, particularly those related to NMDAGluR-dysfunction (191–193). This model therefore may also exhibit schizophrenia-like changes in MMR and could be used as a potential experimental platform to examine the pathology underlying schizophrenia-like reductions in the mismatch response, and potential treatments for such alterations.

CONCLUSION

The above review supports several conclusions regarding the potential of MMN as a tool to study the biological processes taking place in those with (and potentially those at-risk for) schizophrenia.

MEASUREMENT AND REPORTING OF MMN

There are pros and cons to any experimental design and it is the authors' opinion that there is no optimal design for use in schizophrenia studies. To recommend an optimal design, while improving consistency in the literature, would come at the expense of the unique contributions that can be made by novel designs [see Ref. (24) for review] that can enrich our understanding of the perceptual inference within the MMN process and how gain in this signal is controlled. Furthermore, study design is often limited by mundane and yet important considerations of test duration that could render particular paradigms less feasible. However, two recommendations arise from this review. The first is that authors and journals facilitate a closer adherence to publication standards. A failing of the current literature is that a large number of studies (including some by our group) do not adhere to recommended publication standards for ERP research which stipulates the display of the original ERPs from which difference waveforms have been derived (194). By comparing research findings across species and drug studies (as above) the importance of at least reporting standard and deviant ERPs becomes clear. Secondly, while the traditional oddball paradigm provides a robust measure of the reduction in MMN amplitude in schizophrenia, protocols designed to identify constituents of the MMN process (or oddball combined with rigorous controls) introduce the capacity to begin disentangling which components of the process are in fact compromised. This advantage becomes crucial when attempting the translation of this research into animal models (see Translation to Animal Models) and arguably also to pharmacological studies (see How do Pharmacological Manipulations Alter the MMN Process?). Where feasible, future studies should consider the advantage of designs (or analysis techniques) that facilitate the differentiation between adaption effects and something more akin to true contextual deviance detection.

VULNERABILITY TO SCHIZOPHRENIA

Our review of the literature to date indicates limited support for small MMN conferring some vulnerability to schizophrenia but we consider this an open question best addressed by large longitudinal studies. It is the authors' opinion that there is much to gained by continued efforts to understand factors that influence MMN size (using novel designs, pharmacological, and animal research) in parallel to such efforts.

PHARMACOLOGY AND ANIMAL MODELS OF MMN

It seems clear from the pharmacological studies (in animals and humans) that adaptation and sensitivity to contextual deviance may show differential effects in the presence of compromised NMDAGluR function. Pharmacological, like animal studies, require indices of both to be informative about the effect of agents on the MMN process. Similar to schizophrenia studies, animal, and pharmacological studies inconsistently report on standard and deviant effects. While our review of pharmacological studies is more supportive of some agents (e.g., glutamatergic and cholinergic) than others (e.g., monoamines), our knowledge of influences on perceptual inference and learning underlying MMN continues to grow and challenge existing models [e.g., Ref. (98, 195)] and it remains possible that future paradigms may be sensitive to agents that current paradigms are not. In other areas of learning, animal models and pharmacology have provided great insight into schizophrenia [associative learning (196)] and there is good reason to suppose that this will also be true of MMN research as well as offering the potential to examine commonalities in underlying pathology. While there are many challenges in translating the potential of MMN in elucidating the pathophysiology of the schizophrenic illness, we believe the current state of research encourages scientists to pursue the many numerous potentially fruitful avenues available to achieve this goal.

AUTHOR CONTRIBUTIONS

Juanita Todd, – lead writer and overall editor. Primary contributions Sections "The Potential – Why is there so Much Interest in MMN in Schizophrenia?" "The Measurement of MMN – Is there an Optimal Paradigm with Which to Study MMN in Schizophrenia?" "How do Pharmacological Manipulations Alter the MMN Process?" and "Conclusion." Lauren Harms – Primary contribution Section "Translation to Animal Models." Reference manager. Patricia T. Michie – Primary contributions Sections "The Measurement of MMN – Is there an Optimal Paradigm with Which to Study MMN in Schizophrenia?" and "Does MMN-Reduction Indicate Vulnerability to Schizophrenia?" Ulrich Schall – co-writer of all sections and preparation of **Tables 1–3**.

ACKNOWLEDGMENTS

Our thanks are extended to Ms. Lisa Whitson and Mr. Alexander Provost who sourced many of the papers reviewed for the pharmacology section. Lauren Harms is supported by a National Health and Medical Research Council Project grant (ID1026070). Research referenced in this paper includes that supported by additional National Health and Medical Research Council Project grants (IDs 569259 and 1002995). Ulrich Schall was supported by the Schizophrenia Research Institute utilizing infrastructure funding from the New South Wales Ministry of Health and New South Wales Ministry of Trade and Investment (Australia).

REFERENCES

1. Näätänen R. *In Attention and Brain Function*. Hillsdale, NJ: Lawrence Erlbaum Associates (1992).
2. Winkler I. Interpreting the mismatch negativity. *J Psychophysiol* (2007) **21**(3–4):147–63. doi:10.1027/0269-8803.21.34.147
3. Kujala T, Tervaniemi M, Schroger E. The mismatch negativity in cognitive and clinical neuroscience: theoretical and methodological considerations. *Biol Psychol* (2007) **74**:1–19. doi:10.1016/j.biopsycho.2006.06.001
4. Picton TW, Alain C, Otten L, Ritter W, Achim A. Mismatch negativity: different water in the same river. *Audiol Neurootol* (2000) **5**:111–39. doi:10.1159/000013875
5. Umbricht D, Krljes S. Mismatch negativity in schizophrenia: a meta-analysis. *Schizophr Res* (2005) **76**:1–23. doi:10.1016/j.schres.2004.12.002
6. Alho K. Cerebral generators of mismatch negativity (MMN) and its magnetic counterpart (MMNm) elicited by sound changes. *Ear Hear* (1995) **16**:38–51. doi:10.1097/00003446-199502000-00004
7. Javitt DC, Steinschneider M, Schroeder CE, Vaughan HG Jr, Arezzo JC. Detection of stimulus deviance within primate primary auditory cortex: intracortical mechanisms of mismatch negativity (MMN) generation. *Brain Res* (1994) **667**:192–200. doi:10.1016/0006-8993(94)91496-6
8. Ulanovsky N, Las L, Nelken I. Processing of low-probability sounds by cortical neurons. *Nat Neurosci* (2003) **6**:391–8. doi:10.1038/nn1032
9. Näätänen R, Jacobsen T, Winkler I. Memory-based or afferent processes in mismatch negativity (MMN): a review of the evidence. *Psychophysiology* (2005) **42**:25–32. doi:10.1111/j.1469-8986.2005.00256.x
10. May PJ, Tiitinen H. Mismatch negativity (MMN), the deviance-elicited auditory deflection, explained. *Psychophysiology* (2010) **47**:66–122. doi:10.1111/j.1469-8986.2009.00856.x
11. Garrido MI, Friston KJ, Kiebel SJ, Stephan KE, Baldeweg T, Kilner JM. The functional anatomy of the MMN: a DCM study of the roving paradigm. *Neuroimage* (2008) **42**:936–44. doi:10.1016/j.neuroimage.2008.05.018
12. Garrido MI, Kilner JM, Kiebel SJ, Friston KJ. Dynamic causal modeling of the response to frequency deviants. *J Neurophysiol* (2009) **101**:2620–31. doi:10.1152/jn.90291.2008
13. Ruhnau P, Herrmann B, Schroger E. Finding the right control: the mismatch negativity under investigation. *Clin Neurophysiol* (2012) **123**:507–12. doi:10.1016/j.clinph.2011.07.035
14. Schmidt A, Diaconescu AO, Kometer M, Friston KJ, Stephan KE, Vollenweider FX. Modeling ketamine effects on synaptic plasticity during the mismatch negativity. *Cereb Cortex* (2013) **23**:2394–406. doi:10.1093/cercor/bhs238
15. Friston K. A theory of cortical responses. *Philos Trans R Soc Lond B Biol Sci* (2005) **360**:815–36. doi:10.1098/rstb.2005.1622
16. Winkler I, Karmos G, Naatanen R. Adaptive modeling of the unattended acoustic environment reflected in the mismatch negativity event-related potential. *Brain Res* (1996) **742**:239–52. doi:10.1016/S0006-8993(96)01008-6
17. Lieder F, Stephan KE, Daunizeau J, Garrido MI, Friston KJ. A neurocomputational model of the mismatch negativity. *PLoS Comput Biol* (2013) **9**:e1003288. doi:10.1371/journal.pcbi.1003288
18. Escera C, Alho K, Winkler I, Naatanen R. Neural mechanisms of involuntary attention to acoustic novelty and change. *J Cogn Neurosci* (1998) **10**:590–604. doi:10.1162/089892998562997
19. Schroger E, Wolff C. Attentional orienting and reorienting is indicated by human event-related brain potentials. *Neuroreport* (1998) **9**:3355–8. doi:10.1097/00001756-199810260-00003
20. Schroger E, Wolff C. Behavioral and electrophysiological effects of task-irrelevant sound change: a new distraction paradigm. *Brain Res Cogn Brain Res* (1998) **7**:71–87. doi:10.1016/S0926-6410(98)00013-5
21. Ahveninen J, Jaaskelainen IP, Pekkonen E, Hallberg A, Hietanen M, Naatanen R, et al. Increased distractibility by task-irrelevant sound changes in abstinent alcoholics. *Alcohol Clin Exp Res* (2000) **24**:1850–4. doi:10.1111/j.1530-0277.2000.tb01989.x
22. Escera C, Alho K, Schroger E, Winkler I. Involuntary attention and distractibility as evaluated with event-related brain potentials. *Audiol Neuro Otol* (2000) **5**:151–66. doi:10.1159/000013877
23. Näätänen R, Kujala T, Winkler I. Auditory processing that leads to conscious perception: a unique window to central auditory processing opened by the mismatch negativity and related responses. *Psychophysiology* (2011) **48**:4–22. doi:10.1111/j.1469-8986.2010.01114.x
24. Todd J, Michie PT, Schall U, Ward PB, Catts SV. Mismatch negativity (MMN) reduction in schizophrenia – Impaired prediction-error generation, estimation or salience? *Int J Psychophysiol* (2012) **83**:222–31. doi:10.1016/j.ijpsycho.2011.10.003
25. Javitt DC, Grochowski S, Shelley A, Ritter W. Impaired mismatch negativity (MMN) generation in schizophrenia as a function of stimulus deviance, probability, and interstimulus/interdeviant interval. *Electroencephalogr Clin Neurophysiol* (1998) **108**:143–53.
26. Shelley A-M, Silipo G, Javitt DC. Diminished responsiveness of ERPs in schizophrenic subjects to changes in auditory stimulation parameters: implications for theories of cortical dysfunction. *Schizophr Res* (1999) **37**:65–79. doi:10.1016/S0920-9964(98)00138-8
27. Sato Y, Yabe H, Todd J, Michie P, Shinozaki N, Sutoh T, et al. Impairment in activation of a frontal attention-switch mechanism in schizophrenic patients. *Biol Psychol* (2003) **62**:49–63. doi:10.1016/S0301-0511(02)00113-8
28. Menon RR, Barta PE, Aylward EH, Richards SS, Vaughn DD, Tien AY, et al. Posterior superior temporal gyrus in schizophrenia: grey matter changes and clinical correlates. *Schizophr Res* (1995) **16**:127–35. doi:10.1016/0920-9964(94)00067-I
29. Pantelis C, Velakoulis D, Mcgorry PD, Wood SJ, Suckling J, Phillips LJ, et al. Neuroanatomical abnormalities before and after onset of psychosis: a cross-sectional and longitudinal MRI comparison. *Lancet* (2003) **361**:281–8. doi:10.1016/S0140-6736(03)12323-9
30. Pantelis C, Velakoulis D, Wood SJ, Yucel M, Yung AR, Phillips LJ, et al. Neuroimaging and emerging psychotic disorders: the Melbourne ultra-high risk studies. *Int Rev Psychiatry* (2007) **19**:371–81. doi:10.1080/09540260701512079
31. Harms MP, Wang L, Campanella C, Aldridge K, Moffitt AJ, Kuelper J, et al. Structural abnormalities in gyri of the prefrontal cortex in individuals with schizophrenia and their unaffected siblings. *Br J Psychiatry* (2010) **196**:150–7. doi:10.1192/bjp.bp.109.067314
32. Takahashi T, Wood SJ, Yung AR, Walterfang M, Phillips LJ, Soulsby B, et al. Superior temporal gyrus volume in antipsychotic-naive people at risk of psychosis. *Br J Psychiatry* (2010) **196**:206–11. doi:10.1192/bjp.bp.109.069732
33. Bhojraj TS, Francis AN, Montrose DM, Keshavan MS. Grey matter and cognitive deficits in young relatives of schizophrenia patients. *Neuroimage* (2011) **54**(Suppl 1):S287–92. doi:10.1016/j.neuroimage.2010.03.069
34. Malla AK, Bodnar M, Joober R, Lepage M. Duration of untreated psychosis is associated with orbital-frontal grey matter volume reductions in first episode psychosis. *Schizophr Res* (2011) **125**:13–20. doi:10.1016/j.schres.2010.09.021
35. Rasser PE, Schall U, Todd J, Michie PT, Ward PB, Johnston P, et al. Gray matter deficits, mismatch negativity, and outcomes in schizophrenia. *Schizophr Bull* (2011) **37**:131–40. doi:10.1093/schbul/sbp060
36. Sweet RA, Bergen SE, Sun Z, Marcsisin MJ, Sampson AR, Lewis DA. Anatomical evidence of impaired feedforward auditory processing in schizophrenia. *Biol Psychiatry* (2007) **61**:854–64. doi:10.1016/j.biopsych.2006.07.033
37. Lewis DA, Sweet RA. Schizophrenia from a neural circuitry perspective: advancing toward rational pharmacological therapies. *J Clin Investig* (2009) **119**:706–16. doi:10.1172/JCI37335
38. Sweet RA, Henteleff RA, Zhang W, Sampson AR, Lewis DA. Reduced dendritic spine density in auditory cortex of subjects with schizophrenia. *Neuropsychopharmacology* (2009) **34**:374–89. doi:10.1038/npp.2008.67
39. Deo AJ, Cahill ME, Li S, Goldszer I, Henteleff R, Vanleeuwen J-E, et al. Increased expression of Kalirin-9 in the auditory cortex of schizophrenia subjects: its role in dendritic pathology. *Neurobiol Dis* (2012) **45**:796–803. doi:10.1016/j.nbd.2011.11.003
40. Salisbury DF, Kuroki N, Kasai K, Shenton ME, Mccarley RW. Progressive and interrelated functional and structural evidence of post-onset brain reduction in schizophrenia. *Arch Gen Psychiatry* (2007) **64**:521–9. doi:10.1001/archpsyc.64.5.521
41. Gogtay N, Giedd JN, Lusk L, Hayashi KM, Greenstein D, Vaituzis AC, et al. Dynamic mapping of human cortical development during childhood through early adulthood. *Proc Natl Acad Sci U S A* (2004) **101**:8174–9. doi:10.1073/pnas.0402680101
42. Kasai K, Shenton ME, Salisbury DF, Hirayasu Y, Lee C-U, Ciszewski AA, et al. Progressive decrease of left superior temporal gyrus gray matter volume in

patients with first-episode schizophrenia. *Am J Psychiatry* (2003) **160**:156–64. doi:10.1176/appi.ajp.160.1.156
43. Javitt D, Zukin S. Recent advances in the phencyclidine model of schizophrenia. *Am J Psychiatry* (1991) **148**:1301–8.
44. Kantrowitz J, Javitt D. *N*-methyl-D-aspartate (NMDA) receptor dysfunction or dysregulation: the final common pathway on the road to schizophrenia? *Brain Res Bull* (2010) **30**:108–21. doi:10.1016/j.brainresbull.2010.04.006
45. Javitt DC, Zukin SR, Heresco-Levy U, Umbricht D. Has an angel shown the way? Etiological and therapeutic implications of the PCP/NMDA model of schizophrenia. *Schizophr Bull* (2012) **38**:958–66. doi:10.1093/schbul/sbs069
46. Jacobsen T, Schröger E. Is there a pre-attentive memory-based comparison of pitch. *Psychophysiology* (2001) **38**:723–7. doi:10.1111/1469-8986.3840723
47. Jacobsen T, Schröger E, Horenkamp T, Winkler I. Mismatch negativity to pitch change: varied stimulus proportions in controlling effects of neural refractoriness on human auditory event-related brain potentials. *Neurosci Lett* (2003) **344**:79–82. doi:10.1016/S0304-3940(03)00408-7
48. Maess B, Jacobsen T, Schröger E, Friederici A. Localizing pre-attentive auditory memory-based comparison: magnetic mismatch negativity to pitch change. *Neuroimage* (2007) **37**:561–71. doi:10.1016/j.neuroimage.2007.05.040
49. Jacobsen T, Schröger E. Measuring duration mismtach negativity. *Clin Neurophysiol* (2003) **114**:1133–43. doi:10.1016/S1388-2457(03)00043-9
50. Schröger E, Wolff C. Mismatch response of the human brain to changes in sound location. *Neuroreport* (1996) **7**:3005–8. doi:10.1097/00001756-199611250-00041
51. Shelley AM, Ward PB, Catts SV, Michie PT, Andrews S, Mcconaghy N. Mismatch negativity: an index of a preattentive processing deficit in schizophrenia. *Biol Psychiatry* (1991) **30**:1059–62. doi:10.1016/0006-3223(91)90126-7
52. Catts SV, Shelley AM, Ward PB, Liebert B, Mcconaghy N, Andrews S, et al. Brain potential evidence for an auditory sensory memory deficit in schizophrenia. *Am J Psychiatry* (1995) **152**:213–9.
53. Todd J, Michie PT, Schall U, Karayanidis F, Yabe H, Naatanen R. Deviant matters: duration, frequency, and intensity deviants reveal different patterns of mismatch negativity reduction in early and late schizophrenia. *Biol Psychiatry* (2008) **63**:58–64. doi:10.1016/j.biopsych.2007.02.016
54. Todd J, Whitson LR, Smith E, Michie PT, Schall U, Ward P. What's intact and what's not within the mismatch negativity system in schizophrenia. *Psychophysiology* (in press).
55. Sams M, Alho K, Naatanen R. Sequential effects on the ERP in discriminating two stimuli. *Biol Psychol* (1983) **17**:41–58. doi:10.1016/0301-0511(83)90065-0
56. Cowan N, Winkler I, Teder W, Naatanen R. Memory prerequisites of mismatch negativity in the auditory event-related potential (ERP). *J Exp Psychol Learn Mem Cogn* (1993) **19**:909–21. doi:10.1037/0278-7393.19.4.909
57. Bendixen A, Roeber U, Schroger E. Regularity extraction and application in dynamic auditory stimulus sequences. *J Cogn Neurosci* (2007) **19**:1664–77. doi:10.1162/jocn.2007.19.10.1664
58. Cooper RJ, Atkinson RJ, Clark RA, Michie PT. Event-related potentials reveal modelling of auditory repetition in the brain. *Int J Psychophysiol* (2013) **88**:74–81. doi:10.1016/j.ijpsycho.2013.02.003
59. Baldeweg T, Klugman A, Gruzelier J, Hirsch SR. Mismatch negativity potentials and cognitive impairment in schizophrenia. *Schizophr Res* (2004) **69**:203–17. doi:10.1016/j.schres.2003.09.009
60. Dima D, Frangou S, Burge L, Braeutigam S, James AC. Abnormal intrinsic and extrinsic connectivity within the magnetic mismatch negativity brain network in schizophrenia: a preliminary study. *Schizophr Res* (2012) **135**:23–7. doi:10.1016/j.schres.2011.12.024
61. Javitt DC, Shelley A, Ritter W. Associated deficits in mismatch negativity generation and tone matching in schizophrenia. *Clin Neurophysiol* (2000) **111**:1733–7. doi:10.1016/S1388-2457(00)00377-1
62. Rabinowicz EF, Silipo G, Goldman R, Javitt DC. Auditory sensory dysfunction in schizophrenia: imprecision or distractibility? *Arch Gen Psychiatry* (2000) **57**:1149–55. doi:10.1001/archpsyc.57.12.1149
63. Light GA, Swerdlow NR, Rissling AJ, Radant A, Sugar CA, Sprock J, et al. Characterization of neurophysiologic and neurocognitive biomarkers for use in genomic and clinical outcome studies of schizophrenia. *PLoS One* (2012) **7**:e39434. doi:10.1371/journal.pone.0039434
64. Jansson LB, Parnas J. Competing definitions of schizophrenia: what can be learned from polydiagnostic studies? *Schizophr Bull* (2007) **33**:1178–200. doi:10.1093/schbul/sbl065
65. Gottesman I, Gould T. The endophenotype concept in psychiatry: etymology and strategic intentions. *Am J Psychiatry* (2003) **160**:636–45. doi:10.1176/appi.ajp.160.4.636
66. Umbricht D, Koller R, Schmid L, Skrabo A, Grubel C, Huber T, et al. How specific are deficits in mismatch negativity generation to schizophrenia? *Biol Psychiatry* (2003) **53**:1120–31. doi:10.1016/S0006-3223(02)01642-6
67. Hall M, Rijsdijk F, Kalidindi S, Schulze K, Kravariti E, Kane F, et al. Genetic overlap between bipolar illness and event-related potentials. *Psychol Med* (2007) **37**:667–78. doi:10.1017/S003329170600972X
68. Hall M, Schulze K, Rijsdijk F, Kalidindi S, Mcdonald C, Bramon E, et al. Are auditory P300 and duration MMN heritable and putative endophenotypes of psychotic bipolar disorder? A Maudsley bipolar twin and family study. *Psychol Med* (2009) **39**:1277–87. doi:10.1017/S0033291709005261
69. Kahkonen S, Yamashita H, Rytsala H, Suominen K, Ahveninen J, Isometsa E. Dysfunction in early auditory processing in major depressive disorder revealed by combined MEG and EEG. *J Psychiatry Neurosci* (2007) **32**:316–22.
70. Takei Y, Kumano S, Hattori S, Uehara T, Kawakubo Y, Kasai K, et al. Preattentive dysfunction in major depression: a magnetoencephalography study using auditory mismatch negativity. *Psychophysiology* (2009) **46**:52–61. doi:10.1111/j.1469-8986.2008.00748.x
71. Qiao Z, Yu Y, Wang L, Yang X, Qiu X, Zhang C, et al. Impaired pre-attentive change detection in major depressive disorder patients revealed by auditory mismatch negativity. *Psychiatry Res* (2013) **211**:78–84. doi:10.1016/j.pscychresns.2012.07.006
72. Hall MH, Rijsdijk F, Picchioni M, Schulze K, Ettinger U, Toulopoulou T, et al. Substantial shared genetic influences on schizophrenia and event-related potentials. *Am J Psychiatry* (2007) **164**:804–12. doi:10.1176/appi.ajp.164.5.804
73. Ahveninen J, Jaaskelainen IP, Osipova D, Huttunen MO, Ilmoniemi RJ, Kaprio J, et al. Inherited auditory-cortical dysfunction in twin pairs discordant for schizophrenia. *Biol Psychiatry* (2006) **60**:612–20. doi:10.1016/j.biopsych.2006.04.015
74. Corlett PR, Honey GD, Fletcher PC. From prediction error to psychosis: ketamine as a pharmacological model of delusions. *J Psychopharmacol* (2007) **21**:238–52. doi:10.1177/0269881107077716
75. Fisher DJ, Labelle A, Knott VJ. Auditory hallucinations and the mismatch negativity: processing speech and non-speech sounds in schizophrenia. *Int J Psychophysiol* (2008) **70**:3–15. doi:10.1016/j.ijpsycho.2008.04.001
76. Fisher DJ, Grant B, Smith DM, Borracci G, Labelle A, Knott VJ. Effects of auditory hallucinations on the mismatch negativity (MMN) in schizophrenia as measured by a modified 'optimal' multi-feature paradigm. *Int J Psychophysiol* (2011) **81**:245–51. doi:10.1016/j.ijpsycho.2011.06.018
77. Fisher DJ, Labelle A, Knott VJ. Alterations of mismatch negativity (MMN) in schizophrenia patients with auditory hallucinations experiencing acute exacerbation of illness. *Schizophr Res* (2012) **139**:237–45. doi:10.1016/j.schres.2012.06.004
78. Shinozaki N, Yabe H, Sato Y, Hiruma T, Sutoh T, Nashida T, et al. The difference in mismatch negativity between the acute and post-acute phase of schizophrenia. *Biol Psychol* (2002) **59**:105–19. doi:10.1016/S0301-0511(01)00129-6
79. Zhou Z, Zhu H, Chen L. Effect of aripiprazole on mismatch negativity (MMN) in schizophrenia. *PLoS One* (2013) **8**:e52186. doi:10.1371/journal.pone.0052186
80. Leifker FR, Patterson TL, Bowie CR, Mausbach BT, Harvey PD. Psychometric properties of performance-based measurements of functional capacity: test-retest reliability, practice effects, and potential sensitivity to change. *Schizophr Res* (2010) **119**:246–52. doi:10.1016/j.schres.2010.03.021
81. Burdick KE, Goldberg JF, Harrow M, Faull RN, Malhotra AK. Neurocognition as a stable endophenotype in bipolar disorder and schizophrenia. *J Nerv Ment Dis* (2006) **194**:255–60. doi:10.1097/01.nmd.0000207360.70337.7e
82. Light GA, Braff DL. Mismatch negativity deficits are associated with poor functioning in schizophrenia patients. *Arch Gen Psychiatry* (2005) **62**:127–36. doi:10.1001/archpsyc.62.2.127
83. Light GA, Braff DL. Stability of mismatch negativity deficits and their relationship to functional impairments in chronic schizophrenia. *Am J Psychiatry* (2005) **162**:1741–3. doi:10.1176/appi.ajp.162.9.1741
84. Kiang M, Light GA, Prugh J, Coulson S, Braff DL, Kutas M. Cognitive, neurophysiological, and functional correlates of proverb interpretation abnormalities in schizophrenia. *J Int Neuropsychol Soc* (2007) **13**:653–63. doi:10.1017/S1355617707070816

85. Hermens DF, Ward PB, Hodge MA, Kaur M, Naismith SL, Hickie IB. Impaired MMN/P3a complex in first-episode psychosis: cognitive and psychosocial associations. *Prog Neuropsychopharmacol Biol Psychiatry* (2010) **34**:822–9. doi:10.1016/j.pnpbp.2010.03.019
86. Friedman T, Sehatpour P, Dias E, Perrin M, Javitt DC. Differential relationships of mismatch negativity and visual p1 deficits to premorbid characteristics and functional outcome in schizophrenia. *Biol Psychiatry* (2012) **71**:521–9. doi:10.1016/j.biopsych.2011.10.037
87. Wynn JK, Sugar C, Horan WP, Kern R, Green MF. Mismatch negativity, social cognition, and functioning in schizophrenia patients. *Biol Psychiatry* (2010) **67**:940–7. doi:10.1016/j.biopsych.2009.11.024
88. Green M, Kern R, Braff D, Mintz J. Neurocognitive deficits and functional outcome in schizophrenia: are we measuring the "right stuff?" *Schizophr Bull* (2000) **26**:119–36. doi:10.1093/oxfordjournals.schbul.a033430
89. Barch DM, Carter CS, Macdonald AW III, Braver TS, Cohen JD. Context-processing deficits in schizophrenia: diagnostic specificity, 4-week course, and relationships to clinical symptoms. *J Abnorm Psychol* (2003) **112**:132–43. doi:10.1037/0021-843X.112.1.132
90. Javitt DC, Shelley A-M, Silipo G, Lieberman JA. Deficits in auditory and visual context-dependent processing in schizophrenia: defining the pattern. *Arch Gen Psychiatry* (2000) **57**:1131–7. doi:10.1001/archpsyc.57.12.1131
91. Magleby K. Modal gating of NMDA receptors. *Trends Neurosci* (2004) **25**:231–3. doi:10.1016/j.tins.2004.03.001
92. Zhang W, Howe J, Popescu G. Distinct gating modes determine the biphasic relaxation of NMDA receptor currents. *Nat Neurosci* (2008) **11**:1373–5. doi:10.1038/nn.2214
93. Popescu G. Modes of glutamate receptor gating. *J Physiol* (2012) **590**:73–91. doi:10.1113/jphysiol.2011.223750
94. Wang H, Stradtman G, Xiao-Jung W, Wen-Jun G. A specialised NMDA receptor function in layer 5 recurrent microcircuitry of the adult rat prefrontal cortex. *Proc Natl Acad Sci U S A* (2008) **105**:16791–6. doi:10.1073/pnas.0804318105
95. Wang M, Yang Y, Ching-Jung W, Nao L, Lu E, Mazer J, et al. NMDA receptors subserve persistent neuronal firing during working memory in dorsolateral prefrontal cortex. *Neuron* (2013) **77**:736–49. doi:10.1016/j.neuron.2012.12.032
96. Miyanishi T, Sumiyoshi T, Higuchi Y, Seo T, Suzuki M. LORETA current source density for duration mismatch negativity and neuropsychological assessment in early schizophrenia. *PLoS One* (2013) **8**:e61152. doi:10.1371/journal.pone.0061152
97. Todd J, Myers R, Pirillo R, Drysdale K. Neuropsychological correlates of auditory perceptual inference: a mismatch negativity (MMN) study. *Brain Res* (2010) **1310**:113–23. doi:10.1016/j.brainres.2009.11.019
98. Todd J, Provost A, Cooper G. Lasting first impressions: a conservative bias in automatic filters of the acoustic environment. *Neuropsychologia* (2011) **49**:3399–405. doi:10.1016/j.neuropsychologia.2011.08.016
99. Cirillo M, Seidman L. Verbal declarative memory dysfunction in schizophrenia: from clinical assessment to genetics and brain mechanisms. *Neuropsychol Rev* (2003) **13**:43–77. doi:10.1023/A:1023870821631
100. Kawakubo Y, Kasai K, Kudo N, Rogers MA, Nakagome K, Itoh K, et al. Phonetic mismatch negativity predicts verbal memory deficits in schizophrenia. *Neuroreport* (2006) **17**:1043–6. doi:10.1097/01.wnr.0000221828.10846.ba
101. Kaur M, Battisti RA, Ward PB, Ahmed A, Hickie IB, Hermens DF. MMN/P3a deficits in first episode psychosis: comparing schizophrenia-spectrum and affective-spectrum subgroups. *Schizophr Res* (2011) **130**:203–9. doi:10.1016/j.schres.2011.03.025
102. Price GW, Michie PT, Johnston J, Innes-Brown H, Kent A, Clissa P, et al. A multivariate electrophysiological endophenotype, from a unitary cohort, shows greater research utility than any single feature in the Western Australian family study of schizophrenia. *Biol Psychiatry* (2006) **60**:1–10. doi:10.1016/j.biopsych.2005.09.010
103. Toyomaki A, Kusumi I, Matsuyama T, Kako Y, Ito K, Koyama T. Tone duration mismatch negativity deficits predict impairment of executive function in schizophrenia. *Prog Neuropsychopharmacol Biol Psychiatry* (2008) **32**:95–9. doi:10.1016/j.pnpbp.2007.07.020
104. Yung AR, Yuen HP, Mcgorry PD, Phillips LJ, Kelly D, Dell'olio M, et al. Mapping the onset of psychosis: the comprehensive assessment of at-risk mental states. *Aust N Z J Psychiatry* (2005) **39**:964–71. doi:10.1080/j.1440-1614.2005.01714.x
105. Jessen F, Fries T, Kucharski C, Nishimura T, Hoenig K, Maier W, et al. Amplitude reduction of the mismatch negativity in first-degree relatives of patients with schizophrenia. *Neurosci Lett* (2001) **309**:185–8. doi:10.1016/S0304-3940(01)02072-9
106. Michie PT, Innes-Brown H, Todd J, Jablensky AV. Duration mismatch negativity in biological relatives of patients with schizophrenia spectrum disorders. *Biol Psychiatry* (2002) **52**:749–58. doi:10.1016/S0006-3223(02)01379-3
107. Bramon E, Croft RJ, Mcdonald C, Virdi GK, Gruzelier JG, Baldeweg T, et al. Mismatch negativity in schizophrenia: a family study. *Schizophr Res* (2004) **67**:1–10. doi:10.1016/S0920-9964(03)00132-4
108. Magno E, Yeap S, Thakore JH, Garavan H, De Sanctis P, Foxe JJ. Are auditory-evoked frequency and duration mismatch negativity deficits endophenotypic for schizophrenia? High-density electrical mapping in clinically unaffected first-degree relatives and first-episode and chronic schizophrenia. *Biol Psychiatry* (2008) **64**:385–91. doi:10.1016/j.biopsych.2008.03.019
109. Hong E, Moran L, Du X, O'Donnell P, Summerfelt A. Mismatch negativity and low frequency oscillations in schizophrenia families. *Clin Neurophysiol* (2012) **123**:1980–8. doi:10.1016/j.clinph.2012.03.011
110. Sevik AE, Anil Yagcioglu AE, Yagcioglu S, Karahan S, Gurses N, Yildiz M. Neuropsychological performance and auditory event related potentials in schizophrenia patients and their siblings: a family study. *Schizophr Res* (2011) **130**:195–202. doi:10.1016/j.schres.2011.04.018
111. Brockhaus-Dumke A, Tendolkar I, Pukrop R, Schultze-Lutter F, Klosterkotter J, Ruhrmann S. Impaired mismatch negativity generation in prodromal subjects and patients with schizophrenia. *Schizophr Res* (2005) **73**:297–310. doi:10.1016/j.schres.2004.05.016
112. Atkinson RJ, Michie PT, Schall U. Duration mismatch negativity and P3a in first-episode psychosis and individuals at ultra-high risk of psychosis. *Biol Psychiatry* (2012) **71**:98–104. doi:10.1016/j.biopsych.2011.08.023
113. Jahshan C, Cadenhead KS, Rissling AJ, Kirihara K, Braff DL, Light GA. Automatic sensory information processing abnormalities across the illness course of schizophrenia. *Psychol Med* (2012) **42**:85–97. doi:10.1017/S0033291711001061
114. Shaikh M, Valmaggia L, Broome MR, Dutt A, Lappin J, Day F, et al. Reduced mismatch negativity predates the onset of psychosis. *Schizophr Res* (2012) **134**:42–8. doi:10.1016/j.schres.2011.09.022
115. Higuchi Y, Sumiyoshi T, Seo T, Miyanishi T, Kawasaki Y, Suzuki M. Mismatch negativity and cognitive performance for the prediction of psychosis in subjects with at-risk mental state. *PLoS One* (2013) **8**:e54080. doi:10.1371/journal.pone.0054080
116. Nagai T, Tada M, Kirihara K, Noriaki Y, Hashimoto R, Araki T, et al. Auditory mismatch negativity and P3a in response to duration and frequency changes in the early stages of psychosis. *Schizophr Res* (2013) **150**:547–54 doi:10.1016/j.schres.2013.08.005
117. Perez V, Woods S, Roach B, Ford J, Mcglashan T, Vh S, et al. Automatic auditory processing deficits in schizophrenia and clinically high-risk patients: forecasting psychosis risk with mismatch negativity. *Biol Psychiatry* (2013). doi:10.1016/j.biopsych.2013.07.038
118. Bodatsch M, Ruhrmann S, Wagner M, Muller R, Schultze-Lutter F, Frommann I, et al. Prediction of psychosis by mismatch negativity. *Biol Psychiatry* (2011) **69**:959–66. doi:10.1016/j.biopsych.2010.09.057
119. Oranje B, Van Berckel BN, Kemner C, Van Ree JM, Kahn RS, Verbaten MN. The effects of a sub-anaesthetic dose of ketamine on human selective attention. *Neuropsychopharmacology* (2000) **22**:293–302. doi:10.1016/S0893-133X(99)00118-9
120. Umbricht D, Schmid L, Koller R, Vollenweider FX, Hell D, Javitt DC. Ketamine-induced deficits in auditory and visual context-dependent processing in healthy volunteers: implications for models of cognitive deficits in schizophrenia. *Arch Gen Psychiatry* (2000) **57**:1139–47. doi:10.1001/archpsyc.57.12.1139
121. Kreitschmann-Andermahr I, Rosburg T, Demme U, Gaser E, Nowak H, Sauer H. Effect of ketamine on the neuromagnetic mismatch field in healthy humans. *Cogn Brain Res* (2001) **12**:109–16. doi:10.1016/S0926-6410(01)00043-X
122. Umbricht D, Vollenweider FX, Schmid L, Grubel C, Skrabo A, Huber T, et al. Effects of the 5-HT2A agonist psilocybin on mismatch negativity generation and AX-continuous performance task: implications for the neuropharmacology of cognitive deficits in schizophrenia. *Neuropsychopharmacology* (2003) **28**:170–81. doi:10.1038/sj.npp.1300005
123. Korostenskaja M, Nikulin VV, Kicic D, Nikulina AV, Kahkonen S. Effects of NMDA receptor antagonist memantine on mismatch negativity. *Brain Res Bull* (2007) **72**:275–83. doi:10.1016/j.brainresbull.2007.01.007

124. Heekeren K, Daumann J, Neukirch A, Stock C, Kawohl W, Norra C, et al. Mismatch negativity generation in the human 5HT2A agonist and NMDA antagonist model of psychosis. *Psychopharmacology* (2008) **199**:77–88. doi:10.1007/s00213-008-1129-4
125. Roser P, Haussleiter IS, Chong H-J, Maier C, Kawohl W, Norra C, et al. Inhibition of cerebral type 1 cannabinoid receptors is associated with impaired auditory mismatch negativity generation in the ketamine model of schizophrenia. *Psychopharmacology* (2011) **218**:611–20. doi:10.1007/s00213-011-2352-y
126. Schmidt A, Bachmann R, Kometer M, Csomor PA, Stephan KE, Seifritz E, et al. Mismatch negativity encoding of prediction errors predicts S-ketamine-induced cognitive impairments. *Neuropsychopharmacology* (2012) **37**:865–75. doi:10.1038/npp.2011.261
127. Gunduz-Bruce H, Reinhart RMG, Roach BJ, Gueorguieva R, Oliver S, D'Souza DC, et al. Glutamatergic Modulation of Auditory Information Processing in the Human Brain. *Biol Psychiatry* (2012) **71**:969–77. doi:10.1016/j.biopsych.2011.09.031
128. Harrison PJ, Weinberger DR. Schizophrenia genes, gene expression, and neuropathology: on the matter of their convergence. *Mol Psychiatry* (2005) **10**:40–68. doi:10.1038/sj.mp.4001558
129. Lewis DA, Moghaddam B. Cognitive dysfunction in schizophrenia: convergence of gamma-aminobutyric acid and glutamate alterations. *Arch Neurol* (2006) **63**:1372–6. doi:10.1001/archneur.63.10.1372
130. Javitt DC, Steinschneider M, Schroeder CE, Arezzo JC. Role of cortical *N*-methyl-D-aspartate receptors in auditory sensory memory and mismatch negativity generation: implications for schizophrenia. *Proc Natl Acad Sci U S A* (1996) **93**:11962–7. doi:10.1073/pnas.93.21.11962
131. Umbricht D, Koller R, Vollenweider FX, Schmid L. Mismatch negativity predicts psychotic experiences induced by NMDA receptor antagonist in healthy volunteers. *Biol Psychiatry* (2002) **51**:400–6. doi:10.1016/S0006-3223(01)01242-2
132. Stephan KE, Baldeweg T, Friston KJ. Synaptic plasticity and dysconnection in schizophrenia. *Biol Psychiatry* (2006) **59**:929–39. doi:10.1016/j.biopsych.2005.10.005
133. Jaaskelainen IP, Lehtokoski A, Alho K, Kujala T, Pekkonen E, Sinclair JD, et al. Low dose of ethanol suppresses mismatch negativity of auditory event-related potentials. *Alcohol Clin Exp Res* (1995) **19**:607–10.
134. Jaaskelainen IP, Pekkonen E, Hirvonen J, Sillanaukee P, Naatanen R. Mismatch negativity subcomponents and ethyl alcohol. *Biol Psychol* (1996) **43**:13–25. doi:10.1016/0301-0511(95)05174-0
135. Lin H, Vicini S, Hsu F-C, Doshi S, Takano H, Coulter DA, et al. Axonal 7 nicotinic ACh receptors modulate presynaptic NMDA receptor expression and structural plasticity of glutamatergic presynaptic boutons. *Proc Natl Acad Sci U S A* (2010) **107**:16661–6. doi:10.1073/pnas.1007397107
136. Moran RJ, Campo P, Symmonds M, Stephan KE, Dolan RJ, Friston KJ. Free energy, precision and learning: the role of cholinergic neuromodulation. *J Neurosci* (2013) **33**:8227–36. doi:10.1523/JNEUROSCI.4255-12.2013
137. Harkrider AW, Hedrick MS. Acute effect of nicotine on auditory gating in smokers and non-smokers. *Hear Res* (2005) **202**:114–28. doi:10.1016/j.heares.2004.11.009
138. Baldeweg T, Wong D, Stephan KE. Nicotinic modulation of human auditory sensory memory: evidence from mismatch negativity potentials. *Int J Psychophysiol* (2006) **59**:49–58. doi:10.1016/j.ijpsycho.2005.07.014
139. Dunbar G, Boeijinga PH, Demazieres A, Cisterni C, Kuchibhatla R, Wesnes K, et al. Effects of TC-1734 (AZD3480), a selective neuronal nicotinic receptor agonist, on cognitive performance and the EEG of young healthy male volunteers. *Psychopharmacology* (2007) **191**:919–29. doi:10.1007/s00213-006-0675-x
140. Knott VJ, Bolton K, Heenan A, Shah D, Fisher DJ, Villeneuve C. Effects of acute nicotine on event-related potential and performance indices of auditory distraction in nonsmokers. *Nicotine Tob Res* (2009) **11**:519–30. doi:10.1093/ntr/ntp044
141. Martin LF, Davalos DB, Kisley MA. Nicotine enhances automatic temporal processing as measured by the mismatch negativity waveform. *Nicotine Tob Res* (2009) **11**:698–706. doi:10.1093/ntr/ntp052
142. Inami R, Kirino E, Inoue R, Arai H. Transdermal nicotine administration enhances automatic auditory processing reflected by mismatch negativity. *Pharmacol Biochem Behav* (2005) **80**:453–61. doi:10.1016/j.pbb.2005.01.001
143. Knott VJ, Scherling CS, Blais CM, Camarda J, Fisher DJ, Millar A, et al. Acute nicotine fails to alter event-related potential or behavioral performance indices of auditory distraction in cigarette smokers. *Nicotine Tob Res* (2006) **8**:263–73. doi:10.1080/14622200600576669
144. Solowij N, Michie PT. Cannabis and cognitive dysfunction: parallels with endophenotypes of schizophrenia? *J Psychiatry Neurosci* (2007) **32**:30–52.
145. Murray RM, Lappin J, Di Forti M. Schizophrenia: from developmental deviance to dopamine dysregulation. *Eur Neuropsychopharmacol* (2008) **18**(Suppl 3):S129–34. doi:10.1016/j.euroneuro.2008.04.002
146. Solowij N, Yucel M, Respondek C, Whittle S, Lindsay E, Pantelis C, et al. Cerebellar white-matter changes in cannabis users with and without schizophrenia. *Psychol Med* (2011) **41**:2349–59. doi:10.1017/S003329171100050X
147. Yucel M, Bora E, Lubman DI, Solowij N, Brewer WJ, Cotton SM, et al. The impact of cannabis use on cognitive functioning in patients with schizophrenia: a meta-analysis of existing findings and new data in a first-episode sample. *Schizophr Bull* (2012) **38**:316–30. doi:10.1093/schbul/sbq079
148. Bossong MG, Niesink RJM. Adolescent brain maturation, the endogenous cannabinoid system and the neurobiology of cannabis-induced schizophrenia. *Prog Neurobiol* (2010) **92**:370–85. doi:10.1016/j.pneurobio.2010.06.010
149. Juckel G, Roser P, Nadulski T, Stadelmann AM, Gallinat J. Acute effects of Delta9-tetrahydrocannabinol and standardized cannabis extract on the auditory evoked mismatch negativity. *Schizophr Res* (2007) **97**:109–17. doi:10.1016/j.schres.2007.08.015
150. Stadelmann AM, Roser P, Arning L, Gallinat J, Epplen JT, Juckel G. Acute effects of delta9-tetrahydrocannabinol on the auditory evoked mismatch negativity are modulated by the NRG1 gene. *Pharmacopsychiatry* (2010) **43**:194–5. doi:10.1055/s-0030-1254088
151. Boucher A, Arnold J, Duffy L, Schofield P, Micheau J, Karl T. Heterozygous neuregulin 1 mice are more sensitive to the behavioural effects of Delta9-tetrahydrocannabinol. *Psychopharmacology* (2007) **192**:325–36. doi:10.1007/s00213-007-0721-3
152. Javitt DC, Doneshka P, Grochowski S, Ritter W. Impaired mismatch negativity generation reflects widespread dysfunction of working memory in schizophrenia. *Arch Gen Psychiatry* (1995) **52**:550–8. doi:10.1001/archpsyc.1995.03950190032005
153. Lawler CP, Prioleau C, Lewis MM, Mak C, Jiang D, Schetz JA, et al. Interactions of the novel antipsychotic aripiprazole (OPC-14597) with dopamine and serotonin receptor subtypes. *Neuropsychopharmacology* (1999) **20**:612–27. doi:10.1016/S0893-133X(98)00099-2
154. Shapiro DA, Renock S, Arrington E, Chiodo LA, Liu LX, Sibley DR, et al. Aripiprazole, a novel atypical antipsychotic drug with a unique and robust pharmacology. *Neuropsychopharmacology* (2003) **28**:1400–11. doi:10.1038/sj.npp.1300203
155. Mailman R. GPCR functional selectivity has therapeutic impact. *Trends Pharmacol Sci* (2007) **28**:390–6. doi:10.1016/j.tips.2007.06.002
156. Han M, Huang X-F, Deng C. Aripiprazole differentially affects mesolimbic and nigrostriatal dopaminergic transmission: implications for long-term drug efficacy and low extrapyramidal side-effects. *Int J Neuropsychopharmacol* (2009) **12**:941–52. doi:10.1017/S1461145709009948
157. Mervaala E, Alhainen K, Helkala EL, Partanen J, Jousmaki V, Vayrynen M, et al. Electrophysiological and neuropsychological effects of a central alpha 2-antagonist atipamezole in healthy volunteers. *Behav Brain Res* (1993) **55**:85–91. doi:10.1016/0166-4328(93)90010-N
158. Schreiber H, Stolz-Born G, Pietrowsky R, Kornhuber HH, Fehm HL, Born J. Improved event-related potential signs of selective attention after the administration of the cholecystokinin analog ceruletide in healthy persons. *Biol Psychiatry* (1995) **37**:702–12. doi:10.1016/0006-3223(94)00207-J
159. Kahkonen S, Ahveninen J, Jaaskelainen IP, Kaakkola S, Naatanen R, Huttunen J, et al. Effects of haloperidol on selective attention: a combined whole-head MEG and high-resolution EEG study. *Neuropsychopharmacology* (2001) **25**:498–504. doi:10.1016/S0893-133X(01)00255-X
160. Pekkonen E, Hirvonen J, Ahveninen J, Kaehkoenen S, Kaakkola S, Huttunen J, et al. Memory-based comparison process not attenuated by haloperidol: a combined MEG and EEG study. *Neuroreport* (2002) **13**:177–81. doi:10.1097/00001756-200201210-00040
161. Ahveninen J, Kahkonen S, Pennanen S, Liesivuori J, Ilmoniemi RJ, Jaaskelainen IP. Tryptophan depletion effects on EEG and MEG responses suggest serotonergic modulation of auditory involuntary attention in humans. *Neuroimage* (2002) **16**:1052–61. doi:10.1006/nimg.2002.1142

162. Leung S, Croft RJ, Baldeweg T, Nathan PJ. Acute dopamine D(1) and D(2) receptor stimulation does not modulate mismatch negativity (MMN) in healthy human subjects. *Psychopharmacology* (2007) **194**:443–51. doi:10.1007/s00213-007-0865-1
163. Korostenskaja M, Kicic D, Kahkonen S. The effect of methylphenidate on auditory information processing in healthy volunteers: a combined EEG/MEG study. *Psychopharmacology* (2008) **197**:475–86. doi:10.1007/s00213-007-1065-8
164. Leung S, Croft RJ, Guille V, Scholes K, O'Neill BV, Phan KL, et al. Acute dopamine and/or serotonin depletion does not modulate mismatch negativity (MMN) in healthy human participants. *Psychopharmacology* (2010) **208**:233–44. doi:10.1007/s00213-009-1723-0
165. Nelken I, Ulanovsky N. Mismatch negativity and stimulus-specific adaptation in animal models. *J Psychophysiol* (2007) **21**:214–23. doi:10.1523/JNEUROSCI.6045-11.2012
166. Ulanovsky N, Las L, Farkas D, Nelken I. Multiple time scales of adaptation in auditory cortex neurons. *J Neurosci* (2004) **24**:10440–53. doi:10.1523/JNEUROSCI.1905-04.2004
167. Eriksson J, Villa AE. Event-related potentials in an auditory oddball situation in the rat. *Biosystems* (2005) **79**:207–12. doi:10.1016/j.biosystems.2004.09.017
168. von der Behrens W, Bauerle P, Kossl M, Gaese BH. Correlating stimulus-specific adaptation of cortical neurons and local field potentials in the awake rat. *J Neurosci* (2009) **29**:13837–49. doi:10.1523/JNEUROSCI.3475-09.2009
169. Farley BJ, Quirk MC, Doherty JJ, Christian EP. Stimulus-specific adaptation in auditory cortex is an NMDA-independent process distinct from the sensory novelty encoded by the mismatch negativity. *J Neurosci* (2010) **30**:16475–84. doi:10.1523/JNEUROSCI.2793-10.2010
170. Taaseh N, Yaron A, Nelken I. Stimulus-specific adaptation and deviance detection in the rat auditory cortex. *PLoS One* (2011) **6**:e23369. doi:10.1371/journal.pone.0023369
171. Fishman YI, Steinschneider M. Searching for the mismatch negativity in primary auditory cortex of the awake monkey: deviance detection or stimulus specific adaptation? *J Neurosci* (2012) **32**:15747–58. doi:10.1523/JNEUROSCI.2835-12.2012
172. Ehrlichman RS, Maxwell CR, Majumdar S, Siegel SJ. Deviance-elicited changes in event-related potentials are attenuated by ketamine in mice. *J Cogn Neurosci* (2008) **20**:1403–14. doi:10.1162/jocn.2008.20097
173. Ehrlichman RS, Luminais SN, White SL, Rudnick ND, Ma N, Dow HC, et al. Neuregulin 1 transgenic mice display reduced mismatch negativity, contextual fear conditioning and social interactions. *Brain Res* (2009) **1294**:116–27. doi:10.1016/j.brainres.2009.07.065
174. Ruusuvirta T, Lipponen A, Pellinen E, Penttonen M, Astikainen P. Auditory cortical and hippocampal-system mismatch responses to duration deviants in urethane-anesthetized rats. *PLoS One* (2013) **8**:e54624. doi:10.1371/journal.pone.0054624
175. Imada A, Morris A, Wiest MC. Deviance detection by a P3-like response in rat posterior parietal cortex. *Front Integr Neurosci* (2012) **6**:127. doi:10.3389/fnint.2012.00127
176. Pincze Z, Lakatos P, Rajkai C, Ulbert I, Karmos G. Separation of mismatch negativity and the N1 wave in the auditory cortex of the cat: a topographic study. *Clin Neurophysiol* (2001) **112**:778–84. doi:10.1016/S1388-2457(01)00509-0
177. Umbricht D, Vyssotki D, Latanov A, Nitsch R, Lipp HP. Deviance-related electrophysiological activity in mice: is there mismatch negativity in mice? *Clin Neurophysiol* (2005) **116**:353–63. doi:10.1016/j.clinph.2004.08.015
178. Jung F, Stephan KE, Backes H, Moran R, Gramer M, Kumagai T, et al. Mismatch responses in the awake rat: evidence from epidural recordings of auditory cortical fields. *PLoS One* (2013) **8**:e63203. doi:10.1371/journal.pone.0063203
179. Tikhonravov D, Neuvonen T, Pertovaara A, Savioja K, Ruusuvirta T, Naatanen R, et al. Effects of an NMDA-receptor antagonist MK-801 on an MMN-like response recorded in anesthetized rats. *Brain Res* (2008) **1203**:97–102. doi:10.1016/j.brainres.2008.02.006
180. Tikhonravov D, Neuvonen T, Pertovaara A, Savioja K, Ruusuvirta T, Naatanen R, et al. Dose-related effects of memantine on a mismatch negativity-like response in anesthetized rats. *Neuroscience* (2010) **167**:1175–82. doi:10.1016/j.neuroscience.2010.03.014
181. Roger C, Hasbroucq T, Rabat A, Vidal F, Burle B. Neurophysics of temporal discrimination in the rat: a mismatch negativity study. *Psychophysiology* (2009) **46**:1028–32. doi:10.1111/j.1469-8986.2009.00840.x
182. Ahmed M, Mallo T, Leppanen PH, Hamalainen J, Ayravainen L, Ruusuvirta T, et al. Mismatch brain response to speech sound changes in rats. *Front Psychol* (2011) **2**:283. doi:10.3389/fpsyg.2011.00283
183. Astikainen P, Stefanics G, Nokia M, Lipponen A, Cong F, Penttonen M, et al. Memory-based mismatch response to frequency changes in rats. *PLoS One* (2011) **6**:e24208. doi:10.1371/journal.pone.0024208
184. Lazar R, Metherate R. Spectral interactions, but no mismatch negativity, in auditory cortex of anesthetized rat. *Hear Res* (2003) **181**:51–6. doi:10.1016/S0378-5955(03)00166-7
185. Astikainen P, Ruusuvirta T, Wikgren J, Penttonen M. Memory-based detection of rare sound feature combinations in anesthetized rats. *Neuroreport* (2006) **17**:1561–4. doi:10.1097/01.wnr.0000233097.13032.7d
186. Nakamura T, Michie PT, Fulham WR, Todd J, Budd TW, Schall U, et al. Epidural auditory event-related potentials in the rat to frequency and duration deviants: evidence of mismatch negativity? *Front Psychol* (2011) **2**:367. doi:10.3389/fpsyg.2011.00367
187. Ruusuvirta T, Penttonen M, Korhonen T. Auditory cortical event-related potentials to pitch deviances in rats. *Neurosci Lett* (1998) **248**:45–8. doi:10.1016/S0304-3940(98)00330-9
188. Ruusuvirta T, Koivisto K, Wikgren J, Astikainen P. Processing of melodic contours in urethane-anaesthetized rats. *Eur J Neurosci* (2007) **26**:701–3. doi:10.1111/j.1460-9568.2007.05687.x
189. Näätänen R. The role of attention in auditory information processing as revealed by event-related potentials and other brain measures of cognitive function. *Behav Brain Sci* (1990) **13**:201–33. doi:10.1017/S0140525X00078407
190. Zoladz PR, Campbell AM, Park CR, Schaefer D, Danysz W, Diamond DM. Enhancement of long-term spatial memory in adult rats by the noncompetitive NMDA receptor antagonists, memantine and neramexane. *Pharmacol Biochem Behav* (2006) **85**:298–306. doi:10.1016/j.pbb.2006.08.011
191. Zuckerman L, Weiner I. Maternal immune activation leads to behavioral and pharmacological changes in the adult offspring. *J Psychiatr Res* (2005) **39**:311–23. doi:10.1016/j.jpsychires.2004.08.008
192. Meyer U, Nyffeler M, Yee BK, Knuesel I, Feldon J. Adult brain and behavioral pathological markers of prenatal immune challenge during early/middle and late fetal development in mice. *Brain Behav Immun* (2008) **22**:469–86. doi:10.1016/j.bbi.2007.09.012
193. Vorhees CV, Graham DL, Braun AA, Schaefer TL, Skelton MR, Richtand NM, et al. Prenatal immune challenge in rats: altered responses to dopaminergic and glutamatergic agents, prepulse inhibition of acoustic startle, and reduced route-based learning as a function of maternal body weight gain after prenatal exposure to poly IC. *Synapse* (2012) **66**:725–37. doi:10.1002/syn.21561
194. Picton TW, Bentin S, Berg P, Donchin E, Hillyard SA, Johnson R, et al. Guidelines for using human event-related potentials to study cognition: Recording standards and publication criteria. *Psychophysiology* (2000) **37**:127–52. doi:10.1111/1469-8986.3720127
195. Todd J, Heathcote A, Mullens D, Whitson LR, Provost A, Winkler I. What controls gain in gain control? Mismatch negativity (MMN), priors and system biases. *Brain Topogr* (in press).
196. Hall J, Romaniuk L, Mcintosh AM, Steele JD, Johnstone EC, Lawrie SM. Associative learning and the genetics of schizophrenia. *Trends Neurosci* (2009) **32**:359–65. doi:10.1016/j.tins.2009.01.011

14

Contributions of Experimental Psychiatry to Research on the Psychosis Prodrome

Mitja Bodatsch*, Joachim Klosterkötter and Jörg Daumann

Department of Psychiatry and Psychotherapy, University of Cologne, Cologne, Germany

***Correspondence:**
Mitja Bodatsch, Department of Psychiatry and Psychotherapy, University of Cologne, Kerpener Street 62, Cologne 50924, Germany
e-mail: mitja.bodatsch@uk-koeln.de

In the recent decades, a paradigmatic change in psychosis research and treatment shifted attention toward the early and particularly the prodromal stages of illness. Despite substantial progress with regard to the neuronal underpinnings of psychosis development, the crucial biological mechanisms leading to manifest illness are yet insufficiently understood. Until today, one significant approach to elucidate the neurobiology of psychosis has been the modeling of psychotic symptoms by psychedelic substances in healthy individuals. These models bear the opportunity to evoke particular neuronal aberrations and the respective psychotic symptoms in a controlled experimental setting. In the present paper, we hypothesize that experimental psychiatry bears unique opportunities in elucidating the biological mechanisms of the prodromal stages of psychosis. Psychosis risk symptoms are attenuated, transient, and often only retrospectively reported. The respective neuronal aberrations are thought being dynamic. The correlation of unstable psychopathology with observed neurofunctional disturbances is thus yet largely unclear. In modeling psychosis, the experimental setting allows not only for evoking particular symptoms, but for the concomitant assessment of psychopathology, neurophysiology, and neuropsychology. Herein, the glutamatergic model will be highlighted exemplarily, with special emphasis on its potential contribution to the elucidation of psychosis development. This model of psychosis appears as candidate for modeling the prodrome by inducing psychotic-like symptoms in healthy individuals. Furthermore, it alters pre-attentive processing like the Mismatch Negativity, an electrophysiological component which has recently been identified as a potential predictive marker of psychosis development. In summary, experimental psychiatry bears the potential to further elucidate the biological mechanisms of the psychosis prodrome. A better understanding of the respective pathophysiology might assist in the identification of predictive markers, and the development of preventive treatments.

Keywords: experimental psychiatry, psychosis modeling, PCP/NMDA, mismatch negativity, clinical high-risk, prodrome, schizophrenia

INTRODUCTION

Since more than 10 decades, researchers aim at understanding the neurobiological mechanisms of psychosis. Concomitant with the debut of modern nosology in the late nineteenth century, almost all pioneer thinkers of psychiatry provided theoretical models regarding the underlying biological mechanisms of psychosis even though the experimental techniques at the time did not allow for any empirical evidence. The paradigmatic claim that "all mental disorders are brain disorders" dates back to Griesinger's works (1). Later on, Kraepelin, the ancestor of modern nosology, proposed that "dementia praecox" originates in a misdirected neurodevelopment and insisted on the idea that psychosis is identical to a brain disease (2). Bleuler, who gave birth to the name "schizophrenia," provided a sophisticated theoretical model of disrupted neural association networks contributing to the schizophrenic *Grundsymptome* (3). In this tradition, one of the last hypotheses can be found in the seminal works of the German psychiatrist Gerd Huber, who proposed an elaborated model to trace back subtle psychopathological changes to neurofunctional disturbances of the limbic system (4, 5). Although not all hypotheses of that kind led to fruitful insights, the increasingly elaborated methods of biological psychiatry partially provided empirical evidence for some models in demonstrating, e.g., reductions in brain volume (6), functional aberrations of association cortices (7), and limbic neuropathology (8), thereby justifying the modeling approach as one primary route to guide empirical and experimental work.

However, the empirical work characterized above necessarily represents a kind of "backwards engineering." Always starting from phenomenology, biological psychiatry is principally conditioned to a verification/falsification dichotomy regarding the primary hypothesis. Thus, this backwards approach is limited by the demarcations given by psychopathology and phenomenological nosology.

In this regard, experimental psychiatry, understood as the modern continuation of ancient theoretical modeling, provides a completive approach to the elucidation of the biological mechanisms of psychosis. The experimental evocation of a psychotic syndrome by psychedelics allows for forward predictions on neurofunctional, cognitive, and psychopathological changes (9). Following this route, experimental psychiatry allows for tracing forwards the consequences of targeted manipulations of neurochemical pathways and for the subsequent comparison with empirical and phenomenological findings.

The birth of experimental psychiatry dates back to the seminal studies of Luby and colleagues (10) who demonstrated that a "schizophrenomimetic" drug evokes psychotic symptoms resembling schizophrenia in healthy individuals (10). Following this approach, Domino et al. were able to evoke comparable symptoms in healthy persons by applying the "dissociative" phencyclidine (PCP)-derivate ketamine (11). In the sequel, empirical findings on the neurochemical features of *N*-methyl-D-aspartate receptor (NMDAR) antagonists as PCP and ketamine first supported the dominating hypothesis of dopamine hyperfunction in schizophrenia (11). However, further evidence demonstrating that *N*-methyl-D-aspartate (NMDA) antagonists critically interact with various regulatory mechanisms of corticolimbic functions that are relevant to schizophrenia led to the establishment of the glutamate hypothesis (11). This hypothesis implies that NMDA-mediated dysfunctions play a critical role not only in dopaminergic regulation, which has been reconceptualized as the final common pathway to psychosis, but particularly predict impairments in cortical, sensory, and associative brain regions that contribute to cognitive and negative symptom dimensions (9). Today, it is widely accepted that the glutamate/NMDA pathway represents a discrete pathophysiological aspect of schizophrenia (9, 12, 13).

However, a yet widely neglected aspect of experimental psychiatry represents its potential contribution to the understanding of psychosis development and pre-psychotic, i.e., prodromal stages [but see Ref. (14, 15)]. This aspect, however, may be of particular interest since the neurobiological mechanisms at the very first, subclinical beginning of psychosis development are yet insufficiently understood (16). Thereby, experimental psychiatry may significantly contribute to the identification of targets for preventive treatments.

In the present review, we aim to investigate if and how experimental psychiatry may further elucidate the biological mechanisms of the psychosis prodrome. Thereto, we will firstly give a short overview on the crucial psychopathological, neurocognitive, and neurofunctional findings in the prodrome with special emphasis on neural information processing [functional magnetic resonance imaging (fMRI), electrophysiology]. Secondly, we will exemplarily focus on the well established PCP/NMDA model of psychosis and its potential to mimic the psychosis prodrome.

METHODS

We carried out a computer search of the MEDLINE database. No limits were set regarding the publication date. We used the following Medical Subject Heading (MeSH) categories: (1) (PCP OR NMDA) AND (psychosis OR schizophrenia), (2) [prediction OR ultra-high-risk (UHR) OR clinical high-risk OR at-risk mental state (ARMS) OR basic symptoms (BS)] AND [psychosis OR schizophrenia], and (3) [neurocognition OR cognition OR fMRI OR P50 OR N100 OR sensory gating OR mismatch negativity (MMN) OR P300] AND [UHR OR prodrome] AND [psychosis OR schizophrenia]. Studies on PCP/NMDA were restricted to human subjects. With regard to the psychosis prodrome, studies were included if current at-risk criteria (COPER/COGDIS, UHR) were employed in the respective studies.

THE PSYCHOSIS PRODROME

PSYCHOPATHOLOGY

The prodrome of psychosis is at first a phenomenological concept. It originates in the observation that mental disorders, and particularly schizophrenia, mostly do not appear at a sudden. In general, manifest psychosis represents the severe end of a long-term development in which subtle psychopathological changes appear years before a diagnosis can be validly made (17). Since full-blown psychosis represents a severe disorder with critical long-term consequences, the establishment of prediction and prevention based on prodromal signs of psychosis has become a main goal of clinical research. However, although early clinical signs of psychosis development can validly be traced backwards after an individual has already developed full-blown psychosis, the forward prediction of transition to psychosis is difficult and the respective approaches bear substantial uncertainty regarding their predictions (18, 19). In sum, two predictive approaches are currently implemented.

The BS approach points to subtle, subjectively experienced changes of mental functions that are thought to mark the earliest stages of psychosis development (20, 21). Empirical research has led to two well-defined criteria, pointing either to a collection of highly predictive cognitive and perceptive disturbances (COPER) or to predominantly cognitive disturbances (COGDIS), respectively (22). Subjects qualifying for the COPER criterion developed psychosis in 34.9% within 11 months on average (range 1–37, median 9 months) (23).

The currently most widely used clinical criteria of psychosis prediction point to so called UHR symptoms that are thought to mark the latest stages of psychosis development (24, 25). According to this approach, either attenuated psychotic symptoms or brief, spontaneously remitting psychotic symptoms or a genetic liability in combination with an actual loss of functioning indicate a markedly increased risk for an imminent onset of full-blown psychosis (26). Transition rates in samples identified by the aforementioned criteria amount to 30% on average within the available observation periods (27).

Taken together, the prediction of psychosis development based on clinical criteria inherits significant uncertainty, as mirrored by non-conversion rates of more than 50%, at least within feasible observation periods (27). This observation has led to a paradigm shift in that the aforementioned criteria are thought to identify a "risk-state" probably leading to psychosis rather than a "prodrome" mandatorily leading to manifest psychosis (17).

Although the prospective identification of individuals making the transition to full-blown psychosis thus faces major challenges, it is undoubted that the prodromal development commonly starts from subtle changes in perception and cognition and ends up with attenuated and transient psychotic symptoms, respectively, at the verge of manifest psychosis (28). Furthermore, even though not highly predictive of the further course, negative symptoms appear at very early stages of the prodromal development, thereby even preceding (pre-)psychotic symptoms (29). Besides psychopathology, however, recent research has suggested that the prodrome can also be validly characterized on other domains, i.e., neurocognition and neurofunctioning (28).

NEUROCOGNITIVE FINDINGS

A huge number of studies demonstrated neurocognitive deficits in individuals at-risk and prodromal subjects, respectively. In particular, studies focusing on working memory, executive functions and verbal fluency/learning were able to provide discriminative statistics for the prospective identification of future converters (30–37). Thereby, investigations employing language based tasks demonstrated that verbal fluency deficits precede psychosis onset up to 30 months (30), and that disturbances of working memory can be found up to 64 months prior to psychosis (31). Executive dysfunctions in the prodrome comprise attention and processing speed which appear as well years before psychosis onset (32, 33, 35, 37).

NEUROFUNCTIONAL FINDINGS

Regarding fMRI investigations, yet two studies compared fMRI correlates of neurocognitive functions in converters (i.e., prodromal subjects) to non-converters. Sabb et al. demonstrated a higher activation of temporal lobes, the frontal operculum, the left precentral gyrus, the caudate, and striatal regions of future converters during the semantic logic condition of a language processing task (38). Allen et al. demonstrated an increased activation in future converters, too, with regard to the left superior frontal gyrus, the middle frontal gyrus, parts of the brainstem, and the left hippocampus in a verbal fluency task (39). Taken together with suggestions of a gradual decline in frontal and striatal activation from the clinical risk state to chronic psychosis (40, 41), particularly regions contributing to language processing seem to be involved in prodromal stages (28). Progressive structural changes during transition to psychosis have been found in the superior temporal gyrus (42).

Regarding electrophysiology, the prodrome seems to be characterized by neuronal disturbances in sensory processing domains. Ziermans and colleagues investigated the Pre-Pulse Inhibition (PPI), a startle response, and suggested a differential deficit in converters vs. non-converters (43, 44). Sensory gating measures (P50/N100) seem to be less relevant to the prodromal development since two out of three studies did not find significant differences between converters and non-converters (45–47). The P3 amplitude, which correlates to memory and attentive processes, has been demonstrated to be exclusively disturbed in future converters by one study (48). Of the published studies evaluating the MMN, a correlate of pre-attentive stimulus discrimination presumably sensitive to the stage of illness (49–54), the majority consistently demonstrated MMN deficits in future converters but not in non-converters (55–60). Bodatsch et al. and later on Perez et al. provided evidence that MMN amplitude deficits predict psychosis onset and allow for an estimation of the remaining time until transition (55, 61). Taken together, correlates of sensory processing and pending higher order functions indicate significant disturbances of neural information processing that may characterize the prodrome (28). Thereby, the MMN might be of particular interest regarding future research (62, 63) and early intervention strategies (64).

THE PCP/NMDA MODEL OF PSYCHOSIS

PCP/NMDA AND PHARMACOLOGY

Phencyclidine is a non-competitive antagonist of the NMDA glutamate receptor (NMDAR) (65). Comparable substances are MK801 and ketamine, respectively (66). The binding of PCP at the receptor is state dependent, thereby limited to the open channel state, and shows stereo-selectivity (67, 68). Other channels that can be blocked by PCP are voltage-dependent sodium and potassium channels as well as, with different binding features, the nicotinic acetylcholine receptor (69–71). Interactions with membrane proteins have been identified with regard to opioid receptors, dopamine, and noradrenaline transporters, respectively (72–74). However, the main action site seems to be the NMDAR, since all other effects are less potent and only of minor importance in the clinically relevant doses of PCP (66).

Since NMDA antagonists have been demonstrated to produce schizophrenia-like symptoms, clinical investigations aimed at evaluating the potential therapeutic benefit of glutamatergic agonists (75). Studies investigating naturally occurring agonists employed glycine, D-serine, and D-alanine, respectively (75). The results demonstrate that the combination of one of these agonists with an antipsychotic leads to significant improvements in positive, negative, and cognitive symptom ratings (76–82). In particular, two studies provided preliminary evidence that glycine might lead to partial symptom remission in subjects clinically at-risk of developing psychosis (83). Furthermore, it has been demonstrated that the glutathione precursor *N*-acetyl-cysteine improves MMN deficits in schizophrenia patients (84).

PCP/NMDA AND PSYCHOPATHOLOGY

Since PCP has first been described as "schizophrenomimetic" in the first publications on that topic (10), subsequent research has been able to quantify the respective positive, negative, and cognitive symptoms by psychopathological rating scales (9, 75). Krystal et al. (85) demonstrated that ketamine produces behavior similar to schizophrenia as assessed with the Brief Psychiatric Rating Scale (BPRS) (85). Moreover, individuals suffering from schizophrenia display increases in positive and negative symptom ratings after administration of NMDA antagonists (85, 86). Taken together, the psychopathological observations suggest that NMDA antagonists affect a brain system that is vulnerable to psychotic experiences (9, 75).

However, positive symptoms provoked by ketamine administration have been demonstrated being less severe as those observed in clinical psychosis (85–87). Moreover, some psychopathological characteristics of clinical psychosis seem to be underrepresented in the PCP/NMDA model since, e.g., hallucinations are relatively rare in experimental psychosis (85, 86). However, perception distortion is a typical symptom after ketamine administration (85, 86). In particular, ketamine affects the intensity and integrity of sensory stimuli (85, 88), and salience (85, 88–90), respectively. In turn, negative and disorganized symptoms as alogia and formal thought disorder, respectively, represent specific psychopathological effects of ketamine (91–93).

PCP/NMDA AND COGNITION

N-methyl-D-aspartate antagonists have been demonstrated to produce a wide range of cognitive deficits. Cognitive functions that can be addressed by ketamine comprise predominantly working memory and executive processing (85, 86, 88, 92–96). Moreover, particular performance deficits after administration of subanesthetic doses of ketamine have been shown for learning/cognitive flexibility and verbal fluency (87), which corresponds to the clinical observation of poverty of speech and circumstantiality after ketamine administration (9). The cognitive deficits produced by NMDA antagonists seem to be rather specifically comparable to schizophrenia, since, e.g., a dissociation between disturbed learning ability but intact ability to retain material once learned can be observed in schizophrenia as well as after administration of NMDA antagonists (9, 75, 97).

Taken together, studies demonstrated particularly the induction of working memory impairments and verbal fluency dysfunction in healthy volunteers. These deficits have been pinpointed to ketamine-induced dysfunctions of frontal and temporo-hippocampal parts of the brain (87).

PCP/NMDA AND NEURAL INFORMATION PROCESSING

Deficits in information processing have been reliably demonstrated across methods in schizophrenia. NMDA antagonists have been demonstrated to induce changes in surrogate markers of neural information processing in terms of behavioral and performance changes (9, 15, 75, 87). Furthermore, disturbances of information processing have directly been observed by neurofunctional measures after NMDA antagonist administration. Schizophrenia-like deficits in MMN generation can be induced by local application of NMDA antagonists as well as by systemic administration in healthy individuals (98–102). In contrast, MMN is not modulated by serotonergic or dopaminergic agonists (103, 104). In turn, other brain potentials, e.g., P300, are significantly affected by administration of other psychotomimetic drugs as psilocybin (105). In normal volunteers, however, reduced MMN amplitudes predict susceptibility to ketamine-induced psychosis (98). In schizophrenia, deficits in pre-attentive tone matching might lead to disturbances of higher order functions as the detection of prosody and auditory emotion recognition (9). In turn, in contrast to the results obtained in animal experiments, NMDA antagonists enhance PPI and startle magnitude (106, 107).

With regard to brain imaging studies, it has been demonstrated that ketamine affects metabolic activity in frontal areas, the cingulum, and the thalamus, respectively (90, 108). Furthermore, ketamine induces an increased dopamine release in the striatum of healthy volunteers (109).

DISCUSSION

PCP/NMDA AND THE PRODROME

The PCP/NMDA model of psychosis has been demonstrated to be particularly suited to mimic certain aspects of psychosis (9, 11, 75, 87). These aspects straddle basic neurophysiological aberrations as well as neurocognitive and psychopathological features. The psychopathological symptom patterns observed after NMDA antagonist administration have been shown to be largely comparable to clinical psychosis (85, 86). Cognitive deficits produced by NMDA antagonists can similarly be found in schizophrenia (85, 86, 92, 93, 96). Deficits in neurophysiological measures that have been conceptualized as an endophenotype of psychotic disorders have been specifically evoked by the NMDA antagonist ketamine (98, 99).

Although experimental psychiatry has thus proven its ability to advance the neurobiological understanding of schizophrenia, it still faces many criticism. The neurofunctional and psychopathological changes, respectively, evoked in an experimental setting lack many aspects of clinical psychosis (11). Furthermore, experimental psychiatry falls short of modeling the complex brain network disturbances that underlie schizophrenia (11). The evoked changes are moreover transient, thus not able to mimic long term, reciprocal neurodynamics, and represent in sum only partial aspects of the pathophysiological picture. However, mimicking the vast complexity of psychosis in general or schizophrenia in particular shall certainly not be the goal of experimental psychiatry (11). At the foremost, such a modeling approach would distract any well-defined forward predictions. Instead, experimental psychiatry should aim at providing insights in the effects of particular synaptic functions in psychosis (11).

However, it has yet been almost neglected that particularly these alleged imitations of such models provide some unique opportunities in themselves. Psychosis models promoted our understanding of the crucial pathophysiological features of clinical psychosis. Since the prodrome represents "early psychosis," it can be assumed that the neurobiological properties of the prodrome are at large the very same as in full-blown psychosis, merely at an earlier stage. However, the phenotype of manifest psychosis results not only from the latest differentiation of certain neurobiological alterations, but represents a complex interplay of accumulating developmental factors and progressive pathophysiological changes. This pathophysiological progression defines the later stages of psychosis and makes them distinct from their clinical and biological precursors (110). For example, the pattern of MMN deficits in later stages of schizophrenia has been demonstrated to be different from the early and particularly prodromal stages (111). From a clinical perspective, neurobiological factors at early stages of illness might inform primarily about disease trajectories and prognosis, whereas factors at later stages might inform foremost about persistent pathophysiological mechanisms (110). Experimental modeling of the pre-psychotic stages might thus assist to understand the crucial neurobiological pathways that turn the spontaneously remitting clinical high-risk state into a prodromal development, although these states are clinically indistinguishable (28, 55). However, although models that explicitly address the prodrome of psychosis are yet to come, the existing well established models of psychosis may already provide opportunities for research in this respect.

In synopsis of the literature, the PCP/NMDA model of psychosis displays some properties that brings it close to the prodromal stages of psychosis (see **Table 1** for overview). As in the clinical at-risk state, the produced symptoms might resemble in large parts the full-blown psychotic symptomatology (85, 86), but are, however, transient like at least in some high-risk conditions (brief limited intermittent psychotic symptoms). With regard to psychopathology, it has been demonstrated that the

Table 1 | Comparison of the PCP/NMDA model and the psychosis prodrome.

Domain	Properties of the PCP/NMDA model	Features of the psychosis prodrome
Psychopathology	Positive symptoms less severe than in clinical psychosis Impaired integrity/intensity of sensory perception and aberrant salience Specific negative and disorganized symptoms	Attenuated psychotic symptoms Cognitive and perceptive basic symptoms Negative/disorganized symptoms precede positive symptoms
Cognition	Verbal fluency deficits and working memory impairments	Verbal fluency deficits and working memory impairments predict psychosis onset
Information processing	Dysfunctions of frontal and temporo-hippocampal parts of the brain MMN rather specifically affected	Deficits in frontal cortex, temporal lobes, and hippocampus associated with psychosis onset MMN predicts psychosis onset and allows for estimating the time until transition

positive symptoms induced by NMDA antagonists are less severe than in clinical psychosis (85, 86). This is reminiscent of the attenuated psychotic symptoms that can be found in the prodrome (26). Moreover, changes in the integrity and intensity of sensory perception as well as aberrant salience, as produced by NMDA antagonists (85, 88, 89), might be analogous to the respective BS (21). Besides that, subanesthetic doses of ketamine have been demonstrated to induce particularly negative and disorganized symptoms (91–93) that have been found to precede positive symptoms in the prodromal development (29). Moreover, deficits in verbal fluency and working memory, respectively, which can be evoked by subanesthetic doses of ketamine as well (85, 86, 92–94), have been demonstrated in individuals at-risk and in prodromal stages by neuropsychological and neurofunctional (fMRI) investigations (30–33, 35–39). In clinical studies, the aforementioned cognitive deficits have been demonstrated being predictive of future transition to psychosis in at-risk samples (30–33, 35–37). Finally, the MMN, which has been demonstrated to be predictive of psychosis development (55–58), is rather specifically affected by PCP/NMDA antagonists (9, 75) and altered MMN amplitudes in healthy individuals predicted the individual's susceptibility to PCP induced psychotic experiences (98). The latter aspect suggests that vulnerability as well as resilience to psychotic experiences might be further understood by a detailed elucidation of NMDA antagonist actions in sensory domains. A close relationship between EEG measures, structural brain changes, and glutamate neurotransmission in the psychosis prodrome has already been demonstrated (112, 113). Counterintuitively, however, a PPI deficit as observed in schizophrenia can not be evoked by NMDA antagonists (107), which might illustrate the limitations of modeling. Following the implications of the glutamate hypothesis, at least two studies have yet been able to demonstrate beneficial effects of the naturally occurring agonist glycine in the at-risk state (83).

CONTRIBUTIONS OF EXPERIMENTAL PSYCHIATRY TO THE UNDERSTANDING OF PSYCHOSIS DEVELOPMENT

At least with regard to the PCP/NMDA model of psychosis, some features advocate in favor of the models potential to advance the understanding of psychosis development. As clinical psychosis, however, not all aspects of the prodrome might be sufficiently represented in such a model. In particular, it is yet only speculative if the symptoms provoked by NMDA antagonists are comparable to prodromal psychopathology (21, 24). Moreover, since psychosis development might proceed via different psychopathological syndromes (21, 24, 26) and more than one pathophysiological pathway (110), it is an open question if and which of these could be best mimicked by psychedelic substances. Furthermore, although much of the neurocognitive and neurofunctional disturbances observed in the prodrome might be evoked by NMDA antagonists, the representation might be rather incomplete.

However, the potential contribution of experimental psychiatry to the understanding of the psychosis prodrome should not be underestimated. As in schizophrenia, prodrome modeling might allow for strong forward predictions and assist in the identification of crucial pathophysiological mechanism as illustrated by the glutamate hypothesis (9, 75), which has been significantly promoted by the results of PCP/NMDA research. Regarding the at-risk state of psychosis, the application of glutamatergic agonists might be understood as a logical consequence of the implications derived from the PCP/NMDA model. Experimental psychiatry might thus not only advance basic research, but assist in the identification of targeted pharmacological interventions in putative prodromal stages of illness.

CONCLUSION

A synopsis of the literature shows that the prodrome of psychosis has been almost neglected by experimental psychiatry and the focus has yet been on manifest psychotic disorders. Since prevention of mental disorders became increasingly relevant in the recent decades, it might be fruitful to further evaluate the potential contribution of experimental psychiatry to this goal. As exemplarily illustrated by the PCP/NMDA model of psychosis, however, many aspects advocate that prodromal stages might be validly mimicked by psychedelic substances. In particular, psychopathological as well as neurocognitive and neurofunctional findings in the prodrome seem to be well represented by the PCP/NMDA model. In this regard, future research should aim at comparing the psychopathological properties of putative prodrome models to the respective clinical observations. Furthermore, neurocognitive and neurofunctional effects, respectively, of psychedelics should be evaluated with regard to those deficits that have been demonstrated being predictive of psychosis development.

In summary, experimental psychiatry bears the potential to further elucidate the biological mechanisms of the psychosis prodrome. A better understanding of the respective pathophysiology might assist in the identification of predictive markers, and the development of preventive treatments.

REFERENCES

1. Griesinger W. *Pathologie und Therapie der psychischen Krankheiten, für Ärzte und Studierende.* Stuttgart: Krabbe (1845).
2. Kraepelin E. *Psychiatrie: ein Lehrbuch für Studirende und Aerzte.* Leipzig: J. A. Barth (1899).
3. Bleuler E. *Dementia praecox oder Gruppe der Schizophrenien.* Leipzig: F. Deuticke (1911).
4. Süllwold L, Huber G. Schizophrene Basisstörungen. In: Hippius H, Janzarik W, Müller C, editors. *Monographien aus dem Gesamtgebiete der Psychiatrie.* Berlin: Springer (1986).
5. Klosterkötter J. Basissymptome und Endphänomene der Schizophrenie – Eine empirische Untersuchung der psychopathologischen Übergangsreihen zwischen defizitären und produktiven Schizophreniesymptomen. In: Hippius H, Janzarik W, Müller C, editors. *Monographien aus dem Gesamtgebiete der Psychiatrie.* Berlin: Springer (1988).
6. Levitt JJ, Bobrow L, Lucia D, Srinivasan P. A selective review of volumetric and morphometric imaging in schizophrenia. *Curr Top Behav Neurosci* (2010) **4**:243–81. doi:10.1007/7854_2010_53
7. Maren S, Phan KL, Liberzon I. The contextual brain: implications for fear conditioning, extinction and psychopathology. *Nat Rev Neurosci* (2013) **14**(6):417–28. doi:10.1038/nrn3492
8. Pankow A, Knobel A, Voss M, Heinz A. Neurobiological correlates of delusion: beyond the salience attribution hypothesis. *Neuropsychobiology* (2012) **66**(1):33–43. doi:10.1159/000337132
9. Javitt DC, Zukin SR, Heresco-Levy U, Umbricht D. Has an angel shown the way? Etiological and therapeutic implications of the PCP/NMDA model of schizophrenia. *Schizophr Bull* (2012) **38**(5):958–66. doi:10.1093/schbul/sbs069
10. Luby ED, Cohen BD, Rosenbaum G, Gottlieb JS, Kelley R. Study of a new schizophrenomimetic drug; sernyl. *AMA Arch Neurol Psychiatry* (1959) **81**(3):363–9. doi:10.1001/archneurpsyc.1959.02340150095011
11. Moghaddam B, Krystal JH. Capturing the angel in "angel dust": twenty years of translational neuroscience studies of NMDA receptor antagonists in animals and humans. *Schizophr Bull* (2012) **38**(5):942–9. doi:10.1093/schbul/sbs075
12. Kantrowitz JT, Javitt DC. Thinking glutamatergically: changing concepts of schizophrenia based upon changing neurochemical models. *Clin Schizophr Relat Psychoses* (2010) **4**(3):189–200. doi:10.3371/CSRP.4.3.6
13. Kantrowitz JT, Javitt DC. N-methyl-d-aspartate (NMDA) receptor dysfunction or dysregulation: the final common pathway on the road to schizophrenia? *Brain Res Bull* (2010) **83**(3–4):108–21. doi:10.1016/j.brainresbull.2010.04.006
14. Corlett PR, Honey GD, Fletcher PC. From prediction error to psychosis: ketamine as a pharmacological model of delusions. *J Psychopharmacol* (2007) **21**(3):238–52. doi:10.1177/0269881107077716
15. Corlett PR, Frith CD, Fletcher PC. From drugs to deprivation: a Bayesian framework for understanding models of psychosis. *Psychopharmacology (Berl)* (2009) **206**(4):515–30. doi:10.1007/s00213-009-1561-0
16. Keshavan MS, Berger G, Zipursky RB, Wood SJ, Pantelis C. Neurobiology of early psychosis. *Br J Psychiatry Suppl* (2005) **48**:s8–18. doi:10.1192/bjp.187.48.s8
17. Ruhrmann S, Schultze-Lutter F, Klosterkotter J. Probably at-risk, but certainly ill – advocating the introduction of a psychosis spectrum disorder in DSM-V. *Schizophr Res* (2010) **120**(1–3):23–37. doi:10.1016/j.schres.2010.03.015
18. Ruhrmann S, Klosterkötter J, Bodatsch M, Nikolaides A, Julkowski D, Hilboll D, et al. Chances and risks of predicting psychosis. *Eur Arch Psychiatry Clin Neurosci* (2012) **262**(Suppl 2):S85–90. doi:10.1007/s00406-012-0361-4
19. Ruhrmann S, Schultze-Lutter F, Klosterkötter J. Sub-threshold states of psychosis – a challenge to diagnosis and treatment. *Clin Neuropsychiatry* (2010) **7**(2):72–87.
20. Klosterkötter J, Hellmich M, Steinmeyer EM, Schultze-Lutter F. Diagnosing schizophrenia in the initial prodromal phase. *Arch Gen Psychiatry* (2001) **58**(2):158–64. doi:10.1001/archpsyc.58.2.158
21. Schultze-Lutter F. Subjective symptoms of schizophrenia in research and the clinic: the basic symptom concept. *Schizophr Bull* (2009) **35**(1):5–8. doi:10.1093/schbul/sbn139
22. Klosterkötter J, Schultze-Lutter F, Bechdolf A, Ruhrmann S. Prediction and prevention of schizophrenia: what has been achieved and where to go next? *World Psychiatry* (2011) **10**(3):165–74.
23. Schultze-Lutter F, Klosterkötter J, Picker H, Steinmeyer E, Ruhrmann S. Predicting first-episode psychosis by basic symptom criteria. *Clin Neuropsychiatry* (2007) **4**:11–22.
24. Fusar-Poli P, Borgwardt S, Bechdolf A, Addington J, Riecher-Rossler A, Schultze-Lutter F, et al. The psychosis high-risk state: a comprehensive state-of-the-art review. *JAMA Psychiatry* (2013) **70**(1):107–20. doi:10.1001/jamapsychiatry.2013.269
25. Schultze-Lutter F, Schimmelmann BG, Ruhrmann S, Michel C. 'A rose is a rose is a rose', but at-risk criteria differ. *Psychopathology* (2013) **46**(2):75–87. doi:10.1159/000339208
26. Yung AR, Phillips LJ, McGorry PD, McFarlane CA, Francey S, Harrigan S, et al. Prediction of psychosis. A step towards indicated prevention of schizophrenia. *Br J Psychiatry Suppl* (1998) **172**(33):14–20.
27. Fusar-Poli P, Bonoldi I, Yung AR, Borgwardt S, Kempton MJ, Valmaggia L, et al. Predicting psychosis: meta-analysis of transition outcomes in individuals at high clinical risk. *Arch Gen Psychiatry* (2012) **69**(3):220–9. doi:10.1001/archgenpsychiatry.2011.1472
28. Bodatsch M, Klosterkotter J, Muller R, Ruhrmann S. Basic disturbances of information processing in psychosis prediction. *Front Psychiatry* (2013) **4**:93. doi:10.3389/fpsyt.2013.00093
29. an der Heiden W, Hafner H. The epidemiology of onset and course of schizophrenia. *Eur Arch Psychiatry Clin Neurosci* (2000) **250**(6):292–303. doi:10.1007/s004060070004
30. Lencz T, Smith CW, McLaughlin D, Auther A, Nakayama E, Hovey L, et al. Generalized and specific neurocognitive deficits in prodromal schizophrenia. *Biol Psychiatry* (2006) **59**(9):863–71. doi:10.1016/j.biopsych.2005.09.005
31. Riecher-Rossler A, Pflueger MO, Aston J, Borgwardt SJ, Brewer WJ, Gschwandtner U, et al. Efficacy of using cognitive status in predicting psychosis: a 7-year follow-up. *Biol Psychiatry* (2009) **66**(11):1023–30. doi:10.1016/j.biopsych.2009.07.020
32. Pukrop R, Ruhrmann S, Schultze-Lutter F, Bechdolf A, Brockhaus-Dumke A, Klosterkotter J. Neurocognitive indicators for a conversion to psychosis: comparison of patients in a potentially initial prodromal state who did or did not convert to a psychosis. *Schizophr Res* (2007) **92**(1–3):116–25. doi:10.1016/j.schres.2007.01.020
33. Kim HS, Shin NY, Jang JH, Kim E, Shim G, Park HY, et al. Social cognition and neurocognition as predictors of conversion to psychosis in individuals at ultra-high risk. *Schizophr Res* (2011) **130**(1–3):170–5. doi:10.1016/j.schres.2011.04.023
34. Becker HE, Nieman DH, Dingemans PM, van de Fliert JR, De Haan L, Linszen DH. Verbal fluency as a possible predictor for psychosis. *Eur Psychiatry* (2010) **25**(2):105–10. doi:10.1016/j.eurpsy.2009.08.003
35. Lin A, Yung AR, Nelson B, Brewer WJ, Riley R, Simmons M, et al. Neurocognitive predictors of transition to psychosis: medium- to long-term findings from a sample at ultra-high risk for psychosis. *Psychol Med* (2013) **43**(11):2349–60. doi:10.1017/S0033291713000123
36. Seidman LJ, Giuliano AJ, Meyer EC, Addington J, Cadenhead KS, Cannon TD, et al. Neuropsychology of the prodrome to psychosis in the NAPLS consortium: relationship to family history and conversion to psychosis. *Arch Gen Psychiatry* (2010) **67**(6):578–88. doi:10.1001/archgenpsychiatry.2010.66
37. Shah J, Eack SM, Montrose DM, Tandon N, Miewald JM, Prasad KM, et al. Multivariate prediction of emerging psychosis in adolescents at high risk for schizophrenia. *Schizophr Res* (2012) **141**(2–3):189–96. doi:10.1016/j.schres.2012.08.012
38. Sabb FW, van Erp TG, Hardt ME, Dapretto M, Caplan R, Cannon TD, et al. Language network dysfunction as a predictor of outcome in youth at clinical high risk for psychosis. *Schizophr Res* (2010) **116**(2–3):173–83. doi:10.1016/j.schres.2009.09.042
39. Allen P, Luigjes J, Howes OD, Egerton A, Hirao K, Valli I, et al. Transition to psychosis associated with prefrontal and subcortical dysfunction in ultra high-risk individuals. *Schizophr Bull* (2012) **38**(6):1268–76. doi:10.1093/schbul/sbr194

40. Pantelis C, Yucel M, Bora E, Fornito A, Testa R, Brewer WJ, et al. Neurobiological markers of illness onset in psychosis and schizophrenia: the search for a moving target. *Neuropsychol Rev* (2009) **19**(3):385–98. doi:10.1007/s11065-009-9114-1
41. Fusar-Poli P. Voxel-wise meta-analysis of fMRI studies in patients at clinical high risk for psychosis. *J Psychiatry Neurosci* (2012) **37**(2):106–12. doi:10.1503/jpn.110021
42. Takahashi T, Wood SJ, Yung AR, Soulsby B, McGorry PD, Suzuki M, et al. Progressive gray matter reduction of the superior temporal gyrus during transition to psychosis. *Arch Gen Psychiatry* (2009) **66**(4):366–76. doi:10.1001/archgenpsychiatry.2009.12
43. Ziermans T, Schothorst P, Magnee M, van Engeland H, Kemner C. Reduced prepulse inhibition in adolescents at risk for psychosis: a 2-year follow-up study. *J Psychiatry Neurosci* (2011) **36**(2):127–34. doi:10.1503/jpn.100063
44. Ziermans TB, Schothorst PF, Sprong M, Magnee MJ, van Engeland H, Kemner C. Reduced prepulse inhibition as an early vulnerability marker of the psychosis prodrome in adolescence. *Schizophr Res* (2012) **134**(1):10–5. doi:10.1016/j.schres.2011.10.009
45. Brockhaus-Dumke A, Schultze-Lutter F, Mueller R, Tendolkar I, Bechdolf A, Pukrop R, et al. Sensory gating in schizophrenia: P50 and N100 gating in antipsychotic-free subjects at risk, first-episode, and chronic patients. *Biol Psychiatry* (2008) **64**(5):376–84. doi:10.1016/j.biopsych.2008.02.006
46. Hsieh MH, Shan JC, Huang WL, Cheng WC, Chiu MJ, Jaw FS, et al. Auditory event-related potential of subjects with suspected pre-psychotic state and first-episode psychosis. *Schizophr Res* (2012) **140**(1–3):243–9. doi:10.1016/j.schres.2012.06.021
47. van Tricht MJ, Nieman DH, Koelman JT, Mensink AJ, Bour LJ, van der Meer JN, et al. Sensory gating in subjects at ultra high risk for developing a psychosis before and after a first psychotic episode. *World J Biol Psychiatry* (2012). doi:10.3109/15622975.2012.680911
48. van Tricht MJ, Nieman DH, Koelman JH, van der Meer JN, Bour LJ, de Haan L, et al. Reduced parietal P300 amplitude is associated with an increased risk for a first psychotic episode. *Biol Psychiatry* (2010) **68**(7):642–8. doi:10.1016/j.biopsych.2010.04.022
49. Hermens DF, Ward PB, Hodge MA, Kaur M, Naismith SL, Hickie IB. Impaired MMN/P3a complex in first-episode psychosis: cognitive and psychosocial associations. *Prog Neuropsychopharmacol Biol Psychiatry* (2010) **34**(6):822–9. doi:10.1016/j.pnpbp.2010.03.019
50. Kaur M, Battisti RA, Ward PB, Ahmed A, Hickie IB, Hermens DF. MMN/P3a deficits in first episode psychosis: comparing schizophrenia-spectrum and affective-spectrum subgroups. *Schizophr Res* (2011) **130**(1–3):203–9. doi:10.1016/j.schres.2011.03.025
51. Horton J, Millar A, Labelle A, Knott VJ. MMN responsivity to manipulations of frequency and duration deviants in chronic, clozapine-treated schizophrenia patients. *Schizophr Res* (2011) **126**(1–3):202–11. doi:10.1016/j.schres.2010.11.028
52. Salisbury DF, Kuroki N, Kasai K, Shenton ME, McCarley RW. Progressive and interrelated functional and structural evidence of post-onset brain reduction in schizophrenia. *Arch Gen Psychiatry* (2007) **64**(5):521–9. doi:10.1001/archpsyc.64.5.521
53. Salisbury DF, Shenton ME, Griggs CB, Bonner-Jackson A, McCarley RW. Mismatch negativity in chronic schizophrenia and first-episode schizophrenia. *Arch Gen Psychiatry* (2002) **59**(8):686–94. doi:10.1001/archpsyc.59.8.686
54. Rasser PE, Schall U, Todd J, Michie PT, Ward PB, Johnston P, et al. Gray matter deficits, mismatch negativity, and outcomes in schizophrenia. *Schizophr Bull* (2011) **37**(1):131–40. doi:10.1093/schbul/sbp060
55. Bodatsch M, Ruhrmann S, Wagner M, Muller R, Schultze-Lutter F, Frommann I, et al. Prediction of psychosis by mismatch negativity. *Biol Psychiatry* (2011) **69**(10):959–66. doi:10.1016/j.biopsych.2010.09.057
56. Higuchi Y, Sumiyoshi T, Seo T, Miyanishi T, Kawasaki Y, Suzuki M. Mismatch negativity and cognitive performance for the prediction of psychosis in subjects with at-risk mental state. *PLoS One* (2013) **8**(1):e54080. doi:10.1371/journal.pone.0054080
57. Shaikh M, Valmaggia L, Broome MR, Dutt A, Lappin J, Day F, et al. Reduced mismatch negativity predates the onset of psychosis. *Schizophr Res* (2012) **134**(1):42–8. doi:10.1016/j.schres.2011.09.022
58. Atkinson RJ, Michie PT, Schall U. Duration mismatch negativity and P3a in first-episode psychosis and individuals at ultra-high risk of psychosis. *Biol Psychiatry* (2012) **71**(2):98–104. doi:10.1016/j.biopsych.2011.08.023
59. Murphy JR, Rawdon C, Kelleher I, Twomey D, Markey PS, Cannon M, et al. Reduced duration mismatch negativity in adolescents with psychotic symptoms: further evidence for mismatch negativity as a possible biomarker for vulnerability to psychosis. *BMC Psychiatry* (2013) **13**:45. doi:10.1186/1471-244X-13-45
60. Jahshan C, Cadenhead KS, Rissling AJ, Kirihara K, Braff DL, Light GA. Automatic sensory information processing abnormalities across the illness course of schizophrenia. *Psychol Med* (2012) **42**(1):85–97. doi:10.1017/S0033291711001061
61. Perez VB, Woods SW, Roach BJ, Ford JM, McGlashan TH, Srihari VH, et al. Automatic auditory processing deficits in schizophrenia and clinical high-risk patients: forecasting psychosis risk with mismatch negativity. *Biol Psychiatry* (2013). doi:10.1016/j.biopsych.2013.07.038
62. Light GA, Naatanen R. Mismatch negativity is a breakthrough biomarker for understanding and treating psychotic disorders. *Proc Natl Acad Sci U S A* (2013) **110**(38):15175–6. doi:10.1073/pnas.1313287110
63. Belger A, Yucel GH, Donkers FC. In search of psychosis biomarkers in high-risk populations: is the mismatch negativity the one we've been waiting for? *Biol Psychiatry* (2012) **71**(2):94–5. doi:10.1016/j.biopsych.2011.11.009
64. Nagai T, Tada M, Kirihara K, Araki T, Jinde S, Kasai K. Mismatch negativity as a "translatable" brain marker toward early intervention for psychosis: a review. *Front Psychiatry* (2013) **4**:115. doi:10.3389/fpsyt.2013.00115
65. Anis NA, Berry SC, Burton NR, Lodge D. The dissociative anaesthetics, ketamine and phencyclidine, selectively reduce excitation of central mammalian neurones by N-methyl-aspartate. *Br J Pharmacol* (1983) **79**(2):565–75. doi:10.1111/j.1476-5381.1983.tb11031.x
66. Morris BJ, Cochran SM, Pratt JA. PCP: from pharmacology to modelling schizophrenia. *Curr Opin Pharmacol* (2005) **5**(1):101–6. doi:10.1016/j.coph.2004.08.008
67. Ferrer-Montiel AV, Merino JM, Planells-Cases R, Sun W, Montal M. Structural determinants of the blocker binding site in glutamate and NMDA receptor channels. *Neuropharmacology* (1998) **37**(2):139–47. doi:10.1016/S0028-3908(98)00007-0
68. Zheng X, Zhang L, Wang AP, Araneda RC, Lin Y, Zukin RS, et al. Mutation of structural determinants lining the N-methyl-D-aspartate receptor channel differentially affects phencyclidine block and spermine potentiation and block. *Neuroscience* (1999) **93**(1):125–34. doi:10.1016/S0306-4522(99)00154-2
69. ffrench-Mullen JM, Rogawski MA. Interaction of phencyclidine with voltage-dependent potassium channels in cultured rat hippocampal neurons: comparison with block of the NMDA receptor-ionophore complex. *J Neurosci* (1989) **9**(11):4051–61.
70. Vincent JP, Bidard JN, Lazdunski M, Romey G, Tourneur Y, Vignon J. Identification and properties of phencyclidine-binding sites in nervous tissues. *Fed Proc* (1983) **42**(9):2570–3.
71. Oswald RE, Bamberger MJ, McLaughlin JT. Mechanism of phencyclidine binding to the acetylcholine receptor from Torpedo electroplaque. *Mol Pharmacol* (1984) **25**(3):360–8.
72. Garey RE, Heath RG. The effects of phencyclidine on the uptake of 3H-catecholamines by rat striatal and hypothalamic synaptosomes. *Life Sci* (1976) **18**(10):1105–10. doi:10.1016/0024-3205(76)90145-4
73. Pubill D, Gasulla D, Sureda FX, Camins A, Pallas M, Escubedo E, et al. Characterization of [3H]nisoxetine binding in rat vas deferens membranes: modulation by sigma and PCP ligands. *Life Sci* (1998) **62**(8):763–73. doi:10.1016/S0024-3205(97)01174-0
74. Sokolov BP. Expression of NMDAR1, GluR1, GluR7, and KA1 glutamate receptor mRNAs is decreased in frontal cortex of "neuroleptic-free" schizophrenics: evidence on reversible up-regulation by typical neuroleptics. *J Neurochem* (1998) **71**(6):2454–64. doi:10.1046/j.1471-4159.1998.71062454.x
75. Javitt DC. Glutamatergic theories of schizophrenia. *Isr J Psychiatry Relat Sci* (2010) **47**(1):4–16.
76. Javitt DC, Zylberman I, Zukin SR, Heresco-Levy U, Lindenmayer JP. Amelioration of negative symptoms in schizophrenia by glycine. *Am J Psychiatry* (1994) **151**(8):1234–6.
77. Heresco-Levy U, Javitt DC, Ermilov M, Mordel C, Silipo G, Lichtenstein M. Efficacy of high-dose glycine in the treatment of enduring negative symptoms of schizophrenia. *Arch Gen Psychiatry* (1999) **56**(1):29–36. doi:10.1001/archpsyc.56.1.29

78. Javitt DC, Silipo G, Cienfuegos A, Shelley AM, Bark N, Park M, et al. Adjunctive high-dose glycine in the treatment of schizophrenia. *Int J Neuropsychopharmacol* (2001) **4**(4):385–91.
79. Neeman G, Blanaru M, Bloch B, Kremer I, Ermilov M, Javitt DC, et al. Relation of plasma glycine, serine, and homocysteine levels to schizophrenia symptoms and medication type. *Am J Psychiatry* (2005) **162**(9):1738–40. doi:10.1176/appi.ajp.162.9.1738
80. Tsai G, Yang P, Chung LC, Lange N, Coyle JT. D-serine added to antipsychotics for the treatment of schizophrenia. *Biol Psychiatry* (1998) **44**(11):1081–9. doi:10.1016/S0006-3223(98)00279-0
81. Tsai GE, Yang P, Chang YC, Chong MY. D-alanine added to antipsychotics for the treatment of schizophrenia. *Biol Psychiatry* (2006) **59**(3):230–4. doi:10.1016/j.biopsych.2005.06.032
82. Buchanan RW, Javitt DC, Marder SR, Schooler NR, Gold JM, McMahon RP, et al. The Cognitive and Negative Symptoms in Schizophrenia Trial (CONSIST): the efficacy of glutamatergic agents for negative symptoms and cognitive impairments. *Am J Psychiatry* (2007) **164**(10):1593–602. doi:10.1176/appi.ajp.2007.06081358
83. Woods SW, Walsh BC, Hawkins KA, Miller TJ, Saksa JR, D'Souza DC, et al. Glycine treatment of the risk syndrome for psychosis: report of two pilot studies. *Eur Neuropsychopharmacol* (2013) **23**(8):931–40. doi:10.1016/j.euroneuro.2012.09.008
84. Lavoie S, Murray MM, Deppen P, Knyazeva MG, Berk M, Boulat O, et al. Glutathione precursor, N-acetyl-cysteine, improves mismatch negativity in schizophrenia patients. *Neuropsychopharmacology* (2008) **33**(9):2187–99. doi:10.1038/sj.npp.1301624
85. Krystal JH, Karper LP, Seibyl JP, Freeman GK, Delaney R, Bremner JD, et al. Subanesthetic effects of the noncompetitive NMDA antagonist, ketamine, in humans. Psychotomimetic, perceptual, cognitive, and neuroendocrine responses. *Arch Gen Psychiatry* (1994) **51**(3):199–214. doi:10.1001/archpsyc.1994.03950030035004
86. Malhotra AK, Pinals DA, Weingartner H, Sirocco K, Missar CD, Pickar D, et al. NMDA receptor function and human cognition: the effects of ketamine in healthy volunteers. *Neuropsychopharmacology* (1996) **14**(5):301–7. doi:10.1016/0893-133X(95)00137-3
87. Bubenikova-Valesova V, Horacek J, Vrajova M, Hoschl C. Models of schizophrenia in humans and animals based on inhibition of NMDA receptors. *Neurosci Biobehav Rev* (2008) **32**(5):1014–23. doi:10.1016/j.neubiorev.2008.03.012
88. Oye I, Paulsen O, Maurset A. Effects of ketamine on sensory perception: evidence for a role of N-methyl-D-aspartate receptors. *J Pharmacol Exp Ther* (1992) **260**(3):1209–13.
89. Vollenweider FX, Leenders KL, Oye I, Hell D, Angst J. Differential psychopathology and patterns of cerebral glucose utilisation produced by (S)- and (R)-ketamine in healthy volunteers using positron emission tomography (PET). *Eur Neuropsychopharmacol* (1997) **7**(1):25–38. doi:10.1016/S0924-977X(96)00042-9
90. Vollenweider FX, Leenders KL, Scharfetter C, Antonini A, Maguire P, Missimer J, et al. Metabolic hyperfrontality and psychopathology in the ketamine model of psychosis using positron emission tomography (PET) and [18F]fluorodeoxyglucose (FDG). *Eur Neuropsychopharmacol* (1997) **7**(1):9–24. doi:10.1016/S0924-977X(96)00039-9
91. Adler CM, Malhotra AK, Elman I, Goldberg T, Egan M, Pickar D, et al. Comparison of ketamine-induced thought disorder in healthy volunteers and thought disorder in schizophrenia. *Am J Psychiatry* (1999) **156**(10):1646–9.
92. Krystal JH, Karper LP, Bennett A, D'Souza DC, Abi-Dargham A, Morrissey K, et al. Interactive effects of subanesthetic ketamine and subhypnotic lorazepam in humans. *Psychopharmacology (Berl)* (1998) **135**(3):213–29. doi:10.1007/s002130050503
93. Krystal JH, D'Souza DC, Karper LP, Bennett A, Abi-Dargham A, Abi-Saab D, et al. Interactive effects of subanesthetic ketamine and haloperidol in healthy humans. *Psychopharmacology (Berl)* (1999) **145**(2):193–204. doi:10.1007/s002130051049
94. Ghoneim MM, Hinrichs JV, Mewaldt SP, Petersen RC. Ketamine: behavioral effects of subanesthetic doses. *J Clin Psychopharmacol* (1985) **5**(2):70–7.
95. Radant AD, Bowdle TA, Cowley DS, Kharasch ED, Roy-Byrne PP. Does ketamine-mediated N-methyl-D-aspartate receptor antagonism cause schizophrenia-like oculomotor abnormalities? *Neuropsychopharmacology* (1998) **19**(5):434–44. doi:10.1016/S0893-133X(98)00030-X
96. Adler CM, Goldberg TE, Malhotra AK, Pickar D, Breier A. Effects of ketamine on thought disorder, working memory, and semantic memory in healthy volunteers. *Biol Psychiatry* (1998) **43**(11):811–6. doi:10.1016/S0006-3223(97)00556-8
97. Javitt DC, Grochowski S, Shelley AM, Ritter W. Impaired mismatch negativity (MMN) generation in schizophrenia as a function of stimulus deviance, probability, and interstimulus/interdeviant interval. *Electroencephalogr Clin Neurophysiol* (1998) **108**(2):143–53. doi:10.1016/S0168-5597(97)00073-7
98. Umbricht D, Koller R, Vollenweider FX, Schmid L. Mismatch negativity predicts psychotic experiences induced by NMDA receptor antagonist in healthy volunteers. *Biol Psychiatry* (2002) **51**(5):400–6. doi:10.1016/S0006-3223(01)01242-2
99. Umbricht D, Schmid L, Koller R, Vollenweider FX, Hell D, Javitt DC. Ketamine-induced deficits in auditory and visual context-dependent processing in healthy volunteers: implications for models of cognitive deficits in schizophrenia. *Arch Gen Psychiatry* (2000) **57**(12):1139–47. doi:10.1001/archpsyc.57.12.1139
100. Tikhonravov D, Neuvonen T, Pertovaara A, Savioja K, Ruusuvirta T, Naatanen R, et al. Effects of an NMDA-receptor antagonist MK-801 on an MMN-like response recorded in anesthetized rats. *Brain Res* (2008) **1203**:97–102. doi:10.1016/j.brainres.2008.02.006
101. Javitt DC, Steinschneider M, Schroeder CE, Arezzo JC. Role of cortical N-methyl-D-aspartate receptors in auditory sensory memory and mismatch negativity generation: implications for schizophrenia. *Proc Natl Acad Sci U S A* (1996) **93**(21):11962–7. doi:10.1073/pnas.93.21.11962
102. Ehrlichman RS, Maxwell CR, Majumdar S, Siegel SJ. Deviance-elicited changes in event-related potentials are attenuated by ketamine in mice. *J Cogn Neurosci* (2008) **20**(8):1403–14. doi:10.1162/jocn.2008.20097
103. Umbricht D, Vollenweider FX, Schmid L, Grubel C, Skrabo A, Huber T, et al. Effects of the 5-HT2A agonist psilocybin on mismatch negativity generation and AX-continuous performance task: implications for the neuropharmacology of cognitive deficits in schizophrenia. *Neuropsychopharmacology* (2003) **28**(1):170–81. doi:10.1038/sj.npp.1300005
104. Leung S, Croft RJ, Baldeweg T, Nathan PJ. Acute dopamine D(1) and D(2) receptor stimulation does not modulate mismatch negativity (MMN) in healthy human subjects. *Psychopharmacology (Berl)* (2007) **194**(4):443–51. doi:10.1007/s00213-007-0865-1
105. Kometer M, Schmidt A, Bachmann R, Studerus E, Seifritz E, Vollenweider FX. Psilocybin biases facial recognition, goal-directed behavior, and mood state toward positive relative to negative emotions through different serotonergic subreceptors. *Biol Psychiatry* (2012) **72**(11):898–906. doi:10.1016/j.biopsych.2012.04.005
106. Linn GS, O'Keeffe RT, Lifshitz K, Schroeder C, Javitt DC. Behavioral effects of orally administered glycine in socially housed monkeys chronically treated with phencyclidine. *Psychopharmacology (Berl)* (2007) **192**(1):27–38. doi:10.1007/s00213-007-0771-6
107. Abel KM, Allin MP, Hemsley DR, Geyer MA. Low dose ketamine increases prepulse inhibition in healthy men. *Neuropharmacology* (2003) **44**(6):729–37. doi:10.1016/S0028-3908(03)00073-X
108. Langsjo JW, Kaisti KK, Aalto S, Hinkka S, Aantaa R, Oikonen V, et al. Effects of subanesthetic doses of ketamine on regional cerebral blood flow, oxygen consumption, and blood volume in humans. *Anesthesiology* (2003) **99**(3):614–23. doi:10.1097/00000542-200309000-00016
109. Breier A, Adler CM, Weisenfeld N, Su TP, Elman I, Picken L, et al. Effects of NMDA antagonism on striatal dopamine release in healthy subjects: application of a novel PET approach. *Synapse* (1998) **29**(2):142–7. doi:10.1002/(SICI)1098-2396(199806)29:2<142::AID-SYN5>3.0.CO;2-7
110. Banati R, Hickie IB. Therapeutic signposts: using biomarkers to guide better treatment of schizophrenia and other psychotic disorders. *Med J Aust* (2009) **190**(4 Suppl):S26–32.
111. Todd J, Michie PT, Schall U, Karayanidis F, Yabe H, Naatanen R. Deviant matters: duration, frequency, and intensity deviants reveal different patterns of mismatch negativity reduction in early and late schizophrenia. *Biol Psychiatry* (2008) **63**(1):58–64. doi:10.1016/j.biopsych.2007.02.016
112. Stone JM, Bramon E, Pauls A, Sumich A, McGuire PK. Thalamic neurochemical abnormalities in individuals with prodromal symptoms of schizophrenia – relationship to auditory event-related potentials. *Psychiatry Res* (2010) **183**(2):174–6. doi:10.1016/j.pscychresns.2010.05.004

113. Stone JM, Day F, Tsagaraki H, Valli I, McLean MA, Lythgoe DJ, et al. Glutamate dysfunction in people with prodromal symptoms of psychosis: relationship to gray matter volume. *Biol Psychiatry* (2009) **66**(6):533–9. doi:10.1016/j.biopsych.2009.05.006

15

Neurocognitive Functioning in Schizophrenia and Bipolar Disorder: Clarifying Concepts of Diagnostic Dichotomy vs. Continuum

Carissa N. Kuswanto[1], Min Y. Sum[1] and Kang Sim[1,2]*

[1] *Research Division, Institute of Mental Health/Woodbridge Hospital, Singapore*
[2] *Department of General Psychiatry, Institute of Mental Health/Woodbridge Hospital, Singapore*

***Correspondence:**
Kang Sim, Department of General Psychiatry, Institute of Mental Health/Woodbridge Hospital, 10, Buangkok View, 539747, Singapore
e-mail: kang_sim@imh.com.sg

The Kraepelinian dichotomy posits that patients with schizophrenia (SCZ) and bipolar disorder (BD) present as two separate psychotic entities such that they differ in terms of clinical severity including neurocognitive functioning. Our study aimed to specifically compare and contrast the level of neurocognitive functioning between SCZ and BD patients and identify predictors of their poor neurocognitive functioning. We hypothesized that patients with SCZ had a similar level of neurocognitive impairment compared with BD. About 49 healthy controls (HC), 72 SCZ, and 42 BD patients who were matched for age, gender, and premorbid IQ were administered the Brief Assessment of Cognition battery (BAC). Severity of psychopathology and socio-occupational functioning were assessed for both patients groups. Both BD and SCZ groups demonstrated similar patterns of neurocognitive deficits across several domains (verbal memory, working memory, semantic fluency, processing speed) compared with HC subjects. However, no significant difference was found in neurocognitive functioning between BD and SCZ patients, suggesting that both patient groups suffer the same degree of neurocognitive impairment. Patients with lower level of psychosocial functioning [$F_{(1,112)} = 2.661$, $p = 0.009$] and older age [$F_{(1,112)} = -2.625$, $p = 0.010$], not diagnosis or doses of psychotropic medications, predicted poorer overall neurocognitive functioning as measured by the lower BAC composite score. Our findings of comparable neurocognitive impairments between SCZ and BD affirm our hypothesis and support less the Kraepelinian concept of dichotomy but more of a continuum of psychotic spectrum conditions. This should urge clinicians to investigate further the underlying neural basis of these neurocognitive deficits, and be attentive to the associated socio-demographic and clinical profile in order to recognize and optimize early the management of the widespread neurocognitive deficits in patients with SCZ and BD.

Keywords: schizophrenia, bipolar disorder, Kraepelinian dichotomy, neurocognitive functions, psychosocial functioning, psychotic spectrum

INTRODUCTION

The Kraepelinian dichotomy, a prominent paradigm in psychiatry, has influenced nosology for severe psychiatric disorders such as schizophrenia (SCZ) and bipolar disorder (BD) within diagnostic classification systems including the Diagnostic Statistical Manual of Mental Disorders and the International Classification of Diseases for many decades (1, 2). The paradigm posits that patients with dementia praecox (SCZ) and manic depression (BD) present as two separate psychotic disorders (3, 4). Evidence in support of the Kraepelinian notion includes volumetric neuroimaging differences in brain regions such as the amygdala, hippocampus, and lateral ventricles that appear to be disorder-specific (5–7). In addition, unlike BD, reduced gray matter volumes and neurocognitive neuromotor impairments occur in the prodromal stage of SCZ despite both having early onset of illness during adolescence and recent findings of common genetic predisposition in BD and SCZ (6, 8–13). Furthermore, patients with SCZ are thought to suffer more extensive brain morphological abnormalities and more severe neurocognitive deficits in comparison with patients with BD (14–18). Other than the apparent empirical evidence, the Kraepelinian dichotomy is appealing clinically due to its conceptual and diagnostic simplicity (19, 20).

However, several issues challenge the dichotomous paradigm of psychotic disorders with respect to SCZ and BD. These issues include the overlapping organic basis and blurred boundaries between psychoses from emerging biological data (21, 22), the non-specificity of psychopathological features such as perceptual disturbances and affective symptoms between SCZ and BD, and the shared genetic susceptibility loci uncovered within recent genome-wide association studies (GWAS) (23, 24). Accumulating evidence from clinical observations, antipsychotic treatment, and findings of neurocognitive functioning in SCZ and BD further argued against the Kraepelinian dichotomy. First, clinicians frequently encounter patients who do not fall neatly into either category, such as individuals with schizoaffective disorders and BD patients with prominent psychotic symptoms. Second, dopamine dysregulation has been implicated in both disorders, making antipsychotic drugs useful in the management of SCZ as well as BD (6, 8). Third, with regards to neurocognitive functioning, extant studies have reported poorer neurocognitive functioning in patients with SCZ compared to those with BD, but there are also data suggesting that patients with SCZ are comparable with BD patients in terms of neurocognitive impairments (14, 25–31). These inconsistent findings on neurocognitive functioning may be due to differences in sample size, specific neurocognitive deficits measured, type of scales used, and presence of other confounders including age and premorbid intelligence (26, 27, 30, 32).

Thus, in this study, we aimed to specifically compare and contrast the level of neurocognitive functioning between patients with SCZ and BD as well as identify predictors of poor neurocognitive functioning in these patients. Based on clinical impression within a tertiary psychiatric hospital context and extant data, we hypothesized that patients with SCZ had a similar level of neurocognitive impairment compared with BD and the neurocognitive impairment is associated with particular socio-demographic and clinical factors after taking into account premorbid intelligence, level of education, and psychotropic medications prescribed.

MATERIALS AND METHODS

PARTICIPANTS

The cross-sectional study sample comprised of a total of 163 participants [72 patients diagnosed with SCZ, 42 patients with BD, and 49 healthy controls (HC)] who gave their written informed consent to participate in the study after a detailed explanation of the study procedures. Patients with SCZ and BD were recruited from the outpatient settings of the Institute of Mental Health, Singapore. All diagnoses were confirmed by a psychiatrist (Kang Sim) using information obtained from the existing medical record, clinical history, mental status examination, interviews with the patients and their significant others as well as the administration of the Structured Clinical Interview for DSM-IV disorders – Patient Version (SCID-I/P) (33). All patients were maintained on a stable dose of psychotropic medication for at least 2 weeks prior to the recruitment and did not have their medication withdrawn for the purpose of the study. HC were administered the Structured Clinical Interview for DSM-IV disorders – Non-Patient Version (SCID-I/NP) (34). None of the participants had a history of significant and/or unstable/untreated medical illnesses such as seizure disorder, head trauma, or cerebrovascular accidents. Moreover, no subjects had a current or past history of substance use or alcohol use disorder. This study was approved by the Institutional Review Boards of the Institute of Mental Health, Singapore.

NEUROCOGNITIVE ASSESSMENT

The brief assessment of cognition battery

The Brief Assessment of Cognition (BAC) battery (35) was administered to all subjects. The subjects were randomly assigned to a sequence of BAC version A and B. The BAC scales include:

1. Verbal memory task – a subject was given 5 attempts to remember 15 words and recall as many words as possible;
2. Digit sequencing task – a subject was presented with clusters of numbers of increasing length and then asked to repeat in order from the lowest to highest length;
3. Token motor task – a subject was given 100 plastic tokens and asked to place 2 tokens at a time within a container as quickly as possible within 60 s;
4. Verbal fluency – divided into semantic and letter fluency, whereby a subject was asked to name as many words as possible within a specific category (e.g., supermarket items), and to name words that begin with a specific letter (e.g., F and S) within 60 s, respectively;
5. Symbol coding task – a subject was asked to write matching numbers from 1 to 9 to symbols within 90 s;
6. Tower of London – as an example, a subject was shown two pictures of three balls of different colors arranged on three different pegs, whereby the balls were arranged differently on each picture and the subjects were asked to give the total number of times the balls in one picture needed to be moved in order to end with the arrangement in the other picture.

We divided the token motor task into two measures, namely the number of tokens correctly placed into a container (tokens correct) and the number of tokens left after 60 s (tokens left). Although both measures tap motor speed function, tokens correct measure did not credit the subjects for tokens put into container incorrectly (i.e., not picked up and placed at the same time) which required eye-hand coordination and precision in order to perform the task correctly. Digit sequencing task, token motor task, symbol coding, and Tower of London measured working memory, motor speed, attention, and speed of information processing and executive functioning respectively (35, 36).

Wide range achievement test (reading scale)

The wide range achievement test (WRAT) (37) reading subscale was used to measure premorbid intelligence in all the subjects.

CLINICAL ASSESSMENTS

Global assessment of functioning

The global assessment of functioning (GAF) (38) rated (from 0 to 90) the severity of symptoms, disability, and the total level of social and occupational functioning. The GAF was administered to both SCZ and BD groups.

Positive and negative syndrome scale

The positive and negative syndrome scale (PANSS) (39) allowed characterization and quantification of psychotic psychopathology. The scale has 7 items for positive symptoms, 7 items for negative symptoms, and 16 items for general psychopathology. The PANSS was administered to SCZ and BD patients.

Young mania rating scales

The Young mania rating scales (YMRS) (40) contains 11 items which were used to measure the severity of manic symptoms in BD patients. There are four items that are graded on a 0–8 scale (irritability, speech, thought content, and disruptive/aggressive behavior). The remaining seven items are graded on a 0–4 scale. The YMRS scale was administered to SCZ and BD patients.

STATISTICAL ANALYSES

All statistical tests were performed using PASW for Windows, version 18.0 (SPSS, Inc., Chicago, IL, USA). The normality of distributions of continuous measures was checked with the Kolmogorov–Smirnov one-sample test. Socio-demographic variables were compared using two sample student t-tests and F-test for continuous variables, and chi-square test for categorical variables. Two-way analysis of covariance (ANCOVA) was used to examine for any difference in neurocognitive functioning (BAC task performance) between the groups after adjusting for the covariates described below. We first compared the neurocognitive measures between all three groups, HC vs. SCZ and HC vs. BD, and adjusting for covariates of age, gender, years of education, and premorbid IQ. We then specifically compared the BAC item performance between SCZ and BD patients, by adjusting for premorbid IQ, age, gender, years of education, and clinical characteristics such as the duration of illness, duration of untreated psychosis, GAF scores, PANSS composite scores, YMRS scores, and antipsychotic dose in terms of mean daily chlorpromazine (CPZ) mg equivalents. Stepwise linear regression analyses were performed to determine predictors of neurocognitive functioning in patients including socio-demographic (such as age, gender) and clinical characteristics (such as diagnosis, duration of illness, GAF scores, PANSS composite scores, YMRS scores, and antipsychotic dose). The significance level for statistical tests was set at two tailed $p < 0.05$.

RESULTS

SOCIO-DEMOGRAPHIC CHARACTERISTICS

Across the three subject groups (HC, SCZ, BD), there were significant differences in subject's and mother's years of education but there was no significant difference in age, sex, handedness, and WRAT scores. Compared to patients with BD, patients with SCZ had longer duration of untreated psychosis and lower level of psychosocial functioning as reflected by the lower GAF scores. There was no significant difference in age, gender, handedness, years of education, WRAT scores, age of onset, and duration of illness between SCZ and BD. The socio-demographic and clinical features of the subjects are shown in **Table 1**.

NEUROCOGNITIVE FUNCTIONING

Table 2 showed the neurocognitive profile across the entire subject sample based on the BAC battery administration. HC subjects scored the highest in all BAC items compared to SCZ and BD patients. Compared to HC, patients with SCZ scored lower in BAC tasks of verbal memory, semantic and letter fluency, digit sequencing, tokens left, symbol coding, total BAC score indicating neurocognitive deficits in verbal memory and fluency, working memory, motor speed, and attention. Compared to HC, patients

Table 1 | Demographic and clinical characteristics of the participants.

Characteristic	HC ($n = 49$)		SCZ ($n = 72$)		BD ($n = 42$)		Statistical analysis			
							SCZ vs. BD		All three groups	
	Mean	SD	Mean	SD	Mean	SD	t-test	p	F-test	p
Age	31.9	10.4	31.47	8.29	32.57	9.673	−0.642	0.522	0.191	0.827
Subject's years of education	13.59	1.62	12.31	2.039	12.15	2.291	0.364	0.717	7.849	0.001*
Father's years of education	8.53	4.22	7.62	3.697	7.31	3.317	0.447	0.655	1.454	0.237
Mother's years of education	7.88	4.29	6.93	3.815	4.98	4.129	2.551	0.012*	6.228	0.002*
WRAT scores	49.78	4.25	49.75	5.301	49.88	4.994	−0.13	0.897	0.75	0.474
Duration of illness	–	–	4.77	5.317	3.32	56.39	1.394	0.166	–	–
Age of onset	–	–	26.69	8.073	28.24	9.294	−0.931	0.354	–	–
Duration of untreated psychosis	–	–	1.715	2.206	0.296	0.528	4.094	<0.001*	–	–
Mean daily CPZ mg equivalents	–	–	185.76	197.47	157.38	174.89	0.771	0.442	–	–
GAF scores										
Total	–	–	50.18	18.821	64.9	21.101	−3.852	<0.001*	–	–
Symptoms	–	–	54.36	20.292	64.98	21.39	−2.641	0.009*	–	–
Disability	–	–	51.46	19.092	65.69	19.749	−3.791	<0.001*	–	–
PANSS										
Positive symptoms	–	–	10.79	3.715	8.55	2.839	3.379	0.001*	–	–
Negative symptoms	–	–	8.33	2.116	7.05	0.309	3.906	<0.001*	–	–
General psychopathology	–	–	20.89	3.71	17.79	1.828	5.067	<0.001*	–	–
Total score	–	–	40.01	7.135	33.38	4.120	5.506	<0.001*	–	–
YMRS	–	–	1.56	2.469	3.4	4.607	2.485	0.015*	–	–
	N	%	N	%	N	%	χ^2	p	χ^2	p
Male	28	57.1	38	52.8	17	40.5	1.608	0.205	2.442	0.295
Right-handed	46	93.9	70	97.2	40	97.6	1.148	0.284	1.102	0.576

*BD, bipolar disorder; CPZ, chlorpromazine; GAF, global assessment of functioning; HC, healthy controls; PANSS, positive and negative syndrome scale; SCZ, schizophrenia; WRAT, wide range achievement test; YMRS, young mania rating scale. *p < 0.05.*

Table 2 | Neurocognitive functioning across subjects based on brief assessment of cognition battery (BAC).

BAC domains	HC ($n=49$)		SCZ ($n=72$)		BD ($n=42$)		ANCOVA[a]						ANCOVA[b]	
							All three groups		HC vs. SCZ		HC vs. BD		SCZ vs. BD	
	Mean	SD	Mean	SD	Mean	SD	*F*	*p*	*F*	*p*	*F*	*p*	*F*	*p*
Verbal memory	9.07	1.92	7.60	2.11	7.85	1.91	6.45	0.002**	9.84	0.002**	11.99	0.001**	0.92	0.340
Digit sequencing	21.62	3.01	19.04	4.54	18.68	4.07	4.64	0.011*	7.13	0.009*	9.74	0.002**	0.05	0.942
Tokens correct	76.12	12.90	73.46	69.26	64.55	15.97	0.54	0.587	0.12	0.729	10.44	0.002**	0.63	0.430
Tokens left	19.56	12.96	25.57	12.65	26.00	13.60	3.50	0.033*	6.55	0.012*	3.90	0.051	0.32	0.573
Semantic fluency	24.64	5.82	20.10	5.77	21.17	5.86	6.13	0.003**	12.05	0.001**	5.58	0.020*	0.18	0.674
Letter fluency	13.91	3.71	12.51	4.51	12.21	4.82	4.27	0.016*	6.83	0.010*	7.35	0.008*	0.02	0.895
Symbol coding	64.68	10.43	49.21	11.42	50.55	10.45	27.47	<0.001**	48.31	<0.001**	32.85	<0.001**	0.08	0.773
Tower of London	17.04	2.12	16.17	3.79	16.27	3.49	0.24	0.785	0.36	0.548	0.17	0.683	0.08	0.783
BAC total	277.66	28.25	239.36	77.12	232.60	43.69	6.27	0.002**	8.00	0.006*	28.55	<0.001**	0.36	0.552

*BAC, brief assessment of cognition battery; BD, bipolar disorder; CPZ, chlorpromazine; GAF, global assessment of functioning; HC, healthy controls; SCZ, schizophrenia; WRAT, wide range achievement test. *p < 0.05 **p < 0.01.*

[a]*Adjusted for WRAT, age, gender, and years of education.*

[b]*Adjusted for WRAT, age, gender, years of education, duration of untreated psychosis, duration of illness, GAF (total, symptoms, and disability), antipsychotic dose, and PANSS and YMRS composite scores.*

with BD scored lower in BAC tasks of verbal memory, semantic and letter fluency, digit sequencing, tokens correct, symbol coding, total BAC score indicating almost similar neurocognitive deficits as SCZ in verbal memory and fluency, working memory, motor speed, and attention. After taking into account multiple comparisons (at conservative threshold of $p < 0.005$), patients with SCZ scored lower on tasks of verbal memory, semantic fluency, symbol coding, and patients with BD scored lower on verbal memory, digit sequencing, and symbol coding when compared with HC.

However, there was no significant difference in all neurocognitive domains of BAC when SCZ and BD groups were compared and after controlling for covariates such as demographic characteristics (age, gender, years of education, WRAT scores) and clinical features (duration of untreated psychosis, antipsychotic dose, as well as GAF, PANSS, and YMRS composite scores). We also noted the possibility that a history of psychosis in BD patients may be associated with poorer performance in neurocognitive tasks compared to those BD subjects without history of psychosis (30). Thus, we performed a *post hoc* analysis whereby we compared BD patients with history of psychosis and those without and we found no significant difference in all neurocognitive performance in all BAC domains.

Multivariate linear regression analyses with the overall BAC score as the dependent variable and demographic (age, gender, education) and clinical factors (diagnosis, WRAT scores, GAF scores, PANSS composite scores, YMRS scores, duration of illness, duration of untreated psychosis, antipsychotic dose) as predictor variables revealed that patients with lower level of psychosocial functioning as indicated by lower GAF score [$F_{(1,112)} = 2.023$, $p = 0.046$] and older age [$F_{(1,112)} = -2.190$, $p = 0.031$], but not diagnosis or doses of psychotropic medications, were associated with poorer overall neurocognitive functioning as measured by the lower BAC composite score.

DISCUSSION

There were several main findings in this study. First, patients with BD and SCZ were found to have greater neurocognitive impairments in most of the BAC domains compared to the HC who were matched for age, gender and premorbid intelligence. Second, the extensive neurocognitive impairments found in SCZ were comparable with those observed in patients with BD. Third, the level of psychosocial functioning and age of patients with SCZ and BD were associated with neurocognitive impairment and not diagnosis or antipsychotic dose. Our findings highlighted that both SCZ and BD patients in our study sample suffered largely similar neurocognitive impairments, which support a continuum concept of psychosis rather than the Kraepelinean concept of dichotomous psychotic conditions.

Our findings of comparable and extensive neurocognitive impairments in both SCZ and BD are consistent with some earlier studies reporting findings of specific neurocognitive impairments across the patient groups. For example, BD and SCZ patients scored significantly worse than control subjects in verbal memory task (assessed by the California Verbal Learning Test), which did not differ when both patient groups were compared (25, 29). Likewise, motor speed was also impaired in patients with SCZ/BD during the Grooved Pegboard test when compared with HC (14, 31). Furthermore, other studies have shown comparable impairments in domains of verbal fluency and working memory within both SCZ and BD patients (14, 25, 28). In terms of executive functioning, a number of studies found comparable neurocognitive deficits in both patient groups irrespective of the tests used such as Wisconsin Card Sorting Test (WCST) (14, 29, 41), Trail Making Test B (TMT B) (28, 31), and Tower of Hanoi (29). Overall, our findings add to the literature to support the notion of comparable and pervasive neurocognitive impairments in patients with BD and SCZ (17, 29).

What may be the biological factors that underlie SCZ and BD which may be relevant to the observed neurocognitive impairments? First, recent evidence from large-scale GWAS has pointed to possible common susceptibility genes underlying SCZ and BD which may affect neurocognitive functioning. These common vulnerability cross disorder genes include ZNF804A, CACNA1C, NRGN, and PBRM1 (5, 19, 23, 24, 42–45). A recent study from the Psychiatric Genome Consortium reported that there are 14 genetic loci associated with both SCZ and BD (46), and shared genetic effects between SCZ and BD accounted for 52% of the genetic variance in SCZ and 69% for BD in the Swedish population (44). Second, neuroimaging aberrations of brain morphology and function have been noted. For example, voxel-based morphometry studies found that there was a substantial overlap in gray matter volumetric reductions such as the prefrontal cortex, thalamus, caudate, medial temporal lobe, insula, and the anterior cingulate regions in SCZ and BD (7, 15, 47). Third, while genetic risks for SCZ and BD are associated with different gray matter changes, McDonald et al. (48) suggested that they share white matter endophenotypes with the reduction of white matter volume in the left frontal and temporoparietal regions in both SCZ and BD.

Of note, older age and poorer psychosocial functioning were found to be associated with neurocognitive impairments in our patients. These findings are in line with that of other studies whereby older age was associated with decreased gray matter volume (49) and poorer neurocognitive performance in SCZ, and which can affect psychosocial functioning (50). The lifetime history of psychotic features in BD patients has also been found to worsen subsequent neurocognitive performance such as cognitive flexibility and working memory indicating age related effects on neurocognitive functioning in BD (10, 26, 27, 30, 32, 51). However, in contrast, Gildengers et al. (52) found no difference in the rate of neurocognitive decline between BD and healthy subjects with age.

We found that antipsychotic medication dose was not associated with neurocognitive impairment in SCZ and BD in this study although there is evidence of antipsychotic medications affecting changes in brain structures and neurocognitive performance. Previous studies have reported both improvements in neurocognitive impairments with antipsychotic treatment in SCZ and BD (26) but negative impact on cognition have also been reported in BD (53, 54). In SCZ patients, some studies reported that the administration of typical antipsychotic medication provides only modest-to-moderate gains in multiple cognitive domains (55, 56), while other studies found no correlation between antipsychotic medication dose and neurocognitive functioning in BD and SCZ (9, 18, 57).

Recent data also suggest that neurocognitive deficits may potentially serve as endophenotypical trait markers for BD and SCZ (58–60). Unlike a state marker whereby neurocognitive performance may vary with and be influenced by current clinical states such as affective change and psychotic phenomenology, a trait marker remains stable throughout the illness course and may be related to genetic factors (60, 61). For SCZ, a twin study by Pardo et al. (58) noted preservative errors on the WCST not only in the SCZ twin but also within non-SCZ monozygotic co-twin suggesting a spectrum of genetic liability. Furthermore, clinical symptoms do not seem to play a role in worsening cognitive performance in ultra-high risk of psychosis subjects (62). In BD, Sobzcak et al. (59) found deficits in memory function, psychomotor performance and attention in high risk relatives suggesting potential neurocognitive trait markers for BD. In a recent longitudinal study involving BD patients, the severity of depressive symptoms did not predict change of performance in any cognitive domains and all domains remained stable over the course of 6 years (60).

There are several limitations to the study. First, our sample size was rather small and the study solely recruited patients with remitted SCZ and BD seen at the outpatient setting of a tertiary psychiatric hospital and thus the results may not be generalizable to patients within the inpatient and in non-tertiary psychiatric settings. Second, this was a cross-sectional study and did not allow observations of changes of neurocognitive functioning over the course of time. Third, the administrators of the neurocognitive tests were not blinded to the diagnoses of the subjects. Lastly, we did not examine other biological correlates such as genetic factors, neurophysiological measures but we intend to do so as a follow up study of these findings. These multimodality studies can potentially elucidate biological underpinnings or correlates of these neurocognitive impairments in SCZ and BD.

In conclusion, we found that patients with BD and SCZ suffer widespread neurocognitive deficits involving almost all the examined cognitive domains. The severity of neurocognitive deficits has been found to be significantly associated with various factors such as the level of psychosocial functioning and age but not specific diagnoses or antipsychotic medications. The underlying biological basis of these neurocognitive deficits may be related to factors common to both conditions and awaits better definition. Our findings support the dimensional concept of psychotic spectrum conditions along a continuum rather than the dichotomous concept as proposed by Kraepelin. Although DSM-V (63) still retains the existing nosological boundaries between BD and SCZ, clinicians would have to remain vigilant in managing each case of SCZ or BD by taking into account their clinical, socio-demographic factors, and assessing for the presence of specific neurocognitive impairment so as to better optimize the care and cater for more individually tailored treatment plans for these patients with potentially crippling conditions.

ACKNOWLEDGMENTS

This study was supported by NHG SIG (12003/12004/11003) research grants awarded to Dr. Kang Sim. We would like to thank all of the patients, their families, and our hospital staff for their support of this study.

REFERENCES

1. Möller HJ. Systematic of psychiatric disorders between categorical and dimensional approaches: Kraepelin's dichotomy and beyond. *Eur Arch Psychiatry Clin Neurosci* (2008) **258**(Suppl 2):48–73. doi:10.1007/s00406-008-2004-3
2. Sorias S. Is the neo-Kraepelinian paradigm in a phase of crisis? *Turk Psikiyatri Derg* (2012) **23**:117–29.
3. Berrios GE, Beer D. The notion of a unitary psychosis: a conceptual history. *Hist Psychiatry* (1994) **5**:13–36. doi:10.1177/0957154X9400501702
4. Kraepelin E. *Dementia Praecox and Paraphenia.* Edinburg: Livingstone (1919).
5. Bellivier F, Geoffroy PA, Scott J, Schurhoff F, Leboyer M, Etain B. Biomarkers of bipolar disorder: specific or shared with schizophrenia? *Front Biosci (Elite Ed)* (2013) **E5**:845–63. doi:10.2741/E665

6. Murray RM, Sham P, Van Os J, Zanelli J, Cannon M, McDonald C. A developmental model for similarities and dissimilarities between schizophrenia and bipolar disorder. *Schizophr Res* (2004) **71**:405–16. doi:10.1016/j.schres.2004.03.002
7. Yu K, Cheung C, Leung M, Li Q, Chua S, McAlonan G. Are bipolar disorder and schizophrenia neuroanatomically distinct? An anatomical likelihood meta-analysis. *Front Hum Neurosci* (2010) **4**:189. doi:10.3389/fnhum.2010.00189
8. Demjaha A, MacCabe JH, Murray RM. How genes and environmental factors determine the different neurodevelopmental trajectories of schizophrenia and bipolar disorder. *Schizophr Bull* (2012) **38**:209–14. doi:10.1093/schbul/sbr100
9. Fusar-Poli P, Deste G, Smieskova R, Barlati S, Yung AR, Howes O, et al. Cognitive functioning in prodromal psychosis: a meta-analysis. *Arch Gen Psychiatry* (2012) **69**:562–71. doi:10.1001/archgenpsychiatry.2011.1592
10. Lewandowski KE, Cohen BM, Öngur D. Evolution of neuropsychological dysfunction during the course of schizophrenia and bipolar disorder. *Psychol Med* (2011) **41**:225–41. doi:10.1017/S0033291710001042
11. Napal O, Ojeda N, Sánchez P, Elizagárate E, Peña J, Ezcurra J, et al. The course of the schizophrenia and its impact on cognition: a review of literature. *Actas Esp Psiquiatr* (2012) **40**:198–220.
12. O'Donnell BF. Cognitive impairment in schizophrenia: a life span perspective. *Am J Alzheimers Dis Other Demen* (2007) **22**:398–405. doi:10.1177/1533317507304745
13. Young RC, Murphy CF, Heo M, Schulberg HC, Alexopoulos GS. Cognitive impairment in bipolar disorder in old age: literature review and findings in manic patients. *J Affect Disord* (2006) **92**:125–31. doi:10.1016/j.jad.2005.12.042
14. Depp CA, Moore DJ, Sitzer D, Palmer BW, Eyler LT, Roesch S, et al. Neurocognitive impairment in middle-aged and older adults with bipolar disorder: comparison to schizophrenia and normal comparison subjects. *J Affect Disord* (2007) **101**:201–9. doi:10.1016/j.jad.2006.11.022
15. Ellison-Wright I, Bullmore E. Anatomy of bipolar disorder and schizophrenia: a meta-analysis. *Schizophr Res* (2010) **117**:1–12. doi:10.1016/j.schres.2009.12.022
16. Krabbendam L, Arts B, van Os J, Aleman A. Cognitive functioning in patients with schizophrenia and bipolar disorder: a quantitative review. *Schizophr Res* (2005) **80**:137–49. doi:10.1016/j.schres.2005.08.004
17. Schretlen DJ, Cascella NG, Meyer SM, Kingery LR, Testa SM, Munro CA, et al. Neuropsychological functioning in bipolar disorder and schizophrenia. *Biol Psychiatry* (2007) **62**:179–86. doi:10.1016/j.biopsych.2006.09.025
18. Seidman LJ, Kremen WS, Koren D, Faraone SV, Goldstein JM, Tsuang MT. A comparative profile analysis of neuropsychological functioning in patients with schizophrenia and bipolar psychoses. *Schizophr Res* (2002) **53**:31–44. doi:10.1016/S0920-9964(01)00162-1
19. Craddock N, Owen MJ. The beginning of the end for the Kraepelinian dichotomy. *Br J Psychiatry* (2005) **186**:364–6. doi:10.1192/bjp.186.5.364
20. Craddock N, Owen MJ. Rethinking psychosis: the disadvantages of a dichotomous classification now outweigh the advantages. *World Psychiatry* (2007) **6**:84–91.
21. Arnone D, Cavanagh J, Gerber D, Lawrie SM, Ebmeier KP, McIntosh AM. Magnetic resonance imaging studies in bipolar disorder and schizophrenia: meta-analysis. *Br J Psychiatry* (2009) **195**:194–201. doi:10.1192/bjp.bp.108.059717
22. De Peri L, Crescini A, Deste G, Fusar-Poli P, Sacchetti E, Vita A. Brain structural abnormalities at the onset of schizophrenia and bipolar disorder: a meta-analysis of controlled magnetic resonance imaging studies. *Curr Pharm Des* (2012) **18**:486–94. doi:10.2174/138161212799316253
23. Lee KW, Woon PS, Teo YY, Sim K. Genome wide association studies (GWAS) and copy number variation (CNV) studies of the major psychoses: what have we learnt? *Neurosci Biobehav Rev* (2012) **36**:556–71. doi:10.1016/j.neubiorev.2011.09.001
24. Williams HJ, Norton N, Dwyer S, Moskvina V, Nikolov I, Carroll L, et al. Fine mapping of ZNF804A and genome-wide significant evidence for its involvement in schizophrenia and bipolar disorder. *Mol Psychiatry* (2011) **16**:429–41. doi:10.1038/mp.2010.36
25. Altshuler LL, Ventura J, van Gorp WG, Green MF, Theberge DC, Mintz J. Neurocognitive function in clinically stable men with bipolar I disorder or schizophrenia and normal control subjects. *Biol Psychiatry* (2004) **56**:560–9. doi:10.1016/j.biopsych.2004.08.002
26. Daban C, Martinez-Aran A, Torrent C, Tabarés-Seisdedos R, Balanzá-Martinez V, Salazar-Fraile J, et al. Specificity of cognitive deficits in bipolar disorder versus schizophrenia. *Psychother Psychosom* (2006) **75**:72–84. doi:10.1159/000090891
27. Glahn DC, Bearden CE, Cakir S, Barrett JA, Najt P, Monkul ES, et al. Differential working memory impairment in bipolar disorder and schizophrenia: effect of lifetime history of psychosis. *Bipolar Disord* (2006) **8**:117–23. doi:10.1111/j.1399-5618.2006.00296.x
28. Meesters PD, Schouws S, Stek M, de Haan L, Smit J, Eikelenboom P, et al. Cognitive impairment in late life schizophrenia and bipolar I disorder. *Int J Geriatr Psychiatry* (2013) **28**:82–90. doi:10.1002/gps.3793
29. Sánchez-Morla EM, Barabash A, Martínez-Vizcaíno V, Tabarés-Seisdedos R, Balanzá-Martínez V, Gabranes-Díaz JA, et al. Comparative study of neurocognitive function in euthymic bipolar patients and stabilized schizophrenia patients. *Psychiatry Res* (2009) **169**:220–8. doi:10.1016/j.psychres.2008.06.032
30. Simonsen C, Sundet K, Vaskinn A, Birkenaes AB, Engh JA, Færden A, et al. Neurocognitive dysfunction in bipolar and schizophrenia spectrum disorders depends on history of psychosis rather than diagnostic group. *Schizophr Bull* (2011) **37**:73–83. doi:10.1093/schbul/sbp034
31. Varga M, Magnusson A, Flekkøy K, David AS, Opjordsmoen S. Clinical and neuropsychological correlates of insight in schizophrenia and bipolar I disorder: does diagnosis matter? *Compr Psychiatry* (2007) **48**:583–91. doi:10.1016/j.comppsych.2007.06.003
32. Bora E, Yucel M, Fornito A, Berk M, Pantelis C. Major psychoses with mixed psychotic and mood symptoms: are mixed psychoses associated with different neurobiological markers. *Acta Psychiatr Scand* (2008) **118**:172–87. doi:10.1111/j.1600-0447.2008.01230.x
33. First MB, Spitzer RL, Gibbon M, Williams JBW. *Structured Clinical Interview for DSM-IV Axis I Disorders-Patient Version. (SCID-P).* Washington, DC: American Psychiatric Press (1994).
34. First MB, Spitzer RL, Gibbon M, Williams JBW. *Structured Clinical Interview for DSM-IV Axis I Disorders-non-Patient Version. (SCID-P).* Washington, DC: American Psychiatric Press (2002).
35. Keefe RSE, Goldberg TE, Harvey PD, Gold JM, Poe MP, Coughenour L. The brief assessment of cognition in schizophrenia: reliability, sensitivity, and comparison with a standard neurocognitive battery. *Schizophr Res* (2004) **68**:283–97. doi:10.1016/j.schres.2003.09.011
36. Ueoka Y, Tomotake M, Tanaka T, Kaneda Y, Taniguchi K, Nakataki M, et al. Quality of life and cognitive dysfunction in people with schizophrenia. *Prog Neuropsychopharmacol Biol Psychiatry* (2011) **35**:53–9. doi:10.1016/j.pnpbp.2010.08.018
37. Stone MH, Jastak S, Wilkinson G. *Wide Range Achievement Test.* New York: Harcourt Assessment (1995).
38. American Psychiatric Association. *Diagnostic and Statistical Manual of Mental Disorders, Fourth Edition, Text Revision (DSM-IV-TR).* Washington, DC: American Psychiatric Association (2000).
39. Kay SR, Fiszbein A, Opler LA. The positive and negative syndrome scale (PANSS) for schizophrenia. *Schizophr Bull* (1987) **13**:261–76. doi:10.1093/schbul/13.2.261
40. Young RC, Biggs JT, Ziegler VE, Meyer DA. A rating scale for mania: reliability, validity and sensitivity. *Br J Psychiatry* (1978) **133**:429–35. doi:10.1192/bjp.133.5.429
41. Morice R. Cognitive inflexibility and pre-frontal dysfunction in schizophrenia and mania. *Br J Psychiatry* (1990) **157**:50–4. doi:10.1192/bjp.157.1.50
42. Craddock N, O'Donovan MC, Owen MJ. Genes for schizophrenia and bipolar disorder? Implications for psychiatric nosology. *Schizophr Bull* (2006) **32**:9–16. doi:10.1093/schbul/sbj033
43. Goes FS, Hamshere ML, Seifuddin F, Pirooznia M, Belmonte-Mahon P, Breuer R, et al. Genome-wide association of mood-incongruent psychotic bipolar disorder. *Transl Psychiatry* (2012) **2**:e180. doi:10.1038/tp.2012.106
44. Lichenstein P, Yip BH, Björk C, Pawitan Y, Cannon TD, Sullivan PF, et al. Common genetic determinants of schizophrenia and bipolar disorder in Swedish families: a population-based study. *Lancet* (2009) **373**:234–9. doi:10.1016/S0140-6736(09)60072-6
45. Purcell SM, Wray NR, Stone JL, Visscher PM, O'Donovan MC, Sullivan PF, et al. Common polygenic variation contributes to risk of schizophrenia and bipolar disorder. *Nature* (2009) **460**:748–52. doi:10.1038/nature08185
46. Andreassen OA, Thompson WK, Schork AJ, Ripke S, Mattingsdal M, Kelsoe JR, et al. Improved detection of common variants associated with schizophrenia and bipolar disorder using pleiotropy-informed conditional false discovery rate. *PLoS Genet* (2013) **9**:e1003455. doi:10.1371/journal.pgen.1003455
47. Anderson D, Ardekani BA, Burdick KE, Robinson DG, John M, Malhotra AK, et al. Overlapping and distinct gray and white matter abnormalities

in schizophrenia and bipolar I disorder. *Bipolar Disord* (2013) **15**:680–93. doi:10.1111/bdi.12096

48. McDonald C, Bullmore ET, Sham PC, Chitnis X, Wickham H, Bramon E, et al. Association of genetic risks for schizophrenia and bipolar disorder with specific and generic brain structural endophenotypes. *Arch Gen Psychiatry* (2004) **61**:974–84. doi:10.1001/archpsyc.61.10.974
49. Schuster C, Schuller AM, Paulos C, Namer I, Pull C, Danion JM, et al. Gray matter volume decreases in elderly patients with schizophrenia: a voxel-based morphometry study. *Schizophr Bull* (2012) **38**:796–802. doi:10.1093/schbul/sbq150
50. Rajji TK, Voineskos AN, Butters MA, Miranda D, Arenovich T, Menon M, et al. Cognitive performance of individuals with schizophrenia across seven decades: a study using the MATRICS Consensus Cognitive Battery. *Am J Geriatr Psychiatry* (2013) **21**:108–18. doi:10.1016/j.jagp.2012.10.011
51. Smith MJ, Barch DM, Csernansky JG. Bridging the gap between schizophrenia and psychotic mood disorders: relating neurocognitive deficits to psychopathology. *Schizophr Res* (2009) **107**:69–75. doi:10.1016/j.schres.2008.07.014
52. Gildengers AG, Chisholm D, Butters MA, Anderson SJ, Begley A, Holm M, et al. Two-year course of cognitive function and instrumental activities of daily living in older adults with bipolar disorder: evidence for neuroprogression? *Psychol Med* (2013) **43**:801–11. doi:10.1017/S0033291712001614
53. Arts B, Jabben N, Krabbendam L, van Os J. A 2-year naturalistic study on cognitive function in bipolar disorder. *Acta Psychiatr Scand* (2011) **123**:190–205. doi:10.1111/j.1600-0447.2010.01601.x
54. Donaldson S, Goldstein LH, Landau S, Raymont V, Frangou S. The Maudsley bipolar disorder project: the effect of medication, family history, and duration of illness on IQ and memory in bipolar I disorder. *J Clin Psychiatry* (2004) **64**:86–93. doi:10.4088/JCP.v64n0116
55. Keefe RSE, Bilder RM, Davis SM, Harvey PD, Palmer BW, Gold JM, et al. Neurocognitive effects of antipsychotic medications in patients with chronic schizophrenia in the CATIE trial. *Arch Gen Psychiatry* (2007) **64**:633–47. doi:10.1001/archpsyc.64.6.633
56. Mishara AL, Goldberg TE. A meta-analysis and critical review of the effects of conventional neuroleptic treatment on cognition in schizophrenia: opening a closed book. *Biol Psychiatry* (2004) **55**:1013–22. doi:10.1016/j.biopsych.2004.01.027
57. Rossi A, Arduini L, Daneluzzo E, Bustini M, Prosperini P, Stratta P. Cognitive function in euthymic bipolar patients, stabilized schizophrenic patients, and healthy controls. *J Psychiatr Res* (2000) **34**:333–9. doi:10.1016/S0022-3956(00)00025-X
58. Pardo PJ, Knesevich MA, Vogler GP, Pardo JV, Twone B, Cloninger CR, et al. Genetic and state variables of neurocognitive dysfunction in schizophrenia: a twin study. *Schizophr Bull* (2000) **26**:459–77. doi:10.1093/oxfordjournals.schbul.a033466
59. Sobzcak S, Honig A, Schmitt JAJ, Riedel WJ. Pronounced cognitive deficits following an intravenous L-tryptophan challenge in first-degree relatives of bipolar patients compared to healthy controls. *Neuropsychopharmacology* (2003) **28**:711–9. doi:10.1038/sj.npp.1300055
60. Sarapas C, Shankman SA, Harrow M, Goldberg JF. Parsing trait and state effects of depression severity on neurocognition: evidence from a 26-year longitudinal study. *J Abnorm Psychol* (2012) **121**:830–7. doi:10.1037/a0028141
61. Gopal YV, Variend H. First-episode schizophrenia: review of cognitive deficits and cognitive remediation. *Adv Psychiatr Treat* (2005) **11**:38–44. doi:10.1192/apt.11.1.38
62. Serrani D. Neurocognitive assessment of ultra high risk of psychosis states using the MATRICS battery (measurement and treatment research to improve cognition in schizophrenia). *Rev Psiq Clin* (2011) **38**:130–4. doi:10.1590/S0101-60832011000400003
63. American Psychiatric Association. *Diagnostic and Statistical Manual of Mental Disorders, Fifth Edition (DSM-V)*. Arlington, VA: American Psychiatric Publishing (2013).

16

Relationship Between Glutamate Dysfunction and Symptoms and Cognitive Function in Psychosis

Kate Merritt *, Philip McGuire and Alice Egerton

Department of Psychosis Studies, Institute of Psychiatry, King's College London, London, UK

****Correspondence:***
Kate Merritt, Department of Psychosis Studies, Institute of Psychiatry, King's College London, De Crespigny Park, Denmark Hill, London SE5 8AF, UK
e-mail: kate.merritt@kcl.ac.uk

The glutamate hypothesis of schizophrenia, proposed over two decades ago, originated following the observation that administration of drugs that block NMDA glutamate receptors, such as ketamine, could induce schizophrenia-like symptoms. Since then, this hypothesis has been extended to describe how glutamate abnormalities may disturb brain function and underpin psychotic symptoms and cognitive impairments. The glutamatergic system is now a major focus for the development of new compounds in schizophrenia. Relationships between regional brain glutamate function and symptom severity can be investigated using proton magnetic resonance spectroscopy (1H-MRS) to estimate levels of glutamatergic metabolites *in vivo*. Here we briefly review the 1H-MRS studies that have explored relationships between glutamatergic metabolites, symptoms, and cognitive function in clinical samples. While some of these studies suggest that more severe symptoms may be associated with elevated glutamatergic function in the anterior cingulate, studies in larger patient samples selected on the basis of symptom severity are required.

Keywords: schizophrenia, psychosis, glutamate, NMDA, MRS, spectroscopy, imaging

INTRODUCTION

Accumulating evidence suggests that glutamatergic dysfunction may contribute to the pathogenesis of schizophrenia, and the symptoms and cognitive deficits associated with the disorder (1). The glutamatergic system presents an attractive therapeutic target, as dopaminergic antipsychotics have little effect on negative symptoms or cognitive impairment, yet these features are better predictors of social and functional outcome than positive symptoms (2, 3). Here we briefly review the existing evidence linking abnormal glutamatergic transmission to cognitive, negative, and positive symptoms of schizophrenia.

The observation that administration of antagonists at the *N*-methyl-D-aspartate glutamate receptor complex (NMDAR) such as phencyclidine (PCP) or ketamine to healthy volunteers induces effects which resemble aspects of schizophrenia symptomatology forms a cornerstone of the glutamate hypothesis of schizophrenia (4–6). NMDAR antagonists also worsen positive, negative, and cognitive symptoms in patients with schizophrenia (7, 8). While dopamine-stimulating drugs such as amphetamine also produce positive "psychotic"-like effects, negative-type symptoms, and cognitive deficits are far more prominently elicited by ketamine than amphetamine administration (9). Neuroimaging studies indicate that these effects of ketamine are mediated by changes in activity in the frontal and cingulate cortices and the thalamus (10–13).

While pharmacological studies have provided evidence linking NMDAR dysfunction to these symptom domains, direct associations between glutamatergic function and symptom severity may be provided by neuroimaging studies. In a single photon emission tomography study using the NMDAR radiotracer ^{123}I-CNS-1261 in schizophrenia, the availability of NMDAR in the hippocampus was negatively associated with the severity of symptoms, especially negative symptoms (14). A ketamine challenge study in healthy volunteers using the same radiotracer linked regional NMDAR binding to the induction of negative (but not positive) symptoms, particularly in the thalamus (15). These approaches are currently limited by a lack of availability of suitable radiotracers (1).

An alternative is to use proton magnetic resonance spectroscopy (1H-MRS) to estimate the concentration of glutamatergic metabolites. MRI scanners with field strengths of 3 T or above can resolve glutamate, at least for the most part, from its metabolite glutamine (16). At lower field strengths glutamate and glutamine are reported in combination, as Glx. A limitation of 1H-MRS is that the glutamate concentration estimates are not specific to neuronal glutamate, and that changes in glutamate levels cannot be specifically attributed to altered neurotransmission over other metabolic processes (17). However the majority (~80%) of glutamine synthesis reflects cycling of neurotransmitter glutamate (17), and clinical studies at 4 T in minimally treated patients with schizophrenia have reported higher Gln/Glu ratios (18) or higher glutamine levels (19) in the anterior cingulate cortex (ACC). This is consistent with increased glutamatergic neurotransmission, but could also result from a deficiency in the conversion of glutamine to glutamate. However the majority of 1H-MRS studies in psychosis have used field strengths <4 T and thereby were unable to accurately quantify glutamine concentrations. Thus, the results from these studies at lower field strengths cannot be specifically attributed to changes in glutamate neurotransmission. Nonetheless, increases in frontal glutamatergic neurotransmission in schizophrenia are broadly consistent with the NMDA receptor hypofunction hypothesis, as administration of NMDAR antagonists to rats increases glutamate release as detected by microdialysis (20), and 1H-MRS studies report elevated Gln/Glu ratios (21), or increased glutamate levels with no changes in glutamine (22). 1H-MRS studies with ketamine in man at 4 T reveal increased ACC glutamine (23), and at 3 T reveal increased ACC glutamate (24). One mechanism through which increases in glutamate release may occur is via NMDAR dysfunction on GABA-ergic interneurons, leading to the disinhibition of glutamatergic pyramidal cells, as described by the NMDAR hypofunction hypothesis (25).

Individual 1H-MRS glutamate studies in schizophrenia have produced some inconsistent findings. In general, studies at higher field strengths suggest that frontal glutamine function is elevated in the early stages of psychosis (18, 19), whereas the findings in chronic schizophrenia are more variable (26–30). This could reflect effects of antipsychotic medication. For example, one cross-sectional and one longitudinal study reported higher Glx levels in the PFC of unmedicated, but not medicated schizophrenia, in comparison to controls (31, 32), although longitudinal studies have reported no effect of medication on anterior cingulate glutamate or glutamine levels (18, 33, 34). It could be that symptom severity contributes to variability in glutamatergic metabolites between patients early or late in the illness, as samples involving patients in the early phase of psychosis usually comprise non- or minimally medicated patients who are relatively symptomatic, whereas studies in chronic schizophrenia often involve patients who have been treated for long periods and have less severe or more stable symptoms (1). In relation to this, a recent meta-analysis of 1H-MRS glutamatergic studies in major depressive disorder found lower levels of Glx in the ACC which were only significant when remitted patients were excluded from the analysis (35).

In order to better understand the possible relationships between 1H-MRS glutamate, glutamine, and Glx levels and symptom severity, we identified publications that have reported associations with severity along symptom domains. These included studies in individuals at risk of psychosis, and patients with first-episode psychosis or established schizophrenia (**Table 1**).

RELATIONSHIPS BETWEEN GLUTAMATE FUNCTION AND POSITIVE SYMPTOMS

Several studies have investigated associations between regional glutamatergic metabolite levels and the severity of positive psychotic symptoms (**Table 1**), and most found no association between regional Glx, glutamate or glutamine levels and positive symptom severity, in either high genetic or clinical risk populations (36, 37), first-episode psychosis (18, 19, 37–40) or chronic schizophrenia (26–28, 30, 41–46).

However, many of these studies involved small patient samples, relied on *post hoc* correlational analyses, and patients in whom the severity and/or the variance in severity of symptoms was low, due to either being sub-clinical threshold in the at risk studies or due to the presence of antipsychotic medication in established schizophrenia. A recent study pooling both medicated and unmedicated patients, where unmedicated patients possessed elevated Glx in medial prefrontal cortex (mPFC), detected an association between positive symptom severity and mPFC Glx, although this did not survive correction for multiple comparisons (31). Another study in the PFC found that treatment reduced the level of Glx/Cr in chronic patients, and associated the change in Glx with improvement in total BPRS score (32). Moreover a recent study found that 4 weeks of antipsychotic treatment in first-episode psychosis patients reduced Glx in the striatum, and this was associated with improvement in PANSS score (47).

A notable exception is the study of Ota et al. (48), which directly compared patients experiencing exacerbated psychotic symptoms to healthy controls and stable patients, and found that increases in Glx in inferior parietal white matter were specific to the group currently experiencing exacerbated psychotic symptoms (48). In line with this, our own studies which have compared glutamate levels in patients according to symptom severity have found higher ACC glutamate levels in first-episode psychosis patients who are still symptomatic following treatment compared to those in remission (38) and in patients with treatment-resistant schizophrenia compared to those who respond to medication (49). These differences may be independent of medication effects, as groups either did not differ according to medication (38, 49) or the symptomatic group were actually receiving higher medication doses (48), and as longitudinal studies have not reported changes in cortical glutamate in relation to changes in positive symptoms following antipsychotic treatment (18, 33, 34). This suggests that glutamate and Glx levels may be selectively elevated in patients whose positive symptoms are not well controlled by conventional antipsychotic medication.

RELATIONSHIPS BETWEEN GLUTAMATE FUNCTION AND NEGATIVE SYMPTOMS

We recently reported that greater severity of PANSS negative symptoms was associated with higher levels of glutamate in the ACC in first-episode psychosis (38). Although there were several methodological differences, this contrasts with the study of Reid et al. (26), which reported that negative symptoms were associated with *lower* levels of ACC Glx in chronic schizophrenia. Other studies investigating correlations between ACC glutamatergic metabolites and negative symptoms have found no significant relationship (18, 19, 28, 42, 46, 50). We are not aware of any studies which have specifically compared regional levels of glutamatergic metabolites in patient groups selected according to differences in negative symptom severity.

As listed in **Table 1**, in brain regions other than the ACC many studies have failed to detect significant relationships between negative symptoms and regional glutamate, glutamine, or Glx levels in high genetic or clinical risk groups (36, 37), first-episode psychosis (18, 37, 39, 40), or chronic schizophrenia (27, 30, 31, 41, 44, 45, 48).

A general consideration of studies investigating relationships between glutamate markers and positive and negative symptoms is the scale used to score symptom severity. As detailed in **Table 1**, scores on a number of scales have been used and while these scales are highly correlated there are also some important differences in the clinical items included (51). As most studies examining

Table 1 | Summary of articles reporting high levels of glutamate metabolites associated with greater or lesser severity of symptoms.

Reference	Field strength	Population	*n*	Brain region	Metabolite	Measure	Direction
Tandon et al. (54)	1.5	Familial high risk	23	Thalamus	Glx	SIPS	+
						CSS	NS
				Caudate	Glx	SIPS, CSS	+
				ACC	Glx	SIPS, CSS	NS
Yoo et al. (36)	1.5	GHR	22	ACC, DLPFC, thal	Glx	PANSS, BPRS	NS
de la Fuente-Sandoval et al. (37)	3	ARMS + drug naïve FE	36	Associative striatum, cerebellar cortex	Glu	PANSS, SIPS	NS
de la Fuente-Sandoval et al. (47)	3	FE	24	Associative striatum	Glu	PANSS	+
				Cerebellar cortex	Glu, Glx	PANSS	NS
Egerton et al. (38)	3	FE	32	ACC	Glu/Cr	PANSS negative	+
						PANSS positive	NS
				Thalamus	Glu/Cr	PANSS	NS
Ota et al. (48)	1.5	Chronic (+1 FE)	46	Inferior parietal	Glx	PANSS positive	+
				Middle frontal	Glx	PANSS	NS
Ohrmann et al. (42)	1.5	Chronic	43	ACC, DLPFC	Glx	PANSS, CDSS, CGI	NS
Tayoshi et al. (28)	3	Chronic	30	ACC, basal ganglia	Glu, Gln	PANSS	NS
Wood et al. (30)	3	Chronic	15	Dorsal, rostral cingulate	Glx	PANSS	NS
Kegeles et al. (31)	3	Chronic	32	mPFC (inclu ACC)	Glx	PANSS negative	NS
						PANSS positive	+ #
Szulc et al. (62)	1.5	Chronic	42	Frontal lobe	Glx/Cr	PANSS	+
Ohrmann et al. (41)	1.5	Chronic	39	DLPFC	Glx	PANSS	NS
Ongur et al. (50)	4	Chronic	17	ACC, POC	Gln/Glu	PANSS, MADRS, YMRS	NS
Stanley et al. (39)	1.5	FE 14wk treatment	37	DLPFC	Gln	SANS, SAPS	NS
Bartha et al. (40)	1.5	FE	10	mPFC (inclu ACC)	Glu, Gln	SANS, SAPS	NS
Theberge et al. (19)	4	FE	21	ACC, thal	Glu, Gln	SANS, SAPS	NS
Bustillo et al. (18)	4	FE Min treated	14	ACC, thal	Gln/Glu	SANS, SAPS	NS
Bustillo et al. (43)	4	Chronic	30	Whole brain slice	Glx	SANS	–
						SAPS	NS
Olbrich et al. (67)	2	FE	9	DLPFC	Glu	SANS, BPRS	–
				Hippocampus	Glu	SANS, BPRS	NS
Shirayama et al. (27)	3	Chronic	19	mPFC (inclu ACC)	Gln/Glu	SANS, BPRS	NS
Rowland et al. (44)	3	Chronic	20	mPFC, inferior parietal	Glx	SANS, BPRS	NS
Rowland et al. (46)	3	Chronic	21	ACC, CSO	Glx	SANS, BPRS	NS
Choe et al. (32)	1.5	Chronic	34	PFC	Glx/Cr	BPRS	+
Reid et al. (26)	3	Chronic	26	ACC	Glx	BPRS negative	–
						BPRS positive	NS

(Continued)

Table 1 | Continued

Reference	Field strength	Population	*n*	Brain region	Metabolite	Measure	Direction
Reid et al. (45)	3	Chronic	35	Substantia nigra	Glx/Cr	BPRS	NS
Tandon et al. (54)	1.5	Familial high risk	23	ACC, thal, caudate	Glx	WCST	NS
Rusch et al. (53)	2	FE + Chronic	29	Hippocampus	Glu	WCST	+
Shirayama et al. (27)	3	Chronic	19	mPFC (inclu ACC)	Gln/Glu	WCST, DSDT Stroop, VF, IGT	+ NS
Ohrmann et al. (42)	1.5	Chronic	43	ACC ACC, DLPFC	Glx Glx	WCST AVLT	– NS
Ohrmann et al. (55)	4	FE + Chronic	35	DLPFC	Glx	AVLT	–
Kegeles et al. (31)	3	Chronic	32	mPFC (inclu ACC)	Glx	N-back	NS
Reid et al. (26)	3	Chronic	26	ACC	Glx	RBANS	NS
Reid et al. (45)	3	Chronic	35	Substantia nigra	Glx/Cr	RBANS	NS
Rowland et al. (44)	3	Chronic	20	mPFC, inferior parietal	Glx	RBANS	NS
Rowland et al. (46)	3	Chronic	21	ACC, CSO	Glx	RBANS	NS
Bustillo et al. (43)	4	Chronic	30	Whole brain slice	Glx	Combined neuropsych	–
Yoo et al. (36)	1.5	GHR	22	ACC, DLPFC, thal	Glx	GAF	NS
Tibbo et al. (59)	3	GHR	20	mPFC	Glx/Cr	GAF	–
Egerton et al. (38)	3	FE	32	ACC	Glu/Cr	GAF	+
Egerton et al. (38)	3	FE	32	Thalamus	Glu/Cr	GAF	NS
Shirayama et al. (27)	3	Chronic	19	mPFC (inclu ACC)	Gln/Glu	GAF	NS
Tebartz van Elst et al. (60)	2	Chronic	21	DLPFC	Glu	GAS	+
Aoyama et al. (34)	4	Chronic	17	Thalamus	Total Gln + Glu	LSPR	–

 # Did not survive correction for the six comparisons (PANSS total, positive, and negative symptom subscales in two regions for each neurochemical).
Index: + denotes a positive relationship where higher levels of glutamate were associated with greater symptom severity or worse overall functioning; – denotes a negative relationship where higher levels of glutamate were associated with lesser symptom severity or better overall functioning. NS, not significant; ACC, anterior cingulate cortex; POC, parieto-occipital cortex; DLPFC, dorsolateral prefrontal cortex; MPFC, medial prefrontal cortex; Thal, thalamus; CSO, centrum semiovale; GHR, genetic high risk; RBANS, repeatable battery for the assessment of neuropsychological status; WCST, Wisconsin card sorting test; DSDT, the digit span distraction test; TMT, trail making test; IGT, Iowa gambling task; VF, verbal fluency; AVLT, auditory verbal learning test; BPRS, brief psychiatric rating scale; GAF, global assessment of functioning; CGI, clinical global impression scale; GAS, global assessment scale; SIPS, structured interview for prodromal symptoms; CSS, Chapman schizotypy scales; CDSS, Calgary Depression Scale for Schizophrenia; LSPR, life skills profile rating.

relationships between brain glutamate measures and symptoms have relied on *post hoc* correlational analysis, it is of note that additional items are included on the SAPS/SANS compared to the PANSS, which in turn has additional items compared to the BPRS. Therefore use of the SAPS/SANS may be preferable as they provide a more detailed assessment of symptoms.

RELATIONSHIPS BETWEEN GLUTAMATE MEASURES AND COGNITIVE DYSFUNCTION

Relatively few studies have investigated relationships between glutamate measures and cognitive dysfunction in schizophrenia. The most commonly investigated task has been the Wisconsin card sort test (WCST): in schizophrenia, deficits on this task are associated with abnormal activation in the ACC and DLPFC (52). In a study of 19 patients with chronic schizophrenia at 3 T, poor performance on the WCST was associated with higher Gln/Glu ratios in the mPFC (including the ACC) (27). In contrast, a larger study of 43 patients with chronic schizophrenia at 1.5 T found that ACC, but not DLPFC, Glx levels were positively associated with WCST learning potential (42). In first-episode psychosis, an association between hippocampal, but not DLPFC, glutamate, and WCST errors was reported (53), and in a small sample of 16 genetic high risk individuals, no correlations between WCST performance and Glx levels in the caudate, ACC, or thalamus were detected (54).

Other tasks investigated include the Stroop, digit span distractibility test, auditory verbal learning test (AVLT), N-back task, Iowa gambling task and verbal fluency test (**Table 1**). Of these, there are reports of a positive association between mPFC Gln/Glu ratio and impairments on the digit span distraction test, which probes short-term memory and selective attention (27), and of DLPFC Glx and verbal learning and memory on the AVLT (55). Overall, the findings have been inconsistent and further studies with larger sample sizes are required. While the above studies used a voxel of interest method, using whole brain slice proton echo planar spectroscopy at 4 T in 30 patients Bustillo et al. (43) detected a positive correlation between general cognitive performance in schizophrenia and Glx. Furthermore, subsequent path analyses suggested that the relationship between glutamate and cognitive performance may be associated with negative symptoms and unemployment (43).

The relationship between glutamate and cognition in schizophrenia has been further investigated by combining 1H-MRS with functional magnetic resonance imaging (fMRI) of the blood oxygen level dependent (BOLD) response to measure changes in regional brain activation as participants perform cognitive tasks. In subjects at clinical high risk of developing psychosis, reductions in thalamic glutamate were correlated with an elevated BOLD response in the prefrontal cortex during a verbal fluency task, whereas the converse association was observed in controls (56). In a study by Valli et al. (57), medial temporal lobe glutamate levels were correlated with hippocampal BOLD response during an episodic memory task in controls, whereas this coupling was absent in clinical high risk subjects (57). Finally one study showed that hippocampal Glx was related to inferior frontal gyrus activation during episodic memory in controls, and suggested that the absence of this positive coupling in medicated schizophrenia patients may underlie episodic memory deficits, reflecting the results seen in Valli et al. (57, 58). Further investigation of the relationships between regional levels of glutamatergic metabolites and abnormalities in regional brain activation during cognitive tasks may provide a more sensitive means to characterize the relationship between glutamate and cognition in schizophrenia.

RELATIONSHIPS BETWEEN GLUTAMATE MEASURES AND SOCIAL AND OCCUPATIONAL FUNCTIONING

Several studies have also reported correlations between brain glutamate levels and overall level of social and occupational functioning (**Table 1**). In genetically high risk subjects, lower levels of Glx/Cr in the mPFC were associated with lower levels of overall functioning (59). A longitudinal study at 4 T showed that loss of glutamate and glutamine in the thalamus, but not the ACC, over 7 years since first presentation correlated with impaired social functioning (34). In contrast, in first-episode psychosis higher levels of glutamate in the ACC, but not the thalamus, were associated with worse overall functioning (38), and in chronic schizophrenia higher DLPFC glutamate levels were also associated with worse overall functioning (60). Other studies have found no association between glutamate measures and overall functioning in chronic schizophrenia (27) or genetic high risk subjects (36).

SUMMARY AND FUTURE DIRECTIONS

1H-MRS studies relating regional glutamate measures to symptoms in schizophrenia have produced inconsistent findings. There may be several methodological reasons for this, including differences in the brain region investigated, and between samples such as medication, illness stage, and symptom severity. The use of sub-optimal technical approaches such as low field strengths together with small sample sizes may also underlie the conflicting findings. A recent study at 4 T indicates that elevations in the ratio of Gln/Glu are present in schizophrenia patients, consistent with elevated glutamatergic neurotransmission (18). However the majority of 1H-MRS studies in schizophrenia use field strengths <4 T which cannot reliably measure glutamine, and glutamate and Glx measures cannot be specifically attributed to glutamate neurotransmission (17). The increasing availability of higher field strength scanners may resolve some of the apparent inconsistencies in the literature.

The majority of studies that have investigated relationships between glutamate levels and symptom severity have applied correlational analysis, usually *post hoc* to the main study findings. A few studies have directly compared glutamatergic metabolite levels in patient groups on the basis of symptom severity, specifically those who were or were not currently experiencing symptom exacerbation (48), were or were not in symptomatic remission following initial treatment (38) or did or did not have treatment-resistant illness (49). All found higher levels of glutamate or Glx in the more symptomatic patient group.

The field would benefit from further studies pre-selecting groups of patients who differ in severity of negative symptoms or cognitive impairment, or longitudinal studies comparing within-subjects glutamate levels during periods of illness stability compared to relapse. Studies of the relationships between cognitive dysfunction and glutamate in schizophrenia may benefit from combination with fMRI to determine the efficiency of glutamate in supporting networks that subserve cognitive function. To date there are only a handful of published studies of this type. Finally, relationships between glutamate levels and symptom severity may be indirect; for example Stone et al. showed that hippocampal glutamate may interact with striatal dopamine to determine risk of psychosis (61), and a path analysis has suggested that negative symptoms may be secondary to poor cognition associated with low brain Glx (43).

One question is whether baseline levels of glutamate, glutamine, or Glx are predictive of subsequent outcome or response to treatment in schizophrenia. A recent study showed that elevated frontal Glx at baseline was associated with poor response after 4 weeks of antipsychotic treatment (62). This is consistent with the above findings of glutamatergic elevations in patients with schizophrenia whose symptoms have not responded well to treatment (38, 49).

The suggestion that symptoms that do not respond well to conventional antipsychotic treatment may have a glutamatergic basis (38, 49) warrants further investigation, as compounds that target the glutamatergic system may have particular efficacy in these patients. Meta-analyses conclude that of the agents which may improve NMDA receptor-mediated neurotransmission, the NMDAR co-agonist D-serine and the glycine transporter type 1 inhibitor sarcosine reduce total and negative symptoms as an adjuvant to antipsychotic medication (63, 64). Lamotrigine, which may inhibit glutamate release, blocks the psychomimetic effects of ketamine in healthy volunteers (65) and small trials of lamotrigine in chronic, often treatment-resistant or clozapine-treated patients found that it is beneficial in reducing symptoms (63, 66). Further work is required to determine the relationship between regional glutamate concentrations and the expression of symptoms at different stages of psychotic illness. This area may benefit from meta-analyses of the previously published findings and from new studies selecting patient samples *a priori* on the basis of symptom severity.

REFERENCES

1. Egerton A, Stone JM. The glutamate hypothesis of schizophrenia: neuroimaging and drug development. *Curr Pharm Biotechnol* (2012) **13**(8):1500–12. doi:10.2174/138920112800784961
2. Ventura J, Hellemann GS, Thames AD, Koellner V, Nuechterlein KH. Symptoms as mediators of the relationship between neurocognition and functional outcome in schizophrenia: a meta-analysis. *Schizophr Res* (2009) **113**(2-3):189–99. doi:10.1016/j.schres.2009.03.035
3. Javitt DC. Treatment of negative and cognitive symptoms. *Curr Psychiatry Rep* (1999) **1**(1):25–30. doi:10.1007/s11920-999-0007-z
4. Krystal JH, Karper LP, Seibyl JP, Freeman GK, Delaney R, Bremner JD, et al. Subanesthetic effects of the noncompetitive NMDA antagonist, ketamine, in humans – psychotomimetic, perceptual, cognitive, and neuroendocrine responses. *Arch Gen Psychiatry* (1994) **51**(3):199–214. doi:10.1001/archpsyc.1994.03950030035004
5. Newcomer JW, Farber NB, Jevtovic-Todorovic V, Selke G, Melson AK, Hershey T, et al. Ketamine-induced NMDA receptor hypofunction as a model of memory impairment and psychosis. *Neuropsychopharmacology* (1999) **20**(2):106–18. doi:10.1016/s0893-133x(98)00067-0
6. Malhotra AK, Pinals DA, Weingartner H, Sirocco K, Missar CD, Pickar D, et al. NMDA receptor function and human cognition: the effects of ketamine in healthy volunteers. *Neuropsychopharmacology* (1996) **14**(5):301–7. doi:10.1016/0893-133x(95)00137-3
7. Malhotra AK, Pinals DA, Adler CM, Elman I, Clifton A, Pickar D, et al. Ketamine-induced exacerbation of psychotic symptoms and cognitive impairment in neuroleptic-free schizophrenics. *Neuropsychopharmacology* (1997) **17**(3):141–50. doi:10.1016/S0893-133X(97)00036-5
8. Lahti AC, Koffel B, Laporte D, Tamminga CA. Subanesthetic doses of ketamine stimulate psychosis in schizophrenia. *Neuropsychopharmacology* (1995) **13**(1):9–19. doi:10.1016/0893-133X(94)00131-I
9. Krystal JH, Perry EB, Gueorguieva R, Belger A, Madonich SH, Abi-Dargham A, et al. Comparative and interactive human psychopharmacologic effects of ketamine and amphetamine – implications for glutamatergic and dopaminergic model psychoses and cognitive function. *Arch Gen Psychiatry* (2005) **62**(9):985–95. doi:10.1001/archpsyc.62.9.985
10. Holcomb HH, Lahti AC, Medoff DR, Cullen T, Tamminga CA. Effects of noncompetitive NMDA receptor blockade on anterior cingulate cerebral blood flow in volunteers with schizophrenia. *Neuropsychopharmacology* (2005) **30**(12):2275–82. doi:10.1038/sj.npp.1300824
11. Deakin JFW, Lees J, McKie S, Hallak JEC, Williams SR, Dursun SM. Glutamate and the neural basis of the subjective effects of ketamine. *Arch Gen Psychiatry* (2008) **65**(2):154–64. doi:10.1001/archgenpsychiatry.2007.37
12. De Simoni S, Schwarz AJ, O'Daly OG, Marquand AF, Brittain C, Gonzales C, et al. Test-retest reliability of the BOLD pharmacological MRI response to ketamine in healthy volunteers. *Neuroimage* (2013) **64**:75–90. doi:10.1016/j.neuroimage.2012.09.037
13. Holcomb HH, Lahti AC, Medoff DR, Weiler M, Tamminga CA. Sequential regional cerebral blood flow brain scans using PET with (H2O)-O-15 demonstrate ketamine actions in CNS dynamically. *Neuropsychopharmacology* (2001) **25**(2):165–72. doi:10.1016/s0893-133x(01)00229-9
14. Pilowsky LS, Bressan RA, Stone JM, Erlandsson K, Mulligan RS, Krystal JH, et al. First in vivo evidence of an NMDA receptor deficit in medication-free schizophrenic patients. *Mol Psychiatry* (2006) **11**(2):118–9. doi:10.1038/sj.mp.4001751
15. Stone JM, Erlandsson K, Arstad E, Squassante L, Teneggi V, Bressan RA, et al. Relationship between ketamine-induced psychotic symptoms and NMDA receptor occupancy – a I-123 CNS-1261 SPET study. *Psychopharmacology* (2008) **197**(3):401–8. doi:10.1007/s00213-007-1047-x
16. Snyder J, Wilman A. Field strength dependence of PRESS timings for simultaneous detection of glutamate and glutamine from 1.5 to 7 T. *J Magn Reson* (2010) **203**(1):66–72. doi:10.1016/j.jmr.2009.12.002
17. Rothman DL, De Feyter HM, de Graaf RA, Mason GF, Behar KL. C-13 MRS studies of neuroenergetics and neurotransmitter cycling in humans. *NMR Biomed* (2011) **24**(8):943–57. doi:10.1002/nbm.1772
18. Bustillo JR, Rowland LM, Mullins P, Jung R, Chen H, Qualls C, et al. H-1-MRS at 4 Tesla in minimally treated early schizophrenia. *Mol Psychiatry* (2010) **15**(6):629–36. doi:10.1038/mp.2009.121
19. Theberge J, Bartha R, Drost DJ, Menon RS, Malla A, Takhar J, et al. Glutamate and glutamine measured with 4.0 T proton MRS in never-treated patients with schizophrenia and healthy volunteers. *Am J Psychiatry* (2002) **159**(11):1944–6. doi:10.1176/appi.ajp.159.11.1944
20. Moghaddam B, Adams B, Verma A, Daly D. Activation of glutamatergic neurotransmission by ketamine: a novel step in the pathway from NMDA receptor blockade to dopaminergic and cognitive disruptions associated with the prefrontal cortex. *J Neurosci* (1997) **17**(8):2921–7.
21. Iltis I, Koski DM, Eberly LE, Nelson CD, Deelchand DK, Valette J, et al. Neurochemical changes in the rat prefrontal cortex following acute phencyclidine treatment: an in vivo localized H-1 MRS study. *NMR Biomed* (2009) **22**(7):737–44. doi:10.1002/nbm.1385
22. Kim SY, Lee H, Kim HJ, Bang E, Lee SH, Lee DW, et al. In vivo and ex vivo evidence for ketamine-induced hyperglutamatergic activity in the cerebral cortex of the rat: potential relevance to schizophrenia. *NMR Biomed* (2011) **24**(10):1235–42. doi:10.1002/nbm.1681
23. Rowland LM, Bustillo JR, Mullins PG, Jung RE, Lenroot R, Landgraf E, et al. Effects of ketamine on anterior cingulate glutamate metabolism in healthy humans: a 4-T proton MRS study. *Am J Psychiatry* (2005) **162**(2):394–6. doi:10.1176/appi.ajp.162.2.394
24. Stone JM, Dietrich C, Edden R, Mehta MA, De Simoni S, Reed LJ, et al. Ketamine effects on brain GABA and glutamate levels with 1H-MRS: relationship to ketamine-induced psychopathology. *Mol Psychiatry* (2012) **17**(7):664–5. doi:10.1038/mp.2011.171
25. Homayoun H, Moghaddam B. NMDA receptor hypofunction produces opposite effects on prefrontal cortex Interneurons and pyramidal neurons. *J Neurosci* (2007) **27**(43):11496–500. doi:10.1523/jneurosci.2213-07.2007
26. Reid MA, Stoeckel LE, White DM, Avsar KB, Bolding MS, Akella NS, et al. Assessments of function and biochemistry of the anterior cingulate cortex in schizophrenia. *Biol Psychiatry* (2010) **68**(7):625–33. doi:10.1016/j.biopsych.2010.04.013
27. Shirayama Y, Obata T, Matsuzawa D, Nonaka H, Kanazawa Y, Yoshitome E, et al. Specific metabolites in the medial prefrontal cortex are associated with the neurocognitive deficits in schizophrenia: a preliminary study. *Neuroimage* (2010) **49**(3):2783–90. doi:10.1016/j.neuroimage.2009.10.031
28. Tayoshi S, Sumitani S, Taniguchi K, Shibuya-Tayoshi S, Numata S, Iga J, et al. Metabolite changes and gender differences in schizophrenia using 3-Tesla proton magnetic resonance spectroscopy (H-1-MRS). *Schizophr Res* (2009) **108**(1-3):69–77. doi:10.1016/j.schres.2008.11.014
29. Theberge J, Al-Semaan Y, Williamson PC, Menon RS, Neufeld RWJ, Rajakumar N, et al. Glutamate and glutamine in the anterior cingulate and thalamus of medicated patients with chronic schizophrenia and healthy comparison subjects measured with 4.0-T proton MRS. *Am J Psychiatry* (2003) **160**(12):2231–3. doi:10.1176/appi.ajp.160.12.2231
30. Wood SJ, Yucel M, Wellard RM, Harrison BJ, Clarke K, Fornito A, et al. Evidence for neuronal dysfunction in the anterior cingulate of patients with

schizophrenia: a proton magnetic resonance spectroscopy study at 3 T. *Schizophr Res* (2007) **94**(1-3):328–31. doi:10.1016/j.schres.2007.05.008

31. Kegeles LS, Mao XL, Stanford AD, Girgis R, Ojeil N, Xu XY, et al. Elevated prefrontal cortex gamma-aminobutyric acid and glutamate-glutamine levels in schizophrenia measured in vivo with proton magnetic resonance spectroscopy. *Arch Gen Psychiatry* (2012) **69**(5):449–59. doi:10.1001/archgenpsychiatry.2011.1519
32. Choe BY, Kim KT, Suh TS, Lee C, Paik IH, Bahk YW, et al. 1H magnetic resonance spectroscopy characterization of neuronal dysfunction in drug-naive, chronic schizophrenia. *Acad Radiol* (1994) **1**(3):211–6. doi:10.1016/s1076-6332(05)80716-0
33. Theberge J, Williamson KE, Aoyama N, Drost DJ, Manchanda R, Malla AK, et al. Longitudinal grey-matter and glutamatergic losses in first-episode schizophrenia. *Br J Psychiatry* (2007) **191**:325–34. doi:10.1192/bjp.bp.106.033670
34. Aoyama N, Theberge J, Drost DJ, Manchanda R, Northcott S, Neufeld RWJ, et al. Grey matter and social functioning correlates of glutamatergic metabolite loss in schizophrenia. *Br J Psychiatry* (2011) **198**(6):448–56. doi:10.1192/bjp.bp.110.079608
35. Luykx JJ, Laban KG, van den Heuvel MP, Boks MPM, Mandl RCW, Kahn RS, et al. Region and state specific glutamate downregulation in major depressive disorder: a meta-analysis of H-1-MRS findings. *Neurosci Biobehav Rev* (2012) **36**(1):198–205. doi:10.1016/j.neubiorev.2011.05.014
36. Yoo SY, Yeon S, Choi CH, Kang DH, Lee JM, Shin NY, et al. Proton magnetic resonance spectroscopy in subjects with high genetic risk of schizophrenia: investigation of anterior cingulate, dorsolateral prefrontal cortex and thalamus. *Schizophr Res* (2009) **111**(1-3):86–93. doi:10.1016/j.schres.2009.03.036
37. de la Fuente-Sandoval C, Leon-Ortiz P, Favila R, Stephano S, Mamo D, Ramirez-Bermudez J, et al. Higher levels of glutamate in the associative-striatum of subjects with prodromal symptoms of schizophrenia and patients with first-episode psychosis. *Neuropsychopharmacology* (2011) **36**(9):1781–91. doi:10.1038/npp.2011.65
38. Egerton A, Brugger S, Raffin M, Barker GJ, Lythgoe DJ, McGuire PK, et al. Anterior cingulate glutamate levels related to clinical status following treatment in first-episode schizophrenia. *Neuropsychopharmacology* (2012) **37**(11):2515–21. doi:10.1038/npp.2012.113
39. Stanley JA, Williamson PC, Drost DJ, Rylett RJ, Carr TJ, Malla A, et al. An in vivo proton magnetic resonance spectroscopy study of schizophrenia patients. *Schizophr Bull* (1996) **22**(4):597–609. doi:10.1093/schbul/22.4.597
40. Bartha R, Williamson PC, Drost DJ, Malla A, Carr TJ, Cortese L, et al. Measurement of glutamate and glutamine in the medial prefrontal cortex of never-treated schizophrenic patients and healthy controls by proton magnetic resonance spectroscopy. *Arch Gen Psychiatry* (1997) **54**(10):959–65. doi:10.1001/archpsyc.1997.01830220085012
41. Ohrmann P, Siegmund A, Suslow T, Spitzberg K, Kersting A, Arolt V, et al. Evidence for glutamatergic neuronal dysfunction in the prefrontal cortex in chronic but not in first-episode patients with schizophrenia: a proton magnetic resonance spectroscopy study. *Schizophr Res* (2005) **73**(2-3):153–7. doi:10.1016/j.schres.2004.08.021
42. Ohrmann P, Kugel H, Bauer J, Siegmund A, Kolkebeck K, Suslow T, et al. Learning potential on the WCST in schizophrenia is related to the neuronal integrity of the anterior cingulate cortex as measured by proton magnetic resonance spectroscopy. *Schizophr Res* (2008) **106**(2-3):156–63. doi:10.1016/j.schres.2008.08.005
43. Bustillo JR, Chen HJ, Gasparovic C, Mullins P, Caprihan A, Qualls C, et al. Glutamate as a marker of cognitive function in schizophrenia: a proton spectroscopic imaging study at 4 Tesla. *Biol Psychiatry* (2011) **69**(1):19–27. doi:10.1016/j.biopsych.2010.08.024
44. Rowland LM, Spieker EA, Francis A, Barker PB, Carpenter WT, Buchanan RW. White matter alterations in deficit schizophrenia. *Neuropsychopharmacology* (2009) **34**(6):1514–22. doi:10.1038/npp.2008.207
45. Reid MA, Kraguljac NV, Avsar KB, White DM, den Hollander JA, Lahti AC. Proton magnetic resonance spectroscopy of the substantia nigra in schizophrenia. *Schizophr Res* (2013) **147**(2-3):348–54. doi:10.1016/j.schres.2013.04.036
46. Rowland L, Kontson K, West J, Edden R, Zhu H, Wijtenburg S, et al. In vivo measurements of glutamate, GABA, and NAAG in schizophrenia. *Schizophr Bull* (2012) **39**(5):1096–104. doi:10.1093/schbul/sbs092
47. de la Fuente-Sandoval C, León-Ortiz P, Azcárraga M, Stephano S, Favila R, Díaz-Galvis L, et al. Glutamate levels in the associative striatum before and after 4 weeks of antipsychotic treatment in first-episode psychosis: a longitudinal proton magnetic resonance spectroscopy study. *JAMA Psychiatry* (2013) **70**(10):1057–66. doi:10.1001/jamapsychiatry.2013.289
48. Ota M, Ishikawa M, Sato N, Hori H, Sasayama D, Hattori K, et al. Glutamatergic changes in the cerebral white matter associated with schizophrenic exacerbation. *Acta Psychiatr Scand* (2012) **126**(1):72–8. doi:10.1111/j.1600-0447.2012.01853.x
49. Demjaha A, Egerton A, Murray R, Kapur S, Howes O, Stone J, et al. Antipsychotic treatment resistance in schizophrenia associated with elevated glutamate levels but normal dopamine function. *Biol Psychiatry* (2013). doi:10.1016/j.biopsych.2013.06.011. [Epub ahead of print].
50. Ongur D, Jensen JE, Prescot AP, Stork C, Lundy M, Cohen BM, et al. Abnormal glutamatergic neurotransmission and neuronal-glial interactions in acute mania. *Biol Psychiatry* (2008) **64**(8):718–26. doi:10.1016/j.biopsych.2008.05.014
51. Lyne JP, Kinsella A, O'Donoghue B. Can we combine symptom scales for collaborative research projects? *J Psychiatr Res* (2012) **46**(2):233–8. doi:10.1016/j.jpsychires.2011.10.002
52. Wilmsmeier A, Ohrmann P, Suslow T, Siegmund A, Koelkebeck K, Rothermundt M, et al. Neural correlates of set-shifting: decomposing executive functions in schizophrenia. *J Psychiatry Neurosci* (2010) **35**(5):321–9. doi:10.1503/jpn.090181
53. Rusch N, van Elst LT, Valerius G, Buechert M, Thiel T, Ebert D, et al. Neurochemical and structural correlates of executive dysfunction in schizophrenia. *Schizophr Res* (2008) **99**(1-3):155–63. doi:10.1016/j.schres.2007.05.024
54. Tandon N, Bolo NR, Sanghavi K, Mathew IT, Francis AN, Stanley JA, et al. Brain metabolite alterations in young adults at familial high risk for schizophrenia using proton magnetic resonance spectroscopy. *Schizophr Res* (2013) **148**(1-3):59–66. doi:10.1016/j.schres.2013.05.024
55. Ohrmann P, Siegmund A, Suslow T, Pedersen A, Spitzberg K, Kersting A, et al. Cognitive impairment and in vivo metabolites in first-episode neuroleptic-naive and chronic medicated schizophrenic patients: a proton magnetic resonance spectroscopy study. *J Psychiatr Res* (2007) **41**(8):625–34. doi:10.1016/j.jpsychires.2006.07.002
56. Fusar-Poli P, Stone JM, Broome MR, Valli I, Mechelli A, McLean MA, et al. Thalamic glutamate levels as a predictor of cortical response during executive functioning in subjects at high risk for psychosis. *Arch Gen Psychiatry* (2011) **68**(9):881–90. doi:10.1001/archgenpsychiatry.2011.46
57. Valli I, Stone J, Mechelli A, Bhattacharyya S, Raffin M, Allen P, et al. Altered medial temporal activation related to local glutamate levels in subjects with prodromal signs of psychosis. *Biol Psychiatry* (2011) **69**(1):97–9. doi:10.1016/j.biopsych.2010.08.033
58. Hutcheson NL, Reid MA, White DM, Kraguljac NV, Avsar KB, Bolding MS, et al. Multimodal analysis of the hippocampus in schizophrenia using proton magnetic resonance spectroscopy and functional magnetic resonance imaging. *Schizophr Res* (2012) **140**(1-3):136–42. doi:10.1016/j.schres.2012.06.039
59. Tibbo P, Hanstock C, Valiakalayil A, Allen P. 3-T proton MRS investigation of glutamate and glutamine in adolescents at high genetic risk for schizophrenia. *Am J Psychiatry* (2004) **161**(6):1116–8. doi:10.1176/appi.ajp.161.6.1116
60. Tebartz van Elst L, Valerius G, Buchert M, Thiel T, Rusch N, Bubl E, et al. Increased prefrontal and hippocampal glutamate concentration in schizophrenia: evidence from a magnetic resonance spectroscopy study. *Biol Psychiatry* (2005) **58**(9):724–30. doi:10.1016/j.biopsych.2005.04.041
61. Stone JM, Howes OD, Egerton A, Kambeitz J, Allen P, Lythgoe DJ, et al. Altered relationship between hippocampal glutamate levels and striatal dopamine function in subjects at ultra high risk of psychosis. *Biol Psychiatry* (2010) **68**(7):599–602. doi:10.1016/j.biopsych.2010.05.034
62. Szulc A, Konarzewskaa B, Galinska-Skoka B, Lazarczyka J, Waszkiewicza N, Tarasowb E, et al. Proton magnetic resonance spectroscopy measures related to short-term symptomatic outcome in chronic schizophrenia. *Neurosci Lett* (2013) **547**:37–41. doi:10.1016/j.neulet.2013.04.051
63. Tiihonen J, Wahlbeck K. Glutamatergic drugs for schizophrenia. *Cochrane Database Syst Rev* (2006). doi:10.1002/14651858.CD003730.pub2
64. Singh SP, Singh V. Meta-analysis of the efficacy of adjunctive NMDA receptor modulators in chronic schizophrenia. *CNS Drugs* (2011) **25**(10):859–85. doi:10.2165/11586650-000000000-00000
65. Anand A, Charney DS, Oren DA, Berman RM, Hu XS, Cappiello A, et al. Attenuation of the neuropsychiatric effects of ketamine with lamotrigine – support for

hyperglutamatergic effects of N-methyl-D-aspartate receptor antagonists. *Arch Gen Psychiatry* (2000) **57**(3):270–6. doi:10.1001/archpsyc.57.3.270

66. Chatterton JE, Awobuluyi M, Premkumar LS, Takahashi H, Talantova M, Shin Y, et al. Excitatory glycine receptors containing the NR3 family of NMDA receptor subunits. *Nature* (2002) **415**(6873):793–8. doi:10.1038/nature715
67. Olbrich HM, Valerius G, Rüsch N, Buchert M, Thiel T, Hennig J, et al. Frontolimbic glutamate alterations in first episode schizophrenia: evidence from a magnetic resonance spectroscopy study. *World J Biol Psychiatry* (2008) **9**(1):59–63. doi:10.1080/15622970701227811

Permissions

All chapters in this book were first published by Frontiers; hereby published with permission under the Creative Commons Attribution License or equivalent. Every chapter published in this book has been scrutinized by our experts. Their significance has been extensively debated. The topics covered herein carry significant findings which will fuel the growth of the discipline. They may even be implemented as practical applications or may be referred to as a beginning point for another development.

The contributors of this book come from diverse backgrounds, making this book a truly international effort. This book will bring forth new frontiers with its revolutionizing research information and detailed analysis of the nascent developments around the world.

We would like to thank all the contributing authors for lending their expertise to make the book truly unique. They have played a crucial role in the development of this book. Without their invaluable contributions this book wouldn't have been possible. They have made vital efforts to compile up to date information on the varied aspects of this subject to make this book a valuable addition to the collection of many professionals and students.

This book was conceptualized with the vision of imparting up-to-date information and advanced data in this field. To ensure the same, a matchless editorial board was set up. Every individual on the board went through rigorous rounds of assessment to prove their worth. After which they invested a large part of their time researching and compiling the most relevant data for our readers.

The editorial board has been involved in producing this book since its inception. They have spent rigorous hours researching and exploring the diverse topics which have resulted in the successful publishing of this book. They have passed on their knowledge of decades through this book. To expedite this challenging task, the publisher supported the team at every step. A small team of assistant editors was also appointed to further simplify the editing procedure and attain best results for the readers.

Apart from the editorial board, the designing team has also invested a significant amount of their time in understanding the subject and creating the most relevant covers. They scrutinized every image to scout for the most suitable representation of the subject and create an appropriate cover for the book.

The publishing team has been an ardent support to the editorial, designing and production team. Their endless efforts to recruit the best for this project, has resulted in the accomplishment of this book. They are a veteran in the field of academics and their pool of knowledge is as vast as their experience in printing. Their expertise and guidance has proved useful at every step. Their uncompromising quality standards have made this book an exceptional effort. Their encouragement from time to time has been an inspiration for everyone.

The publisher and the editorial board hope that this book will prove to be a valuable piece of knowledge for researchers, students, practitioners and scholars across the globe.

List of Contributors

Oswald J. N. Bloemen and Therese A. M. J. van Amelsvoort
Department of Psychiatry and Psychology, Maastricht University, Maastricht, Netherlands

Geor Bakker and Wilhelmina A. M. Vingerhoets
Department of Psychiatry and Psychology, Maastricht University, Maastricht, Netherlands
Department of Nuclear Medicine, Academic Medical Centre, University of Amsterdam, Amsterdam, Netherlands

Heekyung Lee
Graduate Program in Neural and Behavioral Science, Downstate Medical Center, State University of New York, Brooklyn, NY, USA

Dino Dvorak
Graduate Program in Biomedical Engineering, Downstate Medical Center, State University of New York and New York University Polytechnic School of Engineering, Brooklyn, NY, USA

André A. Fenton
The Robert F. Furchgott Center for Neural and Behavioral Science, Downstate Medical Center, State University of New York, Brooklyn, NY, USA
Center for Neural Science, New York University, New York, USA

Maria R. Dauvermann, Heather C. Whalley, Liana Romaniuk, Eve C. Johnstone, Stephen M. Lawrie and Thomas W. J. Moorhead
Division of Psychiatry, Royal Edinburgh Hospital, University of Edinburgh, Edinburgh, UK

André Schmidt
Department of Psychiatry, University of Basel, Basel, Switzerland
Medical Image Analysis Center, University Hospital Basel, Basel, Switzerland

Graham L. Lee
McGovern Institute for Brain Research, Massachusetts Institute of Technology, Cambridge, MA, USA

Daniel H. Mathalon and Judith M. Ford
Department of Psychiatry, University of California San Francisco, San Francisco, CA, USA
Mental Health Service (116D), San Francisco VA Medical Center, San Francisco, CA, USA

Neil Roberts
Clinical Research Imaging Centre, QMRI, University of Edinburgh, Edinburgh, UK

Brian J. Roach
Mental Health Service (116D), San Francisco VA Medical Center, San Francisco, CA, USA

Rebecca K. Blais, Savita Bhakta and Mohini Ranganathan
Department of Psychiatry, Yale University School of Medicine, New Haven, CT, USA

Kyung-Heup Ahn, Edward B. Perry Jr. and Deepak Cyril D'Souza
Department of Psychiatry, Yale University School of Medicine, New Haven, CT, USA
Schizophrenia Biological Research Center (116A), VA Connecticut Healthcare System, West Haven, CT, USA
Abraham Ribicoff Research Facilities, Connecticut Mental Health Center, New Haven, CT, USA

Hyun-Sang Cho
Department of Psychiatry, Yale University School of Medicine, New Haven, CT, USA
Department of Psychiatry, Yonsei University College of Medicine, Seoul, South Korea

Oliver Gruber
Center for Translational Research in Systems Neuroscience and Psychiatry, Clinic for Psychiatry and Psychotherapy, University Medical Center Göttingen, Göttingen, Germany

Antonella Chadha Santuccione and Helmut Aach
Medical Affairs - Psychiatry, Roche Pharma AG, Grenzach-Wyhlen, Germany

Lorenz Deserno and Florian Schlagenhauf
Max Planck Institute for Human Cognitive and Brain Sciences, Leipzig, Germany
Department of Psychiatry and Psychotherapy, Charité - Universitätsmedizin Berlin, Berlin, Germany

Rebecca Boehme and Andreas Heinz
Department of Psychiatry and Psychotherapy, Charité - Universitätsmedizin Berlin, Berlin, Germany

Rune A. Kroken and Tore Drønen
Division of Psychiatry, Haukeland University Hospital, Bergen, Norway

Kristiina Kompus
Department of Biological and Medical Psychology, University of Bergen, Bergen, Norway

Else-Marie Løberg
Division of Psychiatry, Haukeland University Hospital, Bergen, Norway
Department of Biological and Medical Psychology, University of Bergen, Bergen, Norway

Renate Grüner
Department of Radiology, Haukeland University Hospital, Bergen, Norway
Department of Physics and Technology, University of Bergen, Bergen, Norway

Kenneth Hugdahl
Division of Psychiatry, Haukeland University Hospital, Bergen, Norway
Department of Biological and Medical Psychology, University of Bergen, Bergen, Norway
Department of Radiology, Haukeland University Hospital, Bergen, Norway
NORMENT Center of Excellence, University of Bergen, Bergen, Norway

Silje Skrede
NORMENT Center of Excellence, University of Bergen, Bergen, Norway
Dr. Einar Martens' Research Group for Biological Psychiatry, Centre for Medical Genetics and Molecular Medicine, Haukeland University Hospital, Bergen, Norway
Department of Clinical Science, K.G. Jebsen Centre for Psychosis Research, University of Bergen, Bergen, Norway

Erik Johnsen
Division of Psychiatry, Haukeland University Hospital, Bergen, Norway
Department of Clinical Medicine, University of Bergen, Bergen, Norway

Jonathan P. Roiser
Institute of Cognitive Neuroscience, University College London, London, UK

Rebekah Wigton
Psychosis Studies, Cognition and Schizophrenia Imaging Lab, Institute of Psychiatry, King's College London, London, UK

Karl J. Friston
Wellcome Trust Centre for Neuroimaging, University College London, London, UK

Eileen M. Joyce
Institute of Neurology, University College London, London, UK

James M. Kilner
Wellcome Trust Centre for Neuroimaging, University College London, London, UK
Institute of Neurology, University College London, London, UK

Maria A. Mendez
Department of Forensic and Neurodevelopmental Sciences, Institute of Psychiatry, King's College London, London, UK

Nicholas Hon
Department of Psychology, National University of Singapore, Singapore

Naomi R. Driesen and Youngsun T. Cho
Department of Psychiatry, Yale University School of Medicine, New Haven, CT, USA

Genevieve Yang
Department of Psychiatry, Yale University School of Medicine, New Haven, CT, USA
Interdepartmental Neuroscience Program, Yale University, New Haven, CT, USA

David C. Glahn
Department of Psychiatry, Yale University School of Medicine, New Haven, CT, USA
Olin Neuropsychiatry Research Center, Institute of Living, Hartford Hospital, Hartford, CT, USA

Alan Anticevic
Department of Psychiatry, Yale University School of Medicine, New Haven, CT, USA
NIAAA Center for the Translational Neuroscience of Alcoholism, New Haven, CT, USA
Abraham Ribicoff Research Facilities, Connecticut Mental Health Center, New Haven, CT, USA
Interdepartmental Neuroscience Program, Yale University, New Haven, CT, USA
Olin Neuropsychiatry Research Center, Institute of Living, Hartford Hospital, Hartford, CT, USA
Department of Psychology, Yale University, New Haven, CT, USA

Michael W. Cole
Department of Psychology, Washington University in St. Louis, St. Louis, MO, USA

Grega Repovs
Department of Psychology, University of Ljubljana, Ljubljana, Slovenia

Aleksandar Savic
Department of Psychiatry, University of Zagreb School of Medicine, Zagreb, Croatia

John D. Murray and Xiao-Jing Wang
Center for Neural Science, New York University, New York, USA

John H. Krystal
Department of Psychiatry, Yale University School of Medicine, New Haven, CT, USA
NIAAA Center for the Translational Neuroscience of Alcoholism, New Haven, CT, USA
Abraham Ribicoff Research Facilities, Connecticut Mental Health Center, New Haven, CT, USA
Department of Neurobiology, Yale University School of Medicine, New Haven, CT, USA

Shinsuke Koike
Office for Mental Health Support, Division for Counseling and Support, The University of Tokyo, Tokyo, Japan
Department of Neuropsychiatry, Graduate School of Medicine, The University of Tokyo, Tokyo, Japan

Yukika Nishimura and Kiyoto Kasai
Department of Neuropsychiatry, Graduate School of Medicine, The University of Tokyo, Tokyo, Japan

Ryu Takizawa
Department of Neuropsychiatry, Graduate School of Medicine, The University of Tokyo, Tokyo, Japan
Social, Genetic and Developmental Psychiatry Centre, Institute of Psychiatry, King's College London, London, UK

Noriaki Yahata
Department of Youth Mental Health, Graduate School of Medicine, The University of Tokyo, Tokyo, Japan

Vaibhav A. Diwadkar, Neil Bakshi, Gita Gupta, Patrick Pruitt and Richard White
Department of Psychiatry and Behavioral Neurosciences, Wayne State University, Detroit, MI, USA

Simon B. Eickhoff
Institute of Clinical Neuroscience and Medical Psychology, Heinrich-Heine University Düsseldorf, Düsseldorf, Germany
Institute of Neuroscience and Medicine (INM-1), Research Center Jülich, Jülich, Germany

Tim B. Ziermans
Department of Clinical Child and Adolescent Studies, Leiden University, Leiden, Netherlands
Department of Neuroscience, Karolinska Institutet, Stockholm Brain Institute, Stockholm, Sweden

Juanita Todd, Lauren Harms and Patricia T. Michie
School of Psychology, University of Newcastle, Callaghan, NSW, Australia
Priority Research Centre for Brain and Mental Health, University of Newcastle, Callaghan, NSW, Australia
Schizophrenia Research Institute, Darlinghurst, NSW, Australia
Hunter Medical Research Institute, Newcastle, NSW, Australia

Ulrich Schall
Priority Research Centre for Brain and Mental Health, University of Newcastle, Callaghan, NSW, Australia
Schizophrenia Research Institute, Darlinghurst, NSW, Australia
Hunter Medical Research Institute, Newcastle, NSW, Australia
School of Medicine and Public Health, University of Newcastle, Callaghan, NSW, Australia

Mitja Bodatsch, Joachim Klosterkötter and Jörg Daumann
Department of Psychiatry and Psychotherapy, University of Cologne, Cologne, Germany

Carissa N. Kuswanto and Min Y. Sum
Research Division, Institute of Mental Health/ Woodbridge Hospital, Singapore

Kang Sim
Research Division, Institute of Mental Health/ Woodbridge Hospital, Singapore
Department of General Psychiatry, Institute of Mental Health/Woodbridge Hospital, Singapore

Kate Merritt, Philip McGuire and Alice Egerton
Department of Psychosis Studies, Institute of Psychiatry, King's College London, London, UK

Index

www.ingramcontent.com/pod-product-compliance
Lightning Source LLC
LaVergne TN
LVHW082158200926
848484LV00008B/2183